T3-BQR-797

T3-BQR-797

◆

CHILD
MALTREATMENT

A CLINICAL
GUIDE AND REFERENCE

G. W. Medical Publishing, Inc.

Mosby–Year Book, Inc.

St. Louis Baltimore Berlin Boston Carlsbad Chicago London Madrid
Naples New York Philadelphia Sydney Tokyo Toronto

CHILD MALTREATMENT

A CLINICAL GUIDE AND REFERENCE

JAMES A. MONTELEONE, M.D.
Professor of Pediatrics and Gynecology
St. Louis University School of Medicine
Director of the Division of Child Protection
Cardinal Glennon Children's Hospital
St. Louis, Missouri

ARMAND E. BRODEUR, M.D., M.RD., L.L.D., F.A.C.R., F.A.A.P.
Professor Emeritus of Radiology and Pediatrics
St. Louis University School of Medicine
Emeritus Director of Pediatric Radiology
Cardinal Glennon Children's Hospital
Director of Radiology
Shriners Hospital for Crippled Children—St. Louis Unit
St. Louis, Missouri

G. W. Medical Publishing, Inc.
St. Louis 1994

Vol. 1

Publisher: Glenn E. Whaley

Design Director: Glenn E. Whaley

Developmental Editor: Elaine Steinborn

Editors:
  –Joan C. Reinbott
  –Linda Wendling
  –Terry Eynon

Production Manager: Angela M. Blackwell

  –Book Design/Page Layout: Angela M. Blackwell
  –Print/Production Coordinator: Charles J. Seibel, III
  –Cover Design: D. Scott Tjaden
  –Production: Christine Bauer
  –Production: Glen Peterson

Indexer: Linda Caravelli

Printed in the United States of America

G. W. Medical Publishing, Inc.
2601 Metro Blvd., St. Louis, Missouri 63043

Library of Congress Cataloging in Publication Data
  Child maltreatment
        p.   cm
      Includes bibliographical references and indexes.
      Contents: [v. 1.]. A clinical guide and reference / [edited by]
  James A. Montelione, Armand E. Brodeur -- [v. 2] A comprehensive
  photographic reference identifying potential child abuse / [edited
  by] James A. Montelione.
      ISBN 1-878060-20-1 (set). -- ISBN 1-878060-10-4 (v. 1). -- ISBN
  1-878060-13-9 (v. 2)
      1. Child abuse--Diagnosis. 2. Battered child syndrome--Atlases.
  3. Battered child syndrome--Diagnosis. 4. Child abuse--Reporting.
  I. Monteleone, James A. II. Brodeur, Armand E.
      [DNLM: 1. Child Abuse. 2. Child Abuse--atlases. WA 320 C53483
  1994]
  RA1122.5.C49   1994
  618.92--dc20
  DNLM/DLC
  for Library of Congress   94-28160
                                                           CIP

96-95 / 9 8 7 6 5 4 3 2

CONTRIBUTORS

Pasquale J. Accardo, M.D.
Professor of Pediatrics
St. Louis University School of Medicine
Medical Director, Knights of Columbus Developmental Center
Cardinal Glennon Children's Hospital
St. Louis, Missouri

Richard C. Barry, M.D.
Professor of Pediatrics
St. Louis University School of Medicine
Director of Emergency Care Services
Cardinal Glennon Children's Hospital
St. Louis, Missouri

Karen M. Bly, R.N., M.Ed.
Nurse/Counselor
Child Protection Unit
Cardinal Glennon Children's Hospital
St. Louis, Missouri

John R. Brewer, M.D.
Associate Clinical Professor of Pediatrics
St. Louis University School of Medicine
Medical Director of Grace Hill Neighborhood Health Clinics
St. Louis, Missouri

Armand E. Brodeur, M.D., M.Rd., L.L.D., F.A.C.R., F.A.A.P.
Professor Emeritus of Radiology and Pediatrics
St. Louis University School of Medicine
Emeritus Director of Pediatric Radiology
Cardinal Glennon Children's Hospital
Director of Radiology
Shriners Hospital for Crippled Children
St. Louis Unit
St. Louis, Missouri

Mary E. S. Case, M.D.
Associate Professor, Department of Pathology
St. Louis University Health Sciences Center
St. Louis, Missouri
Chief Medical Examiner
St. Louis, St. Charles,
Jefferson and Franklin Counties, Missouri

Kevin Coulter, M.D.
Associate Clinical Professor
Department of Pediatrics
University of California, San Francisco
Medical Director
Center for Child Protection
San Francisco General Hospital
San Francisco, California

Oscar A. Cruz, M.D.
Assistant Professor of Ophthalmology
St. Louis University School of Medicine
Director of Pediatric Ophthalmology
Cardinal Glennon Children's Hospital
St. Louis, Missouri

Cassandra K. Dolgin, B.A., J.D.
Member of the Missouri Bar
St. Louis, Missouri

Timothy J. Fete, M.D.
Assistant Professor of Pediatrics
St. Louis University School of Medicine
Director of the Division of General Academic Pediatrics
Cardinal Glennon Children's Hospital
St. Louis, Missouri

Allan D. Friedman, M.D., M.P.H.
Associate Professor and Vice-Chairman
Department of Pediatrics
St. Louis University School of Medicine
St. Louis, Missouri

Joseph Giangiacomo, M.D.
Professor of Ophthalmology
University of Missouri at Columbia
Columbia, Missouri

Sheilah Glaze, M.S.W., L.C.S.W.
Medical Social Worker
Cardinal Glennon Children's Hospital
St. Louis, Missouri

Jesse A. Goldner, M.A., J.D.
Professor of Law
Director of the Center for Health Law Studies
St. Louis University School of Law
Professor of Pediatrics
Professor of Law in Psychiatry
St. Louis University School of Medicine
St. Louis, Missouri

Michael Graham, M.D.
Associate Professor of Pathology and Director of the
Division of Forensic and Environmental Pathology
St. Louis University School of Medicine
St. Louis, Missouri
Chief Medical Examiner for the City of St. Louis, Missouri
Deputy Chief Medical Examiner for St. Louis, St. Charles, and
Jefferson Counties, Missouri

E. Richard Graviss, M.D.
Professor of Pediatrics and Radiology
St. Louis University School of Medicine
Director, Diagnostic Imaging
Cardinal Glennon Children's Hospital
St. Louis, Missouri

Gregory D. Launius, M.D.
Instructor, Department of Radiology
St. Louis University School of Medicine
St. Louis, Missouri

Atchawee Luisiri, M.D.
Associate Professor of Radiology
St. Louis University School of Medicine
St. Louis, Missouri

Sandra H. Manske, R.N., M.A., J.D.
Member of the Missouri Bar
St. Louis, Missouri

Vicki McNeese, M.S.
Staff Psychologist
Cardinal Glennon Children's Hospital
Adjunct Instructor of Psychology
St. Louis University
St. Louis, Missouri

James A. Monteleone, M.D.
Professor of Pediatrics and Gynecology
St. Louis University School of Medicine
Director of the Division of Child Protection
Cardinal Glennon Children's Hospital
St. Louis, Missouri

Wayne I. Munkel, M.S.W., L.C.S.W.
Medical Social Consultant
Department of Social Service
Cardinal Glennon Children's Hospital
St. Louis, Missouri

Peggy S. Pearl, Ed.D.
Professor, Department of Consumer and Family Studies
Southwest Missouri State University
Springfield, Missouri

Anthony J. Scalzo, M.D.
Associate Professor of Pediatrics
Division of Emergency Medicine
St. Louis University School of Medicine
Clinical Toxicologist
Director of Regional Poison Control Center
Cardinal Glennon Children's Hospital
St. Louis, Missouri

Michael J. Silberstein, M.D.
Associate Professor of Radiology
St. Louis University School of Medicine
St. Louis, Missouri

Thomas R. Weber, M.D.
Professor of Surgery
St. Louis University School of Medicine
Director of Pediatric Surgery
Cardinal Glennon Children's Hospital
St. Louis, Missouri

Barbara Y. Whitman, Ph.D.
Associate Professor of Pediatrics
St. Louis University School of Medicine
Director, Family Services and Family Studies
Knights of Columbus Developmental Center
Cardinal Glennon Children's Hospital
St. Louis, Missouri

James J. Williams, M.D.
Staff Pediatrician
The Permanente Medical Group
Redwood City, California
Attending Pediatrician
San Francisco General Hospital
San Francisco, California

FOREWORD

The abuse and misuse of children is not unique to any time or location. Indeed, infanticide, the ultimate outcome of violence against children, has, throughout various times in history, been an accepted procedure to rid society of deformed and sickly newborns as well as children who were felt to impose an economic hardship to a family unit or community.

In America, the medical profession's role in identifying child abuse was noted in 1946 when Dr. Caffey, a radiologist, described the specific association between healed fractures, subdural hematomas, and child abuse. It was not until 1962, however, when Dr. C. Henry Kempe and his associates published their sentinel paper in the *Journal of the American Medical Association*, that medical professionals recognized the battered child syndrome. Over the next three decades, researchers and practitioners gathered data and advanced the body of scientific knowledge concerning the various etiologies of abuse (psychological, social learning, sociological, cultural, and others), tools/methods to facilitate victim-sensitive interviews (anatomically detailed dolls, puppets, drawings, computer programs, videotaping, etc.), the techniques to enhance the identification of abuse (colposcopy, scrologic and immunologic analyses, diagnostic imaging, etc.), and subsequently modalities which address post-assessment interventions (play therapy, art therapy, formal psychological testing, court testimony, etc.).

The various disciplines dealing with abused children represent an interactive and dynamic community of professional groups, including social service, medical, judicial, law enforcement, mental health, and government systems. Each discipline has a specific role both in responding to the violence and interacting with other members of the community — it is the availability and coordination of these independent systems in responding to victims that define the nature and the parameters of the overall response. This lesson is aptly portrayed in this book. Drs. Monteleone and Brodeur and their co-authors have integrated more than 30 years of experience as members of the Cardinal Glennon Child Protection Team with the training and skills they acquired as active participants in the closely knit St. Louis Interagency Task Force.

Many recent books dealing with child abuse and neglect focus on a single aspect of child abuse. Others, in their efforts to reach a broad audience, have omitted crucial information. Drs. Monteleone and Brodeur are to be congratulated. These two physicians and their co-authors have successfully written an exhaustive two-volume reference book to meet the needs of the various disciplines. This text will guide the reader on his or her journey from the initial chapters on the identification and reporting of child abuse, through the more technically complex sections on the medical aspects of diagnosis, to the final chapters focusing on court testimony and the prevention of child abuse.

This comprehensive resource is published as a two-volume set complete with colored illustrations and diagrams. The information is provided in a manner which should hold the interest of both the dilettante and the seasoned professional. In summary, the single criticism noted by this reader is that the authors should have written their very valuable textbook sooner. This text should be considered recommended reading for each of the various disciplines involved in the field of child abuse and neglect regardless of whether the learner is entry level or emeritus.

Howard B. Levy, M.D.
Department of Pediatrics
Grant Hospital of Chicago

PREFACE

This reference was created to help physicians diagnose child maltreatment, recognize those children at high risk for abuse and neglect, and realize strategies for prevention and intervention in abuse cases. Although the text is approached from a medical point of view, the information contained will also be beneficial to other health care professionals, social service workers, attorneys, law enforcement workers, state agencies, and others who might be involved with abused children. Information concerning physical and psychological abuse, neglect, and sexual abuse, as well as their legal aspects, is collected here in a single volume.

In the mid-1980's the St. Louis Child Abuse Network was involved in a project to review deaths and catastrophic injuries in children that resulted from abuse. The results of that study were released to the media and presented at several medical conferences but were not published. This study was unique in that it collected data not only on severely abused children and their families but also on control groups of mildly abused and nonabused children and their families. Along with other studies at the time, it showed the value of reviewing not only the circumstances of the deaths of abused children, but also the circumstances of suspicious deaths. In 1992 the State of Missouri enacted legislation providing for the establishment of death review teams throughout the state. We share the information about how to set up a death review mechanism in this text.

In the past, books focused on the social aspects of child abuse. But many practitioners believe that the social aspects of child abuse should be the domain of social agencies. Most clinicians want to be able to recognize abuse and to know what to do after they decide they have reason to suspect abuse. While the "why" and the "who" are important, the "how" and "what" are foremost in their minds and must be addressed.

Recent books written on sexual abuse in children give only passing mention of the importance of the child's disclosure and interview, focusing rather on the physical examination and the physician's role in the process. We believe the most important aspect of evaluating the sexually abused child in particular is her or his disclosure, because all of the other elements depend on what the child says. The physical examination should not stand alone; it has proven inadequate because 60% to 70% of the children who have been sexually abused have no physical findings of abuse. In addition, an effective interview determines the "credibility" of the child's statement. Current texts on abuse lack information concerning this vital component.

The contributors to this reference are experts in their fields. Since we felt strongly that no one person could effectively address all aspects of child abuse, we sought specific expertise in each area. These individuals have been involved in child protection activities for significant periods of time and are acknowledged as extremely competent by both their peers and the legal system.

Our laws allow parents broad freedom with regard to child rearing, and this book is not challenging parental rights. We must, however, in our schools, through the media, and in our churches teach parenting skills, proper forms of discipline, normal child behavior, proper toilet training techniques, and effective communication methods. The primary caregiver must have these skills. Clinicians must know when to step in and instruct families in these skills with the goal of preventing child abuse. It is hoped that this book will prove valuable in these endeavors.

James A. Monteleone
Armand E. Brodeur

TABLE OF CONTENTS

◆

CHILD MALTREATMENT

A CLINICAL
GUIDE AND REFERENCE

IDENTIFYING, INTERPRETING, AND REPORTING INJURIES

JAMES A. MONTELEONE, M.D.
ARMAND E. BRODEUR, M.D.

A 3-year-old girl was taken to the emergency room after she had fallen down the stairs. She was unconscious and unresponsive. On physical examination, she was found to have ecchymotic areas on her face, chest, abdomen, back, and thighs. All of the injuries were acute and of the same age. CT scan of the head revealed a massive occipital subdural hematoma, and an abdominal CT revealed a laceration of the liver. A social service consult was requested and the incident was reported to the hot line.

The mother was 19 years old and single. She was living with a paramour. The Division of Family Services stated that the child had a similar episode six months earlier when the case was opened. The previous incident had been substantiated as abuse and the child was returned home with the understanding that the paramour would move out of the home. In describing the current incident, the mother said that she and the paramour had gotten "stoned" and the child was thrown against the wall, kicked, and slapped. The child survived, but she was permanently mentally incapacitated. She is presently living in a vegetative state in a chronic rehabilitative state hospital.

The mother and paramour were found guilty of child abuse and sentenced to prison.

Child abuse involves every segment of society and crosses all social, ethnic, religious, and professional lines. The definition of child abuse can range from a narrow focus, limited to intentional inflicted injury, to a broad scope, covering any act that impairs the developmental potential of a child. Included in the definition are neglect (acts of omission) and physical, psychological, or sexual injury (acts of commission) by a parent or caretaker. Intent is not considered in reporting abuse; protection of the child is paramount.

According to the United States Department of Health and Human Services report (1980), the national incidence of countable child maltreatment was 9.8 children per 1,000 population. This totaled about 625,100 children. In 1988 this agency reported that 16.3 children per 1,000 population, or 1,025,900 children, were maltreated. Whether these data reflect an increase in the occurrence of child maltreatment or an increase in the ability of professionals to recognize and report cases is arguable.

We live in a violent society. Children are often the targets of that violence. The violence is most apt to occur in the home and be perpetrated by a family member. Some studies suggest that people who were abused as children are more apt as adults to become perpetrators of abuse than are those who were not abused as children. Social factors—poverty, unemployment, and isolation—are major factors increasing the risk of child abuse (Gelles, 1982).

The diagnosis of the classic battered child who presents with multiple injuries in differing stages of healing is easy for the experienced physician. Determining, with certainty, whether a single injury is accidental or intended is difficult. Inflicted injury is diagnosed when the physician is certain that a single injury in a child could not have been the result of the circumstance described by the caretaker. This decision is based on the physician's clinical experience and reliance on studies in the literature.

Effective strategies to deal with and prevent abuse must involve many disciplines. No one individual, whether pediatrician, radiologist, psychiatrist, nurse, social worker, or juvenile officer, can have all of the answers and consistently make correct decisions without the input from other professionals on the team.

Previously, references dealing with child abuse have concentrated on the social factors—the *who* and the *why* of child abuse. This reference, while not ignoring the who and why, emphasizes the *what* and the *how*: *what* is abuse, *what* to do when one suspects abuse, and *how* to do it.

♦ IDENTIFYING CHILD ABUSE

NORMAL CHILD DEVELOPMENT AND BEHAVIOR

In evaluating injuries, the age of the child is crucial. Infants who are basically immobile and who are receiving good care rarely suffer injury. When they reach the mobile stage and are learning to walk or crawl, single bruises are generally found as a result of their many falls. Multiple bruises, involving multiple body areas, require multiple impacts and the history should reflect multiple incidents.

With some exceptions, a child cannot roll over until at least 4 months of age, often not until about 6 months of age. A child will not crawl until about 10 months or walk until about a year old. He will not run well until age 2, and cannot ride a tricycle until about 3. It is also about this time that the child climbs the stairs alternating feet *(see Denver Developmental Screening Test, p. 23).*

Accidental injuries require specific motor skills on the part of a child. A fall from a bed is not possible before the child can roll over; a fall down the stairs is not plausible until the child can crawl. The ability to turn a circular-motion hot water knob and turn on the tap is not possible until approximately 2 years of age. Therefore a 2-month-old infant cannot roll over, let alone crawl, to a radiator to sustain a burn or get into a toxin, and a 2-year-old who has severe buttock burns could not have ridden a tricycle into a space heater.

Occasionally an injury is blamed on a sibling. This explanation is feasible, since children often are abusive to their siblings. However, the evaluator must determine if the injury could have occurred as described and if the sibling is developmentally mature enough to have initiated the injury. It may be necessary to test the child or sibling to see if the action attributed to him or her is possible.

Explanations of injuries must be evaluated using common sense or a sound knowledge of the consequences of routine accidents in the home. For example, a 17-month-old cannot burn his buttocks by climbing onto a space heater and sitting on the top without burning his hands and legs in the climb—assuming he can climb. Similarly, a 5-month-old cannot spontaneously sustain a severe rectal tear and dilated anus, nor can he suffer multiple skull fractures and internal abdominal injuries in a fall from the couch. Finally, a fractured femur does not generally occur when a 5-month-old tangles his leg in a blanket while rolling over.

CONDITIONS THAT MAY BE CONFUSED WITH ABUSE

A number of conditions over the years have been mistaken for child abuse and have been reported to state protective agencies. It is important that mandated reporters know these conditions and make an effort to identify them. Although it is tragic to miss recognizing a child who has been abused, it is equally tragic to falsely accuse a caretaker of abuse, especially when the child is ill and the allegations add to the caretaker's concerns for the child. A number of systems can be involved: the skin, involving easy bruisability and burns; the skeletal system, with fractures and other bony changes; the eye; and the central nervous system. A list of those conditions that have been reported or that the authors have encountered is given in **Table 1-1**.

Table 1-1. Conditions Which Have Been Mistaken for Abuse

Conditions Manifested by Unusual Skin Lesions or Burns
Mongolian spots
Phytophotodermatitis
Dermatorrhexis of Ehlers-Danlos syndrome
Car seat burns
Staphylococcal scalded skin syndrome
Chickenpox (mistaken for cigarette burns)
Impetigo (mistaken for cigarette burns)
Chemical burns

Conditions Manifested by Bone Abnormalities
Congenital syphilis affecting the skeletal system
Fatigue fractures from exercise
Physical therapy (passive exercise)
Cardiopulmonary resuscitation
Vitamin C or D deficiencies
Skin or skeletal anomalies associated with chromosomal disorders
Copper deficiency
Rickets
Caffey's disease

Conditions Which Cause Easy Bruisability
Vitamin K deficiency from liver disease
Type I Ehlers-Danlos syndrome
Salicylate toxicity
Osteogenesis imperfecta
Folk medicine (cupping, spooning, coining)
Bleeding disorders
Schönlein-Henoch purpura
Purpura fulminans of meningococcemia
Ecchymotic lesions of hypersensitivity vasculitis
Erythema multiforme
Platelet aggregation disorders
Disseminated intravascular coagulation

Conditions Manifested as Eye Hemorrhages
Aneurysm
Motor vehicle accident
Thoracic compression and hypoxia
Valsalva effect with subconjunctival hemorrhages
"Red eye"

Conditions Manifested as CNS Hemorrhages
Aneurysm
Brain tumor
Hemorrhagic disease of the newborn
Folk medicine (fallen fontanelle)

Self-inflicted Injuries
Depression
Mental retardation
Cornelia De Lange syndrome
Lesch-Nyhan syndrome
Familial dysautonomia
Factitious illness
Temper tantrums
Head-bangers
Toddler's fracture

(From Bays, 1993; Oates, 1984; and Wheeler and Hobbs, 1988.)

FOLK MEDICINE

Physicians should become familiar with folk medicine practices in their community and work with organizations that sponsor immigrants in order to educate these individuals concerning acceptable medical care. Among the practices that have been found are the following:

Cao Gio is a form of folk medicine practiced by Southeast Asians. The healers follow traditional folk medicine when they rub a coin or a spoon heated in oil on an ill child's neck, spine, and ribs. The practice can cause a burn or abrasion (Gellis and Feingold, 1976).

In *Caida de Mollera* (fallen fontanelle), which is practiced by Hispanics, an attempt is made to elevate the fontanelle in children dehydrated from diarrhea and vomiting by holding the child upside down (Guarnaschelli et al., 1972). Retinal hemorrhages may result.

Some states have legislation declaring that it is acceptable to treat an ill child with prayer instead of medical care, provided the religious treatment is in accord with the tenets and practices of a recognized religion, such as Christian Science. However, certain states have removed the faith healing exemptions from child endangering and neglect statutes, and other states may follow.

ACCIDENTAL VERSUS INFLICTED INJURIES

Differentiating accidental injuries from inflicted injuries is important in the management of injured children. Errors in diagnosis are both catastrophic and costly for the child and the family. If inflicted injury is not recognized, the child is left in the care of persons who may injure him again. If the diagnosis of inflicted injury is incorrect, parents are wrongfully accused and investigated, and the child and parents may be separated.

A caretaker rarely reports to an emergency room or physician's office stating that he has abused his child. He will try to convince the staff that the injury resulted from an accident initiated by the child. In order to diagnose abuse one must first believe that abuse is a possibility and effectively eliminate the potential of an accident having produced the presenting injury(ies).

Children are forward moving and frontal explorers; therefore, most accidental injuries involve only one plane of the body, the frontal plane. Specific frontal locations affected are the forehead, nose, chin, palms, elbows, and shins—areas where the bone is close to skin.

Palmar hand injuries can be accidental, occurring when breaking a fall or when exploring a dangerous object, such as a hot iron or a piece of machinery. However, both the palms and the backs of the hands are common areas where punishment is inflicted, and the physician should be alert to the possibility of abuse when there are injuries in these areas.

Injuries to the buttocks, genitalia, abdomen, back, and lateral areas of the body, especially the sides of the face, are frequently indicative of abuse. Abdominal bruising is unusual even with blunt trauma. Genital and perianal bruising is usually intentional.

The evaluator must determine if the injury could have occurred as described. Then it must be determined if this particular child is developmentally mature enough to have caused the injury. If the parents state that the child sustained the injury by doing something that he is not developmentally able to do or if the injury is too severe to be caused by the incident described, then the history given is incorrect and the evaluator must conclude that the injury was nonaccidental.

Why does an abusive injury or situation go unrecognized? Several reasons may be cited:

1. The mandated reporter may not be able to accept that a parent could abuse a child.

2. The examiner may not want to get involved or interfere in what he believes is, rightfully, a family situation.

3. If the examiner lacks proper training in observation, abuse may be overlooked.

4. In general, people tend to believe what they are told and base decisions on that belief.

5. Finally, perhaps most often, when the severely injured child presents to the emergency room, medical staff members concentrate on the problem at hand—respiratory arrest, cardiac arrest, shock, or convulsions—and miss the larger question of overall etiology.

♦ INTERPRETING ABUSE INJURIES

CUTANEOUS INJURIES

Skin injuries are the most common and easily recognized manifestations of maltreatment of children. Human bites are strong indicators of abuse. Bruises can vary from superficial injuries, such as first-degree burns and abrasions, to deeper injuries, ranging from lacerations to second- and third-degree burns. Patterns and locations of these injuries are clues to suspecting child abuse.

HUMAN BITES

Human bites are intentional and are common injuries in abuse. Trube-Becker (1977) reported 48 autopsied child abuse cases and noted that 11 of the 48 showed human bite marks. He found evidence of bites on the limbs, abdomen, and cheeks. Recognizing human bite marks is particularly important in child abuse cases because forensic dentists can study them and help determine the perpetrator of these injuries (Levine, 1984). Sims et al. (1973) reported three cases of human bite marks occurring in child abuse that were used to identify the perpetrator.

Human bite marks can be easily overlooked if one is unaware of their characteristics. The location of bite marks on infants tends to differ from the location on older children. Bite marks around the genitalia or buttocks are usually seen in infants and are inflicted as punishment. Older children have bites associated with assault or sexual abuse; they are generally multiple, random, and well-defined and may be associated with a sucking mark. The sucking mark may be the only indicator noted if sexual abuse has occurred.

Figure 1-1. *Bite injury showing three components.*

There are three components of a human bite to look for: the bite mark, the suck mark, and the thrust mark (**Figure 1-1**). Bite marks are ovoid areas with tooth imprints, and shape and size are significant. The suck mark is caused by a pulling of the skin into the mouth, creating a negative pressure. The thrust mark is caused by the tongue as it pushes against the skin, which is trapped behind the teeth. The inner portion of the bite mark may show no abnormality or may contain the suck or thrust mark. These two marks are similar in appearance in that each resembles a contusion in the center of the mark. To accurately identify a bite mark, each component must be recognized.

The anterior teeth give the human bite mark its configuration, which is the shape of the dental arch. Generally, no one tooth stands out (in contradistinction to the canines in animal bites), and the marks are irregular in size, shape, and position. The incisor teeth leave narrow rectangles, the canines leave triangular shapes, and the premolars make circular marks. The canines are more likely to be recognizable in bites from adults than in bites from children.

Early recognition of a human bite mark is critical to preserve valuable information. The body should not be washed or an autopsy begun before the marks have been photographed. A measuring device, such as a ruler, should be placed in the field to be photographed and thereby document the size of the mark. A child's bite can be distinguished from an adult's bite by measuring arch and tooth widths. Moorees (1959) found that the difference between a 5-year-old child's arch width and an adult's is approximately 4.4 mm for the maxilla and 2.5 mm for the mandible. The cumulative widths of the six upper teeth of the child were 10 mm smaller than those of the adult. In the lower arch, the differences were approximately 7 mm. If puncture marks from the canines are visible in the bite, it is possible to distinguish bites of permanent teeth (older than age 8) from primary teeth bites because the distance of separation is greater than 30 mm.

BRUISES

The skin can be a window to deeper injuries. Hemorrhage into deep subcutaneous tissues, such as muscle, will work its way to the surface. The accumulation of blood under the skin will be evident for a number of days, changing color as it ages. A fresh injury is red to blue, with the blue color caused by blood outside the vessels and the red component due to vasodilation with arterial blood visible in vessels; in 1 to 3 days it becomes deep black or purple; in 3 to 6 days the color changes to green and gradually brown; in 6 to 15 days it passes from green to tan to yellow to faded; and finally it disappears. The younger the child, the quicker the color resolves (Wilson, 1977).

Figure 1-2. Child with multiple bruises involving multiple surfaces, on inaccessible places, and in various stages of healing.

Multiple bruises or bruises in inaccessible places are indications that the child has been abused (**Figure 1-2**). In addition, babies who are not mobile do not usually have bruising. The toddler who is learning to walk typically has frontal bruising, as stated earlier. Severe bruising is unlikely. In the older child (age 2 to 5), some parts of the body, such as the knees, shins, foreheads, and elbows, are bruised often because these portions of the body are contact points.

Bruises, ecchymoses, and hematomas are the result of abuse when they occur in areas of the body that are unlikely to be injured accidentally. Multiple bruises and bruises of the buttocks or the genital area are usually not accidental. Bruises in different stages of healing are the result of repeated trauma and indicate abuse when the parents give a history describing a single accident. **A significant discrepancy between the physical findings and the history is the cardinal sign of abuse.**

Figure 1-3. Loop marks caused by whipping with extension cord.

Bruises that take the shape of a recognizable object are generally not accidental. Loop marks are caused by a flexible object, such as a belt, electric cord, or clothesline, folded on itself and used to beat the child (**Figure 1-3**). Multiple curvilinear loop marks on the child are pathognomonic of abuse. These bruises are usually ecchymotic, but can be lacerations or abrasions. A hand imprint on a child's face after a slap and finger and thumb marks on an arm or leg where the child was grabbed or squeezed are inflicted injuries. Belt buckles and other synthetic objects used to inflict punishment leave recognizable imprints on the

Figure 1-4. *Circular bruising of wrist caused by restraints.*

child's skin. Rope burns, bruises, or scars around the arms, ankles, neck, or waist are evidence that the child was tied (**Figure 1-4**). Many of these injuries leave long-lasting scars. There have been incidences when the penis is tied to prevent bed-wetting or pinched as punishment for soiling (**Figure 1-5**). At autopsy, ligatures around the neck may be identified as a series of small hemorrhages seen in the trachea.

Parents can claim that a child suspected of abuse bruises easily. Coagulation studies, including platelet count, prothrombin time, and partial thromboplastin time, should be ordered in an abuse workup when the child has bruises. Bleeding time is a good screening test in some patients with platelet dysfunction. For completeness, coagulation studies should be ordered for all children presenting with marked bruising. Bleeding disorders, such as hemophilia, are usually diagnosed at an early age but occasionally a mild form does not manifest until the child is older. The usual age for a bleeding disorder to become evident is when the child begins to walk and cruise, or with the eruption of the first tooth. This, coincidentally, is also the age when child abuse occurs frequently. It is important to note that hemophilia is a stress-producing disease, and hemophiliac children are at increased risk for being abused. Their tendency for easy bruising can mask an intentional injury.

Figure 1-5. *Ecchymosis of glans penis caused by pinching. Child was disciplined for soiling himself.*

HAIR LOSS

Hair loss (alopecia) can be a manifestation of child maltreatment. Traumatic alopecia occurs when parents pull their child's hair, frequently using the hair as a handle to grab the child and jerk or drag him. Pulling can cause hemorrhage under the galea aponeurotica, which has a rich supply of blood vessels. This accumulation of blood can be an important clue in differentiating between abusive and nonabusive loss of hair. Alopecia can also be a sign of latent syphilis.

Traumatic alopecia is defined as the forceful pulling of hair or the breaking of hair shafts by friction, traction, or other physical trauma. The usual causes of traumatic alopecia are trichotillomania or extreme cosmetic practices. Trichotillomania is conscious or subconscious self-induced alopecia caused by plucking, pulling, breaking, or cutting of the hair. The scalp is the most common site of involvement, but the eyebrows and eyelashes may also be affected. The patient plucks, twirls, or rubs hair-bearing areas, resulting in the loss or breakage of hair shafts. Most affected individuals are under varying degrees of emotional stress. Some have severe psychological problems.

Extreme cosmetic practices that can cause this condition are tight braiding or pony-tails; the use of tight rollers, barrettes, head bands, or rubber bands; hair straightening practices such as teasing or pulling, or frequent brushing with nylon bristles; and the use of hot combs and petrolatum. Other common causes of traumatic alopecia include pressure, as is seen on the occiput of infants who lie on their backs or are in the habit of "head-banging"; prolonged bed rest in one position, as in chronically ill persons or neglected children; thermal or electric burns; repeated vigorous massage; a severe blow to the scalp; and avulsions, such as may occur after abusive hair-pulling.

Alopecia areata is a common disorder characterized by the sudden appearance of sharply defined round or oval patches of hair loss. Recent evidence suggests that an autoimmune process may cause this disorder. Another possible cause of bald patches is fungal infections, for example, ringworm. The diagnosis of alopecia areata is based on its clinical presentation—a sudden appearance and the circumscribed, nonscarring pattern of hair loss. One or more round or oval well-circumscribed and clearly defined patches are usual. Occasionally the initial patches may be atypical, lacking a regular outline or demonstrating scattered long hairs within the bald areas. This will usually distinguish it from other forms of alopecia (Hurwitz, 1981).

FALLS

In most cases, a trivial injury occurs when a child has a routine fall in the home, such as out of bed, from a sofa, off a chair, or down the stairs. There is usually no object, such as a tricycle or stroller, involved; leverage created by such objects and their weight can influence the fall. On some occasions, a single skull fracture, most often parietal, is sustained. None of these fractures is bilateral, diastatic, or greater than 1 mm in width. Intracranial pressure is not increased.

A child, reported to have had a routine fall, may present with a skull fracture, cerebral edema, retinal hemorrhages, subdural hematoma, or epidural hemorrhage. These severe injuries are incongruous with a routine fall, and the inconsistency indicates child abuse. The physician should suspect child abuse whenever the child presents with serious head injury, with or without skull fracture, as a result of a reported fall from a bed, sofa, or crib.

A fall down the stairs, especially when the stairs are not padded, will cause a series of bruises the size and shape of the stair edge. The bruises are usually on multiple body surfaces. Joffe and Ludwig (1988) studied 363 children who fell down stairs and reported that the falls resulted in bony injuries in 7%, head and neck injuries in 73%, extremity injuries in 28%, and truncal injuries in 2%; injury to more than one body part occurred in 2.7%. **No patients had life-threatening injuries and none required admission to an intensive care unit.**

Injuries caused by a fall from a car generally include abrasions. The wounds are usually dirty and contain particulate matter from the road surface and shoulder. The injuries can involve multiple body surfaces because, depending on the speed of the vehicle, the child will roll when he strikes the ground. His clothes should show evidence of the experience. Vehicular accidents are usually reported to the police. In suspicious cases, if the police are unaware of the existence of such an accident, further investigation is warranted.

STUDIES OF FALLS
Falls were the subject of several studies, which are summarized here:

Hall et al. (1989)-Reviewed records from a Medical Examiner's Office and found 18 cases in which a fall of 3 feet or less was associated with fatal head injury. The study was performed as a critique of therapies and practices necessary to prevent fatal outcomes. The authors were not primarily interested in the differentiation between accidental and inflicted injuries. Unfortunately the histories given to explain the falls were not challenged when the children were admitted to the hospital, so explanations for the severe injuries were accepted and the diagnosis of child abuse was not entertained. No other study has concluded that falls of this distance, 3 feet or less, are fatal in children.

Helfer et al. (1977)-Studied 246 children under 5 years of age who fell out of bed, documenting the degree and severity of cerebral injuries. Results from the review of these incidents revealed 85 reports of children who fell to the floor from heights of approximately 90 cm (about 36 inches).

The 85 incidents resulted in the following injuries:

57—no apparent injury; 17—small cuts, scratches, and/or bloody noses; 20—bump and/or bruise; 1— fracture of the skull with no serious sequelae (the child fell off an emergency room cart and had no signs of soft tissue injuries over the site of the fracture). Of the 85 incidents documented, two children had bumps on the forehead, one with a bruise on the back, and one without injury. X-ray films taken following these incidents did not identify any fractures other than the one noted.

Nimityongskul and Anderson (1987)-Using a similar study, concluded that children are not seriously injured in short falls.

Smith et al. (1975)-Studied long falls of children from buildings and found that the shortest falls that resulted in death were from the four-story level (about 30 feet).

Snyder et al. (1977)-Studied 100 falls of children and adults and concluded that life-threatening injury required at least a 15-foot fall. They found just one child death after a presumed 10-foot fall.

Williams (1991)-Reported on 106 infants and children whose injuries resulted from falls that were witnessed by a second person. Only one death occurred, resulting from a 70-foot fall. There were falls of up to 15 feet with no injury, and minor injury or simple fractures were found in 77 patients.

Chadwick et al. (1991)-Examined fatal outcome of injury in 317 infants and children who were seen at a children's trauma center with injuries and a history of a fall. Caretakers of 7 of 100 children who died gave a history of a fall of less than 4 feet. No deaths occurred in 65 children who fell from 5 to 9 feet, and one death occurred in 118 children who fell from 10 to 45 feet. The fall that produced the single death in the long fall group, 10 to 45 feet, was not observed nor was a report of a scene investigation found for the case. Head injuries were the cause of death in all of the children in this study. The head injuries were subdural hematoma, cerebral contusion with brain swelling, or both. All seven patients had fresh subdural bleeding and cerebral edema and one had a skull fracture. The child who presumably fell from the second story had a markedly depressed parietal skull fracture with underlying bleeding. The child survived the head injury but died 6 weeks later from sepsis. Five of the seven fatal cases with short fall histories, less than 4 feet, had evidence of other injuries including old fractures, bruising on the trunk and extremities, genital injury, or more than one impact site on the head.

If the histories of short falls are accepted as explaining the deaths, the conclusion could be reached that the risk of death is greater for children who fall from a distance of less than 4 feet than for those who fall from 5 to 9 feet or from 10 to 45 feet. Chadwick et al. (1991) concluded that the histories given to explain the injuries of the seven fatal falls noted in his study were falsified and emphasized the importance of early reporting to initiate an investigation at the scene. Vital information about the sites is best obtained by trained investigators who examine the alleged fall scenes and interview witnesses as soon as possible.

EXTERNAL HEAD, FACIAL, AND ORAL INJURIES

The head is a common area of injury; approximately 50% of physical abuse patients have head or facial injuries. The reported incidence of intraoral injuries is

Figure 1-6. *Face injury caused by blow to the side of the face. Linear marks are caused by fingers.*

low, most likely because the mouth is often not examined. Detailed dental examinations were performed on 170 physically and sexually abused children who presented to a pediatric emergency department over a 4-month period. Approximately 25% of the physically abused children and 15% of the sexually abused children demonstrated injuries in and around the mouth. The injury patterns differed between the two groups of children (Bernat, 1992).

Many different injuries can be seen in the abused child. As stated earlier, accidental injuries to the face are usually frontal, involving the forehead, nose, chin, and incisor teeth. However, not all frontal injuries are accidental, and a careful history is needed to evaluate its plausibility and consistency with the physical injuries.

Lateral injuries to the face, which are found on the ears, cheeks, temporal and parietal areas (not including single parietal fractures), are highly suspicious for abuse (**Figure 1-6**). Hemorrhages around the ear and ear lobe or inside the ear canal are also important indicators of abuse.

Lacerations, hemorrhage, redness of the soft tissue membranes lining the external auditory canal, or swelling of its cartilage may be evidence of a severe blow to the ear (**Figure 1-7a, b**). Such a blow may cause rupture of the tympanic membrane, with resultant hearing loss or infection secondary to opening of the middle ear chamber. The examiner must look for evidence of a lacerated drum when the membrane has not been perforated by infection or fistula.

The tin ear syndrome results from a slap or other blunt force to the ear (Hanigan et al., 1987). It is identified by bruising and hemorrhage in the helix and antitragus. If sufficient force is generated by the blow, unilateral hemorrhagic retinopathy, cerebral edema, and ipsilateral subdural hematoma may result. The cerebral damage results from the rotational acceleration of the head stretching and tearing the cortical veins. The findings in tin ear syndrome are similar to those found with whiplash or shaken infants (Caffey, 1972).

Frenulum tears can occur through two mechanisms:

1. There may be a direct blow to the mouth. In this case one might see a linear or ragged tear. Besides the torn frenulum, there may be contusions, broken teeth, and facial fractures.

2. At feeding time, the caretaker may force or jam a spoon or bottle into the baby's mouth, ripping the frenulum. Other trauma rarely accompanies this injury.

A frenulum tear can happen accidentally if the child falls and strikes a sharp edge, for example, a coffee table, as is common among toddlers. When a frenulum tear is found in a nonambulatory infant, the case should be evaluated for other evidence of abuse.

Lip injuries are the most frequently seen oral injuries and appear as contusions, lacerations, abrasions, or burns. These injuries are caused when the lip is caught between a blunt force and the teeth. Lip burns are caused by hot liquid or hot objects such as utensils or cigarettes.

Traumatic injuries to the teeth of children are common and often accidental. Teeth injuries can fall into four categories: luxation, intrusion, avulsion, and fracture.

A *luxated* tooth is loosened but remains in the socket. The tooth may be displaced by more than 1 mm in any direction. If one tooth appears to be luxated, all of the teeth must be examined to determine mobility. The patient should be referred to a dentist as soon as possible in cases of luxated teeth.

An *intruded* tooth has been forced into the alveolar bone, and on examination it appears shorter than the rest of the teeth, or, if the causative blow is extreme, the tooth may be driven completely into the alveolar bone and not be visible. Intrusions result from a severe blow to the biting surface of the tooth. Radiographs reveal the extent of the injury.

In *avulsion* the tooth is removed from the socket. This is caused by a blow to the facial surface of the tooth and occurs more commonly with permanent teeth. The examiner must try to locate the missing tooth; it may have been swallowed or aspirated. An oral radiograph is needed to determine if the tooth has been intruded; a chest and abdominal radiograph may be necessary to rule out aspiration or ingestion. The tooth should be saved and a dental consultation obtained.

Fracture of the anterior teeth in children is common and usually not intentional. Fracture may be caused by a sharp blow to the teeth with a hard object and can occur during a fall or when struck. An oral radiograph should be obtained to determine the extent of the injury and locate any missing pieces, which may have been aspirated.

The tongue can be injured with a blow to the jaw, trapping it between the teeth. Most injuries are on the lateral border and appear as cuts or crushed tissue, frequently with jagged indentations. To best examine the tongue, the examiner should ask the patient to extend it as far as possible, then grasp the tongue with a square of gauze and retract it optimally.

If a black eye is present, the history must detail an appropriate injury to that side. It is difficult to break the tissues around the eye without damaging the nose as well, unless the black eye results from a direct blow, as from a fist. It is unlikely that a child will sustain two black eyes as the result of a fall unless the nose is broken also. If the child falls on the center of the face, injury to the nose will occur. This position of contact protects one or both eyes, and they should not be blackened

Figure 1-7. *Injuries to ear, **a,** old, and **b,** recent, caused by a blow to the side of the face. When the injury heals without medical intervention it leaves a distortion of the ear cartilage often called "cauliflower" ear.*

(**Figure** 1-8). Bilateral suborbital bruising can occur secondary to blood seepage into loose tissue areas in cases where there has been a blow to the forehead, possibly from a swing or the corner of a table.

Figure 1-8. Bilateral black eyes, when there is no broken nose, must be caused by at least two blows and cannot be explained by a single incident.

Hemorrhage in the upper eyelid often results when blood seeps down into periorbital tissues after an injury to the forehead or a subgaleal hematoma. Hemorrhage around the entire eye concentrically positioned as the result of a forehead injury is unlikely. Practitioners should be aware of the spontaneous black eye that occurs with malignant neuroblastoma, which may be associated with bony abnormalities palpable on the forehead. There are also rare occurrences of black eye(s) in blood dyscrasia.

CLOSED HEAD INJURY— SHAKEN INFANT SYNDROME

In 1946, Caffey's initial report of the association of multiple fractures with chronic subdural hematomas in infants initiated the recognition of shaken infant syndrome. This syndrome is responsible for at least 50% of the deaths of children caused by nonaccidental trauma and also yields the most severe sequelae of abuse.

In the early 1970s, Guthkelch (1971) and Caffey (1972) concluded that subdural hematoma, interhemispheric subarachnoid hemorrhage, and cerebral contusions in abused children were the result of a whiplash injury to the brain. Early studies were done before the availability of CT scans and therefore emphasized the most severe cases, those who were examined at autopsy. This form of abuse is comparable to those injuries seen in car accidents that result from acceleration-deceleration phenomena. The shaking produces a differential motion between the skull and intracranial structures as the head rotates on the neck. The differential motion causes stretching and tearing of the bridging vessels and the possibility of cerebral contusion or laceration as the brain moves within the skull.

Impact injury probably plays a major role in many closed head injuries. Scalp and subgaleal hemorrhages are often found in children who have died of abusive head trauma, and skull fractures, usually linear, are also common. Hahn et al. (1983) reported findings on 77 children, seen over a 10-year period, who suffered abusive injuries ranging from concussion to irreversible injury and death. Eight percent were believed to have been caused by shaking, 48% were caused by direct trauma to the face and head, and 35% resulted from dropping, throwing, or falling. The remaining children suffered impact trauma that was not directed at the head. Fifty percent had skull fractures, mostly parietal linear fractures. The intracranial injuries noted were 30 subdural hematomas, of which 22 were bilateral; 23 cerebral contusions; and seven concussions.

The low incidence of shaking as an etiology in this group and the frequent finding of concealed impact injury in fatal cases of abuse raise questions about the biomechanics of inflicted head injury. Holbourn (1943) provided the first basis for analyzing head injuries secondary to impact phenomena of the head, but he did not evaluate the effects of acceleration-deceleration forces. Ommaya et al. (1968) noted that rotational injury without direct impact to the head could cause significant injury to the brain and followed a distribution suggested by Holbourn that corresponded to the regions of injury seen in abused infants diagnosed with the shaken infant syndrome. The degree of acceleration needed to cause a given injury is related to the duration of impact. Short duration impacts produce effects dependent on velocity change, not accelerational change alone.

Duhaime et al. (1987) reviewed 48 cases of shaken infants, seen over 8 years, for evidence of impact injury. Sixty-three percent of the patients had physical evidence of blunt impact to the head, as well as findings of retinal hemorrhage, subdural hematoma, subarachnoid hemorrhage, interhemispheric blood, or bilateral chronic subdural effusions. Thirteen percent had blunt extracranial trauma accompanying their intracranial findings, and 24% showed no physical evidence of a blow. Reliable histories were obtained for 40 of the cases and revealed that only one was apparently caused by shaking unassociated with other trauma. Analysis of the 13 fatal cases showed that all had evidence of blunt cranial trauma, but autopsy was necessary to demonstrate this finding in 7 of the 13 cases.

Duhaime et al. (1987) constructed mechanical models approximating the size, weight, and density of a 1-month-old infant. Three varieties of necks were devised and tested, and accelerometers were implanted in the head. Each model was tested at least 20 times, with vigorous shaking, by male and female adults. The occiput of each model was impacted against a metal bar or padded surface. The results showed that both the tangential and the angular accelerations were much higher with impact than with shaking. The authors concluded that, despite significant differences between the neck models, shaking did not generate accelerations great enough to produce concussion, subdural hematoma, or diffuse axonal injury. They determined the accelerations necessary based on estimates derived from the conversion equation proposed by Ommaya et al. (1968). (It should be noted that this conversion equation has not been verified for infants but has been verified in other nonhuman primates. Verification for adult humans has been provided from studies of motor vehicle accidents.)

Impact against a yielding surface will not alter the force delivered to the brain but can minimize the damage to external soft tissues. A boxer may be knocked unconscious, with injury to the brain, after impact from a gloved and cushioned hand yet suffer no facial bruising. In like manner, a child thrown against a soft crib mattress, bed, or carpeted floor can sustain severe brain injuries with no evidence of external damage.

Shaking alone may produce the injuries seen in the shaken infant syndrome. When making this diagnosis, one should emphasize that an impact may have been involved in the injury even though no external evidence of injury is observed (Alexander et al., 1990).

Table 1-2 lists the features in an infant that play an important role in creating shaken infant syndrome. Children under 2 years of age are prone to brain injury during severe shaking and severe shaking with impact because of the disproportionate size of the head compared to the body, the weakness of the cervical muscles, poor head and neck control, the higher water content of the infant brain, and poorer myelination of the brain, large subarachnoid space, and open fontanelles and sutures characteristic of this age.

What makes the shaken infant syndrome more difficult to recognize and diagnose than other forms of infant trauma is the usual absence of external evidence of trauma. In addition, the history given by the caretaker is usually deliberately misleading. The underlying pathophysiology is cerebral anoxia, ischemia, or a combination of both. **Table 1-3** lists the presenting signs and symptoms in an infant suspected to have shaken infant syndrome. The three essential components of the shaken infant syndrome are (1) closed head injury evidenced by altered level

Table 1-2. Mechanism of Shaken Infant Syndrome

Unique Features of Child Less Than 2 Years of Age
Size of head relative to body
Weakness of cervical musculature
Poor control of head and neck
Anatomy of upper cervical spine and foramen magnum
Higher water content of brain
Minor degree of myelination
Large subarachnoid space

Acceleration-Deceleration Phenomena
Rotation of head on neck
Differential motion between skull and intracranial structures
Stretching and tearing of bridging vessels
Cerebral contusion and laceration

Impact

Table 1-3. Presenting Signs and Symptoms of Shaken Infant Syndrome

Altered level of consciousness
Somnolent yet irritable
Coma
Convulsions
Opisthotonic posturing
Respiratory problems
  Arrest
  Hypoventilation
  Cheyne-Stokes
Dead

Table 1-4. Suggested Diagnostic Studies for Shaken Infant Syndrome

History
Optic fundus exam for retinal
  hemorrhages
CT scan (head and abdomen)
MRI in selected cases
Lumbar puncture with precautions
Skeletal survey
Nuclear scan
Drug screen
Routine blood samples
Liver and pancreatic enzymes

Table 1-5. Physical Findings in Shaken Infant Syndrome

Retinal hemorrhages
CNS (closed head) injury
  Bleeding (subdural, epidural,
    subarachnoid, subgaleal)
  Laceration
  Contusion
  Concussion
Bruises–facial, scalp, arms,
  abdomen, back
Soft tissue swelling
Skull fracture(s)
Other fracture(s) (long bones,
  ribs, metaphyseal)
Abdominal injuries
Chest injuries
Hypotension
Tense fontanelle

of consciousness, coma, convulsions, or death; (2) central nervous system injury as evidenced by CNS hemorrhaging, laceration, contusion, or concussion; and (3) retinal hemorrhages. CNS injury can be documented with a CT scan or, if needed to clarify an injury, magnetic resonance imaging (MRI). It should be noted that approximately 40% of these infants have metaphyseal chip fractures of the long bones secondary to traction or shearing (Caffey, 1972). Therefore a skeletal survey should be included in the workup. This should also detect any vertebral injuries (Swischuk, 1969).

One should also look for evidence of impact, frequently indicated by bruises. In addition, routine skull films will help identify fractures, which may be missed by the CT scan if the fracture lies in the same plane as the CT slice. A radionuclide scan can help detect fresh fractures not visible on the routine radiograph.

As in any medical problem, a good history is paramount. It should be remembered that, as in other forms of child abuse, the history in these cases is apt to be misleading, false, or not available. An infant or toddler with a history of, or physical evidence of, altered level of consciousness must be suspected to have head trauma until proven otherwise. If a minor fall is given to explain the injury, child abuse, with closed head injury, should be suspected. As discussed earlier in this chapter, infants under 1 year of age rarely sustain devastating accidental head injury, and accidental severe head injury, as seen in an automobile accident, is usually witnessed.

While giving the central nervous system symptoms adequate attention, the examiner must also be aware that abdominal and/or chest trauma is often present and should be evaluated and treated. The workup of the child includes CT scans of both the head and the abdomen and chest (**Tables 1-4 and 1-5**).

Physical examination of the nude baby is essential to establish the presence of any signs of external trauma such as bruising and should include careful evaluation of hidden places such as the scalp, back, and buttocks. The physician must palpate the various areas of the skin and scalp for soft tissue swelling and the fontanelle for fullness or tension. The examination should also include the genital area. **It must be remembered that the absence of external injury does not rule out a diagnosis of shaken infant syndrome.**

Hypoventilation or Cheyne-Stokes breathing can alert the examiner to central nervous system injury. The neck should be examined for nuchal rigidity. **Most important, the examination must include evaluation of the optic fundi for retinal hemorrhage, which denotes severe trauma and is a necessary component in making the diagnosis of shaken infant syndrome.** Retinal hemorrhages in an infant without a history of severe accidental trauma constitute child abuse until proven otherwise.

As will be discussed in the chapter on the death review process, catastrophic injuries to children are costly in terms of survivor outcome. One third of these children die; one third, although they survive, are mentally and/or physically disabled and often require a lifetime of custodial care; and one third will have a good recovery. As we look at the three outcomes, the third, good recovery, is likely to be the most costly. The survivors often have severe emotional problems and become predators, becoming abusive and ending up in prison (Magid & McKelvey, 1987). Prevention through the early recognition of potential abusers is essential. These children, the apparent survivors, should receive extensive counseling.

DROWNING

Drowning resulting from child abuse is difficult to distinguish from accidental immersion or from sudden and unexpected natural causes. Accidental drownings usually involve toddlers or older children in public areas—swimming pools, drainage ditches, lakes, and rivers—especially in rural areas. In cities, bathtubs are the major sites of accidental childhood drownings. Homicidal drownings usually occur in the home; the victims are young, either infants or toddlers. The pathologic findings of postimmersion syndrome suggest the cause of death. Foreign material in the lungs and injuries of the face are positive correlating factors indicating abuse. However, it is hypothesized that deliberate drowning is underreported and underdiagnosed because of the sparsity of physical evidence and clear criteria on which to base a diagnosis of abuse.

Nixon and Pearn (also as Pearn and Nixon) in 1977 (a,b,c) described several features that serve to differentiate accidental from nonaccidental drowning:

1. Accidental drowning occurs during the usual bath time when more than one child is present in the tub, and generally the older child(ren) left the youngest. The household routine is usually upset, resulting in a lapse of supervision.

2. Nonaccidental drownings or near-drownings occur in the bathtub at an unusual time of day with the drowned child alone in the bath.

3. The parents fit the sociopathologic profile of abusing caretakers, and a precipitating crisis, often a domestic problem, is present.

4. The abused children are older, usually between 15 and 30 months of age, compared with the usual age of 9 to 15 months for accidental drowning.

5. The depth of the bath water ranges from 5 to 35 cm (2 to 14 inches), and those children immersed 5 minutes or more die. Nixon and Pearn found that in cases of deliberate immersion, the child is held under the water until unconsciousness ensues.

6. There is often a history of previous abusive behavior by the parent or guardian or a history of alcohol and drug abuse.

7. There is a delay between the event and calling for help or finding the child, as evidenced by cerebral edema.

8. Postmortem pulmonary features of the postimmersion syndrome, characterized by widespread intraalveolar polymorphonuclear leukocyte infiltrates and edema of hyaline membranes, may be present.

In deaths that occur in the bathtub, the presence of foreign material in the lungs should be noted because it confirms the cause of death as drowning and the location of the drowning. The water from the reported immersion site should be analyzed and matched to that in the lung.

Griest and Zumwalt (1989) reviewed a series of accidental drownings of children between birth and 12 years of age. Irrigation ditch drownings prevailed among the toddler group, whereas lakes, rivers, and swimming pools were the prime location among older children. In bathtub drownings of older children there was a major contributing factor—cerebral palsy and epilepsy. In bathtub drownings of younger children the child was left alone in the tub by the parent or older sibling for a short period of time. In bucket deaths, the child was a toddler who was tall enough to tip himself into the pail, but not large enough to knock it over. The water in the bucket was heavy enough to weigh it down and deep enough to cover the child's nose and mouth.

FETAL ABUSE

Fetal abuse involves a range of behaviors in pregnant women, or their partners, characterized by the nonaccidental performance of acts that can be detrimental to the fetus. These acts include a direct physical assault on the fetus, through the abdominal wall or via the vagina, or a failure to protect the fetus from an indirect assault, as with alcohol, nicotine, or drugs.

The cost of fetal abuse to society is considerable. It has been estimated that the risks to the fetus from maternal alcohol and nicotine abuse outweigh the risks of other medical conditions such as diabetes, toxemia, or Rh incompatibility (Sokol, 1981). No one knows what significance in utero physical assault has on abortion, prematurity, stillbirth, deformity, or mental retardation.

Condon (1985, 1986), in defining fetal abuse, differentiated behaviors directed at the pregnant state, that is, therapeutic or self-induced abortion, from behaviors aimed at the fetus itself. The former behaviors usually occur in early pregnancy, while the latter behaviors more often occur in late pregnancy. These studies showed that parents' attitudes toward "being pregnant" often bear little relationship to those toward the fetus itself, and the dichotomy "wanted" versus "unwanted" pregnancy is not clear-cut, with degrees of ambivalence prevailing. Even a "wanted" fetus may become the victim of abuse.

Although the incidence of fetal abuse is unknown, as with other forms of child abuse, fetal abuse is most likely underreported. Estimates of the incidence of fetal abuse due to alcohol or nicotine have been reported (Kwok et al., 1983; Streissguth et al., 1983). The fetal alcohol syndrome is the third most common known cause of mental retardation in the United States, possibly affecting 1 in 750 live births (Abel & Sokol, 1986). Between one half and two thirds of pregnant women consume some alcohol, and between 2% and 13% of all pregnant women acknowledge heavy consumption (Kwok et al., 1983; Sokol, 1981). A strong association exists between alcohol and cigarette use during pregnancy, with studies revealing that 25% to 35% of pregnant women smoke during pregnancy (Kwok et al., 1983; Streissguth et al., 1983), and 25% of these women smoke more than 20 cigarettes per day.

Until Condon (1985, 1986) reported several cases, no case of physical assault on the fetus through the anterior abdominal wall by the mother had been considered by experienced professionals. Condon noted that, if specific inquiry was made, the impulse to harm the fetus was not uncommon in pregnant women. Although spouse abuse of pregnant women has been reported, only Gelles (1975) speculated that sometimes the fetus was the target in spouse abuse of pregnant women. One such case of fetal assault by an expectant father was noted.

The women involved did not satisfy the criteria for any psychiatric diagnosis, but their behaviors did resemble those of women who subsequently killed their babies shortly after delivery (Condon, 1986).

As stated, the risk of assaultive behavior is greatest in late pregnancy because of the stresses of the third trimester and because of progressive disenchantment, in both partners, with the pregnancy state in the final 2 to 3 months (Condon, 1985). Fetal abuse may be triggered by a woman's perception of rejection by her spouse, family, or doctor, because attention is directed to the fetus and not her. The perceived rejection may be responded to with a physical attack on her "rival," or a more passive neglect or failure to protect. This scenario of neglect can be likened to failure to thrive in the older child wherein poor weight gain and stunted development result.

The initial reactions of the medical community to reports of fetal abuse were that they were isolated, rare phenomena. Condon (1987) presents data, though preliminary, that dispute the rarity of the phenomenon, finding that, after interviewing 112 couples, 8% of pregnant women and 4% of expectant fathers acknowledged that they occasionally experienced an urge to hurt or punish their unborn baby. The male partner was aware of the woman's urge to assault the fetus; 9% of fathers reported that they believed their female partner had experienced an urge to hurt or punish the fetus. When questioned about future child abuse, 8% of the women and 5% of the men acknowledged that they frequently had worries that they might lose their temper after the baby was born and harm the baby. The incidence estimates are probably conservative because the tendency to conceal this urge, based on shame, may result in underreporting. Condon warned that the data are preliminary and must be interpreted with caution. The worth in reporting them derived from the fact that they represent the only systematic attempt to explore expectant parents' feelings of aggression toward their unborn child; they suggest that an urge to hurt or punish the unborn child can be elicited in a significant number of expectant parents, suggesting that the phenomenon is not a clinical rarity.

FETAL ABUSE AND SUBSEQUENT CHILD ABUSE

Is fetal abuse a precursor to later child abuse? In two of Condon's five cases, the abuse continued postnatally. Examining the characteristic low birth weight of abused children, it would seem that a correlation may exist. Smith and Hanson (1974), in a controlled study of abused children, found a fourfold increase in low birth weight, independent of social class. Klaus hypothesized that early maternal-infant separation, forced by a low birth weight, leads to subsequent dysfunctional bonding, predisposing to child abuse. This hypothesis has been challenged (Smith and Hanson, 1974; Herbert et al., 1982; Lamb, 1982). Alternatively, if alcohol abuse during pregnancy constitutes fetal abuse and leads to low birth weight and child abuse occurs frequently among low birth weight children, it could be surmised that fetal abuse is a precursor of child abuse. The use of nicotine during pregnancy may also cause low birth weight and constitute fetal abuse.

Alcohol and nicotine clearly produce effects on the fetus. The possible effects of external physical trauma are speculative at present. The fetus is cushioned by the amniotic fluid and it is unlikely that damage would be caused by external trauma. Abdominal trauma may precipitate labor with resultant prematurity and low birth weight. There is a need for further research in physical fetal abuse.

FETAL ABUSE AND NEONATICIDE

Neonaticide is defined as murder of the baby during the first 24 hours of life. After reviewing the literature, Resnick (1970) concluded that hundreds and possibly thousands of neonaticides occur in the United States each year. Resnick noted that, unlike women who kill their older children, mothers who commit neonaticide are rarely psychotic. Neonaticide is usually committed because the child is not wanted. He went on to say that "passivity" is the most important personality characteristic differentiating women who commit neonaticide from those who obtain abortions. In fetal abuse, it is likely that passive acceptance, or denial, of an unwanted pregnancy is common and consequently elective abortion is not sought. Mothers who commit neonaticide suppress the reality of their pregnancy and make no preparations. They murder the infant when the reality of birth breaks through their defenses.

SUFFOCATION

The number of young children suffocated by their parents is unknown, but smothering is being increasingly reported. The involved families generally have a high incidence of sudden death of other siblings; investigation determines that some of the siblings were also suffocated.

Meadow (1990) reviewed the cases of 27 young children from 27 different families who were suffocated by their mothers. Twenty-four reported previous episodes of apnea, cyanosis, or seizure, and 11 had 10 or more episodes. The episodes began between the ages of 1 and 3 months and continued until discovery or the child died, 6 to 12 months later. The 27 children had 18 older siblings who had died suddenly and unexpectedly in early life. Thirteen of the dead siblings had recurrent apnea, cyanosis, or seizures. Most of them at death were diagnosed as having sudden infant death syndrome (SIDS). Suffocation can also be confused with recurrent apnea, although suffocation has clinical features that may facilitate making the appropriate diagnosis before brain damage or death occurs.

Since many of the dead children and their siblings had an initial diagnosis of SIDS, the features of suffocation must be compared with those of SIDS. The classic features of SIDS are young age, previous good health of the child, lack of previous apnea or other illness, and rarity of a positive family history, together with a thorough, complete autopsy, including metabolic studies, which fails to find another cause of death. In suffocation cases, it is common to find a child more than 6 months old with previous apneic episodes, previous unexplained disorders, and a dead sibling.

Metabolic problems that may present as apparent SIDS include medium chain acyldehydrogenase deficiency (MCAD), type I glycogen storage disease, and carnitine deficiency. Urine chromatography may be difficult if the bladder is empty; other studies can be done on vitreous humor, blood, liver, or other frozen tissue.

There are families who have increased risk for multiple SIDS; therefore, this possibility must be explored. Recurrent SIDS is probably more an environmental problem than a genetic one; there is no increased risk in first cousins or in monozygotic compared with dizygotic twins. Guntheroth et al. (1990) studied 251,124 live births by linked birth and death certificates from Oregon for a 10-year period to determine the risk of recurrence of SIDS. They found five recurrences among 385 subsequent siblings, for a rate of 13/1,000 live births.

In most of Meadow's cases suffocation was suspected when no cause for the apnea was found. Recurrent apnea in a previously healthy child having no viral infection or cardiac, respiratory, metabolic, or neurologic abnormality is rare, and this factor combined with the unexplained death of a sibling led to the diagnosis. It is difficult to diagnose suffocation when it occurs for the first time and when it is a single act rather than repeated.

Suffocation may cause petechial hemorrhages, but it can result in brain damage and death without other findings. Therefore, some deaths classified as SIDS may have been caused by the parents, as careful clinical, pathologic, and psychosocial studies of families have disclosed.

As in the Munchausen Syndrome by Proxy, there are few reports of suffocation of children by men; most acts of suffocation are committed by the natural mother. For more information on the Munchausen Syndrome by Proxy, *see Chapter 13*.

NEGLECT

While not an injury, neglect is a presenting feature in many abuse cases. The symptoms of neglect reflect a lack of both physical and medical care. An unclean baby can be a strong factor in determining neglect, although the ability to accumulate dirt in skin creases and other unreachable places is a natural characteristic of infants and children. There are degrees of uncleanliness. Most babies get dirty during normal play and a bath removes the dirt. The degree of dirtiness that suggests neglect requires several baths to begin to remove it and is accompanied by an offensive odor. Feces and dirt in the skin folds and under the nails may be evidence of failure to provide for the child's basic needs. Diaper rash can be a key to the attentiveness and care attitudes of the parents. The skin of some babies is extremely sensitive and some irritation and excoriation occur. But the diaper rash in these cases shows evidence of being cared for and seldom reaches the point where the skin is denuded, cracked, and bleeding. A baby with a constantly dirty perineum who is left in wet diapers sufficiently long for ammonia burns to occur is not being cared for adequately.

Multiple cat or dog bites and scratches indicate the child may be left unattended for long periods, another factor in neglect. If a parent fails to bring a child to a physician when the child has an infection of the skin and there is evidence that the illness has been present for some time, or if the child's condition is not improving with the treatment prescribed, assuming the diagnosis and treatment are correct, the parents are probably noncompliant, which constitutes medical neglect.

♦ Reporting Suspected Abuse

Mandated reporters include physicians, dentists, podiatrists, nurses, psychologists, speech pathologists, coroners, medical examiners, child day care center employees, childrens' services workers, social workers, and schoolteachers. The physician reporter should be prepared and willing to express an opinion about the cause of the injuries, their seriousness, and the potential danger to the child; he must also be available to the court when needed *(see Chapter 20)*. Although other mandated reporters may be asked to testify, they are less likely to be called than the physician.

Questioning the History

The evaluator must remember that an explanation for an injury should not change when it is questioned or challenged. If the history differs from parent to parent, with different history takers, or when challenged, it is very likely fabricated. Team members must communicate and share information. If the explanations offered differ significantly, further investigation is warranted. For example, a young father told a triage nurse that he found his son unconscious in the back yard at the bottom of the steps. He told the admitting physician the child was convulsing on the floor of the bedroom. The two did not check each other's notes, and the parent was sent home with two other children. Abuse was not diagnosed until 24 hours later when a skeletal survey revealed multiple old and new fractures.

Some parent advocacy groups do not consider any punishment of a child under the guise of discipline as child abuse. These groups consider the intent of the parent when the child was injured. Parents usually believe they are doing what is best for the child. Unfortunately, the injured child is not aware of the good intentions of the parent. As stated earlier, when deciding to report an injury, the mandated reporter concerned about a child's well-being should not be influenced by caretaker intent. The courts, law enforcement, and social services will decide what is best for the child and what influence intent will have.

False Allegations

False reports of child sexual abuse are uncommon and represent only a small proportion of cases (Thoennes & Pearson, 1988). There is concern that many of the reports of sexual abuse determined to be unsubstantiated may be false. Even if false reports are uncommon, they should be a serious concern, not only because of the potential legal consequences of a false accusation, but also because of the distress caused the family and the child.

Alleged abuse of children, physical and sexual, is more common in divorce and separation situations than in stable families. An allegation of abuse is difficult to deal with when made between separated parents and must be carefully evaluated by the professionals involved. It can be a powerful weapon one parent uses against the other or become a ploy to use against each other, calling the authorities at each return of the child, who is trapped in a compromising situation. It can also be a true allegation of abuse and the child and family in need of help.

Hlady and Gunter (1990) reviewed the records of 370 children, of which 41 (11%) were involved in custody disputes; 31 children were female, 10 male; 34 were alleged to be sexually abused, 7 physically abused. More than half were under 4 years of age. Of the 7 physical abuse children, 5 had corroborative evidence; 3

cases alleged neglect in addition. In a population of 110 children not involved in a custody situation, 48 (43.6%) demonstrated physical evidence of abuse. In the 34 children allegedly victims of sexual abuse, 6 (17%) had corroborative physical evidence of abuse. In a custodial group of 219 children reported as victims of sexual abuse, 33 (15%) had corroborative physical evidence.

Sexual abuse is usually secretive, involving two witnesses, abused and abuser. For good reasons, both parties may forget, or want to forget, the experience. Without a confession of guilt, one of those witnesses is lying. Jones (1986) suggested that the system may need to move away from true and false labeling and attempt an assessment based on degrees of probability. He studied 576 cases of sexual abuse reported to the Denver Department of Social Services and found 54% of the reports to be reliable. Nearly 22% were unable to be explored any further because of insufficient evidence. Nearly 17% of the reports were made by adults who were appropriately concerned and were not falsely creating an allegation. These cases were distinct from the fictitious accounts.

The fictitious reports were made by adults and/or their children and were broken down into two groups: 6.25% of the total number of reports were fictitiously made by an adult, and 1.56% by a child, for a total of 7.81% fictitious reports. *Jones made the following conclusions:*

Female teenagers, between 12 and 17 years of age, suffering from post-traumatic stress disorder as a result of documented earlier sexual victimization, made the child generate fictitious allegations.

Two adults involved suffered from major psychoses. Several of the adults were involved in custody disputes.

Adults behind false allegations commonly were victims of sexual abuse when they were children and suffered from psychological aftereffects of the experience.

Jones' study concluded:

1. Fictitious accounts of child sexual abuse, although not common, do occur and involve children of all ages and sexes.

2. To diagnose these cases the evaluator must first accept the possibility that fictitious cases can occur.

3. The diagnosis depends on careful interviews of the child and parents as well as careful search for an explanation for the fictitious report, looking at the family situation and dynamics, and the presence or absence of the post-traumatic stress disorder in the children and parents. It should be noted that in many reliable accounts some of these features also existed.

4. Absence of emotion, threats, or coercion in the child's statement proved helpful in determining when the account was fictitious.

5. A symbiotic mother/child relationship was present in mixed or fused accounts. Fused accounts were made in custody disputes.

6. Those making fictitious accounts require psychological help.

7. Child developmental specialists should be involved in the initial investigation conducted by local social services to help detect fictitious accounts.

Many of the conclusions made by Jones in this study can also be applied to false allegations of abuse other than sexual.

WHAT TO REPORT

Children's hospitals must have a Child Protection Team and must establish guidelines for recognizing and reporting child abuse. No numerical system or lab test is currently available to objectively evaluate abuse. While it may be relatively easy to determine some indicators, assigning a value to each is difficult. What is clearly abuse, what is probably abuse, and what is possibly abuse cannot be easily separated by a numerical system. The human factor remains in the equation, affecting what is reported and what is not. Knowing what and when to report requires a sound knowledge of what child abuse is, a familiarity with child development and behavior, an acquaintance with the child protection system, a knowledge of adult behavior, common sense, and a smattering of physics and biomechanics.

Various common abuse and neglect indicators can be rated on a relative value scale. The tables in this section rate as many of these situations as possible and assign a relative importance to each. It should be noted that these are guidelines only; no list is perfect. If one is to err, we recommend that the reader err on the side of the child. Errors that do not protect the child can be fatal. It is advisable that these lists be made available to clinic and emergency room personnel as reminders of what injuries and situations are suspicious of abuse. A protocol including these lists can be helpful as well as periodic in-service conferences to remind experienced and new personnel of the importance of recognizing abuse (**Tables 1-6, 1-7, and 1-8**).

Table 1-6. Situations which are Possibly Child Abuse and Dictate a Report to the Authorities

Death of an Infant with Unknown Cause and Poor or Questionable History

Evidence of Emotional Abuse
Hair loss
Suicide, runaway
Drug use
Child perpetrator
Child has flat affect passive, failure to thrive

Neglect
Medical treatment delayed (depends on seriousness of condition)
Failure to thrive with no medical condition to explain it
First drug or toxin ingestion with suspicious history
Repeated drug or toxin ingestion
Small child(ren) supervised by child under 12
Severe dehydration, underweight with no medical condition to explain it

Head Injury
Subdural hematoma without appropriate history
Fracture of the skull with suspicious or no history

Thermal Injuries
Burns that involve neglect
Burns with poor or no history

Skeletal Injuries
Fractured long bone with no appropriate history

Bruises
Multiple bruises
Injuries that suggest the use of an instrument
Injuries resulting from discipline in child over 1 year of age

Intrauterine Abuse
Fetal neglect, no prenatal checkups, suspicion of drug or alcohol abuse, poor nutrition
Psychotic mother who gives reason to suspect fetus is in danger
Battered mother

Sexual Abuse
Genital injuries
Child prostitution

Table 1-7. Situations which are Child Abuse and Dictate a Report to the Authorities

Severe Neglect
Abandonment
Long periods with no supervision. Children from
  infancy to 8 years old left unattended
Long delay in obtaining medical help for a serious injury
Maternal deprivation

Head Injury
Evidence of shaken infant syndrome
  –Altered level of consciousness
  –Closed head injury
  –CNS hemorrhaging
  –Retinal hemorrhages
Catastrophic injury explained by routing fall

Deliberate Thermal Injuries
Multiple cigarette burns in varying stages of healing
Glove-and-sock pattern liquid burn
Iron burns (shows iron pattern) on back, back of
  hand, or buttocks or curling iron burns in same areas
Diaper area burns and doughnut-shaped burns
Burns to the back of the hand
Bilateral burns or injuries to hands

Skeletal Injuries
Rupture of the costovertebral junction
Posterior rib fractures

Metaphyseal avulsion fracture
Two or more fractures in different stages of healing
Multiple skull fractures
Long bone fracture in a nonambulating child

Bruises
Bilateral black eyes without broken nose
Skin bruises and lacerations in recognizable shapes,
  such as whip, belt, stick, fist, fingers, buckle,
  rope, or teeth
Circumferential injuries (burns, bruises, lacerations,
  or scars) of the wrists, arms, ankles, legs, and neck
Multiple bruises in inaccessible place, in different
  stages of healing
An injury resulting from discipline in a child less
  than 1 year of age

Trauma
Blunt trauma to abdomen or chest with
  inappropriate or no history
Intrauterine abuse
Crack baby or newborn or other drug-dependent
  mother
Evidence of fetal injury or self-injury

Sexual Abuse
Category IV of sexual molestation *(see Chapter 8)*
Credible disclosure of abuse by child

Table 1-8. Caretaker Indicators

Strong Indicators
Explanation of injury not believable
Explanations are inconsistent/changing story
Paramour in the home
Previously suspected of abuse
Caretaker(s) understates the seriousness of
  child's condition
Caretaker(s) projects blame to third party
Caretaker(s) has delayed bringing child to hospital
Caretaker(s) cannot be located
History of substance abuse
Caretaker(s) unable to function
Child is not up-to-date on immunizations
Child has severe diaper rash, is poorly kept, dirty
Caretaker(s) is psychotic

Nonspecific Indicators
Caretaker(s) is hostile and aggressive
Caretaker(s) is compulsive, inflexible, unreasonable,
  and cold
Caretaker(s) is passive and dependent
Father is unemployed
History of unwanted baby
Caretaker(s) has unrealistic expectations of child
Caretaker(s) is hospital shopper
Frequent visits to the pediatrician without a
  medical reason
Caregiver(s) overreacts to child's misbehavior

DA FORM 5694, MAY 1988
DENVER DEVELOPMENTAL SCREENING TEST
REVISED DDST-R

STO. = STOMACH
SIT. = SITTING

PERCENT OF CHILDREN PASSING

May pass by report →
Footnote no. →
see back of form

©1978 W.K. Frankenburg, M.D.

Date:
Name:
Birthdate:
Hosp. No.:

For use of this form, see HQDA Ltr. 40-88-5, the proponent agency is TSG

♦ **BIBLIOGRAPHY**

Abel, EL, and Sokol, RH: Fetal alcohol syndrome is now leading cause of mental retardation, *Lancet* 8517:1222, 1986.

Alexander, R, et al: Incidence of impact trauma, with cranial injuries ascribed to shaking, *Am J Dis Child* 144(6):724-726, 1990.

Barlow, B, Neiminska, M, Gandli, RP, et al: Ten years of experience with falls from a height in children, *J Pediatr Surg* 18:509-511, 1983.

Bays, J: Conditions mistaken for child abuse, The San Diego Conference on Responding to Child Maltreatment, San Diego, CA, 1993.

Bernat, JE: Dental trauma and bite mark evaluation. In S Ludwig and A Kornberg, eds: *Child abuse*, Churchill Livingstone, New York, 1992, pp. 175-190.

Caffey, J: Multiple fractures in the long bones of infants suffering from chronic subdural hematoma, *AJR* 56:163-173, 1946.

Caffey, J: On the theory and practice: Its potential residual effects of permanent brain damage and mental retardation, *Am J Dis Child* 124:161, 1972.

Caffey, J: The whip-lash-shaken-infant syndrome: Mutual shaking by the extremities with whiplash-induced intracranial intraocular bleedings, linked with residual permanent brain damage and mental retardation, *Pediatrics* 54:396-493, 1974.

Chadwick, DL, Chin, S, Salerno, C, Landsverk, J, and Kitchen, L: Deaths from falls in children: How far is fatal? *J Trauma* 31:1353-1355, 1991.

Condon, JT: The parental-fetal relationship: A comparison of male and female expectant parents, *J Psychosom Obstet Gynecol* 4:271-284, 1985.

Condon, JT: The spectrum of fetal abuse in pregnant women, *J Nerv Ment Dis* 174:509-516, 1986.

Condon, JT: The battered fetus syndrome, *J Nerv Ment Dis* 175:722-725, 1987.

Duhaime, AC, Gennarelli, TK, Thibault, LE, et al: The shaken baby syndrome: A clinical, pathological and biomechanical study, *J Neurosurg* 66:409, 1987.

Ganaway, G: Historical truth versus narrative truth: Clarifying the role of exogenous trauma in the etiology of multiple personality disorder and its variants, *Dissociation* 2:205-220, 1989.

Gelles, RJ: Violence and pregnancy: A note on the extent of the problem and needed services, *Fam Coordinator* 24:81-86, 1975.

Gelles, RJ: The social context of child abuse. In EH Newberger, ed: *Child Abuse*, Little, Brown & Co, Boston, 1982, pp. 25-41.

Gellis, S, and Feingold, M: Cao Gio: Pseudobattering in Vietnamese children, *Am J Dis Child* 130:857-858, 1976.

Gennarelli, TK: Clinical and experimental head injury. In B Aldman and A Chapon, eds: *The Biomechanics of Impact Trauma*, Elsevier Science Publishers, Amsterdam, 1984, p. 103.

Griest, KJ, and Zumwalt, RE: Child abuse by drowning, *Pediatrics* 83:41-46, 1989.

Guarnaschelli, J, Lee, J, and Pitts, FW: Fallen fontanelle (Caida de Mollera): A variant of the battered child syndrome, *JAMA* 222:1545, 1972.

Guntheroth, WG, Lohmann, R, and Spiers, PS: Risk of sudden infant death syndrome in subsequent siblings, *J Pediatr* 116:520-524, 1990.

Guthkelch, AN: Infantile subdural haematoma and its relationship to whiplash injuries, *Br Med J* 2:430, 1971.

Hahn, YS, Raimondi, AJ, McLone, DG, et al: Traumatic mechanisms of head injury in child abuse, *Childs Brain* 10:229, 1983.

Hall, JR, Reyes, HM, Horvat, M, Meller, JL, and Stein, R: The mortality of childhood falls, *J Trauma* 29:1273-1275, 1989.

Hanigan, WC, Peterson, RA, and Njus, G: Tin ear syndrome: Rotational acceleration in pediatric head injury, *Pediatrics* 80:618, 1987.

Helfer, RE, Slovis, TL, and Black, M: Injuries resulting when small children fall out of bed, *Pediatrics* 60:533-535, 1977.

Herbert, TM, Sluckin, W, and Sluckin, A: Mother-to-infant bonding, *J Child Psychol Psychiatry* 23:205-221, 1982.

Hlady, LJ, and Gunter, EJ: Alleged child abuse in custody access disputes, *Child Abuse Negl* 14:591-593, 1990.

Holbourn, AHS: Mechanics of head injuries, *Lancet* 2:438, 1943.

Hurwitz, A, and Castells, S: Misdiagnosed child abuse and metabolic disorders, *Pediatr Nurs* 13:33-36, 1987.

Hurwitz, S: Disorders of hair and nails. In *Clinical Pediatric Dermatology*, WB Saunders Co, Philadelphia, 1981, pp. 361-383.

Joffe, M, and Ludwig, S: Stairway injuries in children, *Pediatrics* 82:457-461, 1988.

Jones, DPH: Reliable and fictitious accounts of sexual abuse in children, *J Interpersonal Violence* Vol. 1: June, 1986.

Junker, F, and Jonker-Bakker, P: Experiences with rituals child sexual abuse: A case study from the Netherlands, *Child Abuse Negl* 15:191-196, 1991.

Kravitz, H, Driessen, G, Gomberg, R, et al: Accidental falls from elevated surfaces in infants from birth to one year of age, *Pediatrics* 44:869-876, 1969.

Kwok, P, Correy, JF, Newman, NM, and Curran, JT: Smoking and alcohol consumption during pregnancy, *Med J Aust* 1:220-223, 1983.

Lamb, M: The bonding phenomenon: Misinterpretations and their implications, *J Pediatr* 101:555-557, 1982.

Lanning, KV: Ritual abuse: A law enforcement view or perspective, *Child Abuse Negl* 15:171-173, 1991.

Levine, LJ: Bite marks in child abuse. In RG Sanger and DC Bloss, eds: *Management of Child Abuse and Neglect: A Guide for the Dental Professional*, Quintessence Publishing, Inc., Chicago, 1984.

Magid, K, and McKelvey, CA: *High Risk: Children Without a Conscience*, Bantam Books, New York, 1987.

Meadow, R: Suffocation, recurrent apnea, and sudden infant death, *J Pediatr* 117:351-356, 1990.

Moorees, CFA: *The Dentition of the Growing Child*, Harvard University Press, 1959.

Nimityongskul, P, and Anderson, L: The likelihood of injuries when children fall out of bed, *J Pediatr Orthop* 7:184, 1987.

Nixon, J, and Pearn, J: Non-accidental immersion in bathwater: Another aspect of child abuse, *Br Med J* 271-272, 1977(a).

Oates, RK: Overturning the diagnosis of child abuse, *Arch Dis Child* 59:665-667, 1984.

Ommaya, AK: The head: Kinematics and brain injury mechanisms. In B Aldman and A Chapon, eds: *The Biomechanics of Impact Trauma*, Elsevier Science Publishers, Amsterdam, 1984, p. 117.

Ommaya, AK, Faas, F, and Yarnell, P: Whiplash injury and brain damage: An experimental study, *JAMA* 204:285, 1968.

Pearn, J, and Nixon, J: Bathtub immersion accidents involving children, *Med J Aust* 211-213, 1977(b).

Pearn, J, and Nixon, J: Prevention of childhood drowning accidents, *Med J Aust* 616-618, 1977(c).

Putman, FW: The satanic ritual abuse controversy, *Child Abuse Negl* 15:175-179, 1991.

Putnam, N, and Stein, M: Self-inflicted injuries in childhood: A review and diagnostic approach, *Clin Pediatr* 24:514-518, 1985.

Resnick, P: Murder of the newborn: A psychiatric review of neonaticide, *Am J Psychiatry* 126:1414-1420, 1970.

Sims, BG, Grant, JH, and Cameron, JM: Bite marks in the "battered baby syndrome," *Med Sci Law* 13:207, 1973.

Smith, MD, Burrington, JD, and Woolf, AD: Injuries in children sustained in free falls: An analysis of 66 cases, *J Trauma* 15:987-991, 1975.

Smith, S, and Hanson, R: 134 battered children: A medical and psychological study, *Br Med J* 3:666-670, 1974.

Snyder, RG, Foust, DR, and Bowman, BM: Study of impact tolerance through free-fall investigation. Prepared for Insurance Institute for Highway Safety by the University of Michigan Highway Safety Research Institute, Final Report 1977.

Sokol, R: Alcohol and abnormal outcomes of pregnancy, *Can Med Assoc J* 125:143-148, 1981.

Streissguth, A, Darby, BL, Barr, HM, and Smith, JR: Comparison of drinking and smoking patterns during pregnancy over a six year interval, *Am J Obstet Gynecol* 145:716-724, 1983.

Swischuk, LE: Spine and spinal cord trauma in the battered child syndrome, *Radiology* 92:733, 1969.

Thoennes, N, and Pearson, J: Summary of findings from the sexual abuse allegations project. In EB Nicholson, ed: *Sexual Abuse Allegations in Custody and Visitation Cases*, American Bar Association, 1988.

Trube-Becker, E: Bite marks on battered children, *Z Rechtsmed* 79:73, 1977.

Wheeler, DM, and Hobbs, CJ: Mistakes in diagnosing non-accidental injury: 10 years' experience, *Br Med J* 296:1233-1236, 1988.

Williams, RA: Injuries in infants and small children resulting from witnessed and corroborated free falls, *J Trauma* 31(10):1350-1352, 1991.

Wilson, EF: Estimation of the age of cutaneous contusions in child abuse, *Pediatrics* 60:751-752, 1977.

Young, WC, Sachs, RG, Braun, BG, and Watkins, RT: Patients reporting ritual abuse in childhood: A clinical syndrome, *Child Abuse Negl* 15:181-189, 1991.

Chapter 2

RADIOLOGY OF CHILD ABUSE

GREGORY D. LAUNIUS, M.D.
MICHAEL J. SILBERSTEIN, M.D.
ATCHAWEE LUISIRI, M.D.
E. RICHARD GRAVISS, M.D.

The role of radiology in child abuse is threefold: (1) identifying traumatic injury; (2) recognizing abusive origin; and (3) employing the optimal imaging modality to document findings. The radiologist's strength lies in identifying the type, extent, and age of the child's injury, as well as in distinguishing between accidental injury and inflicted abuse. This distinction is important, as the recognition of nonaccidental injury opens the door to intervention, thereby breaking the cycle of abuse.

The pediatric radiologist encounters a wide range of injuries resulting from child abuse. The most obvious are the physical injuries from intentionally inflicted trauma. Injury related to child neglect is equally important, since it is more common and harder to detect.

By being aware of the possibility of abuse and alert to its indications, the radiologist is able to identify the traumatic focus. Plain films are most effective in evaluating physical changes to bony structures. However, with the advent of additional modalities, less obvious but significant internal injuries can now be imaged when suspicion is high.

The radiologist plays a key role in the treatment team where he identifies, documents, reports, and testifies in cases of child abuse. In recognizing physical abuse, the radiologist must possess an awareness of the likely mechanism of injury. To this he adds his knowledge of the specificity of radiologic findings and the demographics of child abuse (Cameron, 1978; Merten, 1983).

Often it is the lack of correlation between the type of injury observed, the known mechanism required for its production, and the purported mechanism of injury that allows for the diagnosis of abuse (Swischuk, 1992). Maintaining a high index of suspicion for abuse in his differential diagnosis allows the radiologist to be among the first to note discrepancies between history and radiographic findings. He then selects the appropriate imaging modality to provide the optimal examination to confirm or deny the possibility of nonaccidental injury.

Included in the role of the radiologist is the responsibility to report suspected child abuse to the proper authorities and to work with them to prevent further injury (English & Grossman, 1989). One of the greatest benefits in diagnosing child abuse is the prevention of recurrence. For this reason, meticulous attention to technique and interpretation is essential, and statistically valid, high-quality images must be obtained so that confident testimony can be given (Leonidas, 1983).

It also falls within the radiologist's realm to consider the risk-to-benefit ratio for all examinations. The issue of cost versus diagnostic benefit is subjective and difficult to evaluate, given the implicit ethical considerations. Potential risks from ionizing radiation and complications of contrast or sedation must be weighed against the benefit of preventing further abuse.

In summary, the pediatric radiologist plays a strategic role in the diagnosis of abuse. His awareness of the mechanisms of injury, the optimal imaging modality, and the specificity of findings make him a key member in the team of caregivers of the abused or neglected child (**Table 2-1**).

Table 2-1. Key Plain Film Findings of Abuse

The pathognomonic metaphyseal-epiphyseal fracture, occurring at the ends of long bones, the acromial process of the scapula, and the clavicular ends.

Rib fractures in infants, multiple rib fractures, or posterior location correlate strongly with child abuse. (Rib fractures are uncommon sequelae of delivery or CPR.)

Fractures in multiple stages of healing.

Oblique long bone fractures in children under 18 months are suspicious for nonaccidental injury.

Vertebral fractures in infants are suspicious for abuse and require neurologic and skeletal follow-up.

Infantile subdural hematomas are best assumed to be indicative of nonaccidental injury in the absence of appropriate history and external signs.

Skull fractures which are depressed, cross the midline, or are occipital are suggestive of abuse.

♦ MODALITIES

The radiologist has at his disposal multiple methods of evaluating bony and soft tissue structures, including X-ray films, nuclear medicine, computerized tomography, magnetic resonance imaging, and ultrasound.

X-RAY FILMS

Plain films provide the foundation for imaging nonaccidental injury in children. The radiographic skeletal survey has its highest yield in children under 2 years of age. After age 2, a more directed approach can be used, and after age 5, complete screening is usually unnecessary. Bone abnormalities themselves rarely result in long-term handicapping conditions. In performing radiologic studies for bone injuries the greatest benefit may be derived from documenting and dating abuse in the hope of preventing recurrence.

The skeletal survey should include a two-view chest with bone technique, a two-view skull, lateral lumbar spine, AP pelvis and AP views of the upper and lower extremities, including AP feet and PA hands (Kleinman, 1987). While the number of radiographs will vary with the size of the patient, the use of a single image, formerly called a "babygram," is no longer acceptable (Merten & Carpenter, 1990).

It is of great importance to maintain high technical standards in obtaining films in child abuse. One of the most frequent causes of missed or overdiagnosed cases of child abuse relates to poor quality films.

NUCLEAR MEDICINE

Radiopharmaceuticals can be tagged and delivered to specific organs. Long scan times are required during imaging by the gamma camera. In children, sedation is frequently required. Radiation doses must be specific to each child to minimize exposure (Harcke, 1978). In addition, potassium perchlorate administration is useful to decrease the thyroid dose in technetium studies (Harcke, 1978).

In child abuse, bone imaging is the most commonly requested nuclear study to demonstrate osseous injuries not identified on standard X-rays (Merten &

Carpenter, 1990). Bone scanning demonstrates abnormalities within hours of osseous injury, and can show lesions missed on plain films (Harcke, 1978). These occult injuries may be nondisplaced traumatic fractures, stress fractures, and periosteal reaction. Injuries in regions difficult to evaluate on plain film, such as spine and ribs, can also be well-seen (Merten & Carpenter, 1990; Harcke, 1978).

The high sensitivity of bone scintigraphy is offset by its low specificity. In addition, lesions adjacent to the growth plate can be missed entirely unless asymmetry is noted with the contralateral growth plate (Harcke, 1978). A high degree of technical precision is required as even asymmetric positioning can cause abnormal activity on images.

The bone scan delivers a greater radiation dose than plain films, is less readily available, and costs more (Merten & Carpenter, 1990; Kleinman, 1987). Most nuclear medicine departments are not experienced in imaging children, and long scan times make patient motion a significant problem. Liver/spleen nuclear scanning is useful in evaluating splenic trauma, but the low specificity decreases its value for hepatic injury (Reece & Grodin, 1985).

COMPUTED TOMOGRAPHY

Computed tomography has proven to be cost-effective and useful for evaluation of intracranial and intraabdominal abnormalities (Merten & Carpenter, 1990). In the acute setting, CT is superior to MRI for the relative ease with which imaging can be performed in the unstable patient.

In addition, CT is faster, less expensive, and not affected by rib and vertebral artifact, as is ultrasound (Kirks, 1983). CT is the examination of choice for children with suspected abdominal trauma (Tolia et al., 1990; Kirks, 1983). Specifically, CT facilitates the identification of splenic and hepatic injury in children without significant clinical complaint following blunt trauma.

A head CT is needed for evaluation of any child with a positive skeletal survey (Merten & Carpenter, 1990). It allows specific and sensitive detection of abnormalities such as extra-axial fluid collections, intraparenchymal and intraventricular hemorrhage, and cerebral edema (Reece & Grodin, 1985). CT is the method of choice for acute assessment of intracranial abnormalities and provides rapid, easy follow-up examination (McClelland et al., 1980).

There are, however, some limitations in intracranial CT evaluation. Small hemorrhages can be missed due to volume averaging. Subdural hematomas and fractures that lie in the plane of section can be missed entirely (Ball, 1989). Also, CT is relatively insensitive for the evaluation of small posterior fossa subdural hematomas, due to extensive artifact, unless coronal or thin sections are used (Kleinman, 1987; Zimmerman et al., 1978).

MAGNETIC RESONANCE IMAGING

MR imaging, with its greater anatomic detail, is more sensitive than CT in detecting certain intracranial abnormalities, such as subdural hematomas, parenchymal contusions, and bleeding (Merten & Carpenter, 1990; Sato et al., 1989). MRI has the advantage of multiplanar imaging without ionizing radiation. Coronal planes and absent bone artifact improve sensitivity to posterior fossa hemorrhage and subdurals (Alexander et al., 1986) (**Figure 2-1**).

Long MRI scan times frequently require sedation, as the technique is very sensitive to motion artifact. In the acute setting, it is even more difficult to obtain quality MRI examinations. Consequently, CT remains the modality of choice for intracranial assessment because of its availability and rapidity in the unstable patient.

Figure 2-1. *Coronal T2 weighted image demonstrating bright signal in bilateral subdural hematomas along parietal convexities (arrows).*

MR imaging also allows the relative dating of subdural hemorrhage. This makes it useful in differentiating chronic subdurals with ventricular enlargement from atrophy (Merten & Carpenter, 1990; Ball, 1989). MRI is of greater use in the subacute and chronic phases of CNS evaluation of child abuse. Overall, MRI remains of limited value in nonaccidental injury.

ULTRASOUND

Ultrasound allows the imaging of soft tissues without radiation exposure and is a safe and inexpensive means of examination. Ultrasound examinations are performed rapidly with sedation rarely needed. In children under 2 years, ultrasound can be used to detect intracranial abnormalities, such as ventricular enlargement, cerebral edema, and intracranial hemorrhage. Large extra-axial fluid collections are visible, but smaller collections may be missed.

Ultrasound is often used as a screening tool in suspected nonaccidental abdominal injury, and the examination can be tailored to evaluate specific organs, such as the liver, spleen, pancreas, or kidneys. Evaluation via ultrasound is of particular use in identifying sequelae of abuse, such as pseudocysts and pancreatitis (Merten & Carpenter, 1990). Free fluid or hemorrhage within the abdomen can be readily appreciated using ultrasound, as can retroperitoneal hematoma (Silverman & Kuhn, 1992).

A potential limitation for ultrasound examination is the technical variability that results from the different skill levels of sonographers. In addition, organs can be obscured by ribs, bone, and air artifact (Kleinman, 1987).

◆ DATING SKELETAL INJURY

The capacity to determine the age of a skeletal injury is critical to the radiologic diagnosis of child abuse (Merten & Carpenter, 1990). The differentiation between accidental and inflicted injuries depends as much on the ability to determine *when* as *how* the injury occurred. Dating injuries illuminates discrepancies between the radiographic findings and the history provided. Any incongruity can warn of possible abuse. Radiologic studies are also extremely useful in distinguishing old or healing bone injuries from new ones (McNeese & Hebeler, 1977). The presence of old *and* new fractures, suggesting that abuse took place over a period of time, is a strong indicator of nonaccidental injury in children.

The ability to determine the time of occurrence relies on the accepted radiologic and pathologic correlation for osseous injury. Following bone injury, hemorrhage occurs around the fracture, lifting the periosteum. An acute inflammatory change is initiated within hours and lasts approximately three days (Perper & Wecht, 1980).

In the first four days, histologic studies show that osteogenic granulation tissue has initiated the proliferative phase without radiographically appreciable healing. In this stage, soft tissue edema or a fracture line may be the only radiographic evidence of injury (Perper & Wecht, 1980). It is at this time that the radionuclide bone scan can detect subperiosteal change not yet evident radiographically.

A minimum of five days is required to see visible radiologic changes. In 5 to 14 days a thin layer of subperiosteal new bone will be formed (Kleinman, 1987). By 10 days, the cellular collar which includes osteogenic cells is noted (Perper & Wecht, 1980). Within a week, woven bone is being formed for the temporary repair, which will correspond to the callus which is the body's "splint" for the fracture. This callus calcifies 10 to 15 days after injury and can be difficult to appreciate initially (Swischuk, 1992).

It is not unusual for fracture sites in infants and young children to appear normal six months after injury. This healing process applies to the fracture of a long bone, as well as to metaphyseal injury and rib fractures. However, fractures of the skull are an exception in that no significant healing reaction will occur for a minimum of 4 to 6 weeks (Cameron, 1978).

In summary, the dating of a fracture involves the recognition of soft tissue changes, fracture line visibility, calcification of callus, and ossification of new periosteal bone (Swischuk, 1992). The radiologist is able to correlate the physical and radiologic findings, keeping in mind the age of the injury and the mechanism of production.

♦ MULTIPLE FRACTURES

A maxim in the evaluation of plain films by the radiologist is that multiple fractures at multiple stages of healing are pathognomonic for child abuse (Swischuk, 1992). The concept of multiple fractures includes both injuries of a number of different bones, as well as more than one site of trauma within the same bone (**Figure 2-2**). It is important for the radiologist to remember that although multiplicity of injury is a characteristic finding in nonaccidental injury in childhood, severe accidental trauma is another plausible explanation. Also, certain bone diseases can produce radiologic changes consistent with the multiple fractures of child abuse. Careful history and clinical correlation are essential.

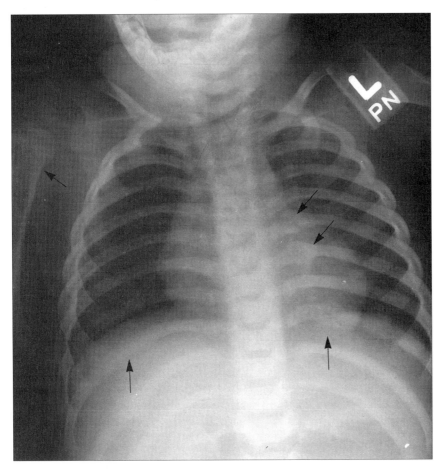

Figure 2-2. AP chest radiograph demonstrates multiple fractures at varying stages of healing. A new right humeral fracture and multiple bilateral healing rib fractures are present.

♦EXTREMITIES

Skeletal injuries, in contrast to intracranial and abdominal injuries, are rarely life-threatening, can cause long-term deformity, and have higher specificity for abuse. The entire axial and appendicular skeleton can be a target for abuse, with the extremities being the most common focus.

The skeletal survey is the primary examination for musculoskeletal trauma. A standard skeletal survey consists of AP views of the extremities, including the hands and feet, AP and lateral skull, AP chest and abdomen, and a lateral thoracolumbar spine. The risk-to-benefit ratio regarding radiation exposure favors the continued use of the skeletal survey (Ellerstein & Norris, 1984).

Physical signs suggesting skeletal injuries in abuse include tenderness, swelling, reduced range of motion, pseudoparalysis, and limb deformity. In the abuse setting these symptoms indicate the need for skeletal survey. Neurological changes should also initiate a skeletal survey, as 70% of abuse-related intracranial injuries have associated fractures (Merten & Carpenter, 1990; McNeese & Hebeler, 1977).

The skeletal survey is most beneficial in younger patients and children with extensive soft tissue injury. This relates to the observation that the younger the child, the greater the chance the fracture is from nonaccidental injury (Elliot, 1979).

Neonatal abuse requires special consideration. In utero conditions such as infection and rickets can cause osseous abnormalities. Injuries related to birth trauma and congenital skeletal dysplasia in the newborn may also present with bones in various stages of repair (Radkowski, 1983).

Fractures are found in slightly over one third of all physically abused children and represent over 80% of the total abuse-related injuries seen by radiology. Dislocations are uncommon in nonaccidental injury. Joint malalignment relates most often to metaphyseal-epiphyseal injury. True dislocations are usually associated with severe trauma. Relative weakness of the metaphyseal-epiphyseal region with resultant propensity for fracture spares the joint space ligaments from dislocating force (Merten & Carpenter, 1990; Kleinman, 1987).

TYPES OF FRACTURES/MECHANISMS OF INJURY

In child abuse, skeletal fractures can be subdivided into those involving the metaphyseal-epiphyseal region and those involving the diaphysis. The metaphyseal-epiphyseal fractures include the classically described corner fracture, bucket handle fracture, and metaphyseal lucency. Recent research has shown that these fractures represent varying appearances of the same injury (**Figure 2-3a,b,c**). They are pathognomonic for abuse as the force required for this type of injury is greater than that of a simple fall or accident (Silverman & Kuhn, 1992). They can occur in any bone adjacent to a growth plate, such as the clavicle or acromial process of the scapula.

Historically, metaphyseal-epiphyseal fractures were thought to represent avulsion of peripheral metaphyseal fragments at a site of fixed periosteal attachment. It is now known that shaking and jerking with attendant accelerating/decelerating forces produce a shearing effect resulting in transverse fractures in the weak, immature primary spongiosum layer. These transverse fractures along with the varying degrees of ossification in the fracture fragments and the projection of the radiograph combine to produce the multiple appearances of the same injury (Kleinman, 1987).

Figure 2-3a. Fracture through the distal femoral metaphysis presents as abnormal lucency (arrows).

Figure 2-3b. Metaphyseal fracture presents as corner avulsion due to projection and thickness of ossified segments involved (arrow).

Figure 2-3c. Fracture across the entire metaphysis combined with nontangential projection produces characteristic "bucket handle" fracture of child abuse.

Fractures of the diaphysis are less specific for abuse than metaphyseal-epiphyseal fractures, but occur four times more often in abused children. Diaphyseal fractures are either oblique (spiral) or transverse. A single long bone fracture, coinciding with either the pathognomonic metaphyseal or multiple rib fracture injury patterns, should be considered nonaccidental without plausible history. Oblique fractures are caused by rotational or torsional forces applied to the limb, and transverse fractures result from a direct blow or a bending force. Torsional forces that produce the spiral fracture can be either accidental or intentionally inflicted. Without appropriate history, lower extremity spiral fractures in children who are not yet ambulatory imply abuse (**Figure 2-4**).

Subperiosteal hematoma is a common diaphyseal injury in child abuse. The loosely attached, highly vascularized periosteum of the diaphysis is easily lifted off the bone by hemorrhage from injury. Initial images show an intact cortex, but may reveal soft tissue edema related to the hemorrhage. Between 5 and 14 days after injury, an unbroken line of calcification reflecting periosteal new bone formation can be seen. Further healing will result in cortical thickening. Researchers have found that in cases of cortical thickening, there is often evidence to suggest rough handling or shaking (Merten & Carpenter, 1990; Tufts et al., 1982; Kleinman, 1987) (**Figure 2-5**).

Figure 2-4. Single bony injury in a 4 1/2-year-old with Crouzon's disease. Films demonstrate oblique diaphyseal fracture with rotational component.

Figure 2-5. Examination demonstrates diaphyseal periosteal reaction (arrows) consistent with healing subperiosteal hemorrhage.

Figure 2-6. *Lateral radiograph demonstrating an oblique fracture of the right femoral diaphysis. Other metaphyseal fractures with varied stages of healing were present. Bucket handle fracture is seen distally (arrow).*

Figure 2-7. *Distal femoral metaphyseal-epiphyseal fracture presenting as a bucket handle fracture in 4-month-old male.*

♦REGIONAL SKELETAL INJURIES

FEMUR

The femur is one of the most frequently fractured long bones in nonaccidental injury. Two peaks in incidence for femoral fracture occur, one at 6 months and the next at 3 years of age (Kleinman, 1987). Femoral shaft fractures are more common than metaphyseal-epiphyseal fractures, but are of lower specificity for abuse (Leonidas, 1983). As age increases, specificity decreases. The rotational mechanism of injury for an oblique fracture is highly suspicious for abuse in non-walking children (Kleinman, 1987). These fractures require correlation with the history, presence of healing, and other injuries before being diagnosed as nonaccidental (**Figure 2-6**).

The distal metaphyseal-epiphyseal complex is fractured more often than the proximal (Kleinman, 1987), with lesions often bilateral due to flailing motion associated with severe shaking (**Figure 2-7**). The multiple growth plates in the proximal femur, with initial nonossification, make fractures in this region difficult to evaluate. Radiographic changes might show only subtle findings of soft tissue injury or abnormal alignment of the shaft relative to the pelvis. Arthrography or bone scintigraphy can aid in evaluating this region. Identification of proximal fractures is important, since proximal growth plate fractures have greater long-term sequelae than their more common distal counterparts.

TIBIA AND FIBULA

Tibial shaft fractures are less common than metaphyseal fractures. In contrast to the femur, metaphyseal-epiphyseal fractures usually involve the proximal tibia

(Kleinman, 1987). Bilateral metaphyseal fractures of the proximal tibia are not uncommon and result from acceleration/deceleration forces produced by shaking (**Figure 2-8**).

The tibial diaphysis is a common location for subperiosteal hemorrhage and subperiosteal reaction. Fracture lines in shaft fractures are not always seen (Kleinman, 1987), and healing reaction can be the only indication of their presence. Rotational stress in a newly walking child is not unusual, is unintentional, and produces the so-called toddler's fracture, which usually occurs between the ages of 9 months and 3 years and should not be confused with abusive injury (Kleinman, 1987; Kirks, 1984) (**Figure 2-9**).

Fibular fractures are rare. Shaft fractures are often found in conjunction with tibial shaft fractures as a result of a direct blow. Distal and proximal fibular metaphyseal fractures are possible but rare (**Figure 2-10**).

Figure 2-8. *The typical location for tibial metaphyseal-epiphyseal fractures is seen in this 3 1/2-month-old female with a bucket handle fracture.*

Figure 2-9. *Extensive tibial periosteal reaction with no fracture ever appreciated in this 7-week-old child with right parietal fracture and subgaleal hematoma.*

Figure 2-10. *AP view of the right tibia and fibula demonstrate healing reaction at a fibular fracture site (arrow-a). Mild tibial periosteal reaction is also present, suggesting evolving subperiosteal hemorrhage. Also noted is a bucket handle tibial metaphyseal fracture (arrow-b).*

FOOT FRACTURES
Foot fractures are not common, but their specificity for abuse is high. They more often involve older children. Of the multiple foot bones, the metatarsal is the most likely site of injury. For this reason, detailed foot views are helpful in the skeletal survey (Merten & Carpenter, 1990; Kleinman, 1987).

HUMERAL SHAFT FRACTURES
Humeral shaft fractures tend to be oblique fractures arising from indirect torsion, such as grabbing the upper extremity distally and pulling or twisting. The less common transverse fracture is usually the result of a direct blow (**Figure 2-11**).

Figure 2-11. An oblique fracture of the left humerus with rotational component is demonstrated in this 2 month-old female with multiple fractures.

Other mechanisms of injury, such as shaking the child by the forearms or pulling the child up, are more often involved in injury to the metaphyseal-epiphyseal complexes. Injuries to the proximal growth plates, as in the femur, are difficult to evaluate because of their nonossified components. Subtle radiographic signs such as metaphyseal lucency or healing reaction may be the first plain film indication of trauma.

Another radiographic finding in metaphyseal-epiphyseal fractures is the displacement of the humerus away from the glenoid cavity (Kleinman, 1987). This occurs with greater frequency in association with severe trauma. An arthrogram can help confirm this finding.

Distinction between fracture separation and elbow dislocation is complicated by the nonossified nature of the distal humeral epiphysis. Statistically, fracture/separation is more common than dislocation. Prior to ossification, the olecranon lies medial to its expected location overlying the distal humerus in epiphyseal separation. After ossification of the capitellum at 3 to 4 months, the capitellar-radial relationship can be used to distinguish dislocation from metaphyseal-epiphyseal complex injury (Silverman & Kuhn, 1992) (**Figure 2-12**).

Supracondylar fractures are typical of accidental injury and are nonspecific for child abuse (Kleinman, 1987). They require correlation with other factors, such as history and degree of healing.

The literature reveals that forearm fractures represent 10% to 20% of all skeletal injuries from child abuse (Kleinman, 1987). This reflects the tendency to grab the upper extremities when shaking and pulling the child. Metaphyseal-epiphyseal injuries are much more common distally than proximally. The bucket handle appearance is rarely seen, with most injuries presenting as metaphyseal lucencies or corner fractures (Merten & Carpenter, 1990).

Diaphyseal fractures of the radius and ulna occur in child abuse and are most often transverse. In these cases, blocking blows with the forearm corresponds to the known mechanism of injury for transverse fractures—that is, direct impact. Periosteal bone formation also presents in the forearm diaphyses as the manifestation of subperiosteal hemorrhage from direct blow or twisting injury (Kleinman, 1987).

HANDS

It is suspected that hand fractures, like foot fractures, occur more frequently than the literature might indicate. This may reflect the failure to obtain quality hand radiographs (Kleinman, 1987). Fractures of the metacarpals can involve both the shafts and the metaphyseal-epiphyseal regions. Fractures or dislocations of the phalanges have been described in child abuse, possibly related to corporal punishment from direct blows.

♦ SPINE INJURIES

Fractures of the spine are infrequently associated with abuse. Those related to nonaccidental injury are often only a part of major trauma and may involve more than one site and level. The area of the spine most often involved is the thoracolumbar region. Abusive spine injuries are usually noted in infants and young children, with half being younger than 1 year. Most of these fractures are related to hyperflexion-hyperextension, either from shaking or direct blows (Merten & Carpenter, 1990; Cameron, 1978; Leonidas, 1983; Kleinman, 1987). Trauma to the spinal cord may occur without apparent bony injury. Swelling of the adjacent soft tissues may be the only plain film indication of spinal cord injury.

Most abusive injuries to the spine involve the vertebral body, and hyperflexion is the common mechanism of injury. Radiographic findings vary from subtle to severe anterior vertebral compression fractures. This often appears as a loss of bone

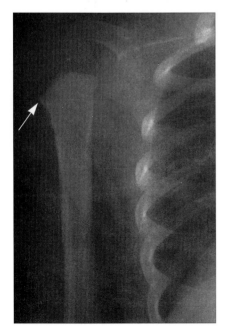

Figure 2-12. Proximal metaphyseal avulsion of the humerus (arrow) is less common than distal metaphyseal involvement in abuse.

on the anterosuperior and, less frequently, the anteroinferior margin of the vertebral body. With healing, sclerosis will be evident at the fracture site. Vertebral fractures are typically in the thoracolumbar spine, and a lateral view of this region in the standard skeletal survey provides optimal visualization (**Figure 2-13**).

Spinal trauma can cause anterior disk herniation with narrowing of the intervertebral disk space. Disturbance of the ring apophysis from disk herniation can alter vertebral body development with long-lasting debilitating effect. Disk space narrowing caused by abuse is less marked than that from infectious diskitis. The anterior corner notching is typically larger in abuse than in diskitis/osteomyelitis. When radiographic findings provide insufficient distinction from abuse, clinical and laboratory findings can help differentiate these entities (Kleinman, 1987).

Fractures of the posterior elements have been described by Kleinman as a result of hyperflexion-hyperextension injuries from shaking. Most often they present as spinous process avulsions at the interspinous ligament attachment. With time, these show progressive calcification and ossification. These avulsion injuries of the posterior elements are stable. Only in rare instances has the unstable "hangman's fracture" been described. This may present as a subtle vertical lucency posterior to the body of C2 (Kleinman, 1987).

Subluxation of one vertebral body in relation to another may also occur in child abuse. Most subluxations are anterior or posterior and are effectively demonstrated on the lateral radiograph. Rare lateral subluxations have been described and would be seen on the AP view of the abdomen-pelvis. Cervical involvement is rare. Cervical pseudosubluxation at C2 is a common variant readily distinguished by means of alignments of the posterior elements. The method developed by Dr. Swischuk for this differentiation is readily available in Keats' *Atlas of Roentgenographic Measurement.* Pseudosubluxation is more common than true subluxation (Keats, 1985).

Bone scintigraphy has been helpful in evaluation of posterior elements and transverse processes but is relatively insensitive for vertebral body fractures (Merten & Carpenter, 1990). Therefore, the modality of choice remains plain films of the skeletal survey (Kleinman, 1987). Identification of spinal fractures requires careful examination of the thoracolumbar spine on the lateral view. Any vertebral fracture in an infant must raise the possibility of inflicted injury with resultant follow-up for abuse both clinically and radiographically.

CHEST

Injury to the bony thorax occurs less frequently than extremity fractures in child abuse. Thoracic injury is of greater diagnostic specificity than extremity fractures

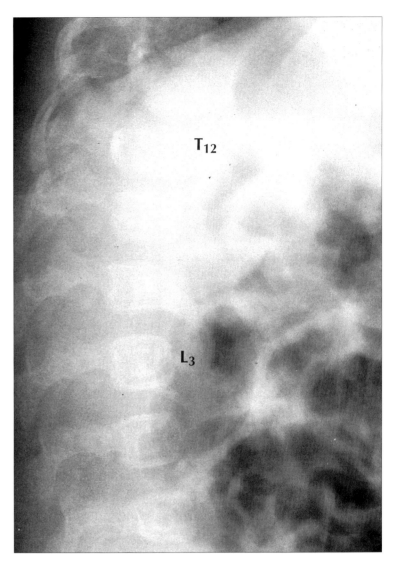

Figure 2-13. Lateral thoracolumbar spine with compression fractures presenting as loss of height of the anterior L1 and L2 vertebral bodies in a child with intracranial injuries and skull fracture.

(Merten & Carpenter, 1990). Most chest injuries involve rib fractures and resultant complications. Accidental fracture of the rib cage is rare in infants and young children, as the rib cage is relatively compliant and resistant to injury from falls and accidental childhood trauma. The typical accidental injury occurs in children older than 2 years; a reversal of this age distribution is seen in abuse, with almost 90% under 2 years. Most rib fractures in abuse are multiple and located posteriorly, next to the costovertebral junction. The next most common fracture site is the lateral rib, with anterior costochondral separations occurring rarely. These last two sites are more often associated with extremely violent trauma.

Excessive squeezing of the chest can cause fractures at points of maximal stress. Ribs articulate with the spine at the costovertebral junction. As the ribs extend posterolaterally away from the spine, they overlie the transverse process. When squeezed, the ribs are bent over the transverse process, and injury can damage the periosteum or produce a fracture. As greater stress is applied, the force is transferred to the lateral and then the anterior ribs. This mechanism accounts for the location and equal age of multiple fractures in a single rib (Kleinman, 1987).

Although squeezing is the most often described mechanism of injury, direct blows to the chest can also cause rib fractures. The fracture occurs at the site of impact, often with an accompanying bruise (Alexander et al., 1990). Rib fractures are often initially invisible. The healing phase can cause asymmetric appearance of the posterior ribs from bone widening and sclerosis in posterior rib fractures. Lateral oblique films can help image lateral fractures. Callus formation may actually reveal the fracture line within the area of rib widening. The difficulty in imaging acute rib fractures has made the high sensitivity of the bone scan of great use in the difficult clinical situation requiring additional documentation of physical abuse.

Rib fractures related to delivery are rare, and incidental rib fractures in a patient with normal bones are highly suspicious for child abuse. The only mitigating factor would be a reasonable history of severe direct trauma to the chest. It should also be noted that although cardiopulmonary resuscitation has been associated with rib fractures in adults, CPR in children rarely, if ever, causes fracture. Children have been known to present to emergency rooms with a supposed history of resuscitation and resultant fractures, and these explanations are often accepted without question (Feldman & Brewer, 1984). In light of this common misconception, unexplained rib fractures, specifically the posterior, are virtually pathognomonic for child abuse.

Underlying intrathoracic injury can result from severe squeezing. While pneumothoraces and subcutaneous emphysema can result from rib trauma, they are an uncommon occurrence. Pneumothoraces are best seen on the upright or decubitus chest radiographs. The decubitus films also reveal pleural fluid collections that may or may not relate to rib fracture. Pleural effusions may be a sign of associated pancreatitis, or they may actually represent a chylothorax. This can be the result of a severe compression injury that disrupts the thoracic lymphatic duct. Chylothoraces in the chest are located on the right, owing to thoracic duct anatomy.

The occurrence of pulmonary contusion as it relates to child abuse has not been well-described in the literature, but given the incidence of rib fractures in child abuse, a higher frequency would not be surprising. Pulmonary infiltrates have been reported from both forced aspiration and as a result of infection related to neglect.

CLAVICLE

The majority of clavicular fractures in abuse are in the mid shaft and are indistinguishable from those of accidental injury. Fractures of the medial one third of the clavicle shaft have a greater specificity for abuse. Avulsion fractures of either the medial or lateral clavicular apophyses are of greater diagnostic specificity for abuse. It is convenient to think of these as metaphyseal-epiphyseal lesions. Clavicle avulsion injuries often result from sudden traction of the associated arm. It is not surprising that they are frequently associated with proximal humeral injury.

Since scapular fractures rarely occur by accident, they are highly suspicious for child abuse. The most frequent site is the acromial apophysis. The next most fractured area is the coracoid process; glenoid fractures are uncommon (Merten & Carpenter, 1990). The rare fracture to the body of the scapula occurs as the result of a direct blow, whereas other scapular injuries are the result of indirect forces. Scapular fractures are difficult to evaluate radiographically, due to the scapula's location behind ribs and its anatomically complex shape. Bone scans can be helpful in the assessment of this difficult region.

STERNUM
Sternal injuries are rare. This may relate to the multiple joints and resultant greater mobility, allowing dispersion of forces. Radiographically, they can present as sternomanubrial joint displacement or as defects along the cartilaginous edge of a sternal ossification center (Kleinman, 1987).

PELVIS
Pelvic fractures are not commonly described in conjunction with nonaccidental injury in children. Occasional literature reports have noted periosteal reaction as subtle evidence of abuse. Kleinman suggests that, given the incidence of femoral fractures, fractures involving the adjacent pelvis should be more common, and careful attention to pelvic films may confirm this observation.

In summary, unexplained rib fractures are specific for abuse, as fractures to the ribs are uncommon in children under 2 years. Clavicular fractures involving the medial and lateral ends have a specificity for abuse equal to metaphyseal-epiphyseal lesion in the long bones. Scapular injuries are rare but highly specific for nonaccidental injury *(see Table 2-1)*.

◆ CRANIOFACIAL INJURIES
Intracranial sequelae are the most serious and significant findings in child abuse. The incidence varies from 10% to 44%, depending on the study, on the children studied, and the modality used (Sato et al., 1989). Central nervous system injury may be the only manifestation of abuse; however, 70% have associated skeletal injuries.

The majority of fatalities in child abuse involve head injury. Morbidity and mortality are most significant in children less than 2 years old (90%). Residual changes can be seen in nearly 80% of those surviving intracranial injury. It is suspected that many cases of mental retardation can be ascribed to child abuse (Merten & Osborne, 1983; Reece & Grodin, 1985; Sato et al., 1989; Ball, 1989).

Important in CNS injury are the ramifications of shaking. As a mechanism of injury, shaking accounts for the presence of intracranial injury in children without apparent external trauma to the head. Acceleration/deceleration and rotational forces result in shearing injury to the intracranial contents. These shearing forces separate structures that have varying degrees of fixation/mobility and can result in retinal hemorrhage, extra-axial fluid collections, hemorrhage/contusion at the gray/white matter junctions, and cerebral edema (Merten & Carpenter, 1990; Merten & Osborne, 1983; McClelland et al., 1980; Ball, 1989). Direct blows to the brain can produce the same findings as shaking, with calvarial and extracranial injury. This is because both direct and indirect (shaking) trauma can produce the same rotation/shearing forces that cause intracranial injury. In many instances, shaking and direct blows occur together.

Figure 2-14. High density adjacent to the falx represents a subtle falcine subdural. Although it is common, the falcine subdural is easily missed.

Several unique anatomic characteristics of the infant cranium make it susceptible to specific types of injuries. These include the increased elasticity from calvarial flexibility and sutural patency, as well as the increased plasticity from immature myelinization. Also, the child's brain floats in a relatively larger cerebrospinal fluid space than that of the adult. This renders the bridging veins vulnerable to tearing, with resultant subdural hematomas (Alexander et al., 1990; Merten & Osborne, 1983). The higher metabolic rate in children and infants, along with a higher vasoreactivity, makes children more susceptible to cerebral edema after intracranial injury (Merten & Osborne, 1983). The large head size of the child, combined with the relatively lax musculature of the neck, accentuates the acceleration/deceleration forces in injuries caused by shaking.

The brain is also injured secondarily through trauma to circulation and respiration. Direct trauma to the blood vessels supplying the brain and subsequent cerebral swelling may compromise brain vascularization. Strangulation with resultant asphyxia is another well-described means of producing cerebral edema (Merten & Osborne, 1983).

SUBDURAL HEMATOMAS

Subdural hematoma was among the earliest described indicators of child abuse and is the most common intracranial sequela of abuse (Merten & Carpenter, 1990; Cameron, 1978; Sato et al., 1989). A rupture of the bridging veins between the brain and the sinuses of the dura can be caused by either direct blows to the head or shaking, with its rotational shearing forces. Subdural hematomas are most common under 24 months of age, with peak occurrence at 6 months (Reece & Grodin, 1985) (**Figure 2-14**). They are most often located within the interhemispheric fissure, given the frequent involvement of the sagittal sinus veins, and can extend over the cerebral convexity. Posterior fossa subdurals can be difficult to evaluate on CT due to technical factors. The shape will depend upon the amount of blood, the speed of hemorrhage, and the location within the brain. As blood accumulates at the site of the tear, it can widen the subdural space, causing further tearing and making the adjacent veins susceptible to more tearing.

The high frequency of bilateral subdurals in child abuse corresponds with the picture expected from the shaking theory of injury. As the child is often grasped symmetrically by the limbs, the shearing forces tend to act symmetrically on the bridging veins (Reece & Grodin, 1985; Guthkelch, 1971).

Small hematomas may be difficult to visualize when at the base of the brain or the vertex. Larger subdurals can easily be identified by the crescent configuration between the brain and the skull. These larger subdurals are encountered less often than the more typical intrahemispheric subdural hemorrhage. With time, subdural hematomas have been known to calcify (Kleinman, 1987). Chronic subdural hematomas are not uncommon, being typically located over the frontal convexities and associated with progressive ventricular enlargement. Cerebral atrophy can develop within a month following injury (Sato et al., 1989; Kleinman, 1987). MRI is superior for the detection of small subdural hematomas, especially in the posterior fossa (Merten & Carpenter, 1990).

MRI assists in dating subdural age by following the levels of hemoglobin breakdown products. Determining the presence of these breakdown products aids in distinguishing subdural collections from atrophy and communicating hydrocephalus. Multiple posttraumatic fluid collections of varying ages indicate repetitive trauma (Merten & Carpenter, 1990; Sato et al., 1989) (**Figure 2-15**). Ultrasound is not helpful for evaluation of small subdural hematomas, but it can be used to follow the progressive changes of large subdural hematomas. Varying echogenicity of extra-axial fluid may indicate injuries of different ages (Kleinman, 1987).

Figure 2-15a. *T1 weighted axial scan with subdural hematoma demonstrates signal (arrow) brighter than CSF and slightly less intense than parenchyma (arrow).* ***b.*** *T2 weighted axial image showing bright subdural signal consistent with subacute age (arrow).*

EPIDURAL HEMATOMAS

Epidural hematomas are not often found in the setting of child abuse. If present, they are typically associated with a skull fracture. Large epidural hematomas have a lenticular shape with mass effect. Small epidural hematomas may resemble subdural hematomas. It may be helpful in differentiating between the two to note that epidurals can cross midline in contrast to subdural fluid collections which do not. Due to arterial bleeding, epidurals constitute neurosurgical emergencies (Merten & Carpenter, 1990; Kleinman, 1987) (**Figure 2-16**).

SUBARACHNOID HEMORRHAGES

Subarachnoid hemorrhages and subdural fluid collections frequently coexist. It can be difficult to differentiate between the two. MRI and CT are equally well-suited to detect subarachnoid hemorrhages. The association of subarachnoid hemorrhage with cerebral edema should raise the possibility of child abuse for the clinician if no other signs of trauma are present (Alexander et al., 1990; Cohen et al., 1986; Alexander et al., 1986).

INTRACRANIAL HEMORRHAGES

Intracranial hemorrhages on CT, though not specific for child abuse, can result from either direct trauma or vigorous shaking. These superficial or deep cerebral contusions/hematomas are not unusual in inflicted trauma and are frequently associated with other intracranial injuries. Contusional tears are often noted in the white matter adjacent to the gray/white matter

Figure 2-16. *CT section demonstrating left parietal epidural with lenticular shape. Associated fracture cannot be seen without alterations in window settings. Mass effect on left lateral ventricle.*

Figure 2-17. A focal area of high density in the right parietal lobe is consistent with hemorrhagic contusion at gray/white matter interface. Right parietal skull fracture is visible on bone windows adjacent to subgaleal hematoma.

Figure 2-18. Seven-month-old infant presenting in full arrest with bilateral subdural hematomas (arrows) and cerebral edema demonstrated by loss of gray/white matter differentiation.

junction. Little bleeding is associated with these changes, which are often microscopic (Merten & Carpenter, 1990; Reece & Grodin, 1985; Kleinman, 1987; Cohen et al., 1986) **(Figure 2-17)**.

CEREBRAL EDEMA

In one study of child abuse, cerebral edema occurred in 65% of patients (Guthkelch, 1971). The overall pattern and appearance of cerebral edema varies, depending on the time between examination and injury. Initially, no findings may be seen; delayed images, days later, may show cerebral edema with a mass effect. A small number of cases with diffuse edema have been described as having a "reversal sign" with the white matter having a higher attenuation than the gray matter on CT, reflecting severe diffuse edema. The reversal sign indicates irreversible brain damage (Cohen et al., 1986).

More typically, cerebral edema results in obliteration of the ventricles from mass effect and loss of the gray-white matter differentiation **(Figure 2-18)**. Cerebral edema results from endothelial damage with resultant increased vascular permeability, possibly related to the child's higher level of vasoreactivity. These edema patterns may be focal or general. The presence of focal edema has a higher specificity for abuse. Cerebral edema or infarction may reflect altered cerebral blood flow as a result of vascular injury, as well as hypoxia from asphyxia, smothering, and strangulation (Merten & Carpenter, 1990; Kleinman, 1987; Guthkelch, 1971). Shaking appears to be a more common mechanism of injury for the marked cerebral edema seen without fracture in child abuse (Kleinman, 1987).

CHRONIC SEQUELAE

Intracranial injury can result in focal or diffuse atrophy. Focal atrophy can be seen as ventricular dilatation with ipsilateral enlargement of the extra-axial spaces. Atrophic changes from abuse may be seen one month after injury, with encephalomalacic and porencephalic changes evident on follow-up, consistent with severe injury. The presence of diffuse ventricular enlargement with widening of the extra-axial spaces can be difficult to distinguish from communicating hydrocephalus or the normally prominent cerebrospinal fluid spaces in infants. The presence of blood within the ventricles is a marker for severe intracranial injury (Merten & Carpenter, 1990; Kleinman, 1987).

SKULL FRACTURES

Statistically, fractures to the skull are the second most common bony injury in child abuse. History suspicious for child abuse and the presence of a skull fracture increase the likelihood of intracranial injury (Harwood-Nash, 1992). Most skull fractures are linear and nondepressed, with comminuted, depressed, and diastatic fractures being less common. The parietal and occipital bones are most typically involved. Depressed fractures, occiput fractures, and fractures crossing the midline carry a greater specificity for nonaccidental injury than simple linear fractures (Harwood-Nash, 1992; Merten & Osborne, 1983) (**Figure 2-19**).

Fractures to the skull may be imaged with CT, bone scan, and plain films. CT is sensitive for detection of fractures, given appropriate slice thickness and window settings. However, fractures in the plane of CT section can be missed. The standard method for evaluation is the two-view skull; radiographs must always be obtained in addition to bone scans to evaluate the abused child.

Figure 2-19. Depressed right parietal skull fracture crosses the coronal suture. Depression is evident on the AP view. Fractures crossing sutures are more common in child abuse than in accidental injury.

Sutural widening is one radiographic sign of increased intracranial pressure, as might be seen in chronic subdural hematomas. In cases of psychosocial dwarfism, however, an interesting variation is seen. The deprived child at the time of diagnosis will have normal appearing sutures. After successful treatment for neglect, the child's brain may grow faster than the skull, resulting in sutural splitting. This widening may be mild to 4 mm in width (Kleinman, 1987) (**Figures 2-20 and 2-21**).

MAXILLOFACIAL INJURIES

Maxillofacial abnormalities are rare, manifesting most often as facial soft tissue injuries. Typically, when fractures occur, they involve older children and are

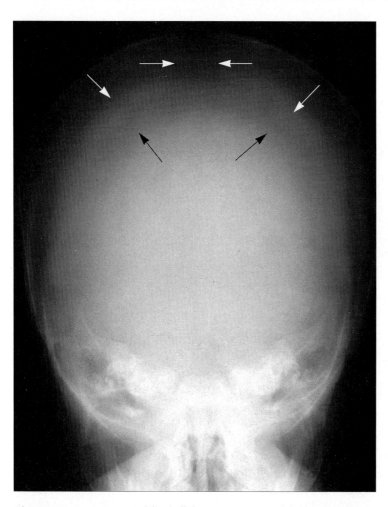

Figure 2-20. *Towne's view of the skull demonstrating sutural diastasis (arrows) suggesting increased intracranial pressure. This 4-month-old infant had bilateral chronic subdural hematomas on CT.*

mandibular. Unexplained facial fractures in infants and children suggest abuse (Merten & Carpenter, 1990; Kleinman, 1987). Blows to the mouth can cause missing teeth or fractures of the mandible. Nasal septal deviation may result from direct trauma to the nose. The only clinical sign might be hemorrhage from the nose (McNeese & Hebeler, 1977). Injuries to the ear often involve the pinna. Subgaleal hematomas or cephalhematomas may result from cases of severe hair-pulling and can be visible on skull films if the soft tissues are hot-lighted (Merten & Carpenter, 1990; McNeese & Hebeler, 1977; Kleinman, 1987). Soft tissue injuries around the orbit called "black eyes" may look identical to the "raccoon eyes" in basilar skull fractures. Appropriate imaging is essential for these situations, as bilateral periorbital hematomas seldom occur without a unique history in the accidental setting (Reece & Grodin, 1985).

Retinal hemorrhage is a specific finding in child abuse not easily explained by impact and is a well-described result of shaking. Specifically, subdural hematomas with retinal hemorrhage should be regarded as the shaking syndrome of child abuse unless another plausible etiology can be determined (Alexander et al., 1990; Swischuk, 1992; Rekate, 1985).

NEUROIMAGING

The modalities of CT, MRI, and ultrasound are available to evaluate intracranial injuries. CT is both sensitive and specific in defining the acute and chronic intracranial abnormalities of abuse. MRI is the most sensitive mode of detecting intracranial injuries (especially shaking trauma). In acute situations, CT is the modality of choice, as it allows the rapid evaluation of both intracranial and calvarial abnormalities in an unstable patient.

The strengths of MRI are apparent in cases of subacute and chronic neural trauma. MRI effectively evaluates the posterior fossa, as it lacks beam-hardening artifact and possesses multiplanar capability. MRI is better than CT at showing nonhemorrhagic contusions of the white matter and other deep cerebral injuries. It is also better than CT in determining the age of extra-axial fluid collections by following changing MRI signals of hemoglobin breakdown products. CT is the primary screening method, with MRI obtained in cases highly suspicious for abuse but with negative head CTs (Merten & Carpenter, 1990; Sato et al., 1989; Kleinman, 1987; Alexander et al., 1986). Neurosonography is of limited use in CNS injury, and is best used for follow-up of ventricle size and gross parenchymal involvement in those patients with open fontanelles (Merten & Carpenter, 1990).

◆ ABDOMINAL INJURIES

In cases of nonaccidental trauma, the abdomen is involved less than the skeleton or the brain. What abdominal injury lacks in frequency it makes up in mortality, with visceral injuries producing a mortality rate of 50% in child abuse (Touloukian, 1968).

Visceral injuries rank second only to head trauma as the leading cause of death from child abuse (Kleinman, 1987).

Abdominal injuries typically occur after the child is ambulatory, that is, older than 2 years. As age increases, a shift occurs in the site of fatal injury from the brain to the abdomen (Kleinman, 1987). Surveys have shown that truly accidental injuries differ in site and severity from inflicted abuse. Accidental injuries usually have specific histories and are brought promptly for treatment. In abuse, the history is more general, such as a fall. In combination with the typically vague symptoms of abdominal injury, this lack of accurate history increases the morbidity and mortality by delaying essential treatment. CT examination has helped bring to light the true prevalence of abuse-related abdominal injury.

LIVER

The liver is the solid visceral organ most often involved in child abuse due to its exposed location next to the epigastric region. This is the site of most direct blows, the usual mechanism for hepatic injury (Merten & Carpenter, 1990). Trauma subsequent to compression and crushing is less common, but has been known to produce burst injuries to the liver. Hepatic injury from rib fracture is rarely seen. In infants, hepatic injuries are not common, as direct blows are rarely administered to children of that age (Cameron, 1978; Kleinman, 1987).

Hepatic contusion, subcapsular hematoma, and hemorrhage occur in child abuse. CT is the study of choice if clinical findings are highly suspicious for hepatic injury. Ultrasound can be used as an initial screening evaluation, as it will provide adequate evaluation of the biliary system, hepatic parenchyma, and the presence of ascites (Kleinman, 1987) (**Figure 2-22**).

Figure 2-21a,b. Initial skeletal survey demonstrated normal sutures in this case of neglect/abuse. Follow-up at 1 month after placement in foster care revealed sutural diastasis from accelerated intracerebral growth and lagging calvarial development, not from raised intracranial pressure.

Historically, the liver/spleen scan has been used to evaluate the abdomen. However, the radionuclide study is of relatively low sensitivity and specificity in child abuse. The frequent difficulty in obtaining an emergent liver/spleen scan also renders it less desirable as an imaging modality in this setting.

Spleen

The spleen is rarely involved in child abuse, secondary to its distance from the epigastric region. Direct blows with their resultant decelerating force are the most common mechanism of splenic injury (Kirks, 1983). Contusions of the spleen and subcapsular hematomas are more common than splenic lacerations in nonaccidental trauma. Ultrasound provides a rapid and safe method of screening; however, CT is more sensitive and specific (**Figure 2-23**).

Figure 2-22. CT scan demonstrates hypodensity in the inferomedial right hepatic lobe, consistent with laceration (arrow-a). A small subcapsular hematoma showing as a crescent of low density along anterior right hepatic lobe (arrow-b).

Figure 2-23. Normal appearing spleen (arrow-a). Area of low density indenting upper left kidney, consistent with splenic hematoma visualized on ultrasound (arrow-b).

Pancreas

Pancreatic disease in children is rare. The pancreas lies over the spine in the epigastrium and is susceptible to compression by a direct blow with subsequent release of pancreatic enzymes due to acinar or ductal rupture. This causes autonecrosis and inflammation of the organ. A resultant mass of necrotic tissue may form a firm, fibrous capsule known as a pancreatic pseudocyst. This may develop rapidly within days of the injury, or it may be gradual and insidious (Kirks, 1983; Kleinman, 1987). In children under 3 years of age, pancreatitis is highly suspicious for abuse (Tolia et al., 1990) (**Figure 2-24**). Symptoms can be mild or severe, and additional physical findings may include elevated serum amylase and ascites. A normal amylase does not exclude a pseudocyst, since amylase levels can return to normal with time (Kleinman, 1987).

Abdominal trauma causes more than half of reported cases of pseudocysts in children, with 30% of these showing concurrent evidence of abuse (Merten & Carpenter, 1990). Radiographic changes of pancreatitis are the well-described, nonspecific sentinel loops and colon cut-off signs. Pancreatic pseudocyst may generate mass effect on adjacent bowel, such as the duodenum or stomach. If the pseudocyst obstructs the bowel, radiographic changes of obstruction may be seen.

Ultrasound is the diagnostic method of choice to evaluate the pancreas and pseudocysts in both the initial and follow-up phases. CT can also be helpful in evaluating injuries to adjacent organs in the retroperitoneum.

In cases of pancreatic involvement, lytic bone lesions from medullary fat necrosis can occur 2 to 10 weeks after injury. Pancreatic enzymes break down medullary fat in bone, producing lytic lesions of variable appearance. The lower extremities, specifically the small bones in the foot, are most often involved, with associated pain and swelling. Spontaneous resolution occurs with residual changes evident up to 1 year later. These lesions should not be mistaken for the bone lesions of leukemia and metastatic neuroblastoma (Wilner, 1982; Kleinman, 1987).

Figure 2-24. Transverse ultrasound view through pancreas demonstrates thickening and inhomogeneity consistent with pancreatitis. The amylase level was 263.

KIDNEY

Nonaccidental trauma rarely results in direct renal injury. In abuse, renal disease is most commonly due to a metabolic imbalance from major trauma, such as shock or myoglobinuria following muscle breakdown. Renal trauma, as in the liver, is rarely caused by rib fracture. Direct blows to the kidney can result in parenchymal tearing and discontinuity of the collecting system, hemorrhage or extravasation into the retroperitoneum. Ectopic renal location can make the kidney more susceptible to injury. If the kidney overlies the spine as in cross-fused ectopia or horseshoe kidney, it is susceptible to the same mechanism that injures the pancreas. CT is the most sensitive and the most specific modality. However, gross screening can be cost-effectively performed with ultrasound.

BLADDER AND URETHRA

The rare occurrence of bladder or urethral involvement may relate to their protected intrapelvic location (Kleinman, 1987). Perforating injury to the bladder is rare. Urethral injury could occur as a result of sexual abuse or inflicted straddle injury.

ESOPHAGUS

Esophageal involvement in child abuse often relates to Munchausen Syndrome by Proxy. Children have been forced to consume dangerous foreign bodies, such as safety pins or glass. Force feeding lye or hot water can cause esophageal ulceration and spasm on the barium swallow with resultant strictures. Such occurrences are rare (Kleinman, 1987).

STOMACH

Stomach distensibility usually spares it from injury from a direct blow or compression. If distended, such as after a meal, perforation can occur, usually along the anterior stomach wall, with resultant pneumoperitoneum. However, this is uncommon, as only 2% of bowel ruptures involve the stomach. Radiographically, findings are nonspecific, except for massive amounts of intraperitoneal air. The clinical presentation is very serious, and may be associated with other visceral injury (Merten & Carpenter, 1990; Kleinman, 1987).

More commonly, the stomach is indirectly involved relating to either duodenal obstruction or gastric atony from starvation or neglect. This atony is a paralytic phenomenon, not a result of mechanical obstruction. In a child who is neither postoperative nor medicated, marked gastric dilatation should raise the suspicion of chronic starvation or neglect (Kirks, 1983).

DUODENUM

The duodenum is often involved in nontraumatic injury because its location over the spine allows it to be trapped and compressed. Involvement of the descending duodenum, which lies to the side of the spine, may be a result of its firm fixation, making it susceptible to compressive blows (Kleinman, 1987).

Being well-vascularized, the duodenum has multiple potential bleeding sites, and intestinal hematoma without appropriate trauma history is classic in cases of child abuse. The areas of hematoma may be diffuse or localized with bleeding in a subserosal location, sparing the mucosa. The majority of small bowel hematomas are found in the duodenum and proximal jejunum, immediately distal to the ligament of Treitz. Duodenal hematomas are typically antimesenteric in location in contrast to the mesenteric location of jejunal and ileal hematomas (Kleinman, 1987).

A hematoma frequently appears on upper GI examinations as a large, smooth, intramural mass that narrows the lumen. In the presence of duodenal hematoma, the plain film may be normal or may show a dilated stomach with a large air/fluid level. Free air or ascites may also be seen from separate concurrent injuries. Circumferential, diffuse bleeding may produce fold-thickening without focal mural defect, known as the stacked coin appearance. This sign is of lower specificity for duodenal hematoma related to abuse.

Over time, the hematomas resolve with varying degrees of mural nodularity. This later stage finding on an upper GI exam may be the only indicator of previous abuse. Ultrasound can be a helpful adjunct in the acute setting of trauma, but upper GI is recommended for confirmation of findings (**Figure 2-25 a,b**).

Figure 2-25a. Following a direct mid-abdominal blow, this patient presented with emesis. Initial upper GI shows wall thickening and duodenal hematomas (arrows).

Direct crushing or compressive forces to the abdomen of the abused child can result in small bowel perforation. Sites susceptible to injury and/or perforation from shearing forces are those fixed in position or at the junction of bowel segments with varying degrees of mobility. This explains why 60% of perforations occur in the proximal jejunum and 30% in the duodenum, followed by the ileum (Kleinman, 1987). Because of the duodenum's retroperitoneal location, plain film signs of free air are often absent (**Figure 2-26**).

The bowel wall can be torn in abuse, allowing gas-forming bacteria to enter the wall. The resultant curvilinear lucency or mottled radiographic appearance of intramural air, pneumatosis intestinalis, can also result from anoxic injury to the wall in abuse (Kleinman, 1987).

COLON

Colonic involvement in nonaccidental injury is most often due to sexual abuse. Rectal perforation may result in free intraperitoneal air evident on plain films. Sexual assaults may utilize foreign objects that may be seen on plain films, and on rare occasions, free intraperitoneal air can be seen following rape. In cases involving major genitorectal trauma, radiology can help assess the acute injury and any resultant sequelae. Sexually abused children may present with vague or unusual abdominal complaints, and it is in the course of evaluating these that the radiologist may meet the patient. The radiologist needs to be aware of physical signs suggesting anogenital trauma, as these may be appreciated when performing examinations for gastrointestinal or voiding disorders.

Figure 2-25b. Follow-up in 5 days shows decrease in intramural hematomas on antimesenteric border.

Figure 2-26. A 26-month-old male presented with vague abdominal complaints; previous lower GI was negative. Upper GI shows duodenal perforation into a walled-off cavity (arrows-a,b,c,d indicate duodenum, arrows-e,f,g,h delineate walled-off cavity).

Colonic injuries are rare from blunt trauma. This may relate to the mobility of the colon and its location either on the edge of the abdomen or in the pelvis. Colonic hematomas and perforation following abuse have been described. This most commonly involves the transverse colon (Kleinman, 1987).

CT examination is the modality of choice for assessing blunt abdominal trauma. Ultrasound is most useful as a screening examination of the abdomen and in pancreatic assessment and follow-up. MRI has limitations in evaluation of the abdomen related to motion artifact. Children with unusual or unexplainable abdominal bruising should always be evaluated for visceral injuries, regardless of whether other injuries are apparent (Cameron, 1978; Kirks, 1983).

♦ DIFFERENTIAL CONSIDERATIONS IN CHILD ABUSE

In diagnosing child abuse, it is important to keep in mind several congenital and acquired diseases that can mimic the bony lesions of nonaccidental injury. Failure to consider these possibilities and eliminate them can result in false diagnosis. These disease entities can usually be differentiated from child abuse by careful physical examination and a thorough history. Certain laboratory tests may also be required to eliminate them from the differential diagnosis.

Accidental trauma can cause fractures that mimic abuse. The toddler's fracture is a well-known example. The rotational stress from a newly walking child may result in a minimally displaced fracture, indistinguishable from an oblique fracture caused by applied stress in abuse. The bone appearance and appropriate history and age help distinguish this specific fracture from abuse. Clavicle fractures are also common injuries that might be mistaken for abuse. Well-described in the perinatal period as a result of birth trauma, these fractures show healing reaction by 14 days. Absence of callus in a clavicle fracture after this time strongly suggests nonaccidental cause (Kleinman, 1987).

Rib fractures related to delivery are uncommon. Those found incidentally weeks after birth when the callus becomes palpable are usually due to abuse unless a plausible history of severe direct trauma is present (Kleinman, 1987). Epiphyseal injuries have been associated with birth trauma related to a breech delivery. These injuries are usually noted in the neonate because of abnormal or absent movement of the afflicted joints. Most long bone fractures from delivery are in the humeral mid-shaft. Fractures of the lower extremity long bones and fractures with varying stages of repair in the newborn are most often related to infection, rickets, or neuromuscular diseases (Radkowski, 1983; Kleinman, 1987).

Many normal variants exist that can be confused with child abuse in infants. Standard radiographic texts or atlases of radiographic variants are helpful to avoid misdiagnosis. A commonly encountered variant is the periosteal reaction due to new bone formation and spurring of the metaphyses in healthy, unabused infants. While the periosteal changes mimic traumatic periostitis, the metaphyseal spurs are not suspicious for abuse unless fragmentation is present. These bony changes occur between 2 and 8 months of life (Kleinman, 1987).

Osteogenesis imperfecta is a frequently mentioned disease entity in the differential diagnosis of child abuse. Abnormalities of collagen production result in weak bones. Four types of osteogenesis imperfecta are recognized with types I, III, and IV most often implicated, as type II is the lethal perinatal form with multiple fractures, blue sclerae, and recessive inheritance. The diagnosis is not complicated by the more severe forms, like type II, but by the types with delayed presentation and subtle bone change. Metaphyseal fractures are typically absent, with long bone fractures more common. Osteopenia with thin bone cortices is typical. Extraskeletal manifestations such as blue sclerae, dentinogenesis imperfecta, or familial inheritance may be of help in the differential diagnosis in infancy (Radkowski, 1983; Kleinman, 1987). The possibility of intentional injury cannot be disregarded in osteogenesis imperfecta, since even children with this disease can be abused (Cameron, 1978).

Children with congenital insensitivity to pain may demonstrate metaphyseal and shaft fractures and periosteal reaction, mimicking abuse even though mineralization is normal. A careful neurologic examination and history are required for this diagnosis. A similar radiographic appearance can occur in children with spinal defects. For example, patients with meningomyeloceles may have altered or absent sensation from the lower extremities and varying degrees of motor involvement allowing repetitive injury resembling abuse (Radkowski, 1983; Kleinman, 1987).

Congenital syphilis produces diffuse symmetric bone changes very similar to child abuse. However, erosions on the medial aspect of the proximal tibia (Wimberger sign) with periosteal new bone formation are diagnostic for syphilis. The spine and epiphyseal ossification centers are spared. Serologic analysis is helpful in eliminating this from consideration (Radkowski, 1983; Kleinman, 1987).

Osteomyelitis can imitate abuse not only by producing periosteal reaction and metaphyseal irregularity, but it can also be multifocal in infancy. Corner fractures are not a part of the radiologic presentation. Clinical tests such as joint tapping and blood cultures can help differentiate this from abuse. Also, infantile meningococcemia has been described as resulting in metaphyseal abnormalities years after the infection. The postulated mechanism is ischemic injury. This makes infantile meningococcemia an important historical question along with metaphyseal abnormalities (Kleinman, 1987; Patriquin et al., 1982).

Infantile cortical hyperostosis (Caffey's disease) is a rare occurrence in young infants, producing painful periosteal reaction. Infants of 2 to 3 months of age present with red and edematous extremities at multiple locations. The periosteal reactions spare the metaphyses. Both flat and tubular bones can be involved. The etiology is unknown, and complete healing occurs. The mandible is involved in more than 95% of cases, making mandibular involvement and the sparing of the metaphyses useful differentiators. A careful and thorough history is also an essential component in differentiating Caffey's disease from abuse (Reece & Grodin, 1985; Radkowski, 1983; Radkowski et al., 1983).

Methotrexate therapy has been known to produce periosteal reactions and metaphyseal-epiphyseal fractures with osteopenia. With current therapy regimens, this is less likely to occur. Long term prostaglandin-E therapy is used to prevent closure of a patent ductus arteriosus. It can produce cortical proliferation in these patients. Bony sequelae involve the long bones and the ribs; patient history can differentiate it from traumatic periostitis (Radkowski, 1983; Radkowski et al., 1983). Vitamin A toxicity can show diaphyseal periosteal reaction; however, metaphyseal-epiphyseal lesions are absent. Epiphyseal abnormalities (cone-shaped epiphyses) may occur with associated limb shortening. Hypervitaminosis-A can be a cause of increased intracranial pressure with sutural widening. Vitamin A blood levels and history of abnormal intake can assist in differentiation from traumatic periostitis (Kleinman, 1987; Radkowski et al., 1983).

Infantile rickets can manifest the bony changes seen in child abuse, but with the addition of osteopenia. Metaphyseal fraying and multiple fractures are common. A typical radiographic finding in rickets is Looser's zones, symmetric transverse stress fractures not found in nonaccidental injury. Diffuse osteopenia with epiphyseal widening and poor epiphyseal definition is typical in rickets and not found in abuse. Radiographic changes of rickets can also be seen in the diseases of biliary atresia, hypophosphatasia, and osteopetrosis (Radkowski, 1983; Kleinman, 1987; Radkowski et al., 1983).

Vitamin C deficiency (scurvy) is less common than rickets and rarely occurs before 6 months. Metaphyseal irregularities and periosteal reaction can simulate abuse, but the associated osteopenia is atypical. The presence of dense metaphyseal bands along with thin dense rings around the epiphyses help differentiate scurvy from abuse. Long bone fractures are also rare (Kleinman, 1987; Radkowski et al., 1983).

Menkes' kinky hair disease is an abnormality of copper absorption with metaphyseal fractures that can mimic the changes of abuse. Periosteal reaction of long bone diaphyses can also be seen. Distinguishing features from child abuse are the presence of multiple wormian bones, kinky hair, and low serum copper.

A significant factor in the misdiagnosis of child abuse is the suboptimal radiograph. This can take the form of an incomplete skeletal survey, poor positioning, and underexposure or overexposure of the radiograph (Merten & Carpenter, 1990). Careful attention must be paid in the initial evaluation to the overall bone density and architecture. Most of the disease entities mentioned above can be eliminated through careful histories, which include social, medical, and dietary assessments. Physical examination and laboratory data can then be useful, especially in patients with a baseline chronic illness. In addition, it is important to remember that a child with a chronic disease can be abused as easily as a healthy child, and in fact is even more prone to abuse (Radkowski, 1983).

♦ CONCLUSION

A certain set of diagnostic guidelines emerges from the literature on radiology's role in child abuse. Its strength lies in detecting type, extent, and age of injury. The motivating force for radiology's contribution is that without recognition and intervention, the abused child "will almost always be abused again, and statistics show that by the third hospitalization, he will be either dead or dying" (Elliot, 1979). A frequent occurrence, often overlooked, is the contribution of the radiologic technologist, who sees both patient and caretaker in a nonthreatening, physician-free environment. The technologist's observations may often assist the radiologist's interpretation. This may vary from reports of cutaneous injury to abnormal behavior by the patient or caretaker.

Perhaps the radiologist's greatest advantage in diagnosing abuse has been stated by Dr. Michael Weller, Department of Radiology, Miller Children's Hospital, Long Beach, California: "The radiologist has black and white film before him and is not swayed by knowledge of the family and preconceptions about them."

◆BIBLIOGRAPHY

Alexander, R, Sato, Y, Smith, W, and Bennett, T: Incidence of impact trauma with cranial injuries ascribed to shaking, *Am J Dis Child* 144(6):724-726, 1990.

Alexander, RC, Schor, DP, and Smith, WL: Magnetic resonance imaging of intracranial injuries from child abuse, *J Pediatr* 6:975-979, 1986.

Ball, WS, Jr: Nonaccidental craniocerebral trauma (child abuse): MR imaging, *Radiology* 173:609-610, 1989.

Brodeur, AE, Silberstein, MJ, and Graviss, ER: *Radiology of the Pediatric Elbow*, GK Hall Medical Publishers, Boston, 1981.

Cameron, JM: Radiological pathological aspects of the battered child syndrome. In SM Smith, ed: *The Maltreatment of Children*, University Park Press, Baltimore, 1978, pp. 69-81.

Cohen, RA, Kaufman, RA, Myers, PA, and Tobin, RB: Cranial computed tomography in the abused child with head injury, *Am J Radiol* 146:97-102, 1986.

Edwards, IK: Court testimony in cases of nonaccidental trauma. In SVW Hilton, DK Edwards, and JW Hilton, eds: *Practical Pediatric Radiology*, WB Saunders Co, Philadelphia, 1984, pp. 487-496.

Ellerstein, NS, and Norris, KJ: Value of radiologic skeletal survey in assessment of abused children, *Pediatrics* 74:1075-1078, 1984.

Elliot, DS: Child abuse: The radiologist's pivotal position, *Appl Radiol* 74-79, 1979.

English, PC, and Grossman, H: Radiology and history of child abuse, *Pediatr Ann* 12(12):870-874, 1989.

Feldman, KW, and Brewer, DK: Child abuse, cardiopulmonary resuscitation, and rib fractures, *Pediatrics* 73(3):339-342, 1984.

Garrow, I, and Werne, J: Sudden apparently unexplained death during infancy. III. Pathologic findings in infants dying immediately after violence, contrasted with those after sudden apparently unexplained death, *Am J Pathol* 29:833-851, 1953.

Gross, RH: Child abuse: Are you recognizing it when you see it? *Contemp Orthop* 92:676-678, 1980.

Guthkelch, AN: Infantile subdural hematoma and its relationship to whiplash injuries, *Br J Med* 2:430-431, 1971.

Harcke, HT, Jr: Bone imaging in infants and children: A review, *J Nucl Med* 19:324-329, 1978.

Harwood-Nash, DC: Abuse to the pediatric nervous system, *Am J Neuroradiol* 13(2):569-575, 1992.

Keats, TE: *Atlas of Roentgenographic Measurement*, Year Book Medical Publishers, Inc, Chicago, 1985, p. 116.

Kirks, DR: Radiological evaluation of visceral injuries in the battered child syndrome, *Pediatr Ann* 12:888-893, 1983.

Kirks, DR: Practical pediatric imaging. In HL Abrams, ed: *Diagnostic Radiology of Infants and Children*, Little, Brown & Co, Boston, 1984, p. 277.

Kleinman, PK: *Diagnostic Imaging of Child Abuse*, The Williams & Wilkins Co, Baltimore, 1987.

Leonidas, JC: Skeletal trauma in the child abuse syndrome, *Pediatr Ann* 12(12):875-881, 1983.

Matin, P: Bone scintigraphy in the diagnosis and management of traumatic injury, *Semin Nucl Med* 13:104-122, 1983.

McClain, PW, Sacks, JJ, Froehlke, RG, and Ewigman, BG: Estimates of fatal child abuse and neglect, United States, 1979 through 1988, *Pediatrics* 91(2):338-343, 1993.

McClelland, CQ, Rekate, H, Kaufman, B, and Perse, L: Cerebral injury in child abuse: A changing profile, *Childs Brain* 7:225-235, 1980.

McNeese, MC, and Hebeler, JR: The abused child—a clinical approach to identification and management, *Clin Symp* 29(5):1-36, 1977.

Meller, JL, Little, AG, and Shermeta, DW: Thoracic trauma in children, *Pediatrics* 74:813-819, 1984.

Merten, DF: Introduction: The battered child syndrome: The role of radiological imaging, *Pediatr Ann* 12:867-868, 1983.

Merten, DF, and Carpenter, BL: Radiologic imaging of inflicted injury in child abuse syndrome, *Pediatr Clin North Am* 37(4):815-836, 1990.

Merten, DF, and Osborne, DS: Craniocerebral trauma in the child abuse syndrome, *Pediatr Ann* 12:12, 1983.

Miller, DS: Fractures among children. I. Parental assault as causative agent, *Minn Med* 42:1209-1213, 1959.

Patriquin, HC, Antoni, T, Jacquier, S, and Marton, D: Late sequelae of infantile meningococcemia in growing bones of children, *Radiology* 141:77-82, 1982.

Perper, JA, and Wecht, CH, eds: *Microscopic Diagnosis in Forensic Pathology*, Charles C Thomas, Springfield, IL, 1980, pp. 3-16.

Radkowski, MA: The battered child syndrome: Pitfalls in radiologic diagnosis, *Pediatr Ann* 12:894-903, 1983.

Radkowski, MA, Merten, DR, and Leonidas, JC: The abused child: Criteria for the radiological diagnosis, *Radiographics* 3:262-297, 1983.

Reece, RM, and Grodin, MA: Recognition of nonaccidental injury, *Pediatr Clin North Am* 32:41-60, 1985.

Rekate, HL: Subdural hematomas in infants, *Neurosurgery* 62:316-317, 1985.

Sato, Y, Yuh, WT, Smith, WL, Alexander, RC, Kao, SC, and Ellerbroek, CJ: Head injury in child abuse: Evaluation with MRI imaging, *Radiology* 173:653-657, 1989.

Silverman, FN, and Kuhn, JP, eds: *Caffey's Pediatric X-ray Diagnosis: An Integrated Imaging Approach*, The C V Mosby Co, St. Louis, 1992, pp. 1814-1816.

Sivit, CJ, and Taylor, BA: Visceral injury in battered children: A changing perspective, *Radiology* 173(3):659-661, 1989.

Starbuck, GW: Recognition and early management of child abuse, *Pediatr Ann* 5:27-41, 1976.

Swischuk, LE: Radiographic signs of skeletal trauma. In S Ludwig and A Kornberg, eds: *Child Abuse: A Medical Reference*, ed 2, Churchill Livingstone, New York, 1992, pp. 151-174.

Teng, CT, Singleton, EB, and Daeschner, CW, Jr: Skeletal injuries of the battered child, *Am J Orthop* 6:202-207, 1964.

Tolia, V, Patel, AS, and Amundson, GM: Pancreatic fracture secondary to child abuse: The role of computed tomography in its diagnosis, *Clin Pediatr* 29(11): 667-668, 1990.

Touloukian, R: Abdominal visceral injuries in battered children, *Pediatrics* 42(4):642-646, 1968.

Tredwell, SJ, Van Peteghem, K, and Clough, M: Pattern of forearm fractures in children, *J Pediatr Orthop* 4:604-608, 1984.

Tufts, E, Blank, E, and Dickerson, D: Periosteal thickening as a manifestation of trauma in infancy, *Child Abuse Negl* 6:359-364, 1982.

Wilner, D: *Radiology of Bone Tumors and Allied Disorders*, WB Saunders Co, Philadelphia, 1982, p. 3621.

Zimmerman, RA, Bilaniuk, LT, and Genneralli, T: Computed tomography of shearing injuries of the cerebral white matter, *Radiology* 127:393-396, 1978.

THORACOABDOMINAL INJURIES ASSOCIATED WITH CHILD ABUSE

RICHARD C. BARRY, M.D.
THOMAS R. WEBER, M.D.

*Case One: A 10-month-old male presented to the Emergency Room with cough and wheezing, and on a routine chest X-ray there were noted multiple healing rib fractures (**Figure 3-1**). Reexamination noted badly bruised buttocks with the outline of a hand. Appropriate further assessment was completed and the case referred immediately to the Division of Family Services for further investigation.*

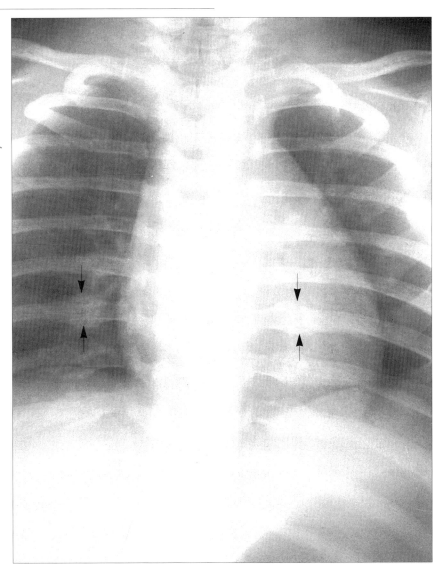

Figure 3-1. *Multiple posterior rib fractures on right.*

*Case Two: A 19-year-old mother rushed into the ER with a pale, lifeless 1-year-old whom she reported would not wake up. The physical examination revealed an obtunded, pale male with extremely precarious vital signs and ecchymotic upper and lower right eyelids as well as old scars on the buttocks in the configuration of an electric cord loop. Further assessment revealed marked anemia and elevated liver enzymes; the CT scan of the abdomen showed a liver laceration and a duodenal hematoma (**Figure 3-2a**). The Division of Family Services was immediately notified for further investigation.*

Figure 3-2a. Multiple posterior rib fractures with pneumothorax on left (arrows).

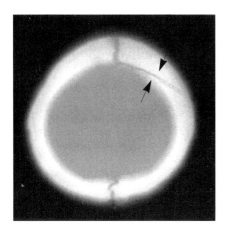

Figure 3-2b. CT scan of head with skull fracture.

Figure 3-2c. Liver laceration (arrows).

Figure 3-2d. Blood in peritoneum (arrows).

Figures 3-2b, 3-2c, and **3-2d** represent the extremes of thoracoabdominal trauma associated with child abuse. The latter case, although not common, is much more serious and life-threatening. The importance of early recognition of an abuse-prone environment cannot be overstressed, not only to prevent the terrible result shown in the second case but also to protect other children who may be in the same immediate setting.

♦UNINTENTIONAL VERSUS ABUSIVE INJURIES

Blunt trauma has been, and continues to be, the primary type of kinetic force (90% to 95% of the cases) associated with thoracoabdominal injury in the pediatric patient, both with accidental and with abusive injuries. Although visceral injuries account for only 2% of all child abuse cases, they are the second leading cause of death after central nervous system trauma. However, many emergency rooms, especially in the inner cities, are seeing an increasing incidence of penetrating injuries primarily due to gunshot wounds and stabbings. In the young patient, up to preteen years, the situation is usually a child caught in the crossfire of a dispute. These truncal penetrations can be rapidly life-threatening and are prone to significant morbidity and mortality. Unfortunately, young children are actually becoming the intended target of gunshots and stabbings as revengeful acts against a parent or relative and, occasionally, due to the impulsive reaction to a child's behavior.

In the preteen and teen years, a significant number of blunt truncal injuries are associated with risk taking, a perceived sense of indestructibility, and the additive use of alcohol, drugs, and motor vehicles. However, it is also in this age group that we see an alarming increase in the number of penetrating wounds, whether inflicted against self or another individual to resolve a dispute, or as an act of revenge. The easy accessibility of weapons, drug activity, and the promise of money are all enticing to the socioeconomically deprived or bored, unsupervised teenager.

Several notable differences in the usual presentation patterns (**Table 3-1**) may be helpful in determining abuse as the cause of thoracoabdominal trauma. In accidental truncal injury due to motor vehicle injury, the child is often brought immediately to the emergency room by ambulance. The child is accompanied by EMS personnel, and usually everyone involved in the incident, including the child, if alert, willingly gives a reasonable and useful history. This is in marked contrast to the abusive setting in which there is often a delay, sometimes until even the caretaker recognizes that the child has reached a life-threatening stage. Unfortunately, the history given by the caretaker in these latter instances will frequently be one of trivial trauma or no history of trauma. This leaves the physician in an extremely difficult position, with a child in a tenuous cardiovascular status, perhaps comatose, and with little or no historical information.

Table 3-1. Differences in Usual Presentation Factors in Child Abuse Versus Accidental Thoracoabdominal Injury		
Presentation Factor	**Accidental**	**Abuse**
Time of presentation after injury	Immediate	Delayed
History		
Present	Available and reliable	Often unavailable or unreliable or inconsistent with the injury.
Past	Unremarkable	Previous abusive episodes and 50% known to DFS.
Age	7.8 years (mean)	2.5 years (mean)
Old inflicted bruises	0%	50% to 90%
Old fractures	Very infrequent	Frequent
Most frequent abdominal organ injured	Spleen	Liver
Multiple visceral injuries	Infrequent	Frequent
Intestinal injury	Infrequent	Frequent
Death	4.5% to 12.5%	12% to 60%

Pediatric child abuse occurs at all ages but primarily in children less than 6 years of age with the peak age range being infancy to about 3 years of age. The older toddler (mean age, 2.5 years) is most likely to be exposed to visceral trauma. On the other hand, accidental blunt thoracoabdominal trauma occurs more often in school-aged children (mean age, 7.8 years), and the majority are related to motor vehicle accidents.

In both accidental and abusive settings, males outnumber females 2:1 to 3:1. In general, the skin is the most common organ to call attention to abuse. Since abuse is usually a repetitive activity, about 50% to 90% of the patients with visceral injuries have multiple old scars or bruises in various stages of healing. The locations and configurations often clearly indicate inflicted injuries. When it comes to the visceral organs, the liver is more likely to be injured with abuse and the spleen with accidental injury; however, there is a fair amount of overlap among solid organ injuries. Abusive settings are more likely to produce multiple organ injuries. Gastrointestinal injuries such as intraluminal hematomas, perforations, and shearing mesentery injuries are more common in abuse (40% to 65%) than in accidents (8% to 15%). This type of injury is more frequently due to a punch or kick to the mid-epigastrium, leading to compression of the liver and the fixed retroperitoneal portion of the duodenum (**Figures 3-3 and 3-4**). These types of injuries can also occur in accidents associated with seatbelt injuries or by hitting the handlebars of a bicycle. Mortality rates associated with visceral injuries range from 12% to 60% in the abusive setting; this relates primarily to the late presentation and the poor or absent history of trauma, leading to further delay in making a final diagnosis. Death rates due to accidental visceral injuries are much lower, ranging from 4.5% to 12.5%. Of course, if head injury is associated with either situation, the death rate markedly increases.

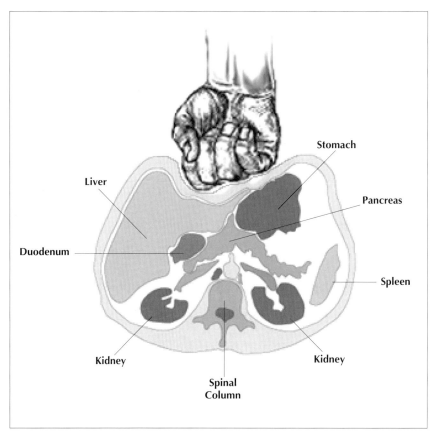

Figure 3-3. Dynamics of blunt trauma to the abdomen.

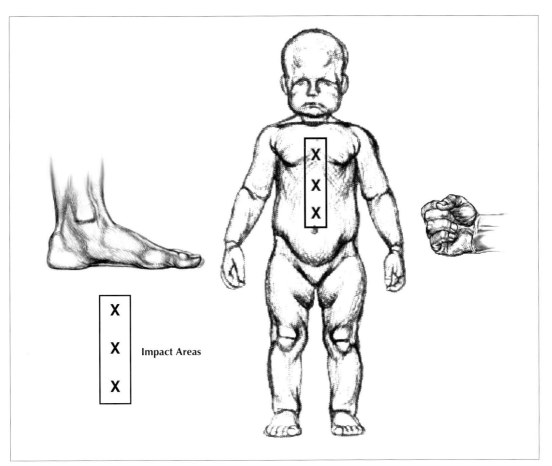

Figure 3-4. Areas of impact with blunt trauma.

X X X (Impact Areas)

♦HISTORY

To reiterate, in significant accidental truncal injuries, presentations are usually immediate and a consistent, reasonable history is given by observers and the caretaker. This is not the case with abuse and, frequently, the accompanying adult, usually the mother, will not be responsible for the injury and may or may not know about the incident. She may not disclose this information out of fear of recrimination or to protect the father or boyfriend. Although the history may not be correct, it often focuses on the site of injury. For example, if there was abdominal trauma, the mother may report that the child has had bilious emesis or report one or more of the following symptoms in her child: stomach pain, swollen abdomen, difficulty in breathing, or tarry, black stools. One should focus on the history to be sure it is consistent with the injury and the child's developmental level. If there are multiple historians, one needs to pay attention to inconsistencies in the histories. Likewise, one should check with other medical personnel to ensure that they received the same information. Multiple instances of changing or varied stories may be the first clues that the child is the victim of abuse. The alert child may not be old enough to verbalize details of what has happened or may not describe the abusive episode because he fears further abuse and trusts the abusive adult caretaker more than unfamiliar medical personnel.

Past family history may actually be more helpful in some situations and may be willingly offered by the mother. For example, she may volunteer that a sibling was previously removed from the home for neglect. The present, abused child may have been seen many times in the past. The records of previous visits should always be reviewed, looking for multiple previous episodes of trauma. Some institutions have computer programs that tabulate the number of visits for trauma each time a patient is seen. This system is to alert the practitioner that this could be an "at-risk" child. One can also assess if the caretaker is meeting minimal health maintenance care by getting routine immunizations and screening studies. It is advisable to contact the hospital social services department and/or the state Division of Family Services to check on previous reports. Approximately 50% of patients with major abusive events, including truncal injuries, are already known to the Division of Family Services. It should be emphasized that responsibility is not only to the immediate patient in medical care but also to other children who may be exposed to these abusive caretakers.

♦ GENERAL APPROACH AND CLINICAL ASSESSMENT

Although the main objective of this chapter is to discuss the approach and evaluation of thoracoabdominal injuries associated with abuse, it should be noted that, not infrequently, other sites may be injured as well, influencing the ability to provide an adequate clinical assessment. A good example is an associated head and neck injury in a child who has been violently shaken with vigorous holding of the trunk, and also has visceral injury as a result of trauma to the trunk. The child's level of consciousness and responses may be markedly depressed due to the head and neck injury, making examination of the truncal area essentially unreliable. All patients, especially those brought to an emergency room setting, should have a rapid cardiopulmonary assessment to determine hemodynamic stability. If the patient is unconscious, obtunded, or pale with poor cardiovascular status, these abnormalities must be rapidly addressed and reversed. Only then should one proceed with further assessment of the child. Unfortunately, abused patients who present at this stage, with truncal injury and associated shock, frequently have a very poor outcome and a significant rise in mortality due to the long delay in seeking medical help. Since the history is often unreliable, one must do a complete clinical assessment, including a good physical examination. The child should be unclothed during that exam, and all surfaces should be viewed.

Examination of the skin is often helpful, even in thoracoabdominal injuries where there may not be obvious fresh or old bruises over the site of actual visceral injury. The presence of scars and bruises in other areas, representing repetitive abuse by their location or patterns, for example, old and recent burns, loop marks, handprints, and other patterns, suggests an abusive situation and further leads the physician to a thorough evaluation of the child.

Alert children who are young and frequently upset and frightened must be made as comfortable as possible to allow for a reliable examination. Often these children appreciate being held in their mothers' laps, which is reassuring and gives a sense of security. A complete physical examination should be performed and, if one suspects there is thoracoabdominal injury, that part of the examination should be performed last. It is important to visualize, listen to, feel, and percuss all appropriate anatomical sites, including soft tissues, solid organs, and bony skeleton, looking for clues to present and previous abuse. If the child is alert and old enough to walk, it is a good idea to see the patient walk, while looking for signs of discomfort and abnormal gait. This is particularly valuable in the toddler and preschool child. When significant physical findings are noted or there is strong suspicion of truncal abuse, these areas should be assessed with appropriate laboratory and imaging studies.

LABORATORY STUDIES

Some or all of the trauma laboratory studies (**Table 3-2**) are frequently obtained on patients suspected of visceral injury due to abuse. Many times these studies are strongly encouraged and freely obtained to provide direction regarding further testing and imaging.

Table 3-2. Laboratory Studies

CBC	Result	Clinical Significance
Hg/Ht	↓	Blood loss versus anemia of other cause
MCV	WNL	Blood loss
	↓	Anemia from previous blood loss or other etiology
WBC	↑(left shift)	Stress reaction versus infection (i.e., peritonitis with perforated bowel, etc.)
Guaiac	⊕Stool	Intraluminal gastrointestinal bleeding
	⊕Gastric	Intraluminal gastrointestinal bleeding
Urine RBC/hemoglobin	> 10	Genital/urinary injury
Myoglobin	⊕	Rhabdomyolysis
AST/ALT	≥ 450/250 IU	Liver injury
Amylase	↑	Pancreatic and/or contiguous bowel/spleen injury
Lytes/BUN/BS	↑BS	Stress response
Creatinine	Abn K	Necrotic bowel, etc.
Blood gases	Persistent decreased CO_2 Persistent metabolic acidosis	
PT/PTT	↑	Potential bleeding problems
CPK - MB Bands	↑	Cardiac injury
Drug screen (urine/serum)	Positive	Caretaker neglectful or intentional poisoning

The complete blood count (CBC) and indices will give a baseline hemoglobin, hematocrit, and white blood cell count; when these are abnormal, blood loss or infection, such as peritonitis, may be present. However, iron deficiency anemia and lead toxicity are common in this age group and, therefore, the total hemogram should be examined to determine if the abnormalities are due to blood loss, lack of production of blood, or both. A strongly positive stool and/or gastric aspirate guaiac test suggests that there is intraluminal gastrointestinal bleeding. Red blood cells or hemoglobin in the urine can suggest renal injury, but their absence does not negate this possibility. The kidneys, because of their location, are relatively well-protected; therefore, if they are damaged, this suggests a vigorous abusive assault.

Aspartate amino transferase (AST) and alanine amino transferase (ALT) can be useful predictors of liver injury. Oldham et al. (1984) found that 44 of 100 patients with blunt abdominal trauma had elevated liver enzymes (AST/ALT). Nineteen of the 44 with abnormal elevation of liver enzymes had abdominal CT scan–proven injuries to the liver. None of the children in this series with negative abdominal CT scans had elevated liver enzyme studies. This suggests that these are extremely reliable tests. Hennes et al. (1990) further refined the predictability of liver enzymes with abdominal trauma by showing that an AST and ALT level equal to or greater than 450 and 250 IU, respectively, identified all patients with liver injury proven by CT scan.

An elevated amylase level indicates traumatic pancreatitis, which is the most common cause of pancreatitis in the young child, but also may suggest injury to the duodenum and spleen due to the proximal location of these structures and their closeness to the pancreas. Child abuse is the most common etiology for duodenal hematoma and is associated with signs and symptoms of duodenal obstruction. Serum electrolytes, blood urea nitrogen (BUN), blood glucose, creatinine, and blood gases should be obtained to assess the total clinical status of the child. A child who remains persistently acidotic, hyperkalemic, and obtunded after appropriate fluid resuscitation suggests possible necrotic bowel, waiting to perforate, or significant rhabdomyolysis. Prothrombin time (PT) and partial thromboplastin time (PTT) are probably not helpful if the child has no history of bleeding disorders and if a reliable history is obtained. However, these studies might help in assessing liver injury and preparing for appropriate infusion therapy if the patient requires operative intervention.

In the child suspected of having cardiac injury, serial creatinine phosphokinase (CPK) isoenzymes with MB bands will often be more useful than repeated electrocardiograms (EKGs). Cardiac injury occurs far less frequently than both abdominal and pulmonary insult. In general, chest trauma is much less common than abdominal injury but should be suspected when respiratory distress is noted. The chest contents can be injured without fracture of the thoracic cage due to the marked plasticity and flexibility of the ribs of the young child. However, if fractured ribs are present, the probability of injury to the chest viscera, as well as to the abdominal contents, is much higher.

Drug screens of urine and serum are often necessary in obtunded or comatose patients without an adequate history. A child may have been given an overdose of a sedative or barbiturate after excessive crying from the pain associated with abusive blows to the abdomen, which might be detected only by laboratory studies.

IMAGING STUDIES

Chapter 2 reviews the studies that are useful in the assessment of individual organs. Some or all of the imaging studies listed in **Table 3-3** can be obtained based on the clinical assessment and relevant correlation of other studies obtained. Spinal, chest, abdominal, and pelvic radiographs are obtained because of their rapid accessibility and are primarily used to find fractures, dislocations, and major abnormalities of the chest and to suggest the need for evaluation of soft tissue structures and organs using more sophisticated imaging. The primary practitioner, who may see this patient in an after-hours setting or in an emergency room and who might be required to make an initial reading of the radiographs, must pay particular attention to the presence of old rib fractures and metaphyseal fractures. Often films of the chest and abdomen will include parts of the appendicular skeleton. However, if there is serious concern regarding appendicular skeletal injuries, then detailed skeletal films and, occasionally, even a radioisotope bone scan may be necessary. It should be remembered that fractures are the next most common sign of abuse after bruises and skin findings. A useful technique in reading the radiographs is to evaluate the X-rays as individual segments, that is, bones, soft tissues, and air shadows, and then assess the whole picture. If one traces and visualizes each skeletal part with a finger, one is less likely to miss old rib fractures or the coincidental healing of a spiral humeral fracture on a chest film. In general, soft tissue integrity of both chest and abdomen is most reliably evaluated by computer tomography. For the abdomen, the use of intraluminal and intravenous contrast allows identification of organ structural integrity, gastrointestinal tract obstruction, perforation, and shearing injury. This imaging modality is helpful in identifying the site of injury and allows for appropriate monitoring and preparedness in incidences of nonoperative management. Diagnostic peritoneal lavage has been relegated to a minor position in pediatric trauma. Although it reliably identifies bleeding, it does not delineate which organ(s) may be involved and whether the patient needs an operation. Most of the care is supportive, with close observation. Diagnostic peritoneal lavage is still used

Table 3-3. Imaging Studies	
Plain Radiographs	Spine
	Chest
	Abdomen
	Pelvis
	Detailed skeletal survey
CT Scans	Abdomen
	Head

when the patient requires emergency neurosurgical operative intervention and there is no time available for an abdominal CT. Arteriography is used for the rare chest vascular injury.

It must be emphasized that in a comatose child, even after abusive head injury is recognized, the abdomen must still be aggressively evaluated to detect major injury, which can suddenly lead to unexpected deterioration.

◆SUMMARY

Thoracoabdominal injury secondary to child abuse is relatively rare but can have very high mortality and morbidity. *Consequently, it is important to be aware of this possibility and to remember the following clues:*

1. Delayed presentation with nonspecific complaints, usually related to the abdomen and chest, with either multiple stories or reports that are inconsistent with the physical findings or the child's development.

2. Past history of that abusive or neglectful incident and previous report to the Division of Family Services.

3. Mean age of 2.5 years.

4. Old inflicted bruises or scars (present in 50% to 90% of cases). Consequently, all young children with nonspecific complaints or injuries should have a rapid but thorough complete physical examination.

5. Generous use of screening trauma laboratory studies, especially SGOT, SGPT, amylase, stool guaiac, hemoglobin, hematocrit, and urine analysis to give direction with regard to the need for CT imaging or other diagnostic studies.

◆BIBLIOGRAPHY

Coant, P, Kornberg, A, Brody, A, and Edwards-Holmes, K: Markers for occult liver injury in cases of physical abuse in children, *Pediatrics* 89(2):274-278, 1992.

Cooper, A, Floyd, T, Barlow, B, Niemirska, M, Ludwig, S, Seidl, T, O'Neill, J, Templeton, J, Ziegler, M, Ross, A, Gandhi, R, and Catherman, R: Major blunt abdominal trauma due to child abuse, *J Trauma* 28(10):1483-1487, 1988.

Evers, K, and DeGaeta, LR: Abdominal trauma, *Emerg Med Clin North Am* 3(3):525-539, 1985.

Feldman, KW, and Brewer, DK: Child abuse, cardiopulmonary resuscitation, and rib fractures, *Pediatrics* 73(3):339-342, 1984.

Fossum, RM, and Descheneaux, KA: Blunt trauma of the abdomen in children, *JFSCS* 36(1)47-50, 1991.

Gornall, P, Ahmed, S, Jolleys, A, and Cohen, S: Intra-abdominal injuries in the battered baby syndrome, *Arch Dis Child* 47:211-214, 1972.

Grosfeld, JL, and Ballantine, TVN: Surgical aspects of child abuse (trauma-x), *Pediatr Ann* 106-120, 1976.

Haller, JA: Injuries of the gastrointestinal tract in children: Notes on recognition and management, *Clin Pediatr* 5(8):476-480, 1966.

Haller, JO, Bass, IS, and Sclafani, SJA: Imaging evaluation of traumatic hematuria in children, *Urol Radiol* 7:211-218, 1984.

Haller, JO, Kleinman, PK, Merten, DF, Cohen, HL, Cohen, MD, Hayden, PW, Keller, M, Towbin, R, and Sane, SM: Diagnostic imaging of child abuse, *Pediatrics* 87(2):262-265, 1991.

Hennes, HM, Smith, DS, Schneider, K, Hegenbarth, MA, Duma, MA, and Jona, JZ: Elevated liver transaminase levels in children with blunt abdominal trauma: A predictor of liver injury, *Pediatrics* 86(1):87-94, 1990.

Hernanz-Schulman, M, Genieser, NB, and Ambrosino, M: Sonographic diagnosis on intramural duodenal hematoma, *J Ultrasound Med* 8:273-276, 1989.

Kaufman, RA, and Babcock, DS: An approach to imaging the upper abdomen in the injured child, *Semin Roentgenol* 14(4):308-320, 1984.

Kaufman, RA, Towbin, R, Babcock, DS, Gelfand, MJ, Fuice, KS, Oldham, KT, and Noseworthy, J: Upper abdominal trauma in children: Imaging evaluation, *AJR* l42:449-460, 1984.

Kirks, DR: Radiological evaluation of visceral injuries in the battered child syndrome, *Pediatr Ann* 12(12):888-893, 1983.

Kleinman, PK, Brill, PW, and Winchester, P: Resolving duodenal-jejunal hematoma in abused children, *Radiology* 160:747-750, 1986.

Kleinman, PK, Marks, SC, Adams, VI, and Blackbourne, BD: Factors affecting visualization of posterior rib fractures in abused infants, *AJR* 150:635-638, 1988.

Kleinman, PK, Raptopoulos, VD, and Brill, PW: Occult nonskeletal trauma in the battered-child syndrome, *Pediatr Radiol* 141:393-396, 1981.

Ledbetter, D, Hatch, E, Feldman, K, Fligner, C, and Tapper, D: Diagnostic and surgical implications of child abuse, *Arch Surg* 123:1101-1105, 1988.

Mayer, T, Walker, M, Johnson, D, and Matlak, M: Causes of morbidity and mortality in severe pediatric trauma, *JAMA* 245(7):719-721, 1981.

McEniery, J, Hanson, R, Grigor, W, and Horowitz, A: Lung injury resulting from a nonaccidental crush injury to the chest, *Pediatr Emerg Care* 7(3):166-168, 1991.

Meller, J, Little, A, and Shermeta, D: Thoracic trauma in children, *Pediatrics* 74(5):813-819, 1984.

Merten, D, and Carpenter, B: Radiologic imaging of inflicted injury in the child abuse syndrome, *Pediatr Clin North Am* 37(4): 815-837, 1990.

Oldham, K, Guice, K, Kaufman, R, Martin, L, and Noseworthy, J: Blunt hepatic injury and elevated hepatic enzymes: A clinical correlation in children, *J Pediatr Surg* 19(4):457-461, 1984.

O'Neill, JA, Meacham, WF, Griffin, PP, and Sawyers, JL: Patterns of injury in the battered child syndromoe, *J Trauma* 13(4):332-339, 1973.

Pena, SDJ, and Medovy, H: Child abuse and traumatic pseudocyst of the pancreas, *J Pediatr* 83(6):1026-1028, 1973.

Philippart, AI: Blunt abdominal trauma in childhood, *Surg Clin North Am*, 57(1)151-163, 1977.

Ramenofsky, ML: Pediatric abdominal trauma, *Pediatr Ann* 16(4)318-326, 1987.

Reece, RM, and Grodin, MA: Recognition of nonaccidental injury, *Pediatr Clin North Am* 32(1):41-60, 1985.

Rodgers, B: Trauma and the child, *Heart Lung* 6(6):1052-1056, 1977.

Sivit, C, Taylor, G, and Eichelberger, M: Visceral injury in battered children: A changing perspective, *Radiology* 173(3):659-661, 1989.

Taylor, GA, and Eichelberger, MR: Abdominal CT in children in neurologic impairment following blunt trauma, *Ann Surg* 210(2):229-233, 1989.

Taylor, GA, Fallat, ME, Potter, BM, and Eichelberger, MR: The role of computed tomography in blunt abdominal trauma in children, *J Trauma* 28(12):1660-1664, 1988.

Chapter 4

OPHTHALMIC MANIFESTATIONS OF CHILD ABUSE

OSCAR A. CRUZ, M.D.
JOSEPH GIANGIACOMO, M.D.

In 1946, Caffey suggested that multiple fractures in long bones of several infants with chronic subdural hematoma were secondary to trauma (Caffey, 1974). Two of these children also had retinal hemorrhage. Caffey recognized that only trauma could explain this spectrum of injuries, yet he failed to implicate intentional trauma and stated that the injuries could be the result of forgotten or relatively minor traumatic episodes.

It was not until 1964 that the ophthalmology profession began to describe the ocular manifestations of child abuse. The first report of abusive injuries in ophthalmic literature was made by G. T. Kiffney. Kiffney reported an abused child who presented with multiple skull fractures, intracranial hemorrhage, and leukokoria (1964). The child had bilateral cataracts and total retinal detachments. Retrospectively, the diagnosis of child abuse was made.

♦PRESENTING SIGNS

The presenting signs of child abuse involve the eyes in 4% to 6% of cases (Friendly, 1971; Jensen et al., 1987), and the spectrum of ocular findings in the battered child syndrome is vast. An ocular injury can be as minor as periorbital edema or as severe as a ruptured globe (**Table 4-1**). The ocular sequelae of abuse can include amblyopia on the basis of monocular cataract, strabismus, or anterior segment injury. Detection of eye injury is difficult when the examination takes place several days after the abuse has occurred. Because nearly 40% of physically abused children have associated ocular trauma, it is imperative that all children suspected of being abused have a thorough dilated ophthalmic examination (Friendly, 1971; Jensen et al., 1987). The presence of positive ocular findings often indicates that the child should have prompt neuroimaging (MRI).

Table 4-1. Ocular Manifestations of the Two Most Common Forms of Child Abuse	
Physical Abuse	Intraocular retinal hemorrhages
	Periorbital ecchymosis
	Vitreoretinal injury other than hemorrhage
	Cataract or subluxated lens
	Hyphema
	Subconjunctival hemorrhage
	Optic nerve injury
	Strabismus or gaze palsy
Sexual Abuse	Sexually transmitted infections

♦ Nonabusive Ocular Injuries

Nonabusive ocular injuries are often seen in newborns, infants, and children. Examples of nonabusive injuries include retinal hemorrhage, resulting from the process of birthing, and thoracic compression needed in CPR (**Table 4-2**). Other than by time, nonabusive hemorrhages cannot be distinguished from retinal hemorrhage resulting from abusive-inflicted injury. Other results of nonabusive ophthalmic injury can include periorbital edema and subconjunctival hemorrhage.

Table 4-2. Common Nonabusive Causes of Retinal Hemorrhage	
Medical Procedures	Birthing process Extracorporeal membrane oxygenation (ECMO) dyscrasia; ethmoglobinopathies
Accidental Trauma	Subdural or subarachnoid hemorrhages secondary to accidental trauma

Retinal Hemorrhage

Retinal hemorrhages can occur in any layer of the retina without being the result of child abuse. The presence of retinal or vitreous hemorrhages in a child younger than 3 years of age who has no medical risk factors has been considered by some to be pathognomonic of nonaccidental injury (Levin, 1991).

Result of Birth Process

Head trauma resulting from birthing has been found to cause retinal hemorrhages in 8% to 50% of otherwise healthy newborns (Von Barsewisch, 1979). Giles found retinal hemorrhages in 40 of 100 newborns examined on the first day of life, but only 20% of these infants still had retinal hemorrhages on the third day of life (Giles, 1960). If retinal hemorrhages are detected in infants over 1 month of age, a cause other than the birth process must be considered (Friendly, 1983).

Result of CPR

Retinal hemorrhages can occur rarely when cardiopulmonary resuscitation (CPR) is administered (Goetting & Sowa, 1990). Sufficient thoracic compression can cause an acute rise in retinal venous pressure and subsequent hemorrhage. Caution must be used when interpreting fundus findings in children who have undergone CPR, as the findings could be the result of nonaccidental trauma.

Periorbital Edema and Subconjunctival Hemorrhage

Periorbital edema and subconjunctival hemorrhage are common ocular manifestations of nonaccidental injury. These injuries are frequently accompanied by bleeding from forehead and scalp contusions. The ophthalmologist then faces the challenge of determining if the physical findings of periorbital edema or subconjunctival hemorrhage (**Figure 4-1 a,b**) are consistent with the history, in particular, of an accidental injury.

Figure 4-1a. *Subconjunctival hemorrhage occurs in 2% to 4% of abused children with ocular manifestations. Direct trauma or increases in thoracic pressure by chest compression can be the cause.* ***b.*** *This is the presumed mechanism of subconjunctival hemorrhage in attempted strangulation.*

The pattern of bruising can be a secondary aid in determining if the injury is nonaccidental. Signs of bilateral ocular trauma suggest inflicted injury because accidents usually involve only one eye (Nelson & Parlato, 1993). With these particular injuries, the large volume of potential tissue space in the periorbital area can lead to significant blood accumulation, and this in turn can lead to marked ecchymotic eyelid swelling. This accumulation of blood often makes the ecchymosis look darker than bruises at other sites, causing the injury to appear older than it actually is. In addition, the increased volume of blood leads to a slower resolution (Levin, 1991).

♦ Abusive Ocular Injuries

The single most common ocular manifestation in child abuse is the presence of retinal hemorrhages (**Figure 4-2**), which have been found in 5% to 23% of physically abused children (Friendly, 1971; Levin, 1990). Eisenbrey's study of victims of head trauma found retinal hemorrhages in 16 of 26 (62%) abused children and in only 1 of 32 (3%) nonabused children. The one child with retinal hemorrhage in the nonabused group was a "newborn infant following a traumatic delivery" (Eisenbrey, 1979).

CURRENT RESEARCH

Retrospective studies of retinal hemorrhage have been flawed by lack of matched controls. They have been limited by the fact that cases of retinal hemorrhages easily could have been missed if routine funduscopic examinations were not performed on all the children. Buys et al. (1992) have produced the only published report of prospective retinal examination of children who suffered head trauma. They examined 78 children between the ages of 4 weeks and 36 months who had sustained head trauma and performed dilated, indirected ophthalmoscopy within 48 hours after the head trauma event occurred. Seventy-five children in their study sustained accidental head injuries and had normal funduscopic examinations. It was determined that three children sustained inflicted head injuries, and all three also had varying degrees of retinal hemorrhage.

Figure 4-2. Retinal hemorrhage.

Billmire and Myers (1985) did a retrospective study of infants younger than 1 year of age who were admitted to the hospital with a head injury. They reported that retinal hemorrhages occurred in 89% of the 28 abused infants but that none occurred in the 54 infants with accidental injuries.

These data support the conclusion that retinal hemorrhages occur only rarely in children younger than 36 months of age after severe head trauma and not at all after moderate or mild head trauma. When a child presents with a head injury and retinal hemorrhages and an absence of an obvious cause, an investigation for child abuse must be considered.

SHAKEN BABY SYNDROME

In infants with shaken baby syndrome (SBS), the incidence of retinal hemorrhage is 50% to 100% (Ludwig & Warman, 1984; Billmire & Myers, 1985; Duhaime et al., 1987). Ludwig and Warman reported that 50% of babies determined to have been shaken had gaze disturbances. These hemorrhages often involve the posterior pole and are bilateral in 58% to 100% of cases (Levin, 1990), although they can be asymmetric. Retinal hemorrhages can be subretinal or intra-retinal predominantly in the bipolar layer or in the nerve fiber layer. Increased severity of retinal hemorrhages in shaken baby syndrome has been correlated with acute neurologic findings (Wilkinson et al., 1989).

Other Vitreoretinal Injuries Resulting From Shaken Baby Syndrome

Retinal dialysis (disinsertion of the retina from its insertion at the ora serrata)
Retinal edema (commotio retinae) in the photoreceptor layer
Central retinal artery occlusion
Exudate
Traction from scarring (gliosis)

PATHOGENESIS

The pathogenesis of retinal hemorrhages in the shaken baby syndrome is a matter of dispute. Many authors believe that the intraocular hemorrhages occur secondary to a sudden rise in retinal venous hydrostatic pressure, which is produced by intracranial hypertension. Greenwall et al. have proposed that hemorrhages secondary to internal splitting of the retina, or traumatic retinoschisis, are caused by tractional forces transmitted from the vitreous, which oscillates violently as the head is shaken (Greenwall et al., 1986). There is both clinical and pathological evidence to support this view (Rao et al., 1988). The time of onset of symptoms occurs quite variably. There is evidence that there can be a delay between the occurrence of an intraocular hemorrhage and the subsequent development of subdural hemorrhage or effusions.

Trerson syndrome is caused by a sudden rise in intracranial pressure due to acute subdural or subarachnoid hemorrhage and is generally characterized by preretinal and vitreous hemorrhage. Purtscher retinopathy, characterized by cotton-wool exudates and retinal hemorrhages, is thought to be produced by increased orbital venous pressure secondary to thoracic compression. This type of hemorrhagic retinal angiopathy occurs with pulmonary compression or contusions or fractures of long bones. When it is seen in association with child abuse, there is a paucity of intracranial hemorrhages (Tomasi & Rosman, 1986). Positive ocular findings indicate that the child should have prompt neuroimaging (CT) or magnetic resonance imaging (MRI).

VITREOUS HEMORRHAGE

Vitreous hemorrhage can also occur in shaken baby syndrome, although its appearance is usually delayed from 2 days to 2 weeks after the shaking episode occurs. Vitreoretinal injury, like retinal hemorrhage, is a vision-threatening injury. Vitreous hemorrhage is acutely associated with retinal or subhyaloid hemorrhage.

PHYSIOLOGY

The repeated violent shaking described in shaken baby syndrome can result in repeated severe acceleration/deceleration of the vitreous, which causes trauma to the retina and retinal blood vessels. Chorioretinal atrophy lesions are typically scalloped areas of the retinal pigment epithelial atrophy that are associated with pigment proliferation and atrophic choroidal changes (**Figure 4-3**).

This mechanism has been proposed as the cause of traumatic retinoschisis (Levin, 1990), while retinal folds are believed to cause the more common retinal hemorrhages (Gaynon et al., 1988; Massicotte et al., 1991). Macular folds have been shown to occur where previous large subhyaloid hemorrhages have resolved (Han & Wilkinson, 1990). Unilateral and bilateral retinal detachment due to abuse is most often rhegmatogenous or due to a tear or a hole in the retina that allows fluid vitreous to track underneath the retina and separate it from the sclera. When vitreous hemorrhage results from giant retinal tears, the visual prognosis is dismal. Chorioretinal atrophy in the extreme periphery of the retina, particularly the inferior temporal quadrant, had been demonstrated in child abuse victims. These lesions typically are scalloped areas of retinal pigment epithelial atrophy that are often associated with pigment proliferation and atrophic choroidal changes. They are nonprogressive and are not associated with any other retinal defect (Nelson & Parlato, 1993).

Figure 4-3. Scattered retinal hemorrhages are a benchmark feature of child abuse.

LENS SUBLUXATION OR DISLOCATION

Trauma is the most common cause of lens subluxation or dislocation in childhood, and there have been a number of reported cases involving abuse (Friendly, 1971). The first step, of course, is to rule out nontraumatic displacement — such as that associated with Marfan syndrome, homocystinuria, aniridia, and congenital glaucoma. Traumatic dislocation is usually unilateral, as opposed to spontaneous ectopia lentis, which is usually bilateral, although it can be markedly asymmetric. The lens is displaced in any direction except upward in reported cases resulting from child abuse. Upward displacement is the most common lens displacement direction seen in Marfan syndrome and is the most common cause of spontaneous ectopia lentis. Findings associated with subluxation of the lens include marked astigmatism, monocular diplopia, cataract, and amblyopia in unilateral cases. Dislocation can also cause all of these complications with the addition of glaucoma.

ANTERIOR CHAMBER INJURY

The anterior chamber includes the cornea, iris, and trabecular meshwork (the outflow system for the aqueous humor); essentially it is the area between the crystalline lens and the cornea. Anterior chamber trauma occurring in abused children ranges from 0% to 5%. Hyphema, or blood in the anterior chamber, is caused by injury to the vessels of the peripheral iris or the anterior ciliary body. Other anterior segment injuries, as well as hyphema, are usually caused by direct blunt trauma and are not the result of shaken baby syndrome.

CORTICAL PATHWAYS INJURY

The cortical visual pathways can be injured as a result of child abuse and are most commonly seen in shaken baby syndrome. These injuries result in a poor visual outcome even when there is no permanent vitreoretinal injury. Cortical injuries result in visual field deficits or reduced visual acuity.

Optic atrophy can be unilateral or bilateral. It results either from direct injury, increased intracranial pressure, or injury secondary to cortical injury with retrograde transsynaptic degeneration. Acute papilledema, almost exclusively bilateral, is a poor prognostic sign. The finding of optic nerve sheath hemorrhages suggests that the hemorrhages found surrounding the optic disc could have originated in the subarachnoid space (Lambert et al., 1986).

OCULAR MANIFESTATIONS IN SEXUAL ABUSE

No case of either isolated ocular manifestations or of ocular manifestations in conjunction with findings at another site have been reported in sexually abused children. However, periorbital ecchymosis, retinal and vitreous hemorrhages, papilledema, and subconjunctival hemorrhage have been reported in children who were beaten *and* sexually abused (San Martin et al., 1981). A more likely ophthalmologic manifestation of sexual abuse, however, is the onset of functional visual loss or other functional ocular complaints such as blinding, transient visual obscurations, and photophobia (Catalano et al., 1986; Vrabec et al., 1989). An ocular manifestation of sexually transmitted disease, such as gonococcal conjunctivitis, should be considered a possible indicator of covert sexual abuse (Levin, 1990).

Gonococcal conjunctivitis is characterized by the acute onset of copious mucopurulent conjunctivitis. Corneal involvement can lead to corneal damage or perforation. Evaluation of the child with gonococcal conjunctivitis must include genital and anal inspection, cultures of the rectum, vagina, or male urethra, and a culture of the throat for *Neisseria gonorrhoeae* and other sexually transmitted disease organisms.

CHILD NEGLECT

The most common form of child neglect encountered by the ophthalmologist includes medical noncompliance. Failure to obtain glasses, adhere to patching regimens, or keep follow-up appointments is a frequent and frustrating experience in the practice of pediatric ophthalmology. Some parents also do not seek medical attention for their child when obvious ocular symptoms are present. It is often difficult to determine whether noncompliance is abusively neglectful or whether inadequate financial or social resources are responsible (Levin, 1991).

◆ TEAM APPROACH

The ophthalmologist must be a part of the multidisciplinary team caring for possible child abuse victims. All ophthalmologists must consider the possibility of child abuse in the differential diagnosis, especially when in the role of primary care provider or when ocular manifestations are the only visible signs of abuse. Careful documentation of the clinical findings in children who have sustained trauma, accidental or deliberate, is critical in establishing the spectrum of physical findings in these patients. Riffenburgh and Sathyavagiswaran (1991) recommend that indirect ophthalmoscopy be included as part of the autopsy in all children who died without an obvious cause of death. The ophthalmologic findings often provide confirmatory evidence in cases where abuse is suspected. The ophthalmologic findings must not be reported in isolation; they need to be documented in conjunction with all of the other physical findings in these children.

♦ BIBLIOGRAPHY

Alexander, RC, Schor, DP, and Smith, WL, Jr: Magnetic resonance imaging of intracranial injuries from child abuse, *J Pediatr* 109:975-979, 1986.

Billmire, ME, and Myers, PA: Serious head injury in infants: Accident or abuse? *Pediatrics* 75:340-342, 1985.

Buys, YM, Levin, AV, Enzenauer, RW, et al: Retinal findings after head trauma in infants and young children, *Ophthalmology* 99:1718-1723, 1992.

Caffey, J: The whiplash shaken infant syndrome: Manual shaking by the extremities with whiplash-induced intracranial and intraocular bleedings linked with residual permanent brain damage and mental retardation, *Pediatrics* 54:396-403, 1974.

Catalona, RA, Simon, JW, Krobel, GB, et al: Functional visual loss in children, *Ophthalmology* 93:385, 1986.

Duhaime, AC, Alario, A, Lewander, W, et al: Head injury in very young children: Mechanism, injury types and ophthalmic findings in 100 hospitalized patients younger than 2 years of age, *Pediatrics* 90:179-185, 1992.

Duhaime, AC, Gennarelli, TA, Thibault, LE, et al: The shaken baby syndrome: A clinical, pathological, and biomechanical study, *J Neurosurg* 66:409-415, 1987.

Eisenbrey, AB: Retinal hemorrhage in the battered child, *Child Brain* 5:40-44, 1979.

Elner, SG, Elner, VM, Arnall, M, and Albert, DM: Ocular and associate systemic findings in suspected child abuse: A necroscopy study, *Arch Ophthalmol* 108:1094-1101, 1990.

Friendly, DS: Ocular manifestations of physical child abuse, *Trans Am Acad Ophthalmol Orolaryngol* 75:318-332, 1971.

Friendly, DS: Ocular aspects of physical child abuse. In RD Harley, ed: *Pediatric Ophthalmology*, WB Saunders Co, Philadelphia, 1983.

Gaynon, MW, Koh, K, Marmor, MF, and Frankel, LR: Retinal folds in the shaken baby syndrome, *Am J Ophthalmol* 106:423-425, 1988.

Giangiacomo, J, and Barkett, KJ: Ophthalmoscopic findings in occult child abuse, *J Pediatr Ophthalmol Strabismus* 22:234-237, 1985.

Giles, MJ: Retinal hemorrhages in the newborn, *Am J Ophthalmol* 49:1005-1011, 1960.

Goetting, MG, and Sowa, B: Retinal hemorrhage after cardiopulmonary resuscitation in children: An etiologic re-evaluation, *Pediatrics* 85:585-588, 1990.

Greenwall, MJ, Weiss, A, Oesterle, CS, and Friendly, DS: Traumatic retinoschisis in battered babies, *Ophthalmology* 93:618-625, 1986.

Han, DP, and Wilkinson, WS: Late ophthalmic manifestations of the shaken baby syndrome, *J Pediatr Ophthalmol Strabismus* 27:299-303, 1990.

Hobbs, CJ: When are burns nonaccidental? *Arch Dis Child* 61:357-361, 1986.

Jensen, AD, Smith, RE, and Olson, MI: Ocular clues to child abuse, *J Pediatr Ophthalmol* 8:270-272, 1987.

Kanter, RK: Retinal hemorrhage after cardiopulmonary resuscitation or child abuse, *J Pediatr* 108:430-432, 1986.

Keen, JH, Lendrum, J, and Wolmann, B: Inflicted burns and scalds in children, *Br Med J* 4:268-269, 1975.

Kiffney, GT, Jr: The eye of the battered child, *Arch Ophthalmol* 72:231-233, 1964.

Kleinmann, PK: Diagnostic imaging in infant abuse, *AJR* 155:703-712, 1990.

Lambert, SR, Johnson, TE, and Hoyt, CS: Optic nerve sheath hemorrhages associated with the shaken baby syndrome, *Arch Ophthalmol* 104:1509-1512, 1986.

Levin, AV: Ocular manifestations of child abuse, *Ophthalmol Clin North Am* 3:249-264, 1990.

Levin, AV: Ophthalmologic manifestations. In S. Ludwig, ed: *Child Abuse, A Medical Reference*, Churchill Livingstone, New York, 1991.

Ludwig, S, and Warman, M: Shaken baby syndrome: A review of 20 cases, *Ann Emerg Med* 13:104-107, 1984.

Massicotte, SJ, Folberg, R, Torczynski, E, et al: Vitreoretinal traction and perimacular retinal folds in the eyes of deliberately traumatized children, *Ophthalmology* 98:1124-1127, 1991.

Neinstein, LS, Goldenring, J, and Carpenter, S: Nonsexual transmission of sexually transmitted diseases: An infrequent occurrence, *Pediatrics* 74:67-76, 1984.

Nelson, LB, and Parlato, CJ: Systemic and ophthalmic manifestations of child abuse. In W Tasman, ed: *Duane's Clinical Ophthalmology*, JB Lippincott Co, Philadelphia, Volume 5, Chapter 44, 1993.

Ommaya, AK, Faas, F, and Yarnell, P: Whiplash injury and brain damage: An experimental study, *JAMA* 204:285-289, 1968.

Podgore, JK, and Holmes, KK: Ocular gonococcal infection with minimal or inflammatory response, *JAMA* 246:242-243, 1981.

Rao, N, Smith, RE, Choi, JH, et al: Autopsy findings in the eyes of fourteen fatally abused children, *Forensic Sci Int* 39:293-296, 1988.

Riffenburgh, RS, and Sathyavagiswaran, L: The eyes of child abuse victims: Autopsy findings, *J Forensic Sci* 36:741-747, 1991.

San Martin, R, Steinkuller, PG, and Nisbert, RM: Retinopathy in the sexually abused battered child, *Ann Ophthalmol* 13:89-91, 1981.

Tomasi, LG, and Rosman, NP: Purtscher retinopathy in the battered child syndrome, *Am J Dis Child* 93:1435-1437, 1986.

Von Barsewisch, B: *Perinatal Retinal Hemorrhages*, Springer-Verlag, Berlin, 1979.

Vrabec, TR, Levin, AV, and Nelson, LB: Functional blinking in childhood, *Pediatrics* 83:967-970, 1989.

Wilkinson, WS, Han, DP, Rappley, MD, and Owings, CL: Retinal hemorrhage predicts neurologic injury in the shaken baby syndrome, *Arch Ophthalmol* 107:1472-1474, 1989.

Chapter 5

HEAD INJURY IN CHILD ABUSE

MARY E. S. CASE, M.D.

In a 1946 paper, Caffey called attention to a correlation between the findings of multiple skeletal fractures and subdural hemorrhage in children he believed to have suffered inflicted trauma (Caffey, 1946). In 1962 Kempe stressed the same correlation Caffey found, and the term "battered child syndrome" was applied to describe the medicosociological phenomenon discovered (Kempe et al., 1962).

Since the early 1960s, considerable data have accumulated concerning abusive pediatric head injuries. Recognition of inflicted versus accidental injuries is accomplished in the light of a vast body of literature and knowledge. This chapter will overview the findings in relation to types of head injury and signs to be sought by the practitioner; Chapter 19 will review head injuries from the perspective of a pathologist.

Head injury resulting from abuse is a significant cause of disability and death in children. It is the leading cause of death from abuse, playing a role in 40% to 75% of abusive deaths. Children with nonfatal head injuries often suffer permanent neurological impairments, previously incorrectly attributed to prenatal or perinatal disorders (Oliver, 1975).

Because head injuries in children differ greatly in many aspects from those occurring in adults, particular mention will be made of these differences in describing the various injuries.

◆EXTERNAL FINDINGS IN ABUSIVE HEAD AND FACE INJURIES

Because of the great disparity in size and strength between the adult and child, an adult does not need a weapon or instrument to inflict injury on the child. Many injuries to the head are inflicted by manual violence and result in observable blunt trauma lesions, particularly bruises or contusions and abrasions; less often lacerations may occur. Instruments may also be used, and gunshot wounds, stab wounds, or impact marks from objects such as hammers, boards, or choppers may be seen in children.

A bruise or contusion is an impact site on the skin's surface over subcutaneous or deeper bleeding. Small blood vessels are torn by the impact, yielding the site of hemorrhage. On the surface, bruises undergo progressive color changes— purple/blue to green to yellow and then to brown—before fading away. When injury is inflicted by belts, cords, hands, bites, or hairbrush bristles, bruises appear in distinctive patterns.

Table 5-1. Population Distribution/St. Louis Study *(January 1977-June 30, 1985)*		
Homicide 70 children	Accident 63 children	Undetermined 27 children
Age	**Homicide***	**Accident†**
Under 1 year of age	45%	39%
1 to 2 years of age	19%	28%
2 to 3 years of age	18%	8%
Older	18%	22%

*82% of the homicide group were under 3 years of age.
†75% of the accident group were under 3 years of age.

Table 5-2. Accident—Marks of Injury – Other than Point of Lethal Impact		
Contusions		
Face	1 on each of 2 children	<1%
Abrasions		
Scratch on nose	1 child	<1%
Scars		
Face	1 child	<1%

Bruises on the face, scalp, or neck of a child are significant lesions that should be noted on physical examination. Fewer than 1% of children who die of accidental causes have bruises unrelated to the lethal injury (**Tables 5-1 and 5-2 and Figures 5-1 and 5-2**). In contrast, 65% of children with lethal inflicted injuries have bruises in areas other than those involved in the fatal injury (**Table 5-3**). When bruises appear on physical examination, the parent or caregiver should be questioned regarding their cause. If the explanation does not adequately account for the bruises, abuse should be suspected. The presence of more than one unexplained bruise on a child's head correlates highly with abuse.

The absence of an external lesion on a child's head does not preclude massive internal injury. A child's scalp is extremely elastic, so even massive impacts may leave no external marks. Clinicians can inspect only the external scalp; when the child dies, a pathologist can evaluate sites of hemorrhage into the subgaleal scalp tissues, noting points of impact (**Figure 5-3a,b**). Microscopic sections from these sites can be evaluated to establish the age of the injury; it is especially important to establish the age if gross differences in age between various sites are noted.

Figure 5-1. Bruises to head and face of abused victim.

Figure 5-2. Bruises to face of abused victim seen Figure 5-1.

Figure 5-3a. Multiple areas of subgaleal hemorrhage visible on inner surface of scalp. These were not evident externally on the scalp.

Figure 5-3b. Large area of subgaleal hemorrhage on inner surface of scalp in which can be discerned multiple overlapping impact sites. No external bruise was evident on the scalp.

It should be noted that on rare occasions the child's head may be massively impacted (e.g., due to direct impact on, swinging, or throwing the child), yet no impact site is discernible on the inner surface of the scalp. When this occurs, the impacting surface is usually broad based. When the scalp and brain show extensive damage, however, further evidence is unnecessary.

◆IMPACT INJURIES

Impact injuries result from a blow to the head by a hand, fist, foot, or other object or by throwing or swinging the child so that the head impacts with a surface. Impacts can be single or multiple and can cause skull fractures, epidural hemorrhage, subdural hemorrhage, and contusions.

SKULL FRACTURES

Approximately 50% of children with fatal abusive head injuries sustain skull fractures (O'Neill et al., 1973). Accidental injuries in children that produce skull fractures can be divided into two categories: significant event injuries and trivial falls.

1. Children may be injured as passengers or pedestrians in motor vehicle accidents, falls from second-story or higher windows, or in disasters such as structural collapses due to tornadoes or earthquakes. These injuries produce skull fractures comparable to what is seen in abusive injury, but the well-documented accidental nature of the event shows that it is not abuse.

2. Falls occur frequently in and around the home. Such falls are commonly from beds, cribs, tables, or couches. Minor falls should not produce major injury, and the physician must be certain the degree of damage correlates with the reported fall. Studies reveal that fewer than 1% of children involved in these trivial home falls sustain a skull fracture. Fractures that do occur are small, linear, and usually parietal; they generally cause no loss of or decrease in consciousness, seizures, or intracranial injury.

Table 5-3. Homicide–Marks of Injury		
Contusions		
Face (26 children)		37%
2 to 5 contusions	13 children	
6 to 30 contusions	6 children	
Neck	4 children	
Scalp (35 children)		50%
2 to 5 contusions	19 children	
6 to 21 contusions	6 children	
Abrasions		
Face (26 children)		37%
2 to 5 abrasions	8 children	
Broom marks (metal wires) on child, multiple sites	1 child	
Comb	1 child	
Hair brush	1 child	
Zipper	1 child	
Neck (5 children)		
Scalp (7 children)		
2 to 5 abrasions	4 children	
Scars		
Face (13 children)		19%

An exception to the benign nature of a minor home fall occurs when a toddler sitting or standing in a walker or heavy toy falls together with the object down a flight of stairs. The added weight of the walker or heavy toy increases the potential for serious or fatal head injury. This type of fall is rare and usually can be verified by the damage done to the walker or toy and often to the stairs.

Two recent studies reviewed skull fracture characteristics to distinguish between accidental and abusive origins (Hobbs, 1984; Meservy et al., 1987). *Hobbs concluded that it was possible to predict an inflicted injury if one or more of the following were present when a minor fall was alleged:*

1. Depressed fracture
2. Diastatic fracture (**Figure 5-4**)
3. Fracture width greater than 3 mm (**Figure 5-5**)
4. Complex configuration fractures
5. Multiple fractures
6. Bilateral fractures (**Figure 5-6**)
7. Nonparietal fractures (**Figure 5-7**)
8. Associated intracranial injury

Figure 5-4. *This photograph illustrates fractures on the left parietal calvarium associated with a very wide diastatic fracture of the sagittal suture.*

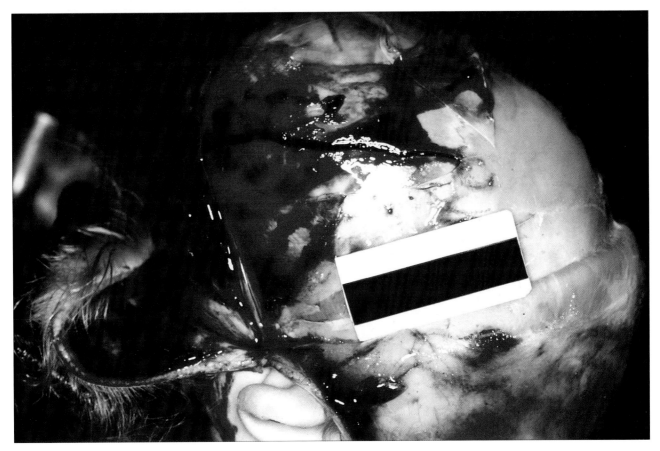

Figure 5-5. *A linear fracture 3 to 4 mm wide, above which is a craniectomy site for removal of subdural blood.*

Figure 5-6. *View of a 9-month-old child's skull base with fractures in each side of the posterior fossa.*

Figure 5-7. *View of a skull base with very wide fracture, 5 to 6 mm, extending from the occipital bone into the posterior fossa.*

Meservy's study concurred with Hobbs' in finding a much higher correlation of multiple fractures, bilateral fractures, and diastatic fractures with abusive injuries than with those caused accidentally.

EPIDURAL HEMORRHAGE

Epidural hemorrhage is less common in children than in adults. Whereas epidural hemorrhage in the adult is usually associated with a fracture that lacerates vessels on the inner table of the skull, in children it may occur when the pliable and poorly ossified skull is deformed in a way that pulls the dura away from the inner table of bone. Vessels may be torn without an associated fracture, with bleeding into the epidural space. Significant force is required to produce such deformation of the skull. Unless a significant accidental event, such as a motor vehicle collision, is reported, epidural hemorrhage in the child is highly suggestive of abuse (Leestma, 1988).

SUBDURAL HEMORRHAGE

Ninety percent of children with fatal inflicted head trauma have subdural hemorrhage. Only 20% of children who sustain massive accidental trauma have subdural hemorrhage; 60% of these have massive crushing injuries with skull fractures and brain lacerations (**Table 5-4**). Therefore in the absence of a major accidental event, subdural hemorrhage in a child is highly indicative of abusive injury. Of those children who sustain massive abusive impacts to the head, the most common intracranial injury is subdural hemorrhage, which is accompanied by skull fracture in 50% of cases (**Figure 5-8**).

Figure 5-8. *This photograph illustrates the calvarium removed and reflected backward into which a large volume of fresh subdural blood has run off the cerebral convexities to be collected in the skull cap.*

Table 5-4. Fatally Head-Injured Children		
Homicide (70 cases)		
Head		
Subdural with fracture	11 (39%)	93%
Subdural without fracture	15 (54%)	
Brain contusions (fracture)	7	
Contusion-tears	2	
Shaking injury	5	
Accident (63 cases)		
Head (10 cases or 16%)		
Subdural with fracture	2	20%
Subdural without fracture	0	
Cervical spine trauma	2	
Penetrating wound	1	
Massive crushing fractures and brain lacerations	6 (60%)	
Some children had more than one type of injury.		

CONTUSIONS

The adult patterns of coup and contrecoup contusions are not commonly seen in children younger than 3 or 4 years. The incomplete myelination of the brain, pliable skull, and very shallow cranial fossae typical of children under 3 years of age account for this paucity of cortical contusions (Merten & Osborne, 1983). When contusions are seen in children as young as 1 1/2 to 2 years old, they are usually associated with overlying fractures and should be considered fracture contusions rather than coup contusions (**Figure 5-9**).

Figure 5-9. *An 18-month-old child who was struck on the head with a heavy ceramic figure, producing frontoparietal fracture with the underlying fracture contusion demonstrated by this photograph.*

Figure 5-10. *Coronal section of a 4-month-old infant with vertical contusion tears in the orbital gyri of the frontal lobes.*

Lindenberg described lesions referred to as contusion tears that usually occur in infants 5 months or younger but can be seen up to age 12 months (Lindenberg & Freytag, 1969). These tears result from an impact that deforms the flexible skull and separates the cortex and subcortical white matter or produces a separation within the cortical layer itself. Tears occur anywhere in the cerebral hemispheres, but most commonly in the frontal and temporal lobes. The tears are poorly delineated by hemorrhage and may be overlooked in a poorly fixed brain (**Figure 5-10**). Since these lesions result from forceful deformation of the head, unless a massive accidental event is associated, their presence is highly suggestive of abusive force.

♦ SHAKEN INFANT SYNDROME

In 1972, Caffey described the practice now known as shaking an infant and the associated findings resulting from this behavior (Caffey, 1972). Although this syndrome is described in Chapters 1 and 19, those aspects related to head injury will be reviewed here.

A child's head and brain differ from those of an adult. First, the child's head represents about 10% of the total body weight compared to about 2% for an adult head (Calder et al., 1984). Also, a child's incompletely myelinated brain is softer in consistency and the thin axonal processes are more vulnerable to shearing forces than the better protected, larger adult brain. The neck muscles of a child are relatively weak and cannot adequately protect against forced whiplash movements of the head. Therefore the top-heavy head can be violently shaken in a whiplash fashion and there is little protection from the neck musculature to resist such movements. Because the skull is not fully ossified, vigorous whiplash movements of the head can cause the head to actually elongate by molding it with the forces of acceleration-deceleration during shaking.

Figure 5-11. Photomicrograph of a section of the superior cerebellar peduncle with numerous retraction bulbs or spheroids. (H & E X200.)

Shaking can occur in several ways. The child is grasped by the trunk or arms and violently shaken back and forth, causing the head to move forward until the chin strikes the chest and then to move backward until the occiput strikes the upper back. The child can also be shaken by grasping the ankles or legs and either shaking or swinging him in a circular motion.

Children at greatest risk for injury from shaking are under 4 years old. Fatal injuries have been observed in children up to 4 years old, but most of these occur in children 2 years or younger.

The pathophysiological consequences of shaking primarily consist of *diffuse axonal injury* produced by the acceleration of the head as it moves rapidly forward and backward (Vowles et al., 1986). As the brain is elongated in a sagittal plane, axonal processes, particularly those that run perpendicular to the sagittal plane, are stretched and can eventually tear. Small blood vessels are also stretched and torn. The structures most affected are the corpus callosum, fornix, corona radiata, and rostrolateral quadrants of the brainstem. The lesions that result from these injuries appear grossly as hemorrhagic foci; microscopically, axonal retraction bulbs or spheroids can be seen (**Figure 5-11**). Silver stains demonstrate varicosities in axonal processes that are damaged but not torn completely, allowing axoplasm to escape and form retraction bulbs. Changes can be observed immediately by electron microscopy or within 12 hours of injury by light microscopy. After several weeks, microglial clusters are seen in these areas. With long-term survival, there is loss of white matter by Wallerian degeneration of the long tracts.

Another finding in shaking is *subdural hemorrhage* resulting from tearing of the bridging veins between the cortex and dura (**Figure 5-12**). Hemorrhage can be unilateral or bilateral and varies from only a few milliliters to larger amounts. Subdural hemorrhage does not cause the brain injury as a space-occupying mass might but indicates that there has been brain acceleration. Experimental studies demonstrate that acceleration without impact can produce subdural hemorrhage (Adams et al., 1985).

Figure 5-12. This photograph demonstrates the few milliliters of subdural blood from over the cerebral convexities collected in the reflected calvarium in a fatally shaken infant.

Retinal hemorrhages are also found in about 80% to 85% of shaken infants. Hemorrhages occur commonly in the retina but also in the uvea or vitreous. In nonfatal suspected abuse cases the eyes should be examined by an experienced ophthalmologist (Greenwald et al., 1986). In fatal cases the eyes are removed at autopsy to document these hemorrhages (**Figure 5-13**).

The whiplash action of the head can also *damage the upper cervical spinal cord*. On rare occasions, fracture of a cervical vertebra occurs (**Figure 5-14**). At autopsy, a posterior neck dissection is done to reveal epidural or subdural hemorrhage of the upper cervical cord (**Figure 5-15**). A recent report demonstrated upper cervical cord contusion from shaking (Hadley et al., 1989).

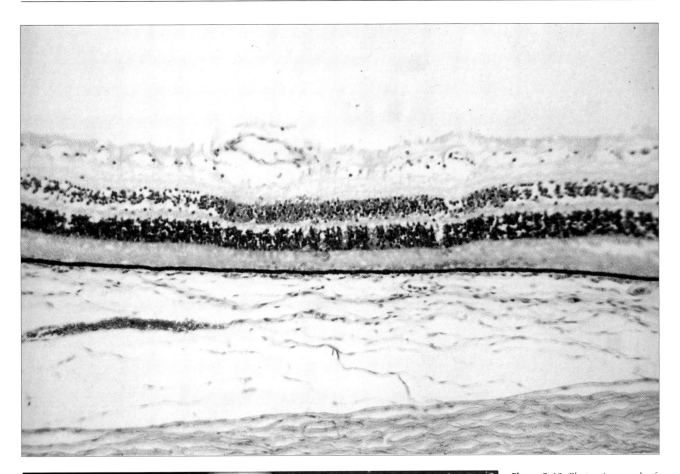

Figure 5-13. Photomicrograph of the retina with hemorrhage from a fatally shaken infant. (H & E X100.)

Figure 5-14. Photograph of a posterior neck dissection demonstrating fracture-dislocation of C1-2 in a shaken infant.

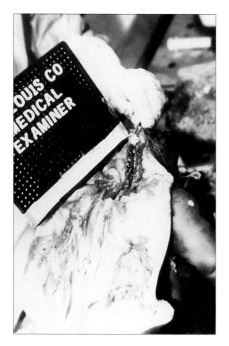

Figure 5-15. *Photograph of a posterior neck dissection in a fatally shaken infant (same child as Figure 5-10) illustrating epidural hemorrhage over the upper cervical cord.*

The act of shaking a child can also result in bruises on the arms or trunk from fingers grasping the child. In addition, there can be avulsion of metaphyseal periosteum in the arms.

♦ Level of Consciousness

Another area in which the child differs from the adult is the rapid development of neurological impairment with severe or fatal head injury. Severely head-injured children very rapidly become unconscious or exhibit a marked decrease in level of consciousness, quickly progressing to unconsciousness. This sequence identifies *when* the injury occurred, since the caretaker should immediately become aware of such a drastic change in the child. It also provides a clue as to *whom* the perpetrator could be, narrowing the focus to those persons present when the injury and change occurred. Of the study of fatally head-injured children shown in Table 5-3, none was conscious on arrival at the hospital and many were already dead.

In children who are shaken to a less than fatal degree, the history frequently includes description of a seizure following the shaking episode. Many children who are neurologically impaired from infancy and were thought to represent prenatal or perinatal hypoxic damage actually suffered repeated shaking to a less than lethal degree but sufficiently to result in loss of extensive axonal connections, leading to permanent brain damage (Benstead, 1983; Frank et al., 1985).

♦ Bibliography

Adams, JH, Graham, DI, and Gennarelli, TA: Contemporary neuropathological considerations regarding brain damage in head injury. In D Becker and JT Povlishock: *Central Nervous System Trauma Status Report*, Prepared for the National Institute of Neurological and Communicative Disorders and Stroke, NIH, Bethesda, 1985, Chapter 4.

Benstead, JG: Shaking as a culpable cause of subdural hemorrhage in infants, *Med Sci Law* 23:242-244, 1983.

Caffey, J: Multiple fractures in the long bones of infants suffering from subdural hematoma, *AJR* 56:163-173, 1946.

Caffey, J: On the theory and practice of shaking infants, *Am J Dis Child* 24:161-169, 1972.

Calder, IM, et al: Primary brain trauma in non-accidental injury, *J Clin Pathol* 37:1095-1100, 1984.

Frank, Y, et al: Neurological manifestations in abused children who have been shaken, *Dev Med Child Neurol* 27:312-316, 1985.

Greenwald, MJ, et al: Traumatic retinoschisis in battered babies, *Ophthalmology* 93:618-625, 1986.

Hadley, MN, et al: The infant whiplash-shake injury syndrome: A clinical and pathological study, *Neurosurgery* 24:536-540, 1989.

Hobbs, CJ: Skull fracture and the diagnosis of abuse, *Am J Dis Child* 59:246-252, 1984.

Kempe, CH, et al: The battered child syndrome, *JAMA* 181:17-24, 1962.

Leestma, JE: Neuropathology of child abuse. In *Forensic Neuropathology*, Raven Press, New York, 1988.

Lindenberg, R, and Freytag, E: Morphology of brain lesions from blunt trauma in early infancy, *Arch Pathol* 87:298-305, 1969.

Merten, DF, and Osborne, DR: Craniocerebral trauma in the child abuse syndrome, *Pediatr Ann* 12:882-887, 1983.

Meservy, CJ, et al: Radiographic characteristics of skull fractures resulting from child abuse, *AJR* 149:173-175, 1987.

Oliver, JE: Microcephaly following baby battering and shaking, *Br Med J* 2:262-264, 1975.

O'Neill, JA, et al: Patterns of injury in the battered child syndrome, *J Trauma* 13:332-339, 1973.

Vowles, D, et al: Diffuse axonal injury in early infancy, *J Clin Pathol* 108:185-189, 1986.

6

Burns and Child Maltreatment

Anthony J. Scalzo, M.D.

When reviewing the literature on the subject of child maltreatment by burning or while providing direct care to a victim of this form of abuse, one is impressed with the notion that "to burn is to brand." Children who are abusively burned are marked or branded with the outward manifestation of parental violence, emotional imbalance, impulsivity, educational and cultural deprivation, and poverty. To intentionally burn a child implies a sustained anger or hostility and appears to be a controlled, premeditated, or even sadistic action (Fowler, 1979).

Others echo these sentiments and suggest that social intervention mechanisms be mobilized to address the multiple problems of the abusively burned child. In terms of severity among the varying forms of abuse, abusive burns should be handled as top priority. The severity of subsequent injuries in burned children suggests that the abusive pattern may be well-ingrained by the time of the burning episode.

The literature attests not only to the physical and emotional trauma but also to the psychological sequelae of abusive burning (Benians, 1988; Bernstein & Cahners, 1979; Green, 1984; Hammond et al., 1989; Leeder, 1979; Libber & Stayton, 1984; McLoughlin & Crawford, 1985; Tarnowski et al., 1989; Weimer et al., 1988). Many victims of house fires die, but victims of scalds often survive with permanent disfigurement, motion disabilities due to contractures, and psychological sequelae. Children who were victims of burns can exhibit aggressive behavior ranging from biting another child to attacking a sibling with an axe. Depression can be manifest by crying without reason, refusal to socialize, or overt attempts at suicide. Withdrawal and other behavioral problems are all aspects of posttreatment adjustment in severely burned children, which was described by a group from the Burn Unit, Cape Town, South Africa, that studied children up to 11 years after the burn event (deWet et al., 1979).

The stigma of the burn does not end when the child is removed from the home of the abusing parent or discharged from the hospital; it may persist for years.

◆ Incidence and Epidemiology

Children 1 to 5 years old comprise the peak age category when burns occur (Demling, 1985). Statistics from the U.S. Consumer Products Safety Commission reveal that 37,000 children under 14 years of age were treated for hot liquid or food and tap water scalds in 1988; nearly half, 16,000 of these children, treated in emergency departments were under 5 years of age. Of the above children, 5,000 were scalded by hot tap water, most often in the bathtub. Although flame injury usually results in a burn involving a larger surface area and therefore is more severe, it is not seen as frequently as scalds. In a study of 520 children treated at a major burn center most burns were of the scald type (47.6%) and occurred in the home (84.6%) (Spear & Munster, 1987) (**Table 6-1**).

Table 6-1. Location and Type of Pediatric Burns	
Baltimore Regional Burn Center	
Place of Accident	
Home	84.6%
Outside	7.6%
Boat/Auto	3.4%
Other	4.0%
Type of Burn	
Scald	47.6%
Flame	29.6%
Grease	6.5%
Flash	5.6%
Contact	5.6%
Electrical	3.9%
Chemical	1.1%

The National Safe Kids Coalition estimates that burns are the third most common form of childhood accidental death in the United States. In *Accident Facts* (National Safety Council, 1979) burns were noted to cause more than 1,300 childhood deaths per year in the United States and ranked behind only motor vehicle and drowning accidents. In 1985 the National Center for Health Statistics (NCHS) revealed that death due to fire and/or burns occurred in 1,461 children ranging in age from birth to 19 years. Other estimates note that 23,638 children were hospitalized and 440,000 were treated for burns, bringing the total cost to society from childhood burn deaths and injuries to approximately $3.5 billion (McLoughlin & McGuire, 1990). Approximately 100,000 children in the United States are hospitalized for the treatment of burn injuries, and several hundred thousand are seen and treated as outpatients (Otherson, 1983). The number of burns not brought to medical attention and those that go unreported as abuse are probably significant.

It is apparent from review of the literature that the victim of abusive burning is usually a young child, 3 to 4 years of age or younger. In one study of 142 inflicted burns (number of patients examined = 892), the average age of the intentionally burned child was 32 months (Hight et al., 1979). The peak age of victims was 13 to 24 months.

Various studies have also linked educationally or culturally deprived maternal background, single or divorced marital status, unemployment, physical abuse of mother (wife battery), and other maternal characteristics, such as isolation, suspiciousness, rigidity, dependence, and immaturity, to increased incidence of abusive burning of children (Ayoub & Pfeifer, 1979; Hight et al., 1979; Joseph & Douglas, 1979; Libber & Stayton, 1984; Rosenberg et al., 1982; Rosenberg & Marino, 1989).

Of all burns, 70% to 90% occur in the home (Feldman, 1980). It is believed that these burns may occur at peak times of stress in the parents' day. In a study of 464 burned children, the risk for burns was highest between 6 p.m. and midnight (Parish et al., 1986). Another study found that the peak hours are in the late afternoon and morning (Feldman, 1980).

Regardless of parental educational deprivation, scald burns occur more often in poorer socioeconomic housing or multi-unit buildings, where units close to the complexes' heating plant receive hotter water than those more distant from the heat source. With poor insulation and inefficient heat sources, the hot water heater's temperature may be increased to satisfy the demands in more distant units, meaning that those units close to the source can receive dangerously hot water. Often these dwellings lack other safety devices, such as smoke detectors, and the families lack the knowledge or resources to install such devices. In the way of prevention, strategies have been presented in such communities to avoid burning episodes (Gallagher, 1982; Haddon, 1980; Katcher et al., 1989; Libber & Stayton, 1984; Maley & Achauer, 1987; McLoughlin & McGuire, 1990; Micik & Miclette, 1985; Murray, 1988; National Safe Kids Campaign, 1990; Webne et al., 1989). Burn prevention issues are discussed later in this chapter.

♦ TYPES OF BURNS AND PHYSICAL CONCEPTS

There are six categories of burn injuries: flame, scald, contact (with hot object), electrical, chemical, and ultraviolet radiation (sun) (McLoughlin & Crawford, 1985). Abusive burns are generally concentrated in the scald and contact categories, although rarer reports of flame (matches, cigarette lighters, or stove), chemical, microwave (actually placing an infant inside a microwave), or even hair dryer-inflicted burns have been reported (Alexander et al., 1987; Ayoub & Pfeifer, 1979; Prescott, 1990; Reece & Grodin, 1985). In reviewing hospital burn admissions, scalds are the most common type of thermal injury seen in children (Feldman et al., 1978). However, if all burn abuse cases are included in the studies, contact burns are more common (Showers & Garrison, 1988; Johnson & Showers, 1985; Keen et al., 1975).

Scald burns result from exposure to a hot liquid. Scalds were the predominant type of burn in both Lenoski and Hunter's (1977) series and Johnson and Showers' (1985) series. Others report that immersion scald burns are more frequently seen than splash, pour, or contact burns.

Scald burns can be superficial, partial, or full thickness; however, the presence of full-thickness, sharply demarcated or symmetrical burns on the buttocks, perineum, genitalia, and distal ends of limbs should alert the professional to the likelihood of child abuse.

Since scalds are the most common cause of burn morbidity, attention must be given to some specific details as to why scalds occur (Caniano et al., 1986). More scald burns occur in the bathroom than in the kitchen (Showers & Garrison, 1988); therefore, hot water temperature in the bathtub, as a physical characteristic, is important. Time of thermal contact and repeated exposure are also important factors in many of these burns. At 49°C (120°F), the lowest setting on most gas water heater thermostats, it takes 5 to 10 minutes to cause full-thickness transepidermal injury to adult skin. However, at 51°C (124°F) it takes 4 minutes. At 52°C (125°F) it takes 2 minutes, and at 54°C (130°F) it takes only 30 seconds to result in a scald. Water at 60°C (140°F), an average temperature for most households, will take 5 seconds to produce a scald burn (Moritz & Henriques, 1947). It is interesting to note that 140°F is generally the recommended intake temperature for many home dishwashers, although some commercial dishwashing detergents will dissolve and sanitize at 130°F. At 70°C (158°F), which is found in some homes, a transepidermal burn will occur in less than 1 second (Robinson & Seward, 1987). Temperature versus time-to-scalding data are given in **Table 6-2 and Figure 6-1**.

It is helpful to remember that children's skin is thinner than adult's skin so serious burning occurs more rapidly and at lower temperatures. Furthermore, hot water exposures of subthreshold time and temperature will result in significant burns if the contact is repeated with little time between exposures. Water at 49°C applied to skin for 3 minutes can be tolerated, but an application of 9 minutes' duration can result in a full-thickness burn (Moritz & Henriques, 1947).

Table 6-2. Temperature Versus Time Burn Chart

Temperature °C	°F	Time to Produce Scald Burn in Adult (less time in children)
49°	120°	5-10 minutes
52°	125°	2 minutes
54°	130°	30 seconds
57°	135°	10 seconds
60°	140°	5 seconds
63°	145°	3 seconds
66°	150°	1-5 seconds
68°	155°	1 second or less
70°	158°	< 1 second

Adapted from Scald Burn Prevention Strategy Manual, Washington, D.C., 1990.

Figure 6-1. *Time versus temperature graph for skin scalding to occur. Adapted from Feldman et al., 1978, based on original work by Moritz & Henriques, 1947.*

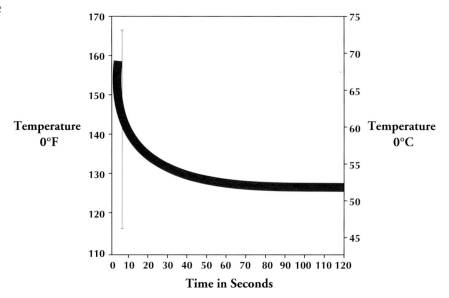

♦Diagnosing the Abusive Burn

The differentiation of inflicted versus accidental injury must begin with definitions. These definitions have both medical and legal implications. The requirement that physicians report abuse, which is law in all 50 states, depends on the physician's ability to recognize abuse and on having a reasonable definition of abuse.

The definition of physical abuse offered here does not exclude reasonable corporal punishment by parents. Physical abuse is: An injury to a child caused by a caretaker, for any reason, including injury resulting from a caretaker's reaction to an unwanted behavior. Injury includes tissue damage beyond erythema or redness from a slap to any area other than the hand or buttocks. Physical discipline should not be used on children who are under 12 months of age. The child should be normal developmentally, emotionally, and physically. Tissue damage includes bruises, burns, tears, punctures, fractures, ruptures of organs and disruption of functions. The use of an instrument on any part of the body is abuse. The injury may be caused by impact, penetration, heat, a caustic, a chemical or a drug (Johnson, 1990).

This definition leaves no confusion defining any physical abuse situation, including burns. An instrument is defined to include devices, gadgets, and implements and mediums of delivery.

All suspicious cases of abuse by burning must be thoroughly investigated. Suspicious burns in a child with prior history of abuse or other physical stigmata of abuse places that child at high risk for lethal abuse.

Incidence of Abusive Burns

The incidence of abusive burns ranges from 4% (Stone et al., 1970) of hospitalized childhood burns to 10% in a more recent study (Showers & Garrison, 1988) or to 28% in specific burn injuries such as tap water scalds (Feldman et al., 1978). During a 12-month period, 84 of 431 burned children (19.5%) were suspected to be abused or neglected (Rosenberg & Marino, 1989). During a 6-year period, 142 of 872 cases of children admitted to a burn center at Children's Hospital of Michigan were found to be nonaccidental (Hight et al., 1979). However, in a study of all pediatric emergency department patients less than 1 year of age, the authors found no incidence of abuse or neglect (Rivara et al., 1988). (It should be noted that most studies reveal the peak age for abusive burning to be over 1 year of age.) Large nationwide studies of overall burns, without specific attention to type, yield 9% to 10% of cases resulting from abuse or neglect.

Comparing it to other forms of abuse, maltreatment by burning has ranked as high as 28% of all types of batterings (Feldman et al., 1978). In a 4-year study at Children's Hospital of Philadelphia, burns accounted for 13% of cases of physical abuse (Ludwig & Fleisher, 1983). More recently, of 256 patients hospitalized for child abuse at a major pediatric center, 56 suffered burns (22%), 53 CNS injuries (22%), 66 failure-to-thrive (26%), and the remainder various other forms of abuse and neglect (Caniano et al., 1986).

Review of the literature over the last 10 to 15 years and clinical experience indicate that the victim of abusive burning is usually 3 to 4 years of age or younger. In Hight's study of 142 of 892 inflicted burns, the average age of the intentionally burned child was 32 months (Hight et al., 1979). The peak age group of victims was 13 to 24 months. Most studies reveal higher rates among male infants and children as compared to adults. One study showed a male:female ratio of 2.5:1 (Libber & Stayton, 1984), while others report a more even distribution (Hight et al., 1979; Showers & Garrison, 1988). The data shown in **Figure 6-2** reveal that although males are more likely to be physically abused (60% compared to 49%), females account for more cases of overall abuse (368,600 compared to 252,500), largely due to the higher incidence of sexual abuse among females.

Percentage of All Abuse

Figure 6-2. Distribution of reported forms of abuse by child's sex. Data from the U.S. Department of Health and Human Services Study of the National Incidence and Prevalence of Child Abuse and Neglect, 1988.

HISTORY AND COMPREHENSIVE EVALUATION

Care for the burn patient's primary medical needs is discussed in books and journals devoted to burn treatment. While these needs are vital, the focus of this book is on identifying abuse and integrating the findings into a plan of action.

Once the patient's medical needs are met, the practitioner directs efforts toward obtaining a careful history outlining the time, nature, extent, and location where the burn occurred. Photographs should be obtained early and a radiologic skeletal survey (humanogram) performed if abuse is suspected, lest the abusive party claim the injuries occurred in the health care facility.

93

Figure 6-3. *Pattern of accidental burn with distribution on anterior trunk. Note that the cooling pattern as water descends results in an "arrow"-shaped configuration.*

The clinician should attempt to determine if the burn is abusive, accidental, or pseudoabusive (due to folk medicine practices) (Asnes & Wisotsky, 1981; Sandler & Haynes, 1978), comparing the history with the physical evidence. First, the patient's developmental skills must be evaluated. Second, the physical aspects of the burn should be analyzed with respect to body anatomic location and compared to the reported cause of the burn. For example, scald burns on the anterior body with a pattern of cooling as it descends (**Figure 6-3**) are consistent with a child pulling a hot liquid from a vessel onto himself. However, a burn located behind the ear, not involving the submental area of the jaw and also avoiding the axilla and back of the shoulder, suggests a liquid thrown from behind (Lung et al., 1977). Scald burns on the buttocks usually occur from forced immersion in hot water, so a history of an accidental fall into the bathtub is suspect. Full-thickness scald burns with a stocking or glove pattern of sharp demarcation on a limb (**Figures 6-4 and 6-5**) or immersion lines with circular or ovoid patterns on the buttocks are not likely to be accidental.

The professional must consider the physical injuries or findings in the context of the history offered. Reliance on a single source for the history or information regarding the injuries can limit the professional's ability to correctly differentiate accidental from suspicious or intentional burns. A cooperative effort between law enforcement, social services, and medical staff is needed. All involved should consider the plausibility of the parents' or guardian's description of how any given injury occurred. This includes scene investigation of serious burns, photographs of the child and the scene of the event, history obtained by several professionals (law enforcement, social workers, nurses, and medical personnel), physical examination, and diagnostic imaging.

Figure 6-4. *Uniform scald of the hand in a 9-month-old girl. This "glove-like" distribution was caused by intentional immersion.*

Figure 6-5. *"Stocking" type burn to the foot. Note the sharp demarcation of the immersion line.*

In suspicious burns, it may be necessary to visit the scene of the burn or analyze photographs taken by police to ascertain if the burn could have occurred in the manner reported. A visit by trained social workers and detectives to the home or scene of the incident can reveal valuable data. This procedure should be requested by medical personnel before final conclusions regarding the etiology of the burn are made. Having the caretaker review the events while walking through the area and demonstrating with a doll the child's position, describing the depth of the water, and so on, helps medical personnel to determine whether the injury was accidental.

An interdisciplinary approach was used in the following case:

CASE HISTORY

A 5-month-old female was admitted through the emergency department. She was in respiratory arrest and required immediate intubation. The mother stated that 2 days before coming to the hospital an adult was pouring hot water near the baby and accidentally spilled it on the child. She treated the burn with cocoa butter. It seemed to be improving. The child's father stated that while he was cleaning the burn with alcohol the baby stopped breathing and had no heart rate. He said that he performed CPR for 2 hours while waiting for the mother to return home so that she could call an ambulance.

PHYSICAL AND LABORATORY FINDINGS

On examination the child was noted to have a deep partial thickness burn of the anterior chest (**Figure 6-6**) with smaller involvement of the chin and forearm. Further examination revealed a distended abdomen, retinal hemorrhages, and a stellate laceration to the vaginal posterior fourchette. Laboratory and radiologic investigation revealed elevated liver transaminases, fracture of the distal femoral metaphysis, fracture of the distal tibial metaphysis (classic "bucket handle" type fracture), and healing fractures of the left sixth through ninth ribs. Computed tomography of the brain revealed a subarachnoid hemorrhage.

EVALUATION

This history is not believable; it is obviously false. Furthermore, such a severe burn in a young infant normally causes a caretaker to seek medical attention immediately. Thinking beyond the emergency at hand and the history given, the emergency staff were able to define a constellation of physical injuries, as well as laboratory and diagnostic imaging findings that could only point to one cause—child abuse.

Figure 6-6. *Deep burn of the anterior chest in a 5-month-old infant who was intubated secondary to respiratory arrest.*

In another case, emergency department staff were given the history that a 23-month-old boy, while riding his tricycle, was caught between a space heater and a wall. The child sustained full thickness (third degree) burns to his buttocks and partial thickness (second-degree) burns to his posterior legs. The family did not seek medical attention for 2 1/2 weeks. After the parents dropped the child off to leave on vacation, he was taken to the emergency department by his grandparents when they noted the injury while bathing him. Analysis of the information gathered at the scene as well as other points of the history led to the conclusion that the burn could not have occurred in the manner reported. The child was unable to ride a tricycle. The temperature of the space heater at the level of the burn would have required 20 minutes to develop a full-thickness burn; only the top of the heater had temperatures hot enough to cause a burn that severe. Using a doll, no position could explain the combination of the buttock and leg burns and their configuration. Investigation revealed that a better source for the burn was the kitchen stove. Measuring the size of the burn and noting its circular configuration, it could be deduced that the circular heating plate of the stove was most likely the source of the buttocks injury. Assuming that the child was intentionally placed on the stove, his calves would align with the hot front door of the stove. This coincided with the tape measurements of the stove and the patient's limb length. In addition, other facts supported abuse as the cause: the child was being toilet trained, the area was typical for disciplinary abuse, there was a long delay before seeking medical assistance, and only a third party, the grandparents, sought help (see Stone's criteria on the following page).

PROTOCOLS AND CRITERIA FOR DETERMINING ABUSE

Many states have comprehensive protocols for determining the likelihood of child abuse. The report of the Task Force for the Study of Non-Accidental Injuries and Child Deaths convened by the Illinois Department of Children and Family

Services, and the Office of the Medical Examiner, Cook County, gives specific details for professionals involved in child health care (Illinois Department of Children and Family Services, 1986). Descriptions should be as detailed and as precise as possible, such as "4x6 cm ovoid-shaped scald of the right posterior buttock with sharp demarcation of edges and uniform burn depth" as opposed to "moderate size burn on the bottom."

Burns themselves are often emotionally as well as physically devastating to the child. Therefore extreme care must be exercised to avoid contributing to the emotional trauma by *incorrectly* accusing a parent of abuse. To effectively develop and use criteria for diagnosing intentional burns, professionals should be familiar with the common manifestations of child abuse and neglect along with those of inflicted burns.

The instruments used to injure children are varied and depend, to some extent, on what is available. A belt, strap, or an adult's hand slapping, grabbing, choking, or pinching accounts for up to 45% of inflicted injuries (Johnson, 1990). When hot objects or water is readily available, the abusive parent chooses these modes.

The full constellation of family psychosocial factors, child's developmental milestones, physical diagnosis, and associated laboratory or radiologic findings may be difficult to collate initially. Several authors have developed guidelines for the clinician, social worker, or nurse to differentiate accidental from abusive or neglectful burns (Ayoub & Pfeifer, 1979; Rosenberg & Marino, 1989; Stone et al., 1970).

When a child presents with a burn and one or more of the following are found to be present, one should consider abuse:

1. Multiple hematomas or scars in various stages of healing
2. Concurrent injuries or evidence of neglect such as malnutrition and failure to thrive (especially suspicious are bone injuries such as old rib fractures and distal tibial, metaphyseal, or spiral fractures)
3. History of multiple prior hospitalizations for "accidental" trauma
4. An inexplicable delay between time of injury and first attempt to obtain medical attention (In some cases, if the parent has medical training, such as an R.N. or M.D., the delay may be because the parents tried to initially care for the burn on their own.)
5. Burns appearing older than alleged day of the accident, similarly indicating ambivalence about seeking care and possibly risking exposure of the abuse
6. An account of the incident not compatible with age and ability of child (An example is that of an infant who "crawled into the hot bathtub" when the infant is only a few months old and developmentally incapable of doing so.)
7. The responsible adults allege that there were no witnesses to the "accident" and the child was merely discovered to be burned, thus hoping to discourage any further inquiry
8. Relatives other than the parents bring the injured child to the hospital or a nonrelated adult brings the child (unless there is good explanation for the parents' absence, such as when a child is being cared for by a baby sitter while the parents are out of town)
9. The burn is attributed to action of a sibling or other child (though this is often a false explanation for abusive burns, it should be noted that siblings can indeed be abusive [Green, 1984])
10. The injured child is excessively withdrawn, submissive, or overly polite, or does not cry during painful procedures

11. There are scalds of the hands or feet, often symmetrical, appearing to be full thickness in depth, suggesting that the extremities were forcibly immersed and held in hot liquid

12. There are isolated burns of the buttocks or perineum and genitalia or the characteristic doughnut-shaped burn of the buttocks, which in children can hardly ever be produced by accidental means

13. The responsible adults give different stories as to the cause of the burn or change their story when questioned

Stone and associates developed this set of criteria after reviewing 26 cases of burn abuse in Chicago (Stone et al., 1970). They noted that males were the victims in 20 of the 26 cases. A large percentage of burns were on the buttocks, perineum, and lower extremities (25 of the 26 cases). Hot liquids were the cause in 15 cases, hot metal surfaces in five, flame in four, and inflicted cigarette burns in one.

Since the palm of the hand and the sole of the foot are thick and relatively resistant to thermal damage, full-thickness burns seen here suggest prolonged immersion and hence inflicted injury (Hight et al., 1979). An exception might be handicapped children, in whom the anesthetic or hypoesthetic areas are thinner skinned and the child may burn unexpectedly and more easily (**Figure 6-7a,b**). However, handicapped children are at increased risk of abuse (Feldman et al., 1981). Sometimes burns or decubitus sores in handicapped children fall into the neglect or pseudoabusive category.

Figure 6-7a,b. *Accidental burn to the legs of an 8 1/2-year-old handicapped child.*

◆ACCIDENTAL BURNS AND CONDITIONS THAT ARE NOT ABUSE

When determining whether an injury is accidental or inflicted, unusual causes of burn injuries should be considered. Unsuspecting parents may expose their children to burn injuries unintentionally.

There were an estimated 656 cases of vaporizer-related injuries in 1979. Two cases of steam vaporizer burns with respiratory involvement have been reported (Colombo et al., 1981). Thermal injury to the lungs from flame or dry hot air is rare; usually the toxic gases from products of pyrolysis (i.e., smoke and other gases) cause inhalation injury. However, inhalation of steam can produce severe pulmonary injury (Moritz et al., 1945) as well as burns to the skin (Colombo et al., 1981).

Another unexpected accidental burn may occur secondary to deck floor tiling such as that used around outdoor pools. These tiles can become very hot after long exposure to the sun (Sheldon & Woodward, 1983).

Inside the home, children have been injured accidentally on hot registers (grating) for floor furnaces (Berger & Kalishman, 1983). In a study conducted on floor register temperatures, a group from New Mexico found that four of the five registers tested exceeded 250°F or 121°C (Berger & Kalishman, 1983). A burn can occur virtually instantaneously at temperatures of this degree. Wall registers may also be sources of accidental burns to children. It may be more likely that hot floor grate registers are sources for accidental rather than inflicted injury. **Tables 6-3 and 6-4** list the estimated sources of burn (U.S. Consumer Product Safety Commission, 1989).

Table 6-3. Heating Units Related to Injury and/or Burns in Children 0 to 4 years of Age (1989)*	
Type of Unit	Estimated Number of Children Treated in U.S. Hospital Emergency Departments
Home radiators	8,925
Fireplaces (all types)	7,174
Kerosene or oil heaters	4,151
Heating systems, not specified	3,948
Coal or wood-burning stoves	2,941
Water heaters	347

Other consumer safety and/or convenience items impact childhood burning. Infant automobile restraint systems are lifesaving and in no way should be discouraged. However, many adults — and health care workers — are not aware how hot the metal parts of the infant car seat can become when left exposed to direct sunlight in hot weather. A 12-week-old infant sustained a 3 cm partial thickness burn to the exposed portion of the anterior thigh from the hot metal turnbuckle adjustment of a car seat (Hankin & Vermeulen, 1980). This case, as well as others cited in the literature of car seat burns (Schmitt et al., 1978; Saitz, 1975), point to the need for advocates for child safety to be aware of unexpected dangers that can cause injuries which may be misdiagnosed as abuse.

The worker must also be aware of unique religious and cultural practices as well as unexpected injuries. Called "pseudoabusive" injuries, burns may be incurred within certain folk medicine customs. For example, in Vietnamese or Cambodian cultures the practice of rubbing a coin or alternatively applying a cup, spoon, or shot glass heated in oil to the skin of an ill child's neck, spine, back, or ribs is termed "coining" ("Cao Gio") or cupping, respectively (Asnes & Wisotsky, 1981; Johnson, 1990; Sandler & Haynes, 1978). These cultures believe that this folk medicine treatment will diminish pain, restore appetite, draw out the fever, and strengthen a weak stomach (Asnes & Wisotsky, 1981). Managing these situations involves education of the families.

Table 6-4. Agents Related to Injury and/or Burns in Children 0 to 4 Years Age (1989)*	
Burn Source	**Estimated Number of Children Treated in U.S. Hospital Emergency Departments†**
Irons	11,745
Hair curlers and curling irons	11,362
Hot water	10,495
Cigarettes, pipes, cigars, or tobacco	6,468
Ranges not specified	5,423
Household products, caustics, drain cleaners, ammonia, oven cleaner	3,155
Gasoline and gasoline cans	2,832
Electrical wiring, outlets, receptacles, and extension cords	2,814
All other ovens	2,690
General home or room fires†	1,592
Light bulbs	1,410
Electric and gas ranges	1,116
Fireworks	1,002
Microwave ovens	817
Cigarette or pipe lighters	713
Hairdryers	368
Matches	209

*Estimates based on U.S. Consumer Products Safety Commission: National Electronic Injury Surveillance System: Product Summary Report—1989, National Injury Information Clearinghouse, Washington, D.C., 1989.

†Does not include deaths at the scene that never arrive at emergency departments.

Common infectious or occasional bullous dermatologic disorders should also be investigated. Most physicians should be familiar with the appearance and associated findings of common impetigo, but sometimes cigarette burns become infected and are difficult to differentiate from circular impetiginous lesions (Raimer et al., 1981). Cigarette burns are usually in clusters and in various stages of healing. Impetiginous lesions usually do not scar, whereas accidental cigarette burns do. Intentional cigarette burns are usually deeper and scar more extensively.

Staphylococcal scalded skin syndrome may be confused with abusive burning, especially since it often involves the inguinal and perigenital area. Scalded skin syndrome is usually generalized rather than localized as in an intentional scald. Also, identifying the staph organism and its response to antibiotics aids in differentiation.

Ischemic, hypoxic-induced injury from various causes can result in the formation of bullae. Although epidermolysis bullosa and related disorders are rare in childhood, they may be present and the clinician should seek dermatologic consultation upon encountering unusual blistering or bullous lesions that lack the other associated features of burns.

Adolescents with preexisting psychiatric illness may present with burns that are self-inflicted, although suicide by this means is rare in Western cultures (Hammond et al., 1988).

♦ABUSIVE BURN PATTERNS

SCALD AND IMMERSION BURNS

Although one study of 131 cases involving abusive forms of burn injury found that contact burns were more common than scald or immersion burns (56% versus 38%) (Showers & Garrison, 1988), the scald is generally considered the most common type of abusive burning (Showers & Garrison, 1988; Johnson & Showers, 1985; Keen et al., 1975). Inflicted scald burns are most frequently caused by hot tap water; a smaller percentage (6%) of the time the liquid is coffee, tea, or cooking grease (Bradshaw et al., 1988; Feldman et al., 1978; Joseph & Douglas, 1979).

Figure 6-8. Two circular burns of skin overlying pubic area in a young toddler. These were caused by inflicted injury from cigarettes.

Immersion burns to the buttocks or genitals are often inflicted by the perpetrator to punish the child for soiling or wetting his or her pants. This occurs in families where the caretakers are rigid in toilet training beliefs. Cigarette burns inflicted in the pubic area as well as blows to the penis with hair brush bristles have also been used to discipline a child during toilet training (**Figure 6-8**).

Depending on the depth of the water, whether in the bath or in the sink, burns may involve the back, buttocks, perineum, and genitalia or may spare these areas and involve "stocking" or "glove-like" burns of the extremities. Children held in a bathtub of shallow water may raise up on their hands and feet or "tripod" themselves in an attempt to protect their buttocks and perineum (Feldman, 1980). This may leave characteristic patterns of full thickness burns to the distal parts of the extremities, especially if the water temperature exceeds 150°F (**Figures 6-9 and 6-10**).

Figure 6-9. Uniform thickness burns to the lower extremities in a 32-month-old girl caused by immersion dipping. This child was burned because she soiled her pants.

Figure 6-10. Posterior aspect of the legs demonstrating a "stocking like" distribution of the burn in the same child as Figure 6-9. Also note the burns to the genital area.

Sometimes the child is held by the head and legs and immersed back first into hot water. A scald as shown in **Figure 6-11** may occur.

Additionally, the child may be forced down against the vessel (tub or sink) and sustain an immersion line burn to the back, part of the buttocks and side, but with a spared area centrally on the buttocks. This so-called doughnut-shaped burn is seen infrequently (**Figures 6-12a,b and 6-13**).

Knowledge of distinctive patterns of burning lead the child protection team to correctly suspect abuse and pursue the correct history for the injury. Phaedrus in 8 A.D. said, "Things are not always what they seem." In the field of child abuse, "things may actually be what they seem," if one questions and obtains the true explanation.

SPLASH BURN INJURIES

Splash burns occur when a hot liquid is thrown or poured onto a victim. The depth of burning is usually less than with the immersion type due to the cooling effect of the liquid as it spreads out or falls secondary to gravity. Splash burns often involve the back, the lateral side of the face, and the posterior shoulder (Lung et al., 1977). The anterior lower side of the face, neck, and shoulder, as well as the front of the chest and trunk, outline a common distribution following an accidental spill from a kettle or saucepan (Coren, 1987; Reece & Grodin, 1985; Rosenberg & Marino, 1989; Yiacoumettes and Roberts, 1977). As the hot liquid drips downward, it often burns in the shape of a "V" ("arrow sign"). This burn pattern occurs when the hot liquid initially contacts the skin and then spreads down the body, cooling as it goes. The edges cool faster than the central tract of hot fluid (**Figure 6-14a,b**). The direction of the "arrow" or combination of "arrow signs" seen with burns in more than one area can aid in making the diagnosis of child abuse. By studying the flow pattern of the hot liquid, clues can be gained that indicate the direction the liquid came from as well as the position of the patient (Feldman, 1980). If the history does not coincide with these physical characteristics, child abuse should be suspected.

Figure 6-11. Uniform thickness scald burn of the entire back on a 2 1/2-year-old girl who was immersed in hot water at 155°F as punishment for soiling her pants.

Figure 6-12a,b. Drawing depicts mechanism by which a child is forcibly held against the bottom of a tub and is burned by hot water in the vessel but has a central area of sparing on the buttocks where skin is in contact with the cooler surface of the vessel.

Figure 6-13. Doughnut-shaped burn of the buttocks in 3 1/2-year-old girl. Note the central area of noninvolved skin. This occurred due to the child being forcibly held against the relatively cooler bottom of a sink while hot water burned the area surrounding the center.

Figure 6-14a,b. Drawing depicting the pattern of burn forming "arrow" signs on the cheek and back. This may occur when hot water is thrown from behind.

The classic arrow sign may not be present, however, with hot grease spills. Grease becomes hotter than water and sticks to the skin rather than running off the surface (Othersen, 1983). It may cause a full-thickness burn to a subcutaneous depth of 0.04 inches (Coren, 1987). The arrow sign may also be absent in forced exposure to running hot water from a faucet. The continuous flow of hot water from the faucet serves as a constant source of heat energy, referred to as an "energy sink." This may cause uniform full-thickness burns without a cooling pattern, as described above. If the child is developmentally old enough to turn on the hot water faucet, he may accidentally sustain such a burn on the anterior surface of his lower trunk and legs. Therefore, when given that history, one must analyze the patterns of the burn, the child's developmental skills, and the presence of other associated findings in order to differentiate abusive from accidental causes of injury.

FLEXION BURNS

Another pattern of abusive burning seen in either of the two types discussed above (immersion or splash) is the flexion burn. In one study this was seen in 5 of 43 burn patients from a series of 712 child abuse cases (Lenoski & Hunter, 1977). This type of burn pattern may occur when a hot liquid is intentionally poured onto the body or the victim is immersed in a hot liquid with the hips or other body parts maximally flexed. The skin within the flexed body area, such as the inguinal crease or popliteal fossa behind the knee, is spared from contact with the burning agent (**Figure 6-15**).

Figure 6-15. Scald burn of 1-year-old child showing spared skin in the inguinal area due to flexion at the hip when the burn occurred.

This may occur in one area or in several areas parallel to each other, yielding alternating areas of burn and spared skin or a "zebra" pattern. Partial contact with grills or repeated application of curling irons to the skin on an area of the body may also give an alternating "zebra" pattern. Additionally, hot water scalds to limbs partially protected by clothes such as socks may yield alternating patterns of burned and spared skin (**Figure 6-16**). These, however, have patterns distinct from scald immersion lines.

CONTACT BURNS

Contact burns comprise a unique group of pattern burns. The health care worker may need to assume the role of a detective in order to accurately diagnose the

Figure 6-16. Hot water scald to the posterior legs of a child who was wearing socks. Note the ribbed pattern from the sock "branded" on the skin.

cause of these inflicted burns. In our experience, curling irons (**Figure 6-17**), steam irons (**Figure 6-18**), cigarettes (**Figure 6-19**) and cigarette lighters, and space heater grills (**Figure 6-20**) are a few of the implements used in abusive burning. Hot plates, light bulbs, and knives also have been used (Feldman, 1980; Green, 1984; Johnson, 1990; Lenoski & Hunter, 1977; Stone et al., 1970).

Figure 6-17. Curling iron burn on the back of the neck of a 3-year-old girl.

Figure 6-18 Inflicted steam iron burn on the lateral surface of the left arm iof a 2-year-old child. Note the sharply demarcated edges and the pattern of steam vent holes "branded" onto the skin. The father claimed that the burn was accidental, but he admitted to spanking the child for "messing her pants."

Figure 6-19 Cigarette burn to the posterolateral arm of a child. This area is unlikely to have been injured accidentally.

Figure 6-20. *Linear pattern of burns caused by a space heater grill intentionally placed on the child's abdomen.*

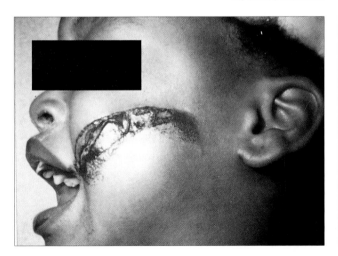

Figure 6-21. *Burn on the left lateral cheek of a child who pulled a hot clothes iron down onto her face by pulling on the cord. Note the irregular shape of the lower half of the burn which is consistent with a hot object contacting the patient's face but then causing a glancing type of injury as it falls.*

Figure 6-22. *Same child as in Figure 6-21. The hot iron fell downward and caused a burn to the anterolateral chest.*

The shape of the object is branded on the child's skin. Tissue destruction, mediated by conduction of heat, in the case of inflicted burns is often uniform in all directions. The shape or pattern of the object or the end of the object is faithfully reproduced in the burn pattern. Such objects can also cause accidental burns, but the patterns are generally nonuniform and appear to be a glancing (brushing against) type of injury. The child in **Figures 6-21 and 6-22** sustained a glancing type injury with a nonuniform burning pattern when she pulled on the cord of an iron, causing it to accidentally fall onto the skin. Here the child

Figure 6-23. *Old clothes iron burn scar of the left buttock with depigmentation. Also note the whip and lash marks on the posterior legs.*

Figure 6-24. *Burn to the palm of the hand in a toddler who reached up to a hot oven door.*

Figure 6-25. *Third-degree burn of the buttocks in an 18-month-old boy who was intentionally set on a hot wood-burning stove as punishment for wetting the bed.*

sustained a partial and irregular burn to the face and then, as the iron continued its fall, to the anterior axilla and chest area. A careful history and analysis of the burn as well as recognition of accidental patterns of burning is essential in a case such as this. This must be compared to the clearly demarcated and inflicted burn pattern seen in Figure 6-18. Additionally, one should be aware of what well-healed iron burns look like years later. **Figure 6-23** shows a well-healed, depigmented iron-shaped burn scar on the left buttock of a child being evaluated for additional signs of abuse, such as old loop and lash marks.

The developmental skill of the child must be considered when evaluating contact burn injuries. Johnson (1990) described the case of a 7-month-old infant with a knife-shaped full-thickness burn to the sole of the foot. The parents said the child accidentally stepped on the hot object. The unlikely occurrence of a hot knife lying on the floor is made even more incredulous by the claim that the 7-month-old stepped on it when the infant could not even stand without support, let alone walk on his own. Similarly, in reference to scald burns, the ability to turn a circular faucet for hot water is achieved beyond infancy and early toddler age; it is unlikely that an accidental burn could be caused this way unless the child is approximately 18 to 24 months old.

Wood-burning stoves are another cause of contact burns, one that is quite prevalent in some areas; it is estimated that 13 million wood stoves are used in the United States (Yanofsky & Morain, 1984). The location of the burn on the body aids in the evaluation of suspected abuse versus accidental injury. The functional position of the hand at the time of the burn yields a recognizable burn pattern (**Figure 6-24**). However, **Figure 6-25** shows a boy who is obviously a victim of abuse with severe burns to the buttocks from a woodstove.

Oppressive toilet training practices account for many abusive burns; for example, an 18-month-old was forced to sit on a hot wood burning stove for having wet the bed. Occasionally, open flames are used to inflict punishment on a child, as shown in **Figure 6-26**. In some older homes, floor heaters made in the 1950s stand approximately 3 feet high with a grid or grill on the top surface. One was involved in the case of an 18-month-old girl with a serious burn (**Figure 6-27**). The history given by her caretaker was that she climbed up and accidentally sat on the heater. This history is not consistent with the burn pattern nor the physics of how the human body sits. The "sitting" part of the buttocks near the inferior gluteal creases and posterior thighs is not burned at all, and there are no burns to the child's hands or knees, as would be expected during climbing. However, the upper buttocks, posterior iliac crest, and sacral areas are "branded" with the grid pattern of the heater's top cover, indicating the child was forcibly held against the hot surface.

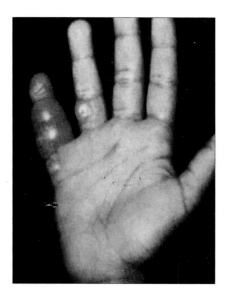

Figure 6-26. *Bullous blister formation on the fourth and fifth fingers of a 2-year-old child whose hand was held over an open flame as punishment.*

Sometimes burns are isolated events, but not infrequently a child will present with multiple old stigmata indicative of child abuse. In addition to the obvious scars, the child may suffer from psychological, emotional, and sexual abuse, as shown in the following case (**Figures 6-28 through 6-30**).

Case History

A 3 1/2-year-old girl was referred to the sexual abuse management clinic after child protection workers in conjunction with a child psychologist discovered evidence of possible sexual abuse. While in day care, she was sexually acting out with the other children and the staff and was constantly masturbating. The child was severely developmentally delayed. With counseling, the child disclosed sexual abuse.

On examination she was noted to have a constellation of old scars from a variety of agents. The child's grandmother stated that the mother had severely disciplined the child and used a graded system of increasingly severe punishment to match the desired level of discipline. First, she used a cigarette to inflict burns or bit the child; next she would burn her repeatedly with a curling iron; and finally she inflicted scalding hot water immersion burns.

♦ PREVENTION

Several authors have presented strategies for injury prevention in the community and in the home (Gallagher, 1982; Haddon, 1980; Katcher et al., 1989; Libber & Stayton, 1984; Maley & Achauer, 1987; McLoughlin & McGuire, 1990; Micik & Miclette, 1985; Murray, 1988; National Safe Kids Campaign, 1990; Webne et al., 1989). Accident prevention theorists conceptualize injury as a disease that is predictable rather than a random event (Haddon, 1980). In 1972 Haddon first described the 10 classic intervention strategies for systematic analysis of injuries; these included the "reduction in the amount of a given hazard brought into being" (Micik & Miclette, 1985). When considering an object as a hazard, one must take into account the triple axis of the injury phenomenon: the host (victim), the vehicle (vector), and the environment. Placing these main points into the context of abusive burns, one would expect fewer bathtub scald burns if there was a maximum water heater temperature of 125°F built into all manufactured units. Antiscald devices are available, which, if installed at the faucet or shower head, will instantly shut off the flow of water if the temperature exceeds a preset value (McLoughlin & McGuire, 1990). Some authors suggest using liquid crystal thermometers to check bathtub water temperature in order to prevent scalds (Katcher et al., 1989). Others who distributed educational pamphlets and liquid crystal thermometers to 12 families found no statistically significant reduction in hot water temperature as a result of the intervention (Webne et al., 1989). This led to the notion that the best preventive measure may be to have hot water heaters installed with preset safe temperatures.

Figure 6-27. *Inflicted pattern burn to the buttocks and sacral area of an 18-month-old girl who was forcibly held against the grid cover of a floor heater.*

Unfortunately, the human host or child victim cannot be modified physically to resist injury, unlike head injury prevention whereby some host modification occurs by using a bicycle helmet. It is also doubtful that we can change the environment for some burns, as people still cook food and boil water in the kitchen and are unlikely to install barriers around such areas to protect small children. However, parents can be educated to unexpected dangers, such as burns from liquids heated in microwave ovens (Puczynski et al., 1983), where skin scalds (James, 1989) and palatal burns (Hibbard & Blevins, 1988) have occurred. Interestingly, water heated in microwaves may not cool off to a safe temperature until some 10 minutes after water that is heated conventionally (James, 1989).

More importantly, we may and should continue to try to change the vector of the trauma, namely the abusive parent. Obviously, this can be an extremely difficult and complex task. Even though studies show a relationship between socioeconomic status and the incidence of burn injuries (Graitcer & Sneizek, 1988; Slater et al., 1987), research is needed in effective ways of rehabilitating the abusive parent. Our system of adjudication may successfully remove children from the home of an abusive parent, but this is certainly not ideal. The child then not only struggles with his or her physical imperfections as a result of the burning process but may also suffer further emotional turmoil due to parental separation.

Figure 6-28. Old cigarette burn to the chin of a 3 1/2 year-old girl who is also shown in Figures 6-29 and 6-30.

Figure 6-29. Multiple linear curling iron burns on the lower posterior leg (more likely non-accidental) of a 3 1/2-year-old girl.

Figure 6-30. Human bite mark on the thigh just above the knee in the child shown in Figure 6-29.

One suggestion is to offer parents anticipating having children a course on child development at a level they can understand. Reporting on their results with a group of well-child classes, some authors found that 76% of the subjects in the experimental group (those whose child care instruction included home fire and burn safety) set their hot water heaters at a safe level, compared to only 23% of those in the control group (Thomas et al., 1984). Such classes might also include counseling regarding child temperament characteristics.

Parents should be discouraged from using infant walkers because children have been able to approach hot objects such as oven doors; reach and pull on cords to pots, fryers, and irons; and pull on tablecloths, thereby sustaining serious burns

(Johnson et al., 1990). Infant walkers have also been related to numerous falls down staircases when parents fail to secure doors or open stairwells.

In cases of accidental trauma, a child's temperament may determine what he does (the "how" of behavior), his motivation (the "why" of behavior), and his competencies or physical abilities (the "what" of behavior) (Zuckerman & Duby, 1985). However, the child's rhythmicity, or lack thereof, with regard to sleep, hunger, or elimination functions as well as the quality of his or her mood (i.e., crying or displeasing behavior) may play even greater roles in abuse or nonaccidental injuries.

It has been suggested that high risk populations should be targeted for abuse prevention strategies (Webne et al., 1989). These strategies include education and counseling of parents to achieve realistic expectations for themselves and their children, income supplementation, employment counseling, and provision of day care services (Reece & Grodin, 1985).

Secondary prevention is also important. High-risk parental signals such as teenage pregnancy, unwanted pregnancy, or substance abuse as well as infant prematurity and childhood developmental disorders should be noted (Johnson, 1990). Furthermore, early intervention may be indicated if one notes undue concern over an unborn baby's sex, a mother's denial of pregnancy or severe depression, lack of eye contact or holding of a baby, parental complaints that diapers are messy and repulsive to clean, and numerous emergency department visits. With regard to the latter, an important caveat in emergency medicine is to always be aware of a "hidden agenda." The parent may present repeatedly to the emergency room with seemingly trivial complaints because she may be asking for help in the only way she knows how. Pediatricians, family practitioners, obstetricians, nurses, and social workers who come into contact with parents and children should be cognizant of these high-risk signals. When possible, they should intervene with counseling, education, and/or referrals to child protection agencies.

One must appreciate the value of *anticipating* injury. Prevention should be the goal toward which our ultimate achievement should aim. When we expect injurious acts or prevent further abuse to a child, we complete the triad of *Anticipation, Recognition,* and *Treatment* and thereby realize the true *ART* of medicine.

♦ BIBLIOGRAPHY

Alexander, RC, Surrell, JA, and Cohle, SD: Microwave oven burns to children, an unusual manifestation of child abuse, *Pediatrics* 79:255-260, 1987.

Asnes, RS, and Wisotsky, DH: Cupping lesions simulating child abuse, *J Pediatr* 99:267, 1981.

Ayoub, C, and Pfeifer, D: Burns as a manifestation of child abuse and neglect, *Am J Dis Child* 133:910, 1979.

Benians, RC: The influence of parental visiting on survival and recovery of extensively burned children, *Burns Incl Therm Inj* 14:31-34, 1988.

Berger, LR, and Kalishman, S: Floor furnace burns to children, *Pediatrics* 71:97-99, 1983.

Bernstein, N, and Cahners, SS: Rehabilitating families of burned children, *Scand J Reconstruct Surg* 13:173-175, 1979.

Bradshaw, C, Hawkins, J, Leach, M, et al: A study of childhood scalds, *Burns Incl Therm Inj* 14:21-24, 1988.

Caniano, DA, Beaver, BL, and Boles, ET: Child abuse: An update on surgical management in 256 cases, *Ann Surg* 203:219-224, 1986.

Colombo, JL, Hopkins, RL, and Waring, WW: Steam vaporizer injuries, *Pediatrics* 67:661-663, 1981.

Coren, CV: Burn injuries in children, *Pediatr Ann* 16:328-339, 1987.

Demling, RH: Burns, *N Engl J Med* 313:1389, 1985.

deWet, B, Cywes, S, Davies, MRQ, et al: Some aspects of post-treatment adjustments in severely burned children, *Burns Incl Therm Inj* 5:321-325, 1979.

Feldman, KW: Child abuse by burning. In CH Kempe and RE Helfer: *The Battered Child*, University of Chicago Press, Chicago, 1980.

Feldman, KW, Clarren, SK, and McLaughlin, JF: Tap water burns in handicapped children, *Pediatrics* 67:560-562, 1981.

Feldman, KW, Schaller, RT, Feldman, JA, et al: Tap water scald burns in children, *Pediatrics* 62:1-7, 1978.

Fowler, J: Child maltreatment by burning, *Burns Incl Therm Inj* 5:83-86, 1979.

Gallagher, SS: A strategy for the reduction of childhood injuries in Massachusetts: SCIPP, *N Engl J Med* 307:1015, 1982.

Graitcer, PL, and Sneizek, JE: Hospitalizations due to tap water scalds, 1978-1985, *MMWR* 37:35, 1988.

Green, AH: Child abuse by siblings, *Child Abuse Negl* 8:311-317, 1984.

Haddon, W, Jr: Advances in the epidemiology of injuries on a basis for public policy, *Public Health Rep* 95:411-421, 1980.

Hammond, J, Nebel-Gould, A, and Brooks, J: The value of speech-language assessment in the diagnosis of child abuse, *J Trauma* 29:1258-1260, 1989.

Hammond, JS, Ward, CG, and Pereira, E: Self-inflicted burns, *J Burn Care Rehabil* 9:178-179, 1988.

Hankin, F, and Vermeulen, F: Infant automobile restraint systems: Beware of the sun, *Pediatrics* 65:625-626, 1980.

Hibbard, RA, and Blevins, R: Palatal burn due to bottle warming in a microwave oven, *Pediatrics* 82:382-384, 1988.

Hight, DW, Bakalar, HR, and Lloyd, JR: Inflicted burns in children, *JAMA* 242:517-520, 1979.

Illinois Department of Children and Family Services, and The Office of the Medical Examiner, Cook County: Protocol for determining if an injury is a result of child abuse or neglect, The Task Force for the Study of Non-Accidental Injuries and Child Deaths, State of Illinois, 1986.

James, MI: Burns from fluid heated in a microwave oven (letter), *Br Med J* 298:1452, 1989.

Johnson, CF: Inflicted injury versus accidental injury, *Pediatr Clin North Am* 37:791-814, 1990.

Johnson, CF, Ericson, AK, and Caniano, D: Walker-related burns in infants and toddlers, *Pediatr Emerg Care* 6:58-61, 1990.

Johnson, CF, and Showers, J: Injury variables in child abuse, *Child Abuse Negl* 9:207-215, 1985.

Joseph, TP, and Douglas, BS: Childhood burns in South Australia: A socio-economic and aetiological study, *Burns Incl Therm Inj* 5:335-342, 1979.

Katcher, ML, Landry, GL, and Shapiro, MM: Liquid crystal thermometer use in pediatric office counseling about tap water burn prevention, *Pediatrics* 83:766-771, 1989.

Keen, JH, Lendrum, J, and Wolman, B: Inflicted burns and scalds in children, *Br Med J* 4:268, 1975.

Leeder, CJ: Families of burn victims receive help through regular group meetings, *Burns* 5:89-91, 1979.

Lenoski, EF, and Hunter, KA: Specific patterns of inflicted burn injuries, *J Trauma* 17:842, 1977.

Libber, SM, and Stayton, DJ: Childhood burns reconsidered: The child, the family, and the burn injury, *J Trauma* 24:245-252, 1984.

Ludwig, S, and Fleisher, G, eds: *Textbook of Pediatric Emergency Medicine*, The Williams & Wilkins Co, Baltimore, 1983.

Lung, RF, Miller, SH, Davis, TS, et al: Recognizing burn injuries as abuse, *Am Fam Physician* 15:134-135, 1977.

Maley, MP, and Achauer, BM: Prevention of tap water scald burns, *J Burn Care Rehabil* 8:62-65, 1987.

McLoughlin, E, and Crawford, JD: Burns, *Pediatr Clin North Am* 321:61-75, 1985.

McLoughlin, E, and McGuire, A: The causes, cost, and prevention of childhood burn injuries, *Am J Dis Child* 144:677-683, 1990.

Micik, S, and Miclette, M: Injury prevention in the community: A systems approach, *Pediatr Clin North Am* 32:251-265, 1985.

Moritz, AR, and Henriques, FC: Study of thermal injury: The relative importance of time and surface temperature in the causation of cutaneous burns, *Am J Pathol* 23:695-720, 1947.

Moritz, AR, Henriques, FC , and McLean, R: The effects of inhaled heat on the air passage and lungs, *Am J Pathol* 21:311, 1945.

Murray, JP: A study of the prevention of hot tapwater burns, *Burns Incl Therm Inj* 14:185-193, 1988.

National Safe Kids Campaign, Children's Hospital National Medical Center, Washington, DC, 1990.

National Safety Council: *Accident Facts,* Washington, DC, 1979.

Otherson, HB: Burns and scalds, *Pediatr Ann* 12:753, 1983.

Parish, RA, Novack, AH, Heimbach, DM, et al: Pediatric patients in a regional burn center, *Pediatr Emerg Care* 2:165-167, 1986.

Prescott, PR: Hair dryer burns in children, *Pediatrics* 86:692-697, 1990.

Puczynski, M, Rademaker, D, and Gatson, RL: Burn injury related to the improper uses of a microwave oven, *Pediatrics* 72:714-715, 1983.

Raimer, BG, Raimer, SS, and Hebeler, JR: Cutaneous signs of child abuse, *J Am Acad Dermatol* 5:203-214, 1981.

Reece, RM, and Grodin, MA: Recognition of non-accidental injury, *Pediatr Clin North Am* 32:41-60, 1985.

Rivara, FP, Kamitsuka, MD, and Quan, L: Injuries to children younger than one year of age, *Pediatrics* 81:93-97, 1988.

Robinson, MD, and Seward, PN: Thermal injury in children, *Pediatr Emerg Care* 3:266-270, 1987.

Rosenberg, NM, and Marino, D: Frequency of suspected abuse/neglect in burn patients, *Pediatr Emerg Care* 5:219-221, 1989.

Rosenberg, NM, Meyers, S, and Shackleton, N: Prediction of child abuse in an ambulatory setting, *Pediatrics* 70:879, 1982.

Saitz, EW: Seat belt buckle burns, *Am J Dis Child* 129:1456, 1975.

Sandler, AP, and Haynes, V: Non-accidental trauma and medical folk belief: A case of cupping, *Pediatrics* 61:921-922, 1978.

Schmitt, BD, Gray, JD, and Britton, HL: Car seat burns in infants: Avoiding confusion with inflicted burns, *Pediatrics* 62:607-609, 1978.

Sheldon, SH, and Woodward, C: Burn injuries secondary to hot floor tiling (letter), *Clin Pediatr* 22:658, 1983.

Showers, J, and Garrison, KM: Burn abuse: A four-year study, *J Trauma* 28:1581-1583, 1988.

Slater, SJ, Slater, H, and Goldfarb, JW: Burned children: A socioeconomic profile for focused prevention programs, *J Burn Care Rehabil* 8:566, 1987.

Spear, RM, and Munster, AM: Burns, inhalation injury and electrical injury. In MC Rogers, ed: *Textbook of Pediatric Intensive Care Medicine*, The Williams & Wilkins Co, Philadelphia, 1987.

Stone, NH, Rinaldo, L, Humphrey, CR, et al: Child abuse by burning, *Surg Clin North Am* 50:1419-1424, 1970.

Tarnowski, KJ, Rasnake, LK, Linsheid, TR, et al: Behavioral adjustment of pediatric burn victims, *J Pediatr Psychol* 14:607-615, 1989.

Thomas, KA, Hassanein, RS, and Christophersen, ER: Evaluation of group well-child care for improving burn prevention practices in the home, *Pediatrics* 74:879-882, 1984.

US Consumer Product Safety Commission. National electronic injury surveillance system: Product summary report, 1989, National Injury Information Clearinghouse, Washington, DC.

Webne, S, Kaplan, BJ, and Shaw, M: Pediatric burn prevention: An evaluation of the efficacy of a strategy to reduce tap water temperature in a population at risk for scalds, *J Dev Behav Pediatr* 10:187-191, 1989.

Weimer, CL, Goldfarb, W, and Slater, H: Multidisciplinary approach to working with burn victims of child abuse, *J Burn Care Rehabil* 9:79-82, 1988.

Yanofsky, NN, and Morain, WD: Upper extremity burns from wood stoves, *Pediatrics* 73:722-726, 1984.

Yiacoumettes, A, and Roberts, M: An analysis of burns in children, *Burns Incl Therm Inj* 3:195-201, 1977.

Zuckerman, BS, and Duby, JC: Developmental approach to injury prevention, *Pediatr Clin North Am* 32:17-29, 1985.

SEXUAL ABUSE: AN OVERVIEW

JAMES A. MONTELEONE, M.D.
SHEILAH GLAZE, M.S.W., L.C.S.W.
KAREN M. BLY, R.N., M.ED.

A 1-month-old boy was admitted to the nursery. The child had been seen by his private pediatrician because of respiratory distress. A routine chest film revealed the child had marble bone disease. The child's mother was 14 years old.

Shortly after admission, the hospital social service department received an anonymous phone call stating that the infant was the result of an incestuous relationship. Since marble bone disease is a rare autosomal recessive disorder, consanguinity was definitely a possibility. The mother was interviewed and she denied the possibility. The Division of Family Services was notified and it stated the family had previously been anonymously reported and the allegation was unsubstantiated.

The infant was scheduled for a bone marrow transplant and, when selecting possible donors, the infant's "grandfather" was a perfect match. The odds of a grandfather being a perfect match are very slim unless he is also the father. With that information, the child's mother was removed from the home. While out of the home, with counseling, she acknowledged that she had been sexually abused by her father and the father subsequently admitted that he had abused her.

This chapter is the first of three dealing with the management of cases involving sexual abuse. These chapters present an overview *(Chapter 7)*, the physical examination procedure *(Chapter 8)*, and the specifics of interviewing these children *(Chapter 9)*. It is the purpose of this chapter to identify and define the components of sexual abuse and to propose a working philosophy for dealing with these cases.

♦ DEFINITION OF SEXUAL ABUSE

Sexual abuse occurs between a child and an adult or older child and is defined as sexual contact or interaction for sexual stimulation and gratification of the adult or older child, who is a parent or caretaker and responsible for the child's care. Sexual abuse is a form of child abuse and must be reported to state child protective services. If the perpetrator is not a caretaker, the sexual activity is sexual assault and may not fall into the category of behaviors reportable to state protective services, but must be reported to a local law enforcement sex crimes unit. The sex crimes unit deals with perpetrators of sex crimes who have no role in the child's care, but are usually known to the victim or the victim's family. The sex offender often pursues this practice as a career and will abuse many children over the course of time.

The long-term effects of sexual abuse are not clearly known (Brassard, 1983). Some children appear to suffer lasting psychological problems, while others are able to cope effectively. Intrafamilial abuse may be passed from one generation to another (American Humane Society, 1981).

ABUSIVE OR ASSAULTIVE ACTS

Sexual abusive or assaultive acts include sexual intercourse, sodomy or anal penetration, oral genital contact, fondling, masturbation, digital penetration or manipulation, and exposure. The acts can be reciprocal or one-sided. Of the acts listed, exposure can be the most difficult to define. Some families are comfortable with nudity in the home; they share bathrooms, share bedrooms, or live in small quarters where privacy is at a premium. Exposure becomes sexual abuse when the person exposing is sexually aroused by the event and does it specifically for that purpose.

CLASSIFICATION OF SEXUAL ABUSE

The acts of sexual abuse can be divided into three categories: assault, incest, and exploitation. Assault and incest are somewhat self-explanatory; exploitation includes prostitution and pornography.

ASSAULT

The perpetrator of a sexual assault is usually male. Sexual assault is usually a one-time event in which the perpetrator forces himself on the child. If the child is examined within a short time of the assault, there is generally physical evidence of trauma, such as tears, blood, and bruises, which constitute dramatic, acute findings of abuse. When dealing with an assault case the child is at greatest risk because the molester is often emotionally unstable. One must make certain the child is protected and does not return to the situation in which the assault took place; the perpetrator must not have access to the child.

INCEST

Incest is defined as sexual intercourse between persons so closely related that they are forbidden by law to marry. Incestuous abuse usually occurs over a long period of time and often involves a conditioning process. The perpetrator is usually male, although female perpetrators are possible and probably underreported. The abuser may not necessarily be related to the child; he may be a stepfather or paramour, but generally is the father figure or provider in the home. Although the classical incestuous relationship involves father and daughter, other common liaisons form between older brother and younger sister, uncle and niece or nephew, and grandfather and granddaughter or grandson.

Classically, there is no evidence of trauma or acute injury. The physical findings are subtle or nonexistent, unless there has been complete penile penetration over a long period. The child usually does not make a disclosure until the abuse has gone on for a number of years, beginning when the child was an infant and continuing with her becoming conditioned and manipulated over many years to accept this as a way of life. Several children in the home may be involved in the abuse.

There is disagreement among authorities, in the classical incestuous situation, whether the child and the perpetrator should be separated during therapy or during the investigation. Some therapists advocate separation. Others believe that as long as the perpetrator admits to the abuse, it is acceptable to allow the abuser to remain in the home and keep the family intact. If possible, the child should remain in the home to avoid being blamed or blaming herself for the disintegration of the family. She may perceive being removed as punishment. The victim must also receive counseling. She often faces alienation, denial, and hostility from mother, father, and siblings. As a result, she may deny that the abuse took place and retract her disclosure.

If the perpetrator does not admit to the abuse, he should be removed from the home so that he cannot manipulate the child further and convince her to retract her disclosure and thus allow the abuse to continue. If the other parent does not accept that the child has been abused, the child should be taken out of the home again so that she will not be influenced to change her mind and deny the truth.

EXPLOITATION
Sexual exploitation, involving prostitution and pornography, is unique in that it often involves a group of participants. It can occur within a family or outside of the home, involving several adults and nonrelated children; then it is referred to as a sex ring. In cases involving families, the whole family—mother, father, and children—can be involved, and the children must be protected and removed from the home situation. This is a pathologic situation in which both parents are often sexually involved with the children and are using the children for prostitution or for pornography. **Exploited children need the greatest intervention and psychiatric help.**

RISK FACTORS
In a review of the data from the 1987 National Survey of Children (Moore et al., 1989), social settings were identified that increased the risk of sexual abuse. Those social conditions are listed in **Table 7-1.** The incidence of abuse was 6% of girls with no risk factor, 9% of girls with one risk factor, 26% of girls with two risk factors, and 68% of girls with three or more risk factors.

♦ SEXUAL ABUSE VICTIMS
Three-fourths of the crimes against children are sex crimes. The American Humane Association estimates that about 4,000 cases of sexual abuse occur annually in each city in the United States. The usual cases of child sexual abuse involve young female children and male caretakers, older male relatives, or other older males with whom they are acquainted. The age difference between the abuser and the victim is 5 years or more. Sex play between age-mates, unless there is coercion, is usually normal. In older studies, females were reported as victims 10 times more often than males (DeVine, 1980). The offenders are male 97% of the time; 50% to 80% are known by the victims. Parents and other relatives are the offenders in 30% to 50% of the cases.

DeFrancis (1969) noted that the average age of female victims, under the age of 16, was 11. The American Humane Association (1981) reported that 72% of incest victims were 13 years or older. In my experience, in over 5,000 victims under 18, the average age was around 5. This may reflect a greater awareness of child sexual abuse in the 1980s, cultural issues, or other, as yet undefined, trends.

Table 7-1. Social Conditions Increasing Risk of Sexual Abuse

Social condition

Lived apart from both biological parents
Raised in poverty
Child handicapped
Alcoholic family member
Drug-abusing family member
Prostitution at home
Transient adults living at home
Mentally ill caretaker
AIDS-related disability of caretaker

Victims of child sexual abuse come from all races, creeds, and socioeconomic levels. Boys are more commonly victimized by someone outside the home, whereas girls are often abused by someone within the home. The children are often threatened with punishment if they do not cooperate. They are told that the activity is a game or something special and fun, but that it must be kept secret.

MALE VICTIMS

A study of 100 patients at the Mayo Clinic (Greenwood et al., 1990) revealed that one in six of the females interviewed admitted to being a victim of sexual abuse; none of the males in a comparable population admitted to abuse. It is possible that a young boy who has a sexual relationship with an adult female may consider it manly and acceptable. If that relationship is with an adult male, the stigmata of homosexuality may arise, so he may not want anyone to know about it or to misinterpret his role in the encounter. Therefore the true incidence of sexual abuse of males is difficult to estimate; many experts feel that it is at least as frequent as the incidence in females, if not higher. Reports suggest that males are 10 times less apt to be abused as females. It is hoped that the true incidence of this problem will be revealed with time.

CHILD VULNERABILITIES

Children have characteristics that make them ideal victims. They are endowed with natural curiosity, even about sex, a taboo subject with which they generally have no experience. A clever child molester can exploit this trait to lower the child's inhibitions and seduce the child into sexual activity. Parents instruct their children to respect and obey adults, so children are easily led by adults. Also, the adult is bigger, stronger, and wiser in the child's eyes. The adult uses these suppositions to influence and control the child's behavior. Most importantly, children crave attention, affection, and approval. Children from broken homes and victims of emotional abuse and neglect are at greatest risk of victimization, trading sex for the missing affection and attention in their lives.

Adolescents can also be exploited by the child molester. An adolescent boy who has been victimized because he rebelliously defies guidelines set by his parents is very unlikely to admit erring.

RESPONSES TO BEING ABUSED

Children who have been sexually abused often act seductively toward adults or act out sexually. A child molester may say that the child seduced him (see later discussion of perpetrators). For this reason, when social services place a sexually abused child in a foster home, the home should be selected with great care and the foster parents must be alerted to the fact that the child has been sexually abused and may behave seductively and act out sexually with others in the home, whether adults or children. The family should be instructed how to deal with the child when he or she demonstrates these behaviors.

♦ THE PERPETRATOR OF SEXUAL ABUSE

The phenomenon of having a sexual attraction for prepubertal children has been defined as **pedophilia** and having a sexual attraction for pubertal children as **ephebephilia**. The term *ephebephile* is rarely used today. For the purpose of this chapter, a pedophile will be defined as an adult who prefers to have sex with children. The pedophile has recurrent, intense sexual urges and sexually arousing fantasies involving children. Although pedophiles prefer to have sex with children, they can and do have sex with adults. Some even have sex with adults specifically to gain access to children.

About 85% of all reported perpetrators are male, and they may come from any profession or trade. It should be noted that this figure may be inaccurate due to the belief that most female child molesters are not reported.

While little is known about female perpetrators, two assumptions are made:

1. Males may be less traumatized by sexual abuse, seeing it as part of coming of age rather than an abusive act.

2. Female/female abuse is probably underreported, with the victims finding the female abuser less frightening than a male abuser and subsequently being less likely to report the abuse. Those females who have been reported were baby sitters, younger girls, and occasionally older women.

Pedophiles and child molesters are not necessarily the same. A child molester sexually molests children, whereas a pedophile has a sexual preference for children and fantasizes about having sex with them, but if he does not act it out, he is not a child molester. Some pedophiles act out their fantasies in legal ways by engaging in sexual activity with adults who look, act, or dress like children. Not all child molesters are pedophiles. A person who prefers to have sex with an adult may decide to have sex with a child. If the sexual fantasies of these individuals do not focus on children, they are not pedophiles.

Groth et al. (1982) divided child molesters into two groups, **regressed** and **fixated**. A regressed individual has a primary sexual orientation toward adults of the opposite sex. Under conditions of stress, this individual may psychologically regress to an earlier psychosexual age and engage in sex with children. Dietz (1983) included the regressed abuser as part of his situational group. The fixated child molester (preferential group of Dietz) has a primary sexual orientation toward children.

Approximately 75% to 80% of abusers are known to their victims. They may be surrogate father figures, especially in families where the father is absent, either physically or emotionally. The child molester usually slowly, consciously or unconsciously, conditions the child. Most do not want to hurt the child. The amount of force or aggression used in their abuse differs. They may be involved in a wide variety of other variant paraphilias, such as exhibitionism, voyeurism, frotteurism, masochism, or sadism.

Araji and Finkelhor (1985) reviewed existing research on pedophilia and noted the following:

1. Children have a special meaning to pedophiles because children lack dominance. They called this emotional congruence.

2. Pedophiles have an unusual pattern of sexual arousal toward children, which they called deviant sexual arousal.

3. Pedophiles seem blocked in their social and heterosexual relationships. This they labeled blockage.

4. Many pedophiles use alcohol or other drugs to lower their inhibitions before abusing children. This was termed disinhibition.

Table 7-2. Classification of Child Molesters

Situational child molesters
    Regressed
    Morally indiscriminate
    Sexually indiscriminate
    Inadequate
 	
Preferential child molesters
    Pedophile

The median age of the pedophile at first conviction is reported as 34.5 years for heterosexuals and 30.2 for homosexuals (Bancroft, 1989). Many begin to abuse children at much younger ages. Lanyon (1986) noted that the child molester is usually a respectable, otherwise law-abiding person, who, because of that respectability, may escape detection and prosecution. Abel et al. (1987) reported that the average child molester is a young, well-educated, middle-class, married, Caucasian (61%) male who is employed in a stable job at a good salary.

Among child molesters, Dietz (1983) proposed two broad categories: **situational** and **preferential**. Lanning (1991) prepared a monograph for law-enforcement officers investigating cases of child sexual exploitation. He reviewed the literature and, following Dietz's recommendations, classified child molesters (**Table 7-2**).

SITUATIONAL CHILD MOLESTERS

The **situational child molester** does not have a true sexual preference for children; sexuality with children may range from a single act to numerous encounters. He abuses not only children but also other vulnerable individuals, such as those who are elderly, sick, or disabled. Four major patterns of behavior are recognized in this category *(see Table 7-2)*.

The **regressed** offender, a subcategory of the situational molester, has low self-esteem and poor coping skills. He turns to children as a sexual substitute. His main criterion is availability. He coerces the child into having sex.

The **morally indiscriminate** individual sexually abuses children as part of a general pattern of abuse. He uses people, and abuses everyone he comes in contact with. He lies, cheats, or steals when it is to his advantage and whenever he thinks he can get away with it. His main criteria are vulnerability and opportunity. He uses force, lures, or manipulation to obtain his victims. His victims usually are strangers or acquaintances, but they can also be his own children.

The **sexually indiscriminate** individual is discriminating in his behavior except when it comes to sex. He is willing to try anything sexual. His main criterion is sexual experimentation. He has sex with children because they are new and different. The children may be his own, and he may also provide them for other adults as part of group sex.

The **inadequate** individual belongs to a group whose pattern of behavior includes psychoses, personality disorders, mental retardation, and senility; he can be classified as the social outcast, the withdrawn, or the unusual. This person becomes sexually involved with children out of insecurity or curiosity. He finds children nonthreatening and ideal for use in fulfilling his sexual fantasies. His sexual activity with children is impulsive.

PREFERENTIAL CHILD MOLESTERS

Preferential child molesters focus their sexual fantasies on children. They have sex with children because they are sexually attracted to and prefer children. Their specific character traits vary, but their sexual behavior is highly predictable. Their problem is a need for frequent and repeated sex with children, so they have the potential to molest large numbers of victims. Three patterns of behavior are recognized in this category (**Table 7-3**).

SEDUCTION

This offender seduces his victims. He courts them, giving them attention, affection, and gifts over a period of time, gradually lowering their sexual inhibitions. His victims are willing to yield to sex for the attention, affection, and gifts they have received. These offenders are often involved with multiple victims at once, in essence a child sex ring, including a group of children in the same class at school, in the same scout troop, or in the same neighborhood. This individual is a master seducer of children because he is able to identify with them. He knows how to talk to children and, more importantly, he knows how to listen to them. He frequently selects children who are already victims of emotional abuse or neglect. His adult status and authority are important in the seduction process.

INTROVERSION

This offender has a preference for children but lacks the personality skills necessary to seduce them. He uses little verbal communication, and usually molests strangers and very young children. He is likely to frequent areas where children congregate, watching them and hoping to find an opportunity to engage them in a sexual encounter. To have access to children, he might marry a woman with children or have his own children.

Table 7-3. Patterns of Behavior

Seduction
Introvesion
Sadism

SADISM

This preferential offender, in order to be aroused and gratified, must inflict pain on the victim. He uses lures or force to access his victims. He is more likely than other preferential child molesters to abduct and murder his victims.

IDENTIFYING PEDOPHILES

A pedophile's sexual behavior is repetitive and predictable. The four major characteristics of the pedophile and the indicators of each are shown in **Table 7-4**. These characteristics can help identify the pedophile, but they are not diagnostic. As in any profile of indicators, no single indicator or group of indicators is sufficient for an absolute identification. Knowledge of the case and common sense should prevail. If enough of these indicators are present, there is cause to believe that the individual is a pedophile. However, it must be reemphasized that not all pedophiles are child molesters.

1. **Long-Term and Persistent Patterns of Behavior** Most of these indicators are self-evident. Several need expanding.
   a. **Sexual abuse in background.** Fortunately the great majority of victims of child sexual abuse do not become offenders; however, most offenders were victims. The pedophile's sexual preference for children usually begins in early adolescence. The pedophile often parallels the patterns of his own abuse on his victims, for example, choosing a victim of the same age as he was when he was abused or choosing the same acts. For this reason all victims of sexual abuse must receive counseling. This should also include any child who is a perpetrator, in order to, hopefully, through therapy, abort a career of abuse.
   b. **Frequent and unexpected moves.** Pedophiles frequently show a pattern of living in one place for several years with a good job and then suddenly moving and changing jobs. When identified, pedophiles are often forced to leave town; this was, and still is, a common way to deal with the problem.
   c. **Multiple victims.** This, along with collecting child pornography, is one of the most important indicators. If a pedophile is caught molesting one child, chances are great that he has molested or attempted to molest other children. A concerted effort should be made to identify the multiple victims.

In 1987 Abel and associates asked 377 child molesters, who had committed sexual acts against children outside of their homes, to reveal the sexual crimes they had committed. The researchers assured confidentiality and immunity from prosecution. These 377 adults had victimized a total of 4,435 girls and 22,981 boys. They acknowledged 5,197 acts of abuse against the girls and 43,100 against the boys. The study also included 203 perpetrators who were sexually involved with children within the home (incest). These 203 incest perpetrators accosted 286 female victims and 75 male victims. They committed a total of 12,927 incestuous acts against the girls and 2,741 against the boys. Fuller (1989) confirmed these findings. Obviously, a single child molester has the potential of committing hundreds of sexual acts on hundreds of children. To stop one abuser can save hundreds of future victims.

   d. **Age and gender specificity.** Most pedophiles prefer children of a specific sex in a specific age range. Pedophiles attracted to young children such as toddlers may not show sex specificity.

Table 7-4. Characteristics of the Pedophile

1. Long-term and persistent patterns of behavior.
   Sexual abuse in background
   Limited social contact as a teenager
   Premature separation from military
   Frequent and unexpected moves
   Prior arrests
   Multiple victims
   Planned, repeated, or high-risk attempts

2. Children as preferred sexual objects.
   Over 25, single, never married
   Lives alone or with parents
   Limited dating relationships if not married
   If married, "special" relationship with spouse
   Excessive interest in children
   Associates and circle of friends are young
   Limited peer relationships
   Age and gender specificity
   Refers to children as objects

3. Well-developed techniques in obtaining victims.
   Skilled at identifying vulnerable victims
   Identifies with children
   Has access to children
   Activities with children often
     excluding adults
   Seduces with attention, affection, and gifts
   Skilled at manipulating children
   Has hobbies and interests appealing to children
   Shows sexually explicit material to children

4. Sexual fantasies focusing on children.
   Youth-oriented decorations in house or room
   Photographing of children
   Collecting child pornography or child erotica

(After K. V. Lanning, 1991.)

119

2. **Well-Developed Techniques in Obtaining Victims**
   a. **Access to children.** This is one of the most important indicators of a pedophile. The pedophile will have a method of gaining access to children. A pedophile may seek employment where he will be in contact with children or where he can specialize in dealing with children.
   b. **Shows sexually explicit material to children.** This is done to misrepresent standards and try to convince the child that these acts are normal.

3. **Sexual Fantasies Focusing on Children**
   a. **Collecting child pornography or child erotica.** As mentioned earlier, this indicator is one of the most significant characteristics of a pedophile. Pedophiles almost always collect child pornography or child erotica. Their collection is their most cherished possession. A search for child pornography is therefore urgent. As soon as legally possible, law enforcement must obtain a warrant to search for child pornography or erotica. If there is a long delay, the pedophile will learn of the investigation and move or hide his collection.

   Another characteristic to be noted about his collection is constancy—he never has enough and he never throws anything away. It is also well-organized. He maintains detailed, neat, orderly records. He is not likely to destroy the collection. He is concerned about the security of his collection, so he hides it in a safe place where he has easy access to it.

THE PEDOPHILE'S DEFENSES

In dealing with pedophiles, the practitioner must be aware of their orientation and their responses to the situation. Evaluation of these responses may be helpful in determining whether abuse has indeed taken place.

DENIAL

Usually the first reaction of a child molester to discovery will be denial. He may act shocked, surprised, or indignant about the allegations. Alternatively, he might admit to an act but deny the intent was sexual gratification.

MINIMIZATION

If the evidence against him rules out denial, the offender may attempt to minimize what he has done. He might claim that it happened on one or two isolated occasions or that he only touched or caressed the victim.

JUSTIFICATION

A child molester typically attempts to justify his behavior, usually blaming the victim and claiming that the victim seduced him, or initiated the sexual activity, or is promiscuous or a prostitute.

FABRICATION

The child molester may create ingenious stories to explain his behavior and dispel any misunderstanding that he is an abuser. The stories range from ludicrous to believable.

MENTAL ILLNESS

The child molester may claim mental illness, stating that he had no control over his actions. He may state that he did not choose to be what he is; it was an act of God and he is the victim.

SYMPATHY

Here the offender expresses regret for what happened. He tries to convince his accusers that he is a good person — law-abiding, God-fearing, and all-American. He pleads for another chance based on his good record and swears that it will never happen again.

ATTACK

The pedophile may decide that the best defense is a good offense. He may harass, threaten, or bribe victims and witnesses. He may attack the reputation of the investigating officer or the motives of the prosecutor. He may become violent.

Guilty, But Not Guilty

This defense involves a plea of nolo contender. The offender states that he is pleading guilty to spare the children the trauma of having to testify or because he has no money to defend himself. This plea saves the offender from acknowledging responsibility for his acts.

It should be noted that after arrest or conviction the offender is at risk for suicide. Family and friends of the accused frequently blame the investigators for the perpetrator's death should a suicide attempt be successful.

◆ Patterns of Abuse

Suzanne Sgroi was the first to point out that sexual encounters between adults and children usually follow a predictable progressive pattern involving engagement, sexual interaction, secrecy, disclosure, and suppression. Perpetrators look for opportunities to be alone with children and engage in sexual activity. After victimization, most perpetrators impose secrecy, which eliminates accountability and enables repetition of the behavior. A suppression phase often follows the disclosure. Others have modified and expanded Sgroi's original theory.

Ritualism and Satanic Worship

Child protection workers often see children who tell of being subjected to sadistic and perverted acts often accompanying sexual abuse. They attribute these acts to ritualism or satanic worship.

Jonker and Jonker-Bakker (1991) reported the results of interviews of 98 children 4 to 11 years of age, and Young et al. (1991), in the same journal, reported the results of interviews of 37 adults who described similar abuse as children. They described sadistic activity such as passing sticks or objects into the vagina, anus, or penis.

The children told of severe physical violence and threats of violence. The children were young when first initiated into these activities. Sex between children was promoted by the abusers. The children described defecation and urination during sexual activity, that they were given drugs and/or alcohol before and during these activities. Some children said that the abusers dressed up with masks, robes, and other unusual clothes. Often the abuse involved more than one child. Pornography was often a prominent feature. These acts were coordinated into a satanic ritual and belief system. The children told of being tortured, witnessing animal and human sacrifice, ingesting body parts and fluids, and taking part in burial ceremonies.

The 37 adults in the Young et al. (1991) report were dissociative disorder patients who came from separate clinical settings and geographical locations. The most frequently reported types of ritual abuse are shown in **Table 7-5**. The clinical syndrome includes dissociative states with satanic overtones, severe post-traumatic stress disorder, survivor guilt, bizarre self-abuse, unusual fears, sexualization of sadistic impulses, indoctrinated beliefs, and substance abuse.

Many child protection workers are skeptical of this form of abuse. Lanning (1991) stated that the problem of discussing ritualistic abuse of children is how to define it. He does not use the term ritualistic abuse because he feels it is misleading and counterproductive as is the use of the word satanic.

Lanning goes on to state that not all ritualistic activity is spiritually motivated and that not all spiritually motivated ritualistic activity is satanic. When a victim describes what might be determined ritualistic activity, several possibilities must be considered. The activity may be part of the excessive religiosity of mentally disturbed offenders, a part of sexual ritualism, or it may be incidental to any real abuse. The offenders may be engaging in ritualistic activity as part of child abuse and exploitation. The motivation may not be to indoctrinate the child into a belief system, but to lower the inhibitions of, control, manipulate, or confuse the child. Lanning warns that labeling this abuse as ritualistic means to apply the same definition to all acts by all spiritual belief systems.

Lanning further states that the idea of secretive individuals regularly killing people as part of a ritual or ceremony and getting away with it is possible but the number of alleged cases has grown so that there are hundreds of victims alleging that thousands of offenders have murdered tens of thousands of people, and there is little or no corroborative evidence. One cannot ignore the lack of physical evidence, that no bodies have been found, that no other physical evidence has been left following alleged violent murders. It would be difficult to successfully commit a large-scale conspiracy crime because the more people involved in any crime conspiracy, the more difficult it is to get away with it. Intra-group conflicts, resulting in individual self-serving disclosures, are likely to occur in any group involved in organized kidnapping, baby breeding, and human sacrifice. The U.S. Department of Justice estimates that 52 to 158 children, the majority being between 14 and 17 years of age, are kidnapped and murdered by strangers each year (Lanning, 1991). There is no evidence, however, to support claims that hundreds to thousands of children are being sacrificed or abused in satanic rituals.

Why would victims describe events that cannot be true? Some of the allegations are impossible. They tell of victims who were cut up and put back together and of sustaining severe injuries that leave no scars. Reports of human sacrifice, cannibalism, and vampirism, though possible, are highly improbable. There may be a genuine phenomenon to explain these allegations with different mechanisms responsible in different cases. The explanation for these claims probably lies in a complex set of dynamics. Ganaway (1989) discussed the psychological issues that might be involved in satanic allegations by adults. Putnam (1991) feels that the material generated by children may be influenced and/or misinterpreted by interviewers. Alternative explanations might involve misperception, offender trickery, or symbolism.

No one can prove with absolute certainty that ritualistic, satanic abuse has not occurred. To totally dismiss these allegations as impossible would be a mistake. Some of the allegations of child pornography are probable and some have been corroborated by medical evidence and by offender confessions.

American law enforcement has been aggressively investigating the allegations of victims of ritualistic abuse. There is little or no evidence of large-scale baby breeding, human sacrifice, and organized satanic conspiracies.

There is great need for research in which criminal, health, and social service agencies are coordinated to study these allegations. It is up to mental health professionals to explain why victims are alleging things that cannot be proven. This area desperately needs study and research by rational, objective social scientists.

Table 7-5. Percentage of 37 Patients Reporting 10 Ritual Abuses in Childhood	
Abuse Reported	**Patients (%)**
Sexual abuse	100
Witnessing and receiving physical abuse/torture	100
Witnessing animal mutilations/killings	100
Death threats	100
Forced drug usage	97
Witnessing and forced participation in human adult and infant sacrifice	83
Forced cannibalism	81
Marriage to Satan	78*
Buried alive in coffins or graves	72
Forced impregnation and sacrifice of own child	60*

Total number of patients = 37. Total female patients = 33. Total male patients = 4.
*Percentages based on 33 female patients.
(From Young et al., 1991.)

This chapter will offer some general tenets that should guide the decisions involved in following a sexual abuse case. Specifically, we will cover principles involved in the history and medical evaluation, behavioral indicators, and the role and philosophy of the sexual abuse management clinic.

♦ THE HISTORY AND MEDICAL EVALUATION

There are three components to consider in evaluating the child suspected to be a victim of sexual abuse. The first, and most important, component is the history or the child's statement of what happened. The second component of the evaluation is assessing the behavioral patterns of the child, comparing them with the behavioral indicators typical of abused children, and then deciding which indicators the child is demonstrating, their importance, and their specificity. The third component of the evaluation is the physical examination. **Neither the physical examination nor the behavioral indicators should stand on their own; they can only support the history given by the child**.

In most medical assessments the history is the most important part of the evaluation of the patient. This is particularly true in the evaluation of a child suspected to be the victim of sexual abuse. Obtaining the child's statement requires an experienced individual who is patient and able to assess the child's developmental skills and the child's credibility. This individual must be able to resist the urge to find out all the details of the abuse before knowing more about the child and the family. **This is both the most difficult phase of the evaluation and the most important**. Every decision that follows hinges on a credible disclosure.

Too much emphasis has been placed on the physical examination. Most sexually abused children show no physical findings, so if one concludes that only those children with positive physical findings are credible, he will be doing a disservice to 60% to 70% of children claiming to be abused. Several physical findings, such as pregnancy in a child under 12 years of age and semen in the vagina, clearly diagnose abuse, but, without a clear statement from the child identifying the perpetrator, the investigation is stymied. The child may even deny abuse. The best option in this situation is to arrange for long-term supportive therapeutic intervention for the child with an experienced therapist who is skilled at talking with abused children. The practitioner must not make the mistake of becoming too anxious and aggressive with this child, too eager to learn all the details of the case, thus placing her in a situation where she has to give an answer. She may give the wrong answer. Patience is essential because it may take several sessions before she is ready to trust the investigator and disclose information about abuse. Alternatively, she may never disclose. The primary concern at this point must be for the safety of the child and the extension of services to ensure that the child receives treatment, if necessary. While the practitioner might prefer to know the identity of the perpetrator, it may be best to be patient and wait for the child to disclose voluntarily.

The nature of the disclosure is important. When gathering background information, it is important to find out the circumstances of the child's disclosure, specifically why she disclosed the information, where the statement was given, and when it was disclosed.

The following vignette illustrates:

> Two siblings are sent to play in the yard. The older boy, Jimmy, is 15 years old, and the younger, Johnny, is 7. Their mother admonishes, "Jimmy, take care of Johnny. I expect you to behave and not to fight. Jimmy, I hold you responsible." There is a disagreement and Jimmy punches Johnny, leaving a considerable bruise. Johnny runs into the house, crying "Jimmy hurt me. He punched me. Look at my arm." Their mother can be certain that Johnny was hurt and that Jimmy was involved. She may not know all of the details, but with time and patience she will soon know.

Use the same set of circumstances and the same disagreement with the same results, but this time the mother is not home. When the upset and injured Johnny runs into the house, he finds no one there. Jimmy follows him into the house and pleads, "Please, don't tell Mom, she'll kill me, she'll ground me." Johnny calms down and Jimmy rewards him with a piece of candy. When Mom comes home, she is none the wiser about the incident until that night, when putting Johnny to bed she sees the bruise left by Jimmy. "How did you get that bruise?" she asks. Johnny, having promised his brother not to tell about the incident, responds, "I don't know, I don't remember." The mother pressures him for an explanation. What does Johnny do? The odds are he will keep his promise and protect Jimmy. If Mom persists, he may well lie. This does not imply that, under similar circumstances, all children will lie. But with these circumstances, with pressure for an answer from the mother, the optimum conditions for disclosure are compromised and the child is placed in a situation in which he may give an improper answer.

An actual case involved the following circumstances:

> A child was brought to the sexual abuse management clinic by the police. She had disclosed that, while at a day care center, a teenage boy employed by the center had injured her when he put a ballpoint pen into her vagina. She made a consistent and convincing disclosure of the incident. On physical examination the vaginal mucosa was erythematous with a small abrasion of the posterior fourchette. There was, to the right of the hymen, a blue dot. The examiner felt there was good evidence that someone had put a ballpoint pen in the child's vagina, as the child had said, leaving a blue dot. The police had the panties she had worn to the center the day before and there was a large spot of blood. It was the blood on the panties which had alerted the mother of the injury. The mother called the police, who arrested the boy. The boy denied he abused the child. Others working with him at the center said that the boy was never alone with the child, or in the bathroom, in which the abuse allegedly occurred. They further said that it would have been impossible to do what the child had described without being seen. The police investigated the bathroom scene and agreed with the center staff that it would have been difficult, if not impossible, to abuse the child in that

location. The police and the sexual abuse management team felt certain the child was abused but wondered if the child might be protecting someone. The mother was asked about the circumstances of the disclosure. She said that she had noted the blood on the child's panties when putting her to bed. The mother asked the child what had happened and who had hurt her. When the child refused to answer, the mother told her that if she did not tell who had hurt her, the child would not be allowed to go to bed. The child then gave her the boy's name and told of the incident. After further investigation, the police felt that the perpetrator was most likely the child's father.

While the nature of the disclosure is important, the nature of the questioning is equally important. Leading, demanding questions can distort the disclosure. Chapter 8 explores this in greater detail, focusing on specific preparation and questions that can be used in interviewing the child.

The investigator must be aware of the child's developmental level, verbal skills, and experiences and realize that young children think in concrete terms. Depending on the age, a child may have limited concepts regarding numbers and times. In addition, children generally have had limited experiences and their vocabulary will reflect this. If the child says, "He peed in my mouth," or "he got pee on me," he may be talking about urine, but he is most likely describing an ejaculation. Depending on the child's age, the child knows only one function for the penis, to urinate; therefore anything coming out of the penis must be urine. The child may say that "he cut me down there with a knife." She may not have been cut with a knife. The child knows how it feels to be cut with a knife and that was how it felt, so she feels that she must have been cut with a knife. What was it that hurt her? It may have been a finger, a fingernail, or a penis, but to the child it felt like a knife.

When a child relates the circumstances of an incident, he concentrates on central or core activity and has limited recollection of peripheral happenings and objects. For example, a 5-year-old girl stated that she had climbed up on an air conditioner and saw the father of a neighbor, her playmate, sexually abusing the child. She described what she saw happening. When asked where this had happened, she said it was in the bedroom. During the investigation of the home it was noted that the air conditioner from which the 5-year-old stated she had observed the abuse overlooked the kitchen. The investigators concluded the child was lying. That may be so, but most likely the child was relating central information and any incidental or peripheral information escaped her attention and memory. The longer the time since the event, the more peripheral details will escape memory. To a lesser degree, even adults miss details of an event.

Children may also have difficulty with number concepts and with how many times something happened. A child may readily count to 10, but when asked to count a number of objects, may not be able to do so. Days of the week, months, and seasons frequently mean nothing to them. The investigator must not depend on either what day of the week the incident happened or how many times when related by a child.

Children do purposely lie. Any parent or teacher can attest to this. Children usually lie to get out of trouble or to avoid trouble. However, the probability that children lie about sexual abuse has been greatly exaggerated. Jones (1986) studied 576 cases of sexual abuse reported to the Denver Department of Social Services; a total of 7.81% of the reports were determined to be fictitious: 6.25% of the total number were fictitiously made by an adult and a mere 1.56% by a child. Children may lie to protect, to deny, or to minimize what has happened. In a related sense, they may withhold information, giving a little bit at a time. Children may also lie with coercion or coaching, more often to deny abuse than to admit it, and with repeated questioning by different interviewers. The child who has been interviewed multiple times may interpret that as disbelief. She tires of telling the same story over and over and may embellish the facts, hoping to convince or please her interrogators.

♦ BEHAVIORAL INDICATORS OF SEXUAL ABUSE

A number of behavioral indicators reveal the possibility of abuse; most are nonspecific and can be seen in any child under stress. No behavioral indicator can provide absolute certainty that abuse has occurred, although several present strong supportive evidence for abuse.

Age-inappropriate knowledge of sex is at the top of the list. If a 3-year-old child gives explicit details of sexual activity, describing ejaculation, fellatio, or anal sex, or states that the abuser used a lubricant such as Vaseline or saliva, the investigator can be confident that the child learned this firsthand. Children may have fantasies that have sexual connotations, but those fantasies do not contain explicit detail regarding sexual acts. Children do not fantasize sexual abuse.

Other strong indicators of abuse are running away and attempting suicide. Platt and Kroth (1979) identified sexual abuse as one of the three main reasons why children run away from home. These authors also reported that 70% of adolescent drug addicts were involved in some form of family sexual abuse, that 75% of adolescent prostitutes were involved in incestuous relationships, and that 50% of the children in a reformatory in Maine and nearly all the children in a Chicago reformatory had been sexually molested before commitment.

Dissociative reaction or multiple personality, a controversial area of child sexual abuse, may explain memory loss and denial. Indications of dissociative reaction may be subtle. At the genital examination the child may suddenly become passive and distant after having been outgoing and relating well. Dissociative reaction can also explain why the child may have trouble remembering details; he has learned to block out unpleasant experiences.

Many children who have been abused show no behavioral indicators. It may be years after the abuse before the child, now an adult, manifests behavior indicators, frequently becoming aggressive or angry and having problems with interpersonal relationships.

♦ THE SEXUAL ABUSE MANAGEMENT CLINIC

The main purpose of the sexual abuse management clinic is to help abused children, make certain the child is safe from further abuse, and help the child and the family cope with and recover from the assault, both emotionally and physically. Too much emphasis has been placed on the legal aspects of abuse and prosecution of the perpetrator. Confessions aside, less than 3% of abuse cases go to trial (Peach, 1991). In my experience less than 10% of rape kits are recovered by the police for use in prosecution, yet great emphasis has been placed on gathering evidence and following legal protocols for interviewing abused children and their families. **It is not appropriate to compromise the child's evaluation and therapy for the slim possibility of legal involvement. The first priority is to take care of the child. Evidence gathering must take second place.**

EMERGENCY ROOM RESPONSIBILITIES

Sexual abuse cases do not belong in the emergency room, an often chaotic environment. Sexually abused children need a calm, nonthreatening environment, as do the parents. Unfortunately, they frequently come to the emergency room in the evening, the busiest time for emergency room personnel. The child usually has just made a statement about the abuse, but the parents cannot reach their physician for advice and therefore they panic. The emergency room should not turn them away, but rather should deal with the situation in an efficient, sensitive manner.

The physical examination should not be postponed if the abuse has occurred recently. If the child has been abused within the past week, it is advisable to arrange for the child to be seen while still in the emergency room or an emergency evaluation may be done in the sexual abuse clinic. If the abuse happened within 72 hours of the examination, a rape kit should be prepared. Rape kits are provided by police forensic departments with standard instructions for their preparation. Any clinic where victims of sexual abuse may be examined should have these kits immediately available.

If the abuse occurred longer than 7 days before, there is no need for an emergency examination, and the evaluator may delay the examination as long as there is certainty that the child is safe.

Personnel in the emergency room may show dismay when they realize there is no advantage to performing a physical examination and no way to obtain physical evidence. They must understand that they may be dealing with a psychiatric emergency, and the family is in crisis and needs reassurance.

The emergency room personnel have the following responsibilities:

1. Be certain the child is safe and will return to a safe environment.

2. Treat any condition that must be treated now; examples include pelvic inflammatory disease, *Neisseria gonorrhoeae* infection, other sexually transmitted diseases, or unrelated infections.

3. Help the family through the crisis. The child may have just disclosed and the family requires immediate emotional support.

4. Make a report to the child abuse hot line, if one has not already been made. If the assault was not by a caretaker, the case should be reported to a sex crimes unit.

5. Involve hospital social services. They will follow up with state services and the hot line, or, if necessary, will initiate the hot line call.

6. Schedule the child to be seen in the sexual abuse management clinic.

The most important considerations are *(1)* the child's safety, *(2)* the perpetrator will not have access to her, *(3)* she will receive emergency psychiatric therapy if needed, and *(4)* any trauma or infection is noted and treated.

♦ PHILOSOPHY OF CARE FOR SEXUALLY ABUSED CHILDREN

To do an effective job when caring for the potentially sexually abused child and feel confident with decisions, it is important that one develop a sound philosophy. Each team should develop a protocol as a guide, including a mission statement and a working philosophy, or position.

The following statements of philosophy were taken from a sexual abuse management protocol. Several have been expanded to provide clarification:

1. The sexual abuse management team is primarily concerned with identification of sexual abuse, crisis intervention, evidence gathering, and long-term therapy for the child and the family.

2. The workup of the sexually abused child is a team effort and should involve all team members. Communication between all team members is essential to ensure a favorable outcome.

3. The team is *not* an arm of the legal system; it is a resource for that system as well as for the state social system and the community.

    The team's function is not to put people in jail or take children away from families; these are functions of the court system. If the team provides the court with good information, the court can make good decisions.

4. Team personnel must guard against having blinders on regarding the possibility of sexual abuse, or they will miss all but the most obvious cases. On the other hand, they must also guard against being too hasty to diagnose sexual abuse. One must remain objective and open-minded in both directions.

5. Sexual abuse management requires special skills. Sexual abuse can have long-lasting psychological effects on the victim and family. Every effort should be made to lessen these sequelae. The sexual abuse clinic experience should not be worse than the actual sexual abuse.

6. Although sexual abuse is unique, it is still similar to other medical problems. Each team member must respect the other's role and allow the process to evolve as in any other medical situation.

7. The evaluation is patient-oriented. The team needs first to deal with the acute situation and to help the patient, yet the needs of others affected by the situation must not be forgotten. At all times confidentiality must be maintained.

8. Sexual abuse is also a medicolegal problem involving gathering evidence. Although this is an important component, it must take second place to the needs of the child and family.

9. No matter how good a team is, it cannot resolve all problems and it cannot be all things to all people. Events and circumstances are not black or white, but are generally gray.

    A significant number of cases, especially those involving preverbal or nonverbal children, fall into a gray zone; the team may be able to decide that something happened but may not be able to determine whether it was sexual abuse or a misunderstanding of a benign event. Although the team may perceive the event as "gray," the family may view it otherwise and will require help in understanding and coping with the situation. Patience is essential.

10. The team cannot expect "justice" in all cases. The legal system must work with, among other things, the reality of admissible evidence and credible witnesses.

    Although everyone, from the family to the medical team to law enforcement personnel to the prosecutor, may believe a child has been abused, for a number of good reasons, not all cases go to court. No sensible prosecutor accepts a case for trial that he does not believe has a reasonable chance for a successful outcome. Families can become so caught up in seeking justice that they become dysfunctional; they can also drag the team into the mire of their cause.

11. Continuous education is a must.

    This can be accomplished in a number of ways, for example, intradepartmental and extradepartmental conferences and meetings, journals, and texts.

12. When dealing with the family and the perpetrator, the team must not judge or confront them.

    Judgment belongs in the courtroom, and confrontation is best handled by state social services and law enforcement personnel.

♦ ADDITIONAL CONCERNS IN CRISIS CENTERS

REGIONAL CENTERS FOR ABUSE MANAGEMENT

The workup of the sexually abused child requires special skills. Just as these children do not belong in an emergency room, neither do they belong in a practitioner's office or in a general medical clinic. Ideally they should be seen in regional centers or child advocacy centers where there is a team of specialists. In that locale one person who is an expert at interviewing the abused child conducts the interview. The center should be equipped so that protective agencies, juvenile court, police, medical personnel, and the prosecuting attorney can witness the interview and have input. All interviews, even those involving the parents and the perpetrator, are carried out in the same setting, with one person asking the questions for all interested parties. The interviews can also be videotaped. In addition, this center should have facilities so that the medical evaluation can be conducted there. Ideally, each state should have enough of these units that they are easily accessible to all and provide 24-hour coverage.

PROTOCOL

To standardize procedures it is advisable to employ a protocol that covers all aspects of the evaluation. It should be noted that no protocol is perfect and followed without exception, and no two cases are alike. Informed judgment must be employed in all evaluations. Nevertheless, a protocol sets the pace for the evaluation. The attorneys involved in the case often request a copy of the protocol that is to be followed and expect the practitioner to defend it.

A suggested protocol table of contents is shown in **Table 7-6**. While this can serve as a guide, each institution must develop a protocol that satisfies the clinic's needs and provides for local laws, hospital practices, etc.

SCREENING PATIENTS

It is often necessary to screen which patients are to be evaluated in the clinic, especially if the number of patients that can be evaluated is limited. The schedule could be filled with patients who are only mildly suspected to have been abused—patients with nonspecific physical and behavioral indicators who have not disclosed information about being abused or who even deny abuse. A common complaint that must be handled comes from a divorced or separated parent, fighting custody, who calls after each visitation because the child cries when seeing the other parent and refuses to go with him or her. On return from visitation if the child gives any signs or symptoms, such as "a red vagina or anus," burning on urination, or suspicious acting-out, the parent demands a complete evaluation. While it is important to respond to cases appropriately, in my experience it is best to handle these calls by phone, employing an experienced person who can evaluate the situation and make referral to the family physician or pediatrician if appropriate. Other referrals that can be made by the abuse center in order to use their resources most effectively include parental counseling to supply education concerning the abuse problem and child or family counseling to handle other problems. As stated earlier, without a credible disclosure from the child, the case may well end up in frustration for all.

The sexual abuse management clinic at my institution accepts no walk-in patients. All cases are screened and the essentials noted. The team meets on a regular basis to discuss each case and prepare a plan before the patient is evaluated. The clinic evaluates only those children who have made a disclosure or who are symptomatic and recommended by a physician who requests further evaluation. Those patients who have specific

---

Table 7-6. Sexual Abuse Management Protocol

Table of Contents

I.   **Mission Statement**
II. **Philosophy**
III. **Statement of Services**
IV. **Referral Process**
V.   **Clinical Process**
    A. Physical Examination
    B. Follow-up Referrals
    C. Parent/Caregiver Interview
    D. Child Interview
        1. Initial interview
        2. Subsequent interviews
        3. Use of dolls and other aids
        4. Videotaping
        5. Probability and Credibility Assessment
VI. **Decision Making**
    A. Pre-evaluation
    B. Case Review
    C. Documentation
    D. Recommendations and Follow-up
VII. **Special Considerations**
    Multiple victim/Multiple Suspects
VIII. **Training of Professionals and Others**
IX. **The Legal System and Testifying**
Appendix
I.   **Colposcopic protocol**
II. **Film Processing and Chain of Custody**
III. **Polaroid Photos**
IV. **Videotaping**
    A. Legal Guidelines
    B. Video cassette processing and chain of custody
    C. Medical Record Protocol on Videotape Cassettes
        1 Protocol for viewing videos
        2. Preparing copies of videos

Clinic Forms
    1. State Form
    2. Parent Interview Form
    3. Child Interview Form
    4. Telephone Screening/Referral Form

behavioral indicators and who have not made any disclosure are interviewed by our therapist or recommended to another experienced counselor before a physical examination is performed.

◆ BIBLIOGRAPHY

Abel, G, Becker, J, Mittleman, M, Cunningham-Rathner, J, Rouleau, J, and Murphy, W: Self-reported sex crimes of nonincarcerated paraphiliacs, *J Interpersonal Violence* 2:3-25, 1987.

American Humane Society: Sexual abuse of children, American Humane Society, 1981.

Araji, S, and Finkelhor, D: Explanations of pedophilia: Review of empirical research, *Bull Am Acad Psychiatry Law* 13:17-37, 1985.

Bancroft, J: *Human Sexuality and Its Problems*, Churchill Livingstone, London, 1989.

Brassard, MR: Sexually abused children: Identification and suggestions for intervention, *School Psychol Rev* 12:93-97, 1983.

Child molesters: A behavioral analysis, ed 3, National Center for Missing and Exploited Children, 1992.

DeFrancis, V: Protecting the child victim of sex crimes committed by adults, final report, Denver, American Humane Association, Children's Division, 1969.

DeVine, RA: Incest: A review of the literature; Sexual abuse of children: Selected readings, US Department of Health and Human Services, DHHS Publication No. (OHDS)78-30161, Nov 1980.

Dietz, PE: Sex offenses: Behavioral aspects. In SH Kadish et al, eds: *Encyclopedia of Crime and Justice*, New York Free Press, New York, 1983.

Ganaway, GK: Historical truth versus narrative truth: Clarifying the role of exogenous trauma in the etiology of multiple personality disorder and its variants, *Dissociation* 2:205-220, 1989.

Greenwood, CL, Tangalos, EG, and Maruta, T: Prevalence of sexual abuse, physical abuse, and concurrent traumatic life events in a general medical population, *Mayo Clin Proc* 65:1067-1071, 1990.

Groth, N, and Birnbaum, H: Adult sexual orientation and attraction to underage persons, *Arch Sex Beh* 7:175-181, 1978.

Jones, DPH: Reliable and fictitious accounts of sexual abuse in children, *J Interpersonal Violence*, June 1986.

Jones, DPH: Ritualism and child abuse, *Child Abuse Negl* 15:163-170, 1991.

Jonker, F, and Jonker-Bakker, P: Experiences with ritualist child sexual abuse: A case study for the Netherlands, *Child Abuse Negl* 15:191-196, 1991.

Lanning, KV: Ritual abuse: A law enforcement view or perspective, *Child Abuse Negl* 15:171-173, 1991.

Lanyon, R: Theory and treatment in child molestation, *J Consult Clin Psychol* 54:176-182, 1986.

Moore, KA, Nord, CW, and Peterson, JL: Nonvoluntary sexual activity among adolescents, *Fam Plann Perspect* 21:110-114, 1989.

Peach, G: Personal communication, 1991.

Platt, JS, and Kroth, RL: The behavioral Q sort as an aid in the responsible modification of adolescent's behavior, *Adolescence* 14:241-246, 1979.

Putnam, FW: The satanic ritual abuse controversy, *Child Abuse Negl* 15:175-179, 1991.

Young, WC, Sachs, RG, Braun, BG, and Watkins, RT: Patients reporting ritual abuse in childhood: A clinical syndrome. Report of 37 cases, *Child Abuse Negl* 15:181-189, 1991.

Chapter 8

PHYSICAL EXAMINATION IN SEXUAL ABUSE

JAMES A. MONTELEONE, M.D.
JOHN R. BREWER, M.D.
TIMOTHY J. FETE, M.D.

A 9-year-old girl was admitted to the hospital via the emergency room. She had been struck by an automobile while running across the street. She had multiple acute abrasions to the hip, head, and arm. She had been unconscious for a short period and it was decided to admit her for observation overnight. A routine urine sample was found to have live sperm. The child denied sexual contact.

Physical findings revealed vaginal changes consistent with chronic sexual abuse.

The family vehemently denied the possibility of abuse. The child was placed in a foster home and after several counseling sessions continued to insist she was never sexually abused. The case was never resolved and the juvenile court returned her to her family.

The physical examination of children suspected to be victims of sexual abuse is not difficult if the parents and child are properly prepared. To prepare them properly, several steps must be taken. First, the practitioner explains to the parents and child what will take place during the examination, giving them an overview of the process. Next, the child and parents, if appropriate, are shown the various instruments that will be employed, including the stethoscope, ophthalmoscope, otoscope, and colposcope. The child may be allowed to examine and even use them. When the child realizes the examination is much like a well-child examination in the family physician or pediatrician's office, he or she usually cooperates.

♦ DEVELOPING RAPPORT

The examiner should spend time getting acquainted with the child to establish rapport. Helping the child talk about special interests, school, sports, or music lessens the tension and enables the child to relax, which is important for the vaginal and anal examinations. The examiner should be patient and friendly. Children are frightened by a hurried or demanding examiner, but they generally respond to and cooperate with one who is pleasant and fun. It is not necessary to wear a lab coat or other hospital and medical garb; such apparel may be frightening for younger children. **Take the time necessary to earn the child's confidence.** Pediatricians are particularly adept at this, having learned through their experience to communicate with children at the child's level and thereby effectively gaining their trust. Above all, **DO NOT make the examination experience worse than the abuse.**

If a nurse will be assisting with the examination, he or she should also help in preparing the child for the examination. The nurse spends time developing a relationship with the child and helps to explain to the child what is going to happen during the examination. This eases the child's fears and ensures better cooperation during the examination.

♦ PROVIDING REASSURANCE

The examiner assures the child that the examination will not cause pain and that he will stop whenever the child wishes. The child must also be assured that the examination is important and necessary.

It is unusual for a child to be badly frightened about or resistive to the examination. **Examining a terrified, resistive child by force is not appropriate.** Rather than force the child to submit to the examination, the child should be sent home and instructions given to the caretaker to reassure the child and return on another day. On the next visit the child is often much more cooperative. However, children younger than 3 years of age frequently cry during any examination procedure.

♦ REVIEWING PREVIOUS RECORDS

If another physician has seen the child, it is important to obtain those medical records. Records from previous hospitalizations can also provide valuable information. The object of such research is old injuries. In particular when the child has physical evidence of injury, it is important to document whether there was a previous accident, perhaps attended by another physician, which might explain the finding, such as a genital injury. This is especially true when you are faced with an impaling injury that evidently happened several years before.

♦ CONDUCTING THE PHYSICAL EXAMINATION

The help of a calm, sympathetic nurse, experienced in the evaluation of the sexually abused child, is essential during the examination. As already stated, the nurse can effectively reassure the child as well as be an advocate for the child during the examination. One other factor must be considered. This examination is very sensitive and the actions of the examiner can be misinterpreted. **During the examination, there MUST always be one other professional in the room in**

addition to the examiner. If possible, the parent of the same sex as the child should also be present during the examination. Occasionally an older child may prefer not to have a parent present during the examination and this request should usually be honored. All adolescents should be given the choice of having a parent present during the examination.

Children who are forced to lie on an examining table for long periods may become apprehensive. Therefore, the examination must be conducted as efficiently as possible.

Since embarrassment is a normal reaction, the examiner must respect the child's need for modesty at all times. An examining gown and sheet are used to cover the child and only the portion of the body that is currently being examined is exposed. In addition, the examination should proceed as quickly as possible. For mutual protection of practitioners and patient, both the examiner and the nurse assisting should wear gloves during the examination.

OBSERVATION

The examination begins with an evaluation of the child's general appearance; this should include looking for evidence of other abuse, such as loop marks or scars from previous injuries or burns; evaluating the status of the child's hygiene; checking nutritional status; assessing congenital anomalies, muscular development, and central nervous system abnormalities; determining whether the child is obese; and measuring vital signs, height, and weight.

Children who have been sexually abused often show signs of physical and emotional abuse. Their demeanor should be observed for signs of depression or dissociative behavior. The child and parents should realize that the examiner is interested in the whole child.

A thorough physical exam should follow with examination of the head, eyes, ears, nose, chest, and abdomen. Details of this examination may be found in pediatric textbooks.

GENITAL EXAMINATION

NORMAL FEMALE ANATOMY

The female external genitalia comprise the mons pubis, the labia majora, the labia minora, the vestibule of the vagina, and the clitoris (O'Rahilly, 1986).

The *mons pubis* is the rounded, median elevation in front of the pubic symphysis. It consists mostly of an accumulation of fat. After puberty, the skin over it is covered with coarse hairs.

The *labia majora* (**Figure 8-2**) are homologous with the scrotum of the male. They are two elongated folds that run downward and backward from the mons pubis. Their outer aspects are covered by pigmented skin containing many sebaceous glands; hair obscures them after puberty. Their inner aspects are smooth and hairless. The labia majora are usually united in front by an anterior commissure. They are not united behind, but the forward projection of the perineal body into the pudendal cleft sometimes gives the appearance of a posterior commissure. This posterior meeting often has a folding, asymmetrical appearance that has been mistaken for abuse.

The *labia minora* (**Figure 8-2**) are the two small folds of skin located between the labia majora, at either side of the opening of the vagina. They end behind by joining the medial aspects of the labia majora and are usually connected with each other by a transverse fold, called the frenulum of the labia. In front, each labium divides into a lateral and a medial part. The lateral parts meet to form a fold over the glans clitoris, called the prepuce of the clitoris. The two medial parts unite below the clitoris to form the frenulum of the clitoris. The labia minora are devoid

Figure 8-1a,b. Normal appearing genital exam (Category I). Crescent shaped hymen (H) with smooth edge except for a small mound (C) with a transverse ridge or rugae behind it, the opposite ridge (R) is better exposed. Other structures shown are the anterior column (B), the anterior hymenal attachment (A), the urethra (U), the labia minora (D) and the fossa navicularis (E).

Figure 8-2. Normal appearing genital exam with a thickened, fimbriated hymen. Other structures shown are the labia majora (L), the labia minora (M), the clitoris (C) and the posterior fourchette (P).

of fat, and the skin covering them is smooth, moist, and pink. They are hidden by the labia majora during childhood, when the labia majora contain less fat and are smaller. At puberty the labia minora change, become more pigmented, often protrude through the labia majora, and lose definition of the posterior ends when they elongate and blend into the vestibular mucosa.

The *vestibule of the vagina* is the area between the labia minora. It contains the openings of the vagina and the urethra. The external urethral orifice is a median slit situated behind the clitoris and immediately in front of the vaginal orifice. The vaginal orifice, larger than the urethral opening, is also a median cleft. Its size and appearance depend on the condition of the hymen. The fossa navicularis is a shallow depression in the vestibule between the vaginal orifice and the frenulum of the labia.

The *clitoris (see Figure 8-2)*, like the penis, consists mainly of erectile tissue and is capable of enlargement as a result of engorgement with blood. Unlike the penis, it does not enclose the urethra. It is located behind the anterior commissure of the labia majora, and most of it is hidden by the labia minora.

The *vagina* has three layers: mucosa, muscular coat, and fibrous coat. The mucosa is lined by stratified squamous epithelium, which is influenced by hormonal change. The mucosa is thick and is marked by a number of transverse ridges, which are more prominent in the lower part of the vagina. These ridges are called vaginal rugae. A longitudinal ridge, termed the anterior column of the rugae, marks the anterior wall, and a similar ridge, termed the posterior column of the rugae, marks the posterior wall. A lower prominence of the anterior column is called the urethral carina or ridge, which is formed by the urethra.

The opening of the vagina into the vestibule is partially closed by the fold called the *hymen*. The hymen varies in size and shape but is often concentric or less often annular (discussed later).

The *anal canal* is the part of the large intestine that extends from the level of the upper aspect of the pelvic diaphragm to the anus. The anus is the terminal orifice of the alimentary canal. Its circumference is called the anal verge. The lower part of the anal canal differs in nerve supply, venous and lymphatic drainage, and type of epithelium above and below this line. The pectinate line marks the lower limit of the anal valves around the circumference of the canal.

Kellogg and Parra (1991) examined the genitalia of 123 normal nonabused female newborns to determine the incidence of variations of the posterior vestibule. The posterior vestibule was defined as the area above the perineum extending internally from the posterior commissure to the posterior hymenal border. They found that 93 (76%) of these children had no white spots or lines in the posterior vestibule, 17 (14%) had white spots in the posterior vestibule just internal to the posterior commissure, and 13 (10%) had white streaks extending from the posterior commissure into the posterior vestibule. In 10 (8%) of the 123 neonates the posterior vestibule was partially concealed by a lip formed by the perineum and posterior commissure positioned anterior to the vestibule.

They determined that such structures are normal anatomical variants and proposed that the white line be designated *linea vestibularis*. This structure is distinct from a median or perineal raphe. The raphe is a flesh-colored, slightly raised, perineal structure, whereas the linea vestibularis is an avascular, flat, posterior vestibule structure.

Posterior vestibule spots and lines are seen macroscopically and occur in the midline. No surrounding neovascularization or thickening of the structures is seen. The lines are distinct and without varying width. The spots occur just internal to the posterior commissure, whereas the line extends from the posterior commissure internally, but not up to the inferior hymenal border.

FINDINGS IN STUDIES OF NONABUSED GIRLS

McCann et al. (1990) examined and photographed with the colposcope a sample of 93 nonabused prepubertal girls between the ages of 10 months and 10 years. Examination techniques included a supine labial separation approach, a supine labial traction method, and a prone knee-chest position. The findings in these children are summarized in **Table 8-1**. It should be noted that probably the only population one can be absolutely certain are not victims of sexual abuse are those in the newborn nursery. The report by Chadwick et al. (1989) was pivotal in describing what are clearly signs of abuse.

In one study of nonabused girls, Berenson et al. (1992) examined 211 girls. The study population consisted of 36% blacks, 33.6% white non-Hispanics, 29.9% Hispanics, and 0.5% Asians. Subjects had a mean age of 21 ± 20.6 (SD) months. Extensive labial agglutination was noted in 5% and partial agglutination in 17%. They noted a significant difference in hymenal configuration by age, with a fimbriated hymen the most common type (46%) in infants aged 12 months or younger and a crescentic hymen the most common (51%) in girls older than 24 months. No significant difference was noted in hymen configuration by race. Hymenal mounds were observed in 7%, hymenal tags in 3%, vestibular bands in 98%, longitudinal intravaginal ridges in 25%, and external ridges in 15% of subjects in whom the anatomy under study could be visualized. Hymenal notches (clefts) occurred superiorly and laterally on the hymenal rim but none were found interiorly on the lower half of the hymen. A narrow rounded hymenal ring with a transection was observed in 1 of 201 subjects and was not considered a normal finding. Transverse hymenal openings, measured only in annular and crescentic hymens, showed a mean that ranged from 2.5 ± 0.8 to 3.6 ± 1.2 mm and varied significantly with age.

Gardner (1992) examined the genitalia of 79 symptom-free young premenarchal girls not thought to have been sexually abused, aged between 3 months and 11 years, 7 months (mean, 5 years, 4 months). Gardner found increased vascularity (44%), midline avascular areas (27%), "ragged" posterior fourchette epithelium (18%), notch configuration of the posterior fourchette (10%), delicate tethers between the hymen and perihymen (14%), hymenal bumps between the 3 and 9 o'clock positions (11%), and asymmetry of the hymenal tissue (9%).

Table 8-1. Genital Findings in Nonabused Girls

Genital findings
  Erythema of the vestibule (56%)
  Periurethral bands (50.6%)
  Labial adhesions (38.9%)
  Lymphoid follicles on the fossa navicularis (33.7%)
  Posterior fourchette midline avascular areas (25.6%)
  Urethral dilation
    With labial traction (90.5%)
    With the supine separation (79.3%)

Hymenal findings
  Mounds (33.8%)
  Projections (33.3%)
  Septal remnants (18.5%)

Intravaginal findings
  Vaginal ridges (90.2%)
  Rugae (88.7%)

The cervix was visualized without a speculum in 69% of the children during the knee-chest examination.

Unusual findings*
  Posterior fourchette friability (4.7%)
  Anterior hymenal clefts (1.2%), (1 child)
  Notches of the hymen (1.2%), (1 child)
  Hymenal septa (2.5%), (2 children)
  Vaginal discharge (2.6%), (2 children)
  Foreign body (1.3%), (1 child)

*The major concern in a study of this type is the lack of certainty about whether the sample contains only nonabused children. The children were screened for behavioral indicators but were not interviewed. (From McCann et al., 1990.)

Figure 8-3. *Enlarged hymenal opening. Horizontal hymenal opening is measured from point A to B, the inner edges of the hymen from 9 to 3 o'clock.*

Figure 8-4. *The points of measurement of the vertical hymenal opening, (A) the anterior hymenal attachment to the hymenal edge (B) at 6 o'clock.*

Normal hymens have three basic configurations or types: fimbriated (denticular, dentelle, or congenital frilly), circumferential (ring, annular, or concentric), and posterior rim (semilunar or crescentic) (Pokorny & Kozinetz, 1988; McCann et al., 1990). Rarer hymen types are cribriform, septate, imperforate, and hymens with lateral or high anterior or posterior openings. Redundant hymenal tissue may form cuffs, wings, or tags.

Dilations of existing blood vessels, which appear as increased vascularity or isolated, single, blood vessels larger than the surrounding vessels located in an area that normally would not contain a large vessel, are usually normal. They should not be mistaken for the injection seen with irritation or infection.

A ridge or furrow may mark the line of union of the two halves of the perineum and is generally an embryonic remnant. Such ridges are usually narrow and can be slightly raised. Those which are extremely broadened can be the result of sexual abuse and stretching of the subcutaneous tissue.

A narrow, smooth, pale-appearing structure may be located in the midline of the posterior fourchette or the fossa navicularis or on the hymen. This can be mistaken for hymenal or vaginal scars. This structure can be identified by position (midline, contiguous with the perineal raphe) and uniformity in shape and contour (scars are usually thickened and retracted).

Small bands of tissue may be seen connecting two opposing surfaces, with the same color and texture as the surrounding tissue. These are periurethral and perihymenal bands. Periurethral bands were present in half of the nonabused children examined by McCann et al. (1990) and were bilateral in 91% of the children. These bands often have a semilunar appearance that creates a false pocket on either side of the urethral meatus. These bands are more commonly found anteriorly. They can appear throughout the vestibule and form an attachment to the hymen. The same structures can be seen in the posterior portion of the vestibule with asymmetry of the fossa navicularis. These bands can be mistaken for synechial bands.

Small (1 to 2 mm) vesicles (**Figure 8-5a,b**) or sacs on the hymen or surrounding tissues that appear to contain lymph-like material are termed *follicles*. The significance of follicles is unknown. McCann suggested that they could be related to irritation but could not confirm that premise because information on potential irritants was not available for their study.

The *hymenal septal remnant* is a small appendage usually midline, attached to the edge of the hymen or lateral to the urethra (**Figure 8-6**). These remnants are detached pieces of septum and often dangle free of the hymen or, on the opposite position on the hymen, appear as a smooth mound on the hymen. They may be mistaken for free bits of torn hymen.

A localized, rounded, smooth-edged, and thickened area of tissue on the edge of the hymen is termed a *hymenal mound* (**Figures 8-1 and 8-5**). These small projections usually mark the spot of the attachment of an intravaginal ridge.

The *hymenal notch* or *cleft* is a concave, smooth-edged indentation on the edge of the hymen. These are usually midline but can also appear on other positions at the rim of the hymen. Their smooth-edged appearance differentiates them from old tears, which are angular at the base. The *anterior hymenal cleft* is a disruption of the usual curl-like configuration of the anterior hymenal attachment site of a crescent-shaped hymen that creates a shallow groove medially.

Rolled hymenal edge is the term applied to a narrow, rolled appearance at the edge of the hymen caused by a thickening of the hymenal rim or by a folding of a floppy hymen on itself *(see Figure 8-10)*. These folds can be straightened out by placing traction on the hymen with labial traction or in the knee-chest position. These folds of the hymen can be mistaken for attenuation of the hymen. For that reason an effort should be made to be certain that any attenuation is not a rolled edge.

Figure 8-5a. Normal vaginal exam demonstrating labial traction technique. b. Enlarged view of patient in a. Note small hymenal mound (arrow), smooth edge of hymen, and normal, lacy vascular pattern. The anterior column can be seen behind the hymen.

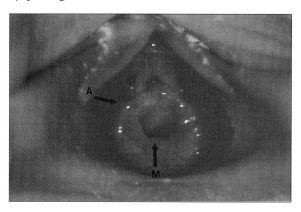

Figure 8-6. Normal appearing genital exam, crescent shaped hymen with small midline mound (M) and hymenal band (A). There is a symmetrical band at 2 o'clock.

Figure 8-7a,b. *Abnormal genital exam with specific findings of abuse (Category III). In the first photo simple separation technique is used. Without magnification this might appear as a normal exam. With labial traction technique the midline healing tear is clearly exposed. Note the follicles at the base of the hymen and the thickened avascular tissue around the injured area.*

Figure 8-8a,b,c. *A progression of photos demonstrating the need to allow the child to relax. This is a 6-month-old chronically abused child with marked anal changes, loss of normal anal landmarks, and destruction of subcutaneous tissue. The child was also vaginally penetrated.*

Figure 8-9. *Normal appearing genital exam with septal remnants A and B. See Figure 8-10.*

Figure 8-10. *Enlarged view of the patient in Figure 8-9. The mound (S) is the posterior attachment and (R) the filamentous anterior remnant of the septum. Note the rolled hymen edge (H).*

Figure 8-11. *Normal appearing genital exam with boggy, estrogen affected hymen in a 1-year-old child.*

Figure 8-12. *Normal appearing genital exam showing small hymenal mound (arrow) and the anterior column (A). The urethral opening diameter is normal.*

Figure 8-13. *Abnormal genital exam, Category II, non-specific findings. The vaginal mucosa and hymenal tissue are inflamed, a non-specific vaginitis. The hymenal edge from 1 o'clock to 4 o'clock remains intact while the limits of the rest of the hymenal edge are distorted and lost.*

As already described, *intravaginal rugae* or *ridges* are narrow longitudinal ridges of mucosa-covered, fibrotic-like tissue that are attached to the inner surface of the hymen and located along either the lateral or the posterior-lateral wall of the vagina (**Figures 8-1 and 8-20**). Intravaginal rugae or ridges are present in most children. They coincide with the projections and mounds on the edges of the hymen. These ridges may be difficult to see without manipulation of the hymen and an attempt to see behind the membrane. The longitudinal ridges are located on the lateral and posterolateral vaginal walls.

Intravaginal columns, as noted, are wide midline longitudinal columns of mucosal tissue on the anterior and posterior walls of the vagina (**Figures 8-1, 8-5b, 8-14**).

CONDUCTING THE EXAMINATION

Because females are most often involved, the following discussion concerning the examination of the genitalia focuses on the female. A brief review of the male examination is given at the end.

An infant or small child can be examined either on the examining table or while on a parent's lap. During the genital and anal examination the nurse assistant or the mother positions the child and separates the child's thighs so that the examiner can see the genital and anal areas.

Figure 8-14. *Abnormal genital exam, Category III, specific findings. The hymenal opening is enlarged, hymenal tissue is attenuated, posterior column (arrow) is visible.*

For a vaginal examination, girls 4 to 5 years of age or older are best examined while they are lying in a supine recumbent position, with knees flexed and heels against the buttocks, in a frog-leg position, on an ordinary examining table. The vulva and vestibule examination may be conducted using one of two techniques: *simple labial*

Figure 8-15. *Normal appearing genital exam. Hymen is thickened, there is a mound (arrow) at the hymenal edge.*

separation, in which light lateral and downward pressure is applied on each side of the perineum, and *labial traction (see Figure 8-7b)*, in which the labia majora are gently grasped between the forefinger and thumb, separated, and pulled toward the examiner. The vulvar vestibule will not be visible if the labia minora are fused by adhesions. This condition may be confused with an imperforate hymen or vaginal agenesis. Adhesions of the labia majora may also limit the visibility of the vestibule. Lack of adequate hygiene is the most common cause of nonspecific vaginitis in girls. Girls with myelomeningocele and paralysis of the lower extremities will show marked vaginal laxity and an enlarged vaginal introitus (Steinhart & Monteleone, 1990). **Table 8-2** lists other conditions to note during the examination.

The vaginal and anal examination should be repeated with the child in the knee-chest position, knees flexed at a 90-degree angle, head turned, and back swayed. The supine knee-chest position, having the child flex her thighs on her abdomen, is often more comfortable for her and also gives excellent exposure.

Examination of a shy or anxious and resistive child can be accomplished with less apprehension if the child is placed in a modified Sims' position, with back to the examiner, head to the examiner's left, the child's left leg extended, and the right knee flexed and thigh drawn to the chest. The child is turned away from the examiner and does not see the examiner so feels less threatened.

Table 8-2. Conditions to Note During the Physical Examination
Evidence of other abuse, such as loop marks and scars
General hygiene
Scars from other injuries
Nutritional status; including height and weight
Anatomic or congenital defects
Difficulty in walking or sitting
Semen on clothing
Grasp marks
Blood stains and/or discharge stains on underwear
Absent or suppressed gag reflex
Extreme compliance, child emotionally distant during examination
Child seductive

The examiner should note the condition of the perineal and anal areas, common sites of dermatologic disorders, nonspecific bacterial inflammation, *Candida*, and eruptions that are part of a general skin disorder such as eczema. Perineal excoriations due to scratching may be evidence of pinworms. Inflammation and scratching may be the sequelae of poor perineal hygiene or nonspecific infection.

The examiner should note vulvar inflammations, eruptions, open lesions, tears, pain, and discharge. The patency of the hymenal orifice is determined, the size of the introital opening measured (if colposcopic photos are taken, this measurement can be determined from the photos), and the form and thickness of the hymen recorded. Usually there is one central opening with a crescent (53.5%) or concentric (34.9%) shaped hymen. There may be two openings, septate hymen (2.5%), or several small openings in the cribriform hymen (1.2%) or the membrane may be imperforate (1.2%) (McCann et al., 1990). McCann and associates were not able to determine the hymenal type in 8% of the study group. It should be noted that transhymenal widths taken with labial traction can be more than 50% wider than those with the supine separation approach.

The configuration and contour of the hymen varies with the age of the child and the method of examination. A redundant-appearing hymen can be changed with traction on the labia or through the use of the knee-chest position. The vertical and horizontal diameters of the introital opening increase with the age of the child (McCann et al., 1990). Maternal hormones also affect the hymen, causing it to be thick and redundant for as long as 2 years after birth and occasionally longer. Similar changes appear as the child reaches puberty, often before breast tissue changes and the appearance of pubic hair.

McCann et al. (1990) compared three separate methods used to examine 172 prepubertal girls for suspected sexual abuse. Their ages ranged from 10 months to 11 years, with a mean of 5 years, 8 months. The techniques used were the supine position with labial separation, the supine position with labial traction, and the knee-chest position. The knee-chest position (98%) and the supine traction method (96%) were superior to the supine separation technique (86%) in opening the vaginal introitus. The largest vertical transhymenal diameters were seen in the knee-chest position and the greatest transverse horizontal diameters were seen in the supine traction procedure. Other soft tissue changes were noted but not quantified. They recommended a multi-method approach to the examination of the sexually abused child to take advantage of the strengths of each technique.

If there is a discharge, the character, consistency, and color should be noted. The presence of any odor should also be recorded, since foreign bodies cause a foul-smelling, blood-streaked, purulent discharge. If there is evidence of infection, dry smears for bacteriologic studies, cultures, and wet slide preparations should be made. Fresh wet smears must be examined immediately for *Trichomonas vaginalis*, clue cells, and *Candida albicans*. The hymen is sensitive and, when cultures are being procured, care should be taken to pass the culture swab beyond the hymen to a less sensitive area.

The examination of the male for sexual abuse is less difficult than the examination of the female. The positive findings in the male are limited to evidence of infection and injury, which are manifested by urethral discharge, bruises, lacerations, bites, ecchymotic areas, and petechiae of the penis. The anal examination of the male is the same as in the female.

COLPOSCOPY

The colposcope has greatly aided the physical examination and enabled the retrieval of added physical findings in sexual abuse cases. It has allowed a better view of genital and anal areas, and, with a camera attached, provides an accurate means of documenting the findings of an examination. If the examiner does not have a colposcope, the naked eye will often suffice or a magnifying lens or otoscope may be employed.

One additional advantage of colposcopic photographs is that they allow the examiner to share observations with colleagues and seek another opinion, sparing the child another examination. These photographs are also valuable as a teaching resource. It should be noted that because of technical difficulties and human error, photographs can be of poor quality, nonexistent, or lost. Therefore, immediately after the examination, drawings should be made and findings described in writing. Preprinted, large, fill-in drawings are useful in providing documentation.

♦ VAGINAL FINDINGS IN SEXUALLY ABUSED GIRLS

ERYTHEMA, INFLAMMATION, AND INCREASED VASCULARITY

In sexual abuse cases, the examiner may see redness of the skin or mucous membranes due to congestion of the capillaries. Normal vaginal mucosa has a pale pink coloration. McCann and associates noted erythema in 56% of the nonabused girls they examined.

INCREASED FRIABILITY

A small dehiscence, or breakdown, with occasional oozing of blood, of the tissues of the posterior fourchette may be precipitated by the examination. This is usually associated with labial adhesions *(see Figure 8-16)*. McCann et al. (1990) noted this to be present in 39.9% of nonabused girls. When the adherent area is large, greater than 2 mm, the suspicion of abuse should be greater.

ANGULATION OF THE HYMENAL EDGE

There may be V-shaped or angular configuration of the edge of the hymen. The hymenal edge should be smooth and round. Angulation often marks a healed old injury. The child with this finding should also be examined in the knee-chest position because if the angulation persists in this position, it is abnormal.

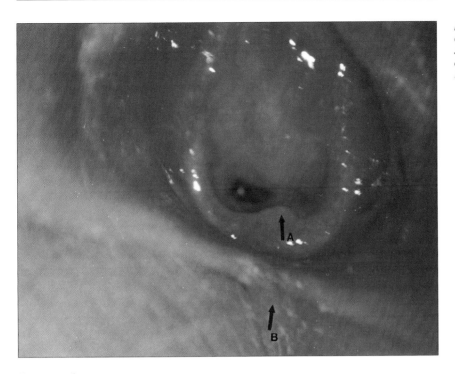

Figure 8-16. Abnormal genital exam, Category III, specific findings. The hymen is attenuated, the posterior column (A) is exposed. There is a breakdown of the friable labial adhesion (B).

LABIAL ADHESIONS

Adherent or fused labia majora are seen posteriorly as a thin central line of fusion. In McCann et al.'s (1990) sample of nonabused children, 38.9% had labial adhesions, more than half of which (19/35) were 2 mm or less in length. These minute adhesions explained the appearance of midline avascular areas and the increase in friability of the tissues of the posterior fourchette. These authors found that traction applied to these small labial adhesions caused them to blanch, producing an avascular appearance. Further traction occasionally caused them to dehisce, producing a small amount of bleeding.

While labial adhesions are a nonspecific finding often seen in girls with no history of sexual abuse, they may also be a manifestation of chronic irritation and can be seen in children who have been abused. McCann et al. (1990) stated that those found in the nonabused girls usually involved the posterior end of the labia majora and generally measured 2 mm in length or less.

URETHRAL DILATION

Urologists have described these changes in adults with urethral intercourse. Monteleone et al. (1988) reported urethral dilatation as an abnormal physical finding in several sexually abused females (**Figures 8-18 and 8-21**). They examined 1,014 children over a period of 2 years in the sexual abuse management clinic, and 234 of these included colposcopic examinations. They graded urethral opening as 1 to 2 mm, +1, up to greater than 8 mm, +4, with gradations between. Of the 234 patients examined colposcopically, 8 received a grade of +1, 8 were +2, 6

Figure 8-17. Abnormal genital exam, Category III, specific findings. Healing injury of the lower half of the hymen and the posterior fourchette. There is early scar tissue along the midline of the hymen. The anterior half of the hymen, though boggy, is normal.

Figure 8-18. Abnormal genital exam, Category III, specific findings. There is scar formation (A) of the hymen at the upper pole, raised and contracted. There is a small opening (D) communicating with the vagina. This may be mistaken for a septum. The mound (C) is normal. The urethral opening (B) is a little more than usually seen with the labial traction technique but is probably normal.

were +3, and 2 were +4. They concluded that mild to moderate urethral dilatation (+1,+2) is probably normal and an artifact of the labial traction technique; higher grades were considered a manifestation of sexual abuse, probably the result of digital manipulation of the urethral orifice. However, they were not able to prove this was the mechanism of the insult. Although several of the children gave histories of digital insertion, none, as would be expected, could state that it involved the urethra. Several had a history of enuresis; none complained of incontinence.

HYMENAL OR VAGINAL TEAR

Deep breaks in the mucosa of the vagina and hymen are referred to as tears. These injuries can be seen with accidental injuries as well as with abuse. Often they occur when a history of impaling is given.

Figure 8-19. Abnormal genital exam, Category III, specific findings. Chronic sexual abuse, hymen at base is totally attenuated, labia minora show permanent thickening and devascularization.

As stated earlier, genital injuries are abuse until proven otherwise. Accidents such as straddle or impaling injuries, usually unilateral, injure anterior or lateral structures, not the interior vaginal introitus (Hobbs & Wynne, 1989). The bony pelvis and labia usually protect the hymen from accidental injury (Enos et al., 1986). Paul (1977) noted that in straddle injuries from falls onto a pointed object, the object rarely penetrates through the hymenal orifice into the vagina. The hymen is usually not torn, and penetration occurs at the lateral margins of the labia minora with the wound entering the vagina through its walls rather than through the hymen. Others concur (Herman-Giddens & Frothingham, 1987; Pokorny & Kozinetz, 1988). Paul stated that violent stretching injury, as seen when a child does a sudden, forceful split on a slippery surface, can cause midline lacerations. These injuries can also be caused during sexual abuse by forceful, sudden abduction of the legs.

DISCHARGE

Vaginal secretions are of various consistencies, colors, and odors. The usual cause of vaginal discharge is a nonspecific vaginitis. Nonspecific vaginitis yields a growth of mixed bacteria not related to a specific disease. Specific vaginitis is a bacterial infection involving such organisms as *Neisseria gonorrhoeae*, *Candida albicans*, and *Trichomonas vaginalis*. Nonspecific vaginitis is seen most often in children between 2 and 7 years of age. The causes of vaginitis are listed in **Table 8-3** (Huffman et al., 1981).

Some genital discharges are not caused by infection or inflammation. It is important to distinguish between those that are inflammatory and those that are not. Most female babies will secrete vaginal fluid during the newborn period, caused by placental and maternal hormones. It is a thick, grayish white, mucoid material that not infrequently becomes blood-stained or grossly bloody. This discharge and bleeding disappear within a week or 10 days after birth. It is a physiologic condition requiring no treatment.

In early puberty girls will have a discharge, usually first noted on the child's underwear. Examination will show vaginal fluid that is curded, thin and milky, or clear mucous in appearance. This is normal and requires no therapy. The menarcheal female often has a clear, sticky discharge during ovulation and a milky discharge before her cycle.

The signs of nonspecific vaginitis are vaginal inflammation and discharge. The child may or may not have symptoms. The only complaint may be a yellowish stain on the child's underpants, noticed by the mother. The character of the discharge, the appearance of the vaginal mucosa, and the child's symptoms do not help to identify the etiologic agent or the type of bacteria causing the infection.

Table 8-3. Etiologic Classification of Vaginitis

Vaginal Infections and Inflammations:
Bacterial

Nonspecific Mixed Infections Secondary to:
    Poor perineal hygiene
    Respiratory infections
    Skin infections
    Intestinal parasitic invasion of vagina
    Foreign bodies in vagina
    Urinary tract infection
    Unknown avenues of infection

Specific infection due to:
    The exanthemas
    Hemophilus vaginalis
        (Corynebacterium vaginalis)
    Hemolytic streptococci
    Corynebacterium diphtheriae
    Neisseria meningitidis
    Neisseria sicca
    Diplococcus pneumoniae
    Shigella flexneri
    Chlamydia
    Gonorrhea (not all types are
        sexually transmitted)

Protozoal Infections
    Trichomoniasis
    Amebiasis
    Other

Mycotic
    Candida
    Other mycotic organisms

(After Huffman et al., 1981.)

Mycoplasmas

Helminthiasis

Hirudiniasis

Viral Infections
    Chickenpox
    Smallpox
    Vaccinia
    Condylomata acuminata
    Herpes

Physical Agents
    Sand
    Other foreign materials

Chemical Agents
    Bubble bath preparations
    Shampoo
    Medications
    Deodorant vulvar sprays

Allergenic Agents
    Nylon or rayon underclothing
    Medications
    Soaps, laundry detergents
    Other allergens

Neoplasia

Granulomatous Diseases

Syphilis

Occasionally nonspecific vaginitis has an acute onset and the vaginal tissues are inflamed and edematous with a profuse, purulent discharge and dysuria. On examination the vulvar mucosa and the outer third of the vagina look hyperemic with a small amount of light gray or clear mucoid discharge. A profuse, purulent, blood-streaked malodorous discharge is typical of a foreign body.

FISSURES
Superficial breaks in the skin or mucous membranes, fissures may ooze blood and be painful. They heal completely and leave no sequelae unless they become infected, in which case they may result in a small scar or an anal tag.

Paradise (1989), in an editorial comment, although finding the study worthy of some praise, found fault because of methodologic uncertainties and limitations in three areas: identifying cases of sexual abuse, the nature of the control group, and the measurement of hymenal orifice diameters and a need to use different measurement techniques. The measurements were taken using supine labial separation only. McCann et al. answered the doubts when they suggested a means in which introital opening could be a reliable parameter in evaluating the abused child. Using the colposcope, they found significant differences in hymenal openings depending on position and methods used to make these measurements (see Table 8-4).

The significance of anteroposterior diameter is doubtful. Annular hymens with tissue encircling the vagina to a full 360 degrees cannot be compared with crescentic hymens in which the hymen is normally absent between 11 and 1 o'clock. Sleevelike or fimbriated hymens should be excluded from comparisons of either horizontal or anteroposterior diameters because of the inability to measure the opening in this type of hymen. This is also true of septate and microperforate hymens.

Clinical reports have expanded our understanding of the healing process; with time, the hymen can completely heal or on occasion contract to a small opening as a result of scar formation.

NEW OR HEALED LACERATIONS

Lacerations are deep breaks in the skin or mucous membranes of the vagina or anus. They often leave scar formation after healing. Fissures and lacerations with scar formation are discussed elsewhere in this chapter.

ENLARGED HYMENAL INTROITAL OPENING

One criterion often used to make a diagnosis of sexual abuse is an enlargement of the hymenal introital opening (Heger & Emans, 1990). Cantwell (1983) stated that a hymenal diameter greater than 4 mm was associated with sexual abuse. White et al. (1989) reported similar findings when they studied 242 females, ages 1 through 12 years, to determine if the vaginal introital diameter was useful in evaluating a child for sexual abuse. The children were divided into three groups: Group I, history of sexual contact and/or *Neisseria gonorrhoeae*; Group II, no history of sexual contact but at risk; and Group III, nonabused. Forty-six percent of children who complained of fondling with penetration had a vaginal introital diameter greater than 4 mm as compared to 14% in those without a history of penetration. Fifty-eight percent of children with more than one encounter had a vaginal introital diameter greater than 4 mm as compared to 29% in those with one encounter. The greatest proportion of children with a vaginal introital diameter greater than 4 mm was observed in the penile-vaginal contact group. These authors believed that a vaginal introital diameter of greater than 4 mm is highly associated with sexual contact in children less than 13 years of age.*

The size of the hymenal opening can vary with increasing age and pubertal development of the child. Other factors such as the position of the child during the measurement, the degree of traction placed on the external genitalia, and the degree of relaxation of the child can influence the measurements. The nature of the abuse and the time elapsed since the abuse can also change genital findings.

Studies by McCann et al. (1990) helped clarify this parameter as a sign of sexual abuse (**Table 8-4**). Horizontal diameters, measured with the labial traction technique or in the knee-chest position, of greater than 10 mm are beyond 2 standard deviations of normal range and can support a diagnosis of sexual abuse. Measurements obtained by simple separation are of limited value unless they are greater than 2 standard deviations beyond normal.

Table 8-4. Size of Hymenal Opening		
Group/Method	**Vertical (mm)**	**Horizontal (mm)**
Preschool (n=50)		
Separation	6.1±2.6 (3.0-13.5)	3.5±1.4 (1.0-7.0)
Traction	7.1±2.3 (3.0-14.0)	5.7±1.6 (1.0-10.0)
Knee chest	7.7±2.4 (3.5-14.0)	4.7±1.5 (2.0-9.0)
Early School Age (n=52)		
Separation	6.0±2.5 (1.0-15.5)	4.0±1.6 (1.0-9.0)
Traction	6.7±2.2 (3.0-15.0)	5.9±1.7 (2.5-10.0)
Knee chest	7.8±2.2 (2.0-13.0)	5.4±1.6 (2.5-8.0)
Preadolescent (n=42)		
Separation	7.0±3.2 (2.5-18.0)	5.0±2.0 (2.0-9.0)
Traction	7.7±2.8 (2.0-17.0)	6.5±2.1 (3.0-10.0)
Knee chest	8.8±2.5 (5.0-15.5)	6.0±2.0 (2.5-11.0)
Transhymenal Diameter (n=144)		
(From McCann et al., 1990.)		

♦ SEXUALLY TRANSMITTED DISEASES

Transmission of sexually transmitted diseases outside the perinatal period by nonsexual means is rare (Paradise, 1989). Gonorrhea or syphilis infections are diagnostic of sexual abuse after perinatal transmission has been ruled out. Herpes type 2, *Chlamydia, Trichomonas,* and condyloma infections are extremely unlikely to be due to anything but abuse, particularly in children beyond infancy.

Chlamydial infections acquired at birth can persist 2 to 3 years in genital, anal, or pharyngeal sites. Untreated trichomonal infections can persist for several months, human papillomavirus can remain latent for up to 8 months of age or longer, and congenital HIV infection may not manifest for months to years. *Chlamydia* is an obligate intracellular organism, and fomite transmission has never been documented. Autoinoculation and fomite transmission may occur with genital warts.

If *Chlamydia, Trichomonas,* genital warts, or HIV infection is diagnosed, even in children younger than 3 years old, an evaluation for sexual abuse is indicated. In one study, 10 of 11 children who presented with venereal warts after age 1 year, including four children younger than 3 years, were proven to have been sexually abused (Herman-Giddens & Frothingham, 1987). Gutman et al. (1991) evaluated 96 children under the age of 13 years who tested positive for HIV and confirmed that 14 (14.6%) had been sexually abused.

For more information on this topic see Chapter 11, Sexually Transmitted Diseases in Abused Children.

SPERM

If the abuse occurred within 72 hours, the examiner should look for the presence of sperm. The survival time of sperm is shortened in prepubertal girls because they lack cervical mucus; if there is a delay before an examination, the likelihood of finding sperm is diminished. Spermatozoa have rarely been detected in vaginal secretions from postpubertal rape victims longer than 12 hours after an assault, although longer survival times have been reported in older subjects. A Wood's lamp helps identify sperm on the clothing or skin. However, sperm is not the only substance that fluoresces under Wood's lamp, so fluorescence is a nonspecific finding. Wood's lamp is not a sensitive screening tool and should be used with caution.

To improve the detection of sexual abuse in children, Gabby et al. (1992) recommend that the p30-enzyme-linked immunosorbent assay be used because of its potential as a more sensitive assay than those in current clinical use. A semen glycoprotein of prostatic origin, p30 has been detected in vaginal fluid 47 hours after intercourse. Herr et al. (1986) described the binding of a monoclonal antibody, mouse antihuman sperm-5 (MHS-5), to a sperm-coating peptide secreted by human seminal vesicles. This reaction does not depend on the presence of sperm and has been used to identify seminal fluid in forensic specimens as old as 6 months. Although MHS-5 binding decreases when diluted with cervical secretions, it is a specific and sensitive technique for detecting seminal fluid.

Acid phosphatase activity is also nonspecific unless the level is very high or specific for prostatic acid phosphatase. Prostatic acid phosphatase activity has been found up to 22 hours after sexual assault and up to 30 hours after voluntary intercourse (Graves et al., 1985). Testing for acid phosphatase should not be the only method used to screen for the presence of semen; spermatozoa are detectable in specimens with no acid phosphatase activity.

A vaginal swab should be obtained and preps made for examination and for the rape kit. It is important to follow the instructions supplied with the kit exactly.

Evidence should be stored securely and a written record kept to establish the chain of evidence, that is, every person-to-person transfer, to document that no tampering or mix-up occurred during the process. DNA fingerprinting, the isolation of a characteristic deoxyribonucleic acid in semen or blood, can establish the identity of a perpetrator with a high degree of certainty from these preparations (Kirby, 1990).

◆STUDIES OF VAGINAL FINDINGS IN SEXUALLY ABUSED CHILDREN

Muram (1989) examined female victims of sexual abuse in which the perpetrator confessed to the abuse. In this study, 30 individuals confessed to sexually assaulting 31 girls, mean age 9.1 years (range 1 to 17 years). In 18 cases (58%) the offender admitted to vaginal penetration. Specific findings were observed in 11 of these 18 (61%) girls. Only 3 of 13 (23%) girls in which penetration was denied showed specific findings. Importantly, in 2 of 18 girls (11%) in which penetration was admitted, the examiner described normal-appearing genitalia and 5 (28%) showed nonspecific abnormalities. Assuming that the perpetrators' reports of penetration are accurate, these data indicate that penetration is possible without leaving physical evidence. Muram classified his findings into the following four categories:

Category 1. Normal appearing genitalia.

Category 2. Nonspecific findings. Abnormalities of the genitalia that could have been caused by sexual abuse, but are also seen in girls who are not victims of sexual abuse. Included in this category are redness or inflammation of the external genitalia, increased vascular pattern of the vestibular and labial mucosa, presence of purulent discharge from the vagina, small skin fissures or lacerations in the area of the posterior fourchette, and agglutination of the labia minora.

Category 3. Specific findings. The presence of one or more abnormalities strongly suggesting sexual abuse. Such findings include recent or healed lacerations of the hymen and vaginal mucosa, hymenal opening of one or more centimeters, proctoepisiotomy (a laceration of the vaginal mucosa extending to involve the rectal mucosa), and indentations on the vulvar skin indicating teeth marks (bite marks). This category also includes patients with laboratory confirmation of a venereal disease (e.g., gonorrhea).

Category 4. Definitive findings. Any presence of sperm.

A hymenal tear was the most common finding in girls who described penile or digital penetration. Of 18 girls who described vaginal penetration, 11 were found to have a hymenal tear, 5 had an irritated and inflamed perineal area, and 2 prepubertal girls had normal-appearing genitalia.

Normal-appearing genitalia was the most common finding in girls who denied penile or digital penetration. Of 13 girls who denied vaginal penetration, 7 were found to have normal-appearing genitalia, 3 were found to have an irritated and inflamed perineal area, and 3 were found to have a hymenal tear.

Of the 31 victims, 21 were evaluated within 1 week of the assault. Irritation and inflammation were noted in 9 of them. No inflammatory reaction was noted in any of the 10 victims who were evaluated 1 week or more after the assault, emphasizing the need for physical evaluation as soon after the assault as possible.

Woodling and Heger (1986) reported that 75% of children who told of painful genital or anal penetration by a penis, finger, or instrument had overt or subtle findings of sexual abuse. The acute findings included abrasions, avulsions, transections, contusions, ecchymoses, petechiae, and focal edema. Chronic or old injuries presented as focal scarring, hymenal deformity, healed microtransections, synechiae, hymenal thickening with scarring, and neovascularization. An additional 5% to 10% of cases were corroborated with colposcopic examination.

Finkel (1989) followed the healing process in 7 children who had experienced acute genital and anal trauma. He noted that superficial wounds which heal by the process of regeneration do not form granulation tissue and have a different healing chronology than wounds that form granulation tissue. Superficial lacerations and abrasions healing by regeneration progress through four stages: (1) thrombosis and inflammation, (2) regeneration of epithelium over denuded surface, (3) multiplication of new cells, and (4) differentiation of new epithelium. This process proceeds at a variable rate but epithelium will generally cover a wound at a rate of 1 mm per 24 hours. Wound healing by the process of regeneration can be complete within 48 to 72 hours. Differentiation of new epithelium is usually complete by 5 to 7 days. When reexamined, 5 of the 7 children had epithelial healing and no changes apparent to the naked eye or at 10X magnification. Superficial labial and anal trauma healed at similar rates.

When the injuries are more serious and deeper, the healing process involves repair, the formation of granulation tissue, and a subsequent scar. Wound healing by repair follows the same steps as regeneration but includes organization and wound contraction. Progressive contraction of the wound with time changes the appearance of the granulation tissue. Initially, the granulation tissue is red. With time, the cellular and vascular components of the forming scar tissue decrease, with color and volume changes of the scar tissue as it matures. Most scars will mature in 60 days. When scar tissue is seen in the process of maturing or having matured, a history of significant injury should be sought.

This study showed that if physical evidence of abuse is to be found in cases where superficial injuries are involved, the child must be examined within 5 to 7 days after the assault. Yet most children do not immediately disclose incidents of sexual abuse. Many victims do not have an examination for weeks, months, or even years after the abuse occurred. By then the injuries have healed and the physical examination reveals few abnormalities.

To emphasize this point, three children who incurred genital injuries as a result of sexual assaults were followed up on a longitudinal basis (McCann et al., 1992). The follow-up period ranged from 14 months to 3 years. Signs of the acute damage disappeared rapidly, and the wounds healed without complications. Following resolution of the injuries, the changes remained stable throughout the prepubertal years. The most persistent findings were irregular hymenal edges and narrow rims at the point of the injury. Over time the jagged, angular margins smoothed off. Disruption of the hymen exposed underlying longitudinal intravaginal ridges whose hymenal attachments created mounds or projections. There was little scar formation. Injuries to the posterior fourchettes healed with minimal scar tissue and left slight evidence of trauma. With the onset of puberty, the hymenal changes were obscured by the hypertrophy of the membrane.

♦PHYSICAL FINDINGS ASSOCIATED WITH ANAL SEXUAL ABUSE

Anal assaults comprise a significant proportion of child sexual abuse attacks. Genital injuries or abnormalities are more often recognized as possible signs of abuse, while anal and perianal injuries may be dismissed as being associated with common bowel disorders such as constipation or diarrhea.

The anal sphincter and anal canal are elastic and allow for dilatation. Digital penetration usually does not leave a tear of the anal mucosa or sphincter. Penetration by a larger object may result in injury varying from a little swelling of the anal verge to gross tearing of the sphincter. If lubrication is used and the sphincter is relaxed, it is possible that no physical evidence will be found. Even penetration by an adult penis can occur without significant injury. After penetration, sphincter laxity, swelling, and small mucosal tears of the anal verge may be observed as well as sphincter spasm. Within a few days the swelling subsides and the mucosal tears heal. Skin tags can form as a result of the tears. Repeated anal penetration over a long period may cause a loose anal sphincter and an enlarged opening.

In the differential diagnosis of anal sexual abuse, the practitioner must be aware of nonabuse-related conditions. Perianal abnormalities are often seen in children with Crohn disease or Hirschsprung disease. The anal canal gapes in children with significant constipation. The distended rectum, with a normal anorectal reflex, initiates the gaping. Stool is often seen in the anal canal. Small fissures can also be seen. These children may have trouble with fecal soiling, which causes reddening of the perianal area. Unfortunately, children who were anally abused often suffer from functional constipation, which results in a damaged anal sphincter and fecal soiling. The pain and injury that follow the anal assault may cause spasm of the sphincter and result in functional constipation.

Muram (1989) examined 310 prepubertal children who were determined to be sexually abused (**Table 8-5**). Muram found normal-appearing perianal and anal regions in 150 of 175 children (85%) who denied anal assault, and in 11 of 70 (16%) who described such assault. Giving a detailed history of anal abuse increased the likelihood of finding anal abnormalities, and anal and perianal abnormalities were found in 59 of the 70 children (84%) who gave a clear history of anal assault. The examination was most often normal when the child denied that anal assault

Table 8-5. Anal and Perianal Findings in 310 Prepubertal Children Who Were Victims of Sexual Abuse

Finding	Frequency
Normal appearing perineum	206 (66%)
Abnormal findings	104 (34%)
Anal gaping*	61
Skin tags	44
Rectal tears	33
Sphincter tears	15
Human papillomavirus	4
Perineal scarring	2
Bite marks	1

Anal gaping–relaxation of the anal sphincter to a diameter ≥ 1 cm when the glutei were separated. (Most evaluators would use a diameter of > 2 cm when palpable stool in the rectum is absent on digital examination.)

had occurred; 25 of 175 (15%) who denied such abuse showed abnormalities. In this study children who had normal results of the genital examination were more likely to have anal abnormalities. This was probably influenced by the large number of males in the study group. Muram showed that failure to document perianal abnormalities in two thirds of the patients demonstrates the limitations of the physical examination in validating allegations of sexual abuse and emphasizes the importance of the child's statement.

PERIANAL ERYTHEMA

Reddening of the skin overlying the perineum as well as the inner aspects of the thighs and labia generally indicates that there has been intracrural intercourse (penis between legs and laid along the perineum). Erythema in this area, however, also results from diaper rash, poor hygiene, or after scratching and irritation from pinworms.

McCann et al. (1990) found perianal erythema in 40.5% of the children they examined. The mean radius of the erythema as measured from the interior edge of the anal verge to the outer border of the color change was 1.5 cm with a maximum width of 3 cm. They found a significant difference in the percentage of males (57%) with perianal erythema as compared to the females (32%).

SWELLING OF THE PERIANAL TISSUES

Circumferential perianal swelling appears as a thickened ring around the anus and has been called the tire sign. It is an acute sign and can reflect traumatic edema.

LAXITY AND REDUCED TONE OF THE ANAL SPHINCTER

Sphincter tone should be assessed by exerting gentle traction on the sphincter. While some doctors prefer digital examination when assessing children who have been abused and anally penetrated, it would seem unwise to assess anal sphincter tone by digital penetration.

SHORTENING OR EVERSION OF THE ANAL CANAL

When there has been anal abuse the anorectal junction becomes approximated to the anal orifice. This is associated with laxity and reduced anal tone. This finding occurs only in the first 2 or 3 years of life and reflects repeated anal intercourse *(see Figure 8-8a,b,c)*.

ANAL DILATATION

Forensic physicians use a variety of terms to describe anal dilatation, including reflex anal dilatation, reflex relaxation of the anus, the lateral buttock traction test, and the "0" sign. McCann et al. (1989) noted anal sphincter dilatation in 49% of the children they examined. The anteroposterior diameter of the orifice varied from less than 0.1 cm to 2.5 cm with a mean of 1.0 cm. In 91% of the subjects with anal dilatation, the anteroposterior diameter was less than 20 mm. The percentage of children with anal dilatation of 20 mm or greater without presence of stool in the rectal ampulla was 1.2%. Stool was seen in 44% of the cases in which dilatation took place. The horizontal diameters of the anal orifice ranged from less than 0.1 to 2 cm with a mean of 0.57 cm.

In those with dilatation, 30% opened within 30 seconds, 55% had their initial dilatation before 2 minutes, and 5% dilated after 4 minutes. None of the anuses that opened after 4 minutes had an orifice greater than 15 mm in the anteroposterior plane. The mean time required for the initial dilatation was 65 seconds, while the mean time for the anus to reach maximum dilatation was 2 minutes, 11 seconds. The anus remained open once the sphincters dilated in 38% of the children, while the anus opened and closed intermittently in 62% of the subjects in which dilatation occurred. Anal dilatation of 20 mm or greater without the presence of stool in the rectal ampulla was unusual.

Figure 8-20. *Abnormal genital exam, Category III, specific findings. Attenuated hymen, exposing posterior ridge (arrow).*

Figure 8-21. *Abnormal genital exam, Category III, specific findings. There is a loss of hymenal tissue at 10 to 11 o'clock. The urethral opening is abnormally enlarged and patulous.*

Figure 8-22. Abnormal genital exam, Category II, non-specific findings. Hymen irregular and thickened, probably due to early estrogen effect. Hymenal opening slightly enlarged. Urethral opening +2, but rim is thickened and avascular.

FISSURES

Breaks in the skin/mucosal covering of the rectum, anus, and anal skin occur as a result of overstretching and frictional force exerted on the tissues. This can occur following the passage of a hard stool or abusive traumatic penetration of the anus. Tiny superficial cracks in the anal verge or perianal skin often result from scratching with pinworms or with excoriation from acute diarrhea or diaper rash.

LARGE TEARS

Large breaks in the skin extending into the anal canal or across the perineum are usually painful and can cause anal spasm. Tears often heal with scarring and leave a skin tag at the site of the trauma. McCann et al. (1990) found anal skin tags or folds located anterior to the anal orifice in the midline equally in preschool, school-aged, and preadolescent children. They found no differences between the races; however, no tags were found in the males. Skin tags/folds posterior to the anus were not seen.

Figure 8-23. Abnormal anal exam, Category II, non-specific findings. Chronic anal changes, especially from 9 to 1 o'clock where there is swelling and a breakdown of the mucosa, deep fissures and erythema. This is secondary to the congenital, anatomic abnormality, anterior displacement of the anus. Note the small perineum. This child was 12 months old and had been treated by her physician for anal fissures since 6 months of age. The problem was complicated by an older sibling who had genital warts and was sexually abused.

VENOUS CONGESTION

Purple to blue discoloration around the anal margin corresponds to areas of venous congestion. The veins can extend as a ring around the whole anal circle, or be limited to a segment. Venous congestion can be seen in the normal anus following excess traction, as from long periods in the knee-chest position. In the McCann et al. (1989) study venous engorgement was seen in approximately three fourths of all the children who remained in the knee-chest position for 4 minutes or longer. Moderate to marked venous congestion at the outset of the examination was not seen.

Venous congestion is not specific for injury from abuse. McCann et al. (1989) found venous congestion present in 7% of the subjects initially, in 52% at the midpoint, and in 73% of the children by the end of the examination. No hemorrhoids were found in any of the children.

SKIN CHANGES

Paul reported that repeated acts of penetration will lead to changes in the anal verge skin *(see Figure 8-21)*. Repeated friction and stretching of the fibers of the corrugator cutis and muscle results in thickening and smoothing away of the anal skin folds. The skin appears smooth, pink, and shiny, with a loss of normal fold pattern. The presence of these skin changes suggests chronicity of abuse.

Scars are evidence of earlier trauma. Paul states that the skin edges are pulled apart once the anal verge skin has split, leaving a triangular break in the continuity of the anal verge with the apex of the triangle pointing into the anal canal. The scar is often fan-shaped, radiating from the anal orifice, and appears as a pale thickened area distorting the normal folds. A skin tag is sometimes found, as well as linear scars. Healing is hampered by infection, passage of stools, or further abuse.

Smooth areas on or near the verge were observed in 26% of the children in the McCann et al. study (1989). These areas were always in the midline, at either the 6 o'clock or the 12 o'clock position. In 47% (8 of 17) of the children with this finding, the smooth area was associated with a depression. Midline depressions without a smooth zone were detected anterior to the anus in 7 (41%) of the patients with this finding.

In that same study, perianal scars were found in 4 of the 240 children evaluated. Three of the lesions were located in the midline at the 12 o'clock position posterior to the rectum. The other one was at the 2 o'clock location and was observable by using the prone, knee-chest position. No fissures, abrasions, lacerations, or hematomas were found in any of the subjects. Perianal skin tags/folds and scars outside the midline were not seen. A prominent anal verge was also an unusual finding.

FUNNELLING

Funnelling is a traditional sign of chronic anal sexual abuse but its presence in children has been questioned. The appearance of funnelling or a hollowing-out of the perianal area is caused by loss of fat tissue or fat atrophy of the subcutaneous area. Although this is often associated with chronic anal sex, it has also been described to occur in nonabused children.

HEMATOMA AND/OR BRUISING

Subcutaneous accumulations of old and new blood and bruising are strong indicators of trauma. It would be very unlikely for these to occur without a history to explain them. These injuries are not likely to be accidental.

ANAL WARTS

Anal warts can occur as an isolated physical finding or in conjunction with other signs consistent with abuse, either anal or genital. Anogenital warts are frequently associated with human papillomavirus types 6 and 11, and less commonly 16 and 18. DNA HPV typing should assist assessment when the question of nonvenereal transmission (e.g., from hand warts) is raised.

Anal warts in children under age 2 years whose mother has a history of genital warts are most likely not the result of abuse. If no history of genital warts is elicited, the family should be evaluated for their presence. In children over 4 years of age with new genital warts, abuse should be considered and the child carefully interviewed by an experienced evaluator. Evaluation of genital warts is difficult in the nonverbal child. *See Chapter 11, Sexually Transmitted Diseases in Abused Children,* for further information on this topic.

PIGMENTATION

McCann et al. (1990) found increased perianal pigmentation in 29.5% of nonabused children in their sample. The degree of pigmentation was minimal in 84%, moderate in 13.6%, and great in 2.2%. The mean radius of the pigmentation was 1.6 cm, with the maximum width being 4 cm. An analysis of variance revealed a significant difference between the races for the presence of increased pigmentation. Of the white children, 22% had this finding as compared to 53.3% of the black and 57.6% of the Hispanic children. The black children had the greatest incidence in the amount of perianal pigmentation, with 17.6% having a moderate to marked degree as compared to 5.1% for the Hispanic and only 2.5% of the white children.

ANAL ASYMMETRY WHEN DILATED

McCann et al. (1989) in their study of nonabused children noted that the anal orifice had a symmetrical oval configuration in 89% of the children whose anus dilated open. In 9% of the subjects the anus was round in appearance, and in 3% it was irregular; 6 children had minimal asymmetry of their anal orifice as it opened and closed intermittently. Marked irregularity of the anal orifice during dilatation was unusual.

◆ NORMAL EXAMINATIONS IN SEXUALLY ABUSED CHILDREN

The physical examination is usually normal in children who have been sexually abused. Even with a confession of penetration by the perpetrator, the examination can be normal (Kerns & Ritter, 1992; Muram, 1989). Many types of sexual molestation do not involve penetration and will not leave physical findings. In addition, a significant number of rapes occur without ejaculation or damage to the hymen (Camps, 1968). The anal sphincter is pliant and, with care and lubrication, can easily allow passage of a penis or an object of comparable diameter without injury. The hymen is elastic and penetration by a finger or penis, especially in an older child, may cause no injury or may only enlarge the hymenal opening.

Bays and Chadwick (1993) have summarized data from 21 studies of reported medical findings in children who were allegedly sexually abused. Normal examinations were reported in 26% to 73% of girls and 17% to 82% of boys. Diagnostic evidence (Category III or IV) of sexual abuse was found in 3% to 16% of the victims. Bays and Chadwick give several explanations for the wide range in percentages of positive and negative findings. Higher rates of physical findings occurred in earlier studies when only the most severe cases came to light. Criteria for what constitutes physical evidence of molestation have changed in the last 20 years as information from clinical studies on abused and nonabused children has been compiled and disseminated.

An absence of physical findings in sexually abused children can be explained in a number of ways. The sooner the examination occurs after the abusive event, the more likely it will reveal positive findings. In two studies comparing timing of examinations, 36% of children examined within 24 hours of a penetrating sexual assault had evidence of genital trauma whereas 13% seen after 24 hours had positive findings (Rimza & Niggemann, 1982). Muram (1989) found irritation and inflammation of the genitalia in 21 of 31 child sexual abuse victims seen within 1 week of the assault, while no findings were noted in victims after a week or more.

Evidence of ejaculate is difficult to find if the child has washed, urinated, or defecated and if more than 72 hours has elapsed since the assault (DeJong & Finkel, 1990; Paradise, 1990; Tipton, 1989).

Injuries can heal rapidly. Hymenal healing occurs in 6 to 30 days and can be complete. Teixeira (1981) examined 500 patients for sexual abuse. He found single, partial hymenal tears healed as soon as 9 days after injury, while extensive tears took up to 24 days to heal. Finkel (1989) followed seven children with acute genital and anal trauma. Six children healed with no residual trauma in 7 to 13 days. Others have also reported complete healing of acute anal and genital injuries from sexual abuse (McCann, 1988; McCann et al., 1992).

At puberty, estrogen stimulates the hymen, causing thickening and proliferation, which can obscure injuries (McCann et al., 1992).

Groth and Burgess (1977) noted that 34% of rapists had erectile or ejaculatory dysfunction. The study was in adult women but may also apply to child molesters.

♦ PHYSICAL FINDINGS IN RAPE VICTIMS

Certain types and locations of hymenal injuries are often seen after abuse. McCann et al. (1990) observed that the hymenal membrane at its midline (6 o'clock position) attachment along the posterior rim of the introitus, during actual or attempted penetration, is the portion of the hymen most likely to be damaged. A narrowed (attenuated) hymen at this position is usually indicative of an injury. Mounds, projections, or notches on the edge of the hymen and the exposure of intravaginal ridges strengthen the possibility of abuse.

McCann et al. (1992) followed three girls with healing injuries resulting from an assault and found that a narrow hymenal rim at the point of injury persisted. The original injuries occurred along the posterior or lateral hymenal rim, between 5 and 9 o'clock. Teixeira (1981) examined 500 rape victims and found that the hymen ruptured most commonly at the 5 to 7 o'clock position. He noted that 310 of the victims had hymenal ruptures, 193 (62%) of which revealed tears in the 5 to 7 o'clock area. He noted that ectopic coitus, or penile impact without penetration, resulted in lesions of the fourchette and partial ruptures. Herman-Giddens and Frothingham (1987) generally concurred with the above study and found that attempted forced vaginal penetration generally resulted in hymenal tears and fissures between the 3 and 9 o'clock positions and may extend across the vestibule and fourchette.

♦ A CLASSIFICATION OF PHYSICAL FINDINGS IN SEXUAL ABUSE EXAMINATIONS

The National Child Sexual Abuse Summit Meeting in 1985 (Tipton, 1989) concluded that some specific physical findings are strongly indicative of sexual abuse beyond reasonable doubt, as follows :

1. Clear-cut tears, fresh or old; scars; significant distortion of the normal shape of the hymen and/or hymenal bruising.

2. Lacerations, scars, bruises, and healing abraded areas, often accompanied by neovascularization, of the posterior fourchette.

3. Anal dilation greater than 15 mm transverse diameter with gentle buttock traction with the child in knee-chest position. Large anal scars in the absence of a history that could explain the scars.

The authors have used the classification of physical findings in sexual abuse as listed in **Table 8-6**. The categories were suggested by Muram. We have expanded the classification and have placed several conditions Muram had in Category III into Category IV.

Table 8-6. Classification of Sexual Abuse Physical Findings

I. **Normal appearing exam**
The majority (60% or more) of abused children fall into this category.
   Mounds
   Clefts
   Bands
   Septal remnants
   Urethral dilation (mild)

II. **Nonspecific findings of sexual abuse**
(often seen in children who have not been sexually abused)
   Condylomata (Human Papilloma Virus, HPV)
      (in children under 2 years, may upgrade with a strong history or with supportive physical findings (hymenal tear, attenuation, etc.)
   Hymenal thickening or edema*
   Injection, erythema, vaginitis (nonspecific), areas of increased vascularity*
   Bacterial vaginosis with clue cells*
   Rounding of hymenal edges
   Labial adhesions
      (depending on history, could be Category III)
   Urethral dilation (moderate)
   Narrowing of hymen (greater than 2 mm)
   Enlargement of the hymenal opening
      (with no other findings)*
   Thickening of the perianal tissue
   Increased pigmentation
   Venous pooling
      (after prolonged knee-chest position)
   Funneling, fat atrophy

III. **Specific (suspicious/highly suspicious) for sexual abuse**
   Hymenal and vaginal tears
   Hymenal scars (usually are retracted), mounted linear avascular areas

Herpes II
Chlamydia trachomatis†
Trichomonas vaginalis
Reflex anal dilation in absence of stool in antrum and greater than 20 mm
Hymenal transections
Hymenal narrowing, flattening (less than 2 mm)
Hymenal attenuation (narrowing or flattening)
Synechiae (lower pole, 3 to 9 o'clock; may be confused with bands of tissue extending from the vaginal wall caused by stretching with labial traction)
Severe rounding of hymenal margin with loss of vascularity
Perianal skin tags/folds outside the midline
Anal scars outside the midline
Marked irregularity of the anal orifice during dilation, persistence of a prominent anal verge
Urethral dilation (severe)
Pelvic inflammatory disease (PID)

IV. **Conclusive of sexual abuse**
(Children under 12 years; older children may be sexually active)
   Neisseria gonorrhoeae†
   Treponema pallidum (syphilis)†
   Sperm, seminal fluid, acid phosphatase activity in discharge (must be very high if nonspecific assay, or prostatic specific)
   Pregnancy
   HIV† (no history to explain)

A nonspecific finding can become a specific finding when a child gives a clear history of recent sexual abuse, especially when describing pain.

†Nonneonatal.

♦CONDITIONS THAT CAN BE MISTAKEN FOR SEXUAL ABUSE

Bays and Jenny (1990) described a number of dermatologic, congenital, traumatic, and infectious physical findings that can be mistaken for sexual abuse (**Table 8-7**). The most common dermatologic condition confused with trauma from sexual assault is lichen sclerosis. It can present in a variety of ways from mild irritation of the labia and vaginal mucosa to dramatic findings such as subepidermal hemorrhages of the genital or anal area involving the labia and vaginal mucosa and/or the anus. A punch biopsy may be necessary to make the diagnosis. The diagnosis is usually suspected when a lighter, "halo" area is noted at the periphery of the reddened or hemorrhagic area.

Table 8-7. Conditions Which Can be Mistaken for Sexual Abuse
Lichen sclerosis et atrophicus
Accidental straddle injuries
Accidental impaling injuries
Nonspecific vulvovaginitis and proctitis
Group A β-streptococcal vaginitis and proctitis
Diaper dermatitis
Foreign bodies
Lower extremity girdle paralysis as in myelomeningocele
Defects which cause chronic constipation, Hirschsprung disease, anteriorly displaced anus
Chronic gastrointestinal disease, Crohn disease
Labial adhesions
Anal fissures

Congenital hemangiomas, streptococcal infections, straddle injuries, and urethral caruncle or prolapse (Johnson, 1991) are other conditions that produce physical findings which can be confused with sexual abuse. We have seen three cases of shigella vaginitis that had been reported as sexual abuse because the children presented with vaginal bleeding and severe vaginal mucosal edema.

Anal changes from Crohn's disease, hemolytic uremic syndrome, postmortem anal dilation, neurogenic patulous anus, lichen sclerosis, and chronic constipation (Bays & Jenny, 1990) may also be mistaken for sexual abuse. Bays and Jenny warned that fissures and anal dilation can be particularly troublesome because they are found both in constipated and in sexually abused children. One study reported 6% to 26% of constipated children had anal fissures, and 15% to 18% had anal dilation. In that study sexually abused children revealed a higher percentage with anal dilation (42%) and fissures (53%) (Hobbs & Wynne, 1989). In a comparable study of 171 children referred for gastrointestinal complaints, 8 (4.7%) revealed anal or perianal abnormalities. One of 30 children referred for constipation had an anal fissure. No child had anal dilation or distortion of the anal opening (Lazar & Muram, 1989). The authors suggest that perianal abnormalities should raise suspicions of possible sexual abuse and be investigated.

◆ QUESTIONS THAT ARE OFTEN ASKED

Can a child be born without a hymen to explain the physical findings described?

There is no documented case of an infant girl born without a hymen. In two studies (Jenny et al., 1987; Mor & Merlob, 1988) 26,199 newborn girls were examined; all had hymens.

Can excessive masturbation or the use of tampons explain abnormal vaginal findings?

Masturbation and tampons do not cause injury to the hymen or internal genital structures. There is no evidence that use of tampons causes trauma to the hymen (Dickinson, 1945; Cowell, 1981; Stewart, 1990). Masturbation in girls usually involves clitoral or labial stimulation and does not cause hymenal injury (Hobbs & Wynne, 1989; Tipton, 1989).

Labbe (1990) described 10 boys with urinary tract infections apparently caused by the boys injecting water into their own urethras while bathing. No genital injuries were described. However, similarly, no injuries were seen in 38 infants with neurogenic bladder whose parents or caretakers catheterized them every 4 to 6 hours during the day for a mean of 28 months (Joseph et al., 1989).

Children who masturbate excessively or insert foreign objects into body orifices usually show no genital or anal injuries. Hyman et al. (1990) examined 97 mentally retarded individuals between 11 months and 21 years old whose behaviors included excessive masturbation and insertion of foreign objects into various body orifices. None had evidence of genital or anal injury.

Can a child contract a sexually transmitted disease by merely sharing the same bed, toilet seat, or towel with an infected individual?

In general, as the title implies, sexually transmitted diseases are sexually transmitted *(see discussion of sexually transmitted diseases in this chapter).*

Can horseback riding, gymnastics, or dancing cause permanent genital changes?

Injuries can occur with physical activities. When such injuries involve the genitalia, the event is very dramatic and will be reported immediately. If a physician finds hymenal changes after a child has disclosed sexual abuse or during a routine examination, injury from one of these activities is not being investigated because it would not be a reasonable explanation for the changes.

◆ BIBLIOGRAPHY

Bays, J, and Chadwick, D: Medical diagnosis of the sexually abused child, *Child Abuse Negl* 17:91-110, 1993.

Bays, J, and Jenny, C: Genital and anal conditions confused with child sexual abuse trauma, *Am J Dis Child* 144:1319-1322, 1990.

Berenson, AB, Heger, AH, Hayes, JM, Bailey, RK, and Emans, SJ: Appearance of the hymen in prepubertal girls, *Pediatrics* 89:387-394, 1992.

Bergeron C, Ferenczy, A, and Richart, R: Underwear: Contamination by human papillomaviruses, *Am J Obstet Gynecol* 162:25-29, 1990.

Chadwick, DL, Berkowitz, CD, Kerns, DL, McCann, J, Reinhart, MA, and Strickland, SL: *Color Atlas of Child Sexual Abuse*, produced by the California Medical Association's Maternal, Perinatal and Child Care Subcommittee on Child Abuse, Year Book Medical Publishers, Inc, Chicago, 1989.

DeJong, AR, and Finkel, MA: Sexual abuse of children, *Curr Probl Pediatr* XX:490-567, 1990.

Finkel, MA: Anogenital trauma in sexually abused children, *Pediatrics* 84:317-322, 1989.

Fleming, KA, Venning, V, and Evans, M: DNA typing of genital warts and diagnosis of sexual abuse of children, *Lancet* 11:454, 1987.

Gabby, T, Winkleby, MA, Boyce, WT, Fisher, DL, Lancanster, A, Sensabaugh, GF, and Crim, D: Sexual abuse of children: The detection of semen on skin, *Am J Dis Child* 146:700-703, 1992.

Gardner, JJ: Descriptive study of genital variation in healthy, nonabused premenarchal girls, *J Pediatr* 120:251-257, 1992.

Graves, HCG, Sensabaugh, GF, and Blake, ET: Postcoital detection of a male-specific semen protein: Application to the investigation of rape, *N Engl J Med* 312:338, 1985.

Heger, A, and Emans, SJ: American Academy of Pediatrics: Introital diameter as the criterion for sexual abuse, *Pediatrics* 85:222-223, 1990.

Herman-Giddens, ME, and Frothingham, TE: Prepubertal female genitalia: Examination for evidence of sexual abuse, *Pediatrics* 80:203-208, 1987.

Herr, JC, Summers, TA, McGee, RS, Sutherland, WM, Sigman, M, and Evans, RJ: Characterization of a monoclonal antibody to a conserved epitope on human seminal vesicle-specific peptides: A novel probe/marker system for semen identification, *Biol Rep* 35:773, 1986.

Hobbs, CJ, and Wynne, JM: Sexual abuse of English boys and girls: The importance of anal examination, *Child Abuse Negl* 13:195-210, 1989.

Huffman, JW, Dewhurst, CJ, and Capraro, VJ: *The Gynecology of Childhood and Adolescence*, ed 2, WB Saunders Co, Philadelphia, 1981.

Hyman, SL, Fisher, W, Mercugliano, and Cataldo, MF: Children with self injurious behavior, *Pediatrics* 85:437-441, 1990.

Kellogg, ND, and Parra, JM: Linea vestibularis: A previously undescribed normal genital structure in female neonates, *Pediatrics* 87:926-929, 1991.

Kerns, DL, and Ritter, ML: Medical findings in child sexual abuse cases with perpetrator confessions, (Abstract) *Am J Dis Child* 146:494, 1992.

Kirby, LT: *Fingerprinting: An Introduction*, Stockton Press, New York, 1990.

McCann, J: Patterns of healing in cases of sexual abuse, Paper presented at symposium *Health Sciences Response to Child Maltreatment*, San Diego, CA, January, 1988.

McCann, J, Voris, J, and Simon, M: Genital injuries resulting from sexual abuse: A longitudinal study, *Pediatrics* 89:307-317, 1992.

McCann, J, Voris, J, Simon, M, and Wells, R: Perianal findings in prepubertal children selected for nonabuse: A descriptive study, *Child Abuse Negl* 13:179-193, 1989.

McCann, J, Voris, J, Simon, M, and Wells, R: Comparison of genital examination techniques in prepubertal girls, *Pediatrics* 85:182-187, 1990.

McCann, J, Wells, R, Simon, M, and Voris, J: Genital findings in prepubertal girls selected for nonabuse: A descriptive study, *Pediatrics* 86:428-439, 1990.

Monteleone, J, Brewer, J, Scalzo, A, Doerhoff, F, Munkel, W, Heaney, S, Bowen, K, Scherzinger, P, and LaRock, T: Urethral dilatation as a physical finding in sexual abuse (abstract). VII International Congress on Child Abuse and Neglect Book of Abstracts. FP106, 1988.

Muram, D: Anal and perianal abnormalities in prepubertal victims of sexual abuse, *Am J Obstet Gynecol* 161:278-281, 1989.

Muram, D: Child sexual abuse: Relationship between sexual acts and genital findings, *Child Abuse Negl* 13:211-216, 1989.

Neinstein, LS, Goldenring, J, and Carpenter, S: Nonsexual transmission of sexually transmitted diseases: An infrequent occurrence, *Pediatrics* 74:67-76, 1984.

O'Rahilly, R: *Anatomy: A Regional Study of Human Structure*, ed 5, WB Saunders Co, Philadelphia, 1986.

Pacheco, BP, Di Paola, G, Ribas, JM, Vighi, S, and Rueda, NG: Vulvar infection caused by human papilloma virus in children and adolescents without sexual contact, *Adolesc Pediatr Gynecol* 4:136-142, 1991.

Paradise, JE: Predictive accuracy and the diagnosis of sexual abuse: A big issue about a little tissue, *Child Abuse Negl* 13:169-176, 1989.

Paradise, JE: The medical evaluation of the sexually abused child, *Pediatr Clin North Am* 37:839-862, 1990.

Paul, DM: The medical examination in sexual offenses against children, *Med Sci Law* 17:251-258, 1977.

Pokorny, SF, and Kozinetz, CA: Configuration and other anatomic details of the prepubertal hymen, *Adolesc Pediatr Gynecol* 1:97-103, 1988.

Steinhart, G, and Monteleone, JA: Unreported observation, 1990.

Teixeira, WRG: Hymenal colposcopic examination in sexual offenses, *Am J Forensic Med Pathol* 3:209-214, 1981.

Tipton, AC: Child sexual abuse: Physical examination techniques and interpretation of findings, *Adolesc Pediatr Gynecol* 2:10-25, 1989.

White, S, Ingram, DL, and Lyna, PR: Vaginal introital diameter in the evaluation of sexual abuse, *Child Abuse Negl* 13:217-224, 1989.

Woodling, BA, and Heger, A: The use of the colposcope in the diagnosis of sexual abuse in the pediatric age group, *Child Abuse Negl* 10:111-114, 1986.

Sexual Abuse– The Interview

Vicki McNeese, M.S.

In recent years, child sexual abuse has captured the attention of professionals and the general public. This is largely due to the highly publicized stories of children sexually molested by the very adults entrusted with their care and well-being. Yet despite our increased awareness and understanding of the dynamics of child sexual abuse, it continues to be a difficult, if not painful, topic for many to contemplate and discuss. Recent attention focused on child sexual abuse clearly depicts the potentially significant effects on and vulnerability of the alleged victim, the perpetrator, and their respective families, as well as on evaluators charged with investigating such allegations. It has become increasingly important to develop stringent standards for evaluation of sexual abuse allegations. Only through a comprehensive investigation of allegations, which includes objective, thorough, and well-documented interviews, can those involved best be protected.

In order to conduct objective, reliable, and child-sensitive interviews, professionals need an awareness and understanding of child development, the history and dynamics of sexual abuse, as well as a working knowledge of the continuing evolution of the evaluation process. Armed with this information, an evaluator can benefit from others' past experiences, positive and negative; assess potential pitfalls and risks to all those involved; and more confidently and comfortably address the challenging task at hand—the child interview.

♦ HISTORY

In the late 1970s and early 1980s, the growing battle against child sexual abuse, while not without opponents, seemed to be a safe and well-supported endeavor. However, as the momentum to identify and protect alleged victims of child sexual abuse grew, investigatory practices and disposition of such cases were increasingly called into question by critics. Hechler (1988) in *The Battle and the Backlash* described the mounting problems in the "child sexual abuse war." He identified clearly drawn lines between professionals regarding the prevalence of child sexual abuse, the credibility of children's statements, and the competence and objectivity of professionals who evaluate allegations of child sexual abuse.

♦ PREVALENCE

The dramatic increase in reports of child sexual abuse in the past decade has caused professionals to ask if current statistics indicate an epidemic of child molestation or if greater public awareness and acceptance have resulted in increased reporting. Since the victims of child sexual abuse often delay reporting or may never disclose their victimization, the true incidence of child sexual abuse is difficult, if not impossible, to ascertain.

Results of a national study *(The National Study of the Incidence and Severity of Child Abuse and Neglect, 1981)* and a privately conducted survey *(Los Angeles Times Poll, 1985)* estimate that approximately one in four girls will be sexually victimized by age 18 (Finkelhor & Hotaling, 1984; Finkelhor, 1986; and Finkelhor et al., 1990). Boys were initially considered to be less at risk for child sexual abuse; however, current epidemiological studies suggest that the incidence of sexual victimization of male children is notably higher than previously believed (Pescosolido, 1989). Childhood sexual abuse was reported by 16% of the males surveyed by the *Los Angeles Times* (1985). These findings, if extrapolated to the general population, suggest that one in six boys will experience sexual victimization. It has been proposed that victimization of boys may be comparable to that of girls, although, due to societal and gender expectations, males are less likely to report their victimization experiences. As a result, male victims are often not identified and thus do not receive appropriate intervention services.

As previously noted, there is considerable controversy and debate in the field of child sexual abuse regarding the accuracy of prevalence statistics. Many professionals contend that child sexual abuse continues to be underreported due to its nature of secrecy and lack of physical findings. On the other hand, critics of current practices cite significant problems in the investigatory process, particularly inadequate interviews conducted by overzealous and poorly trained evaluators, which leads to an overdiagnosis of child sexual abuse.

All professionals involved in evaluating allegations of child sexual abuse must attend to and objectively assess the criticism raised by colleagues. Rather than being viewed as forsaking the vigorous identification and protection of child victims of sexual abuse, honest consideration of criticisms can be used to ensure that evaluation practices are of the highest caliber. A comprehensive, well-documented evaluation by a competent evaluator will, in fact, serve to identify and protect a victimized child, as well as safeguard the rights of others involved. It should never be advocated that professionals, in our well-intended efforts to believe and protect a child, knowingly conduct a biased evaluation.

The evaluation of alleged victims of child sexual abuse is rapidly changing. Wherever possible, professionals responsible for assessing alleged victims and their families must be informed of recent findings in the disciplines of medical and mental health care as well as legal practice. Some clinicians responsible for a multiplicity of cases may feel ill-prepared to assess allegations of child sexual abuse. Even evaluators who feel confident in their knowledge of child development, as well as their ability to effectively communicate with children, are less confident in assessing the validity and credibility of a child's statement regarding sexual victimization. This is especially true if the alleged victim is a young child, developmentally delayed, and/or in any other way hindered in relating experiences and possible trauma.

Evaluators involved in interviewing children about child sexual abuse need to gather accurate information without suggesting particular responses to a child. A well-conducted interview should increase the likelihood that a child will be able to disclose any previous abusive experience and diminish the likelihood of obtaining false or inaccurate information. At the same time an objective, thorough, and well-documented interview will minimize the likelihood of erroneous conclusions.

It is critical that evaluators responsible for assessing allegations of sexual victimization of a child have knowledge and understanding specific to the field of child sexual abuse. Areas of particular concern include risk factors, the process of victimization, dynamics that may hinder a child's disclosure, and currently accepted techniques for evaluating alleged victims.

♦ RISK FACTORS

While any child is a potential victim of sexual abuse, Finkelhor (1986) has examined characteristics such as age, sex, ethnicity, and family relations to identify specific factors that may increase the risk for sexual victimization. His findings indicate that girls are at greater risk than boys. In general, children seem to be most vulnerable to sexual victimization during pre-adolescence, particularly between the ages of 8 and 12 years. Other risk factors cited include family disruptions; parental conflict, absence, or unavailability; and presence of a "nonbiological related father" (Finkelhor et al., 1990).

In recent years, the literature concerning child sexual abuse has also started to examine and document the vulnerability of children when a sibling, cousin, or nonrelated child in the home is engaging in sexually reactive or abusive behaviors (Johnson, 1988). DeJong (1989) concluded that sexual interactions among siblings and cousins are common and that reported cases are usually abusive. Evaluators need to be aware of the potential risk to children who have unsupervised or minimally supervised contact with a child or adolescent who is sexually acting out. A history of sexual victimization in the parents' family of origin and/or a previous sexual abusive experience may also increase a child's risk for sexual victimization.

♦ VICTIMIZATION PROCESS AND DISCLOSURE INHIBITORS

Child sexual abuse should be viewed as a *process* rather than an isolated event. Most children who are abused recognize that something is wrong, but some lack the maturity to identify what that is or know how to respond to it (Fay et al., 1991). In assessing cases of possible sexual abuse, it is important that evaluators recognize and understand the process of victimization, including reasons children don't tell or delay disclosure of abuse. Findings reported by Berliner and Conte (1990) suggest that the victimization process involves three overlapping processes: sexualization of the relationship, justification of the sexual contact, and maintenance of the child's cooperation. Results of this study indicate that virtually all children who disclose a history of sexual abuse say they wish they would have told someone earlier.

One of the most common, compelling, and obvious reasons children often don't "tell" is fear (Smith, 1985). Child victims of sexual abuse not only fear physical repercussions, but also fear potential loss of home and/or the love and attention of a nonoffending parent. The offender is usually considerably larger and stronger than the child and wields overt or covert authority. From this perspective, even a vague threat of violence might be sufficient intimidation to leave a child feeling powerless and afraid (Tobin & Farley, 1990). In assessing suspected victims of abuse, recognition of the power differentiation between an offender and a child victim is a key consideration.

Victims of sexual abuse often feel ashamed or guilty and find few safe opportunities to disclose their victimization. Although shame is a powerful factor in maintaining a child's silence, ignorance of personal boundaries and appropriate physical contacts, especially in young children, also contribute to a child's silence or delayed disclosure. Often by the time a child recognizes the abusive nature of a trusted adult's behavior, the child is likely experiencing feelings of responsibility, shame, and/or isolation—feelings that further inhibit disclosure of victimization experiences. It should be noted that some offenders, rather than using threats, secure a child's compliance and silence through bribes and/or special privileges.

All too often a child's safety depends solely on his or her ability to report the sexually victimizing experience. A frustration for many professionals in the field of child sexual abuse is a child's denial of sexual abuse in the face of overwhelming physical and/or corroborating evidence.

Literature as well as clinical experience emphasizes that a child's disclosure of sexual abuse is a dynamic process. Sorensen & Snow (1991) explored this phenomenon and outlined a process with definable phases and characteristics. Their findings suggest that disclosure follows a progression that may include denial, tentative disclosure, active disclosure, recantation, and reaffirmation. These authors report that denial is a frequent response when a child is too frightened, threatened, or insecure to acknowledge his or her victimization experience. Conclusions of the study reveal that 72% of the children in confirmed cases of sexual abuse initially denied any history of abuse. In only 11% of the cases examined did children actively disclose when they were first questioned.

Recognition of a disclosure progression challenges the common assumption that children can immediately make a disclosure with questioning. These findings have far-reaching implications for investigative procedures and suggest that evaluation protocols which provide more than a single opportunity for disclosure are most likely to facilitate collection of reliable and accurate information. While steps in the process of disclosure are identifiable and share common elements, it is important to recognize that the process for any individual child may be highly idiosyncratic.

◆ BEHAVIORAL INDICATORS

Children may manifest various behavioral changes in response to stress and/or trauma. The particular stress to which a child is reacting may be a divorce, death in the family, the family's relocations (which may necessitate multiple changes in the child's life), a significant illness or injury, physical maltreatment, and/or sexual victimization. Stress-related behaviors often observed in children include but are not limited to sleeping and eating disturbances, increased somatic complaints, regressed behaviors, anxiety and/or depression, changes in academic performance, and aggressive behaviors (Sgroi et al., 1983) (**Table 9-1**).

Table 9-1. Nonspecific Stress-Related Behaviors Observed in Children and Adolescents

In assessing stress-related behaviors the abruptness of onset, severity, and chronicity are factors that should be carefully considered. Abrupt and severe behavioral changes may be particularly indicative of emotional distress and/or possible trauma.

1. Sleep disturbances (e.g., nightmares, night terrors, fear of the dark or sleeping alone, trouble falling asleep and/or frequently awakening during the night, or excessive sleeping).

2. Changes in eating behaviors (e.g., loss of or sudden increase in appetite with resulting weight loss or gain).

3. Regressive behaviors (child's behavior regresses to earlier developmental level, such as clinging and separation difficulties, thumbsucking, and/or diminished bladder and/or bowel control in a child who had been successfully toilet trained).

4. Hyperactivity/hypervigilance/insecure behaviors.

5. Excessive and/or inappropriate fears (e.g., fear of a particular or familiar place, person, or activity not previously noted).

6. Hostile, aggressive, or acting out behaviors/play.

7. Varied and repeated somatic complaints with no known physical etiology.

8. Change/decline in academic performance, school avoidance, poor peer relations.

9. Behaviors suggestive of or in response to a high level of anxiety and/or depression (e.g., excessive crying, expressed feelings of hopelessness, withdrawal from family and friends, diminished interest in previously anticipated activities, decline in personal appearance, suicidal ideation and/or gesture, and substance abuse).

10. Delinquent and/or runaway behaviors.

Research in the area of child sexual abuse (Gomes-Schwartz et al., 1985; Finkelhor & Browne, 1985; Conte & Schuerman, 1987) has consistently concluded that children who have a history of child sexual abuse exhibit more symptoms than children who have no known history of sexual victimization. However, recent studies indicate that there does not appear to be any significant difference in stress-related symptom presentation between child sexual abuse and other types of trauma that children experience (Beitchman et al., 1991). The presence of nonspecific stress-related behaviors is an important factor in the overall evaluation of a child, although evaluators must be cautious when interpreting children's behaviors. Evidence of stress-related behaviors should not be a primary determinant in the belief that a child has been abused. Similarly, the absence of such behavioral reactions should not lead a professional to conclude that a child has not been abused. While most children who have been sexually abused do display some nonspecific stress-related behaviors, other sexually victimized children exhibit no significant observable behavioral reactions. Stress-related behaviors in children should alert a professional to a child's feelings of distress and possible trauma, and should be assessed further. Sexually abused children may have an increased prevalence of certain traits, but these traits may also be found in children without histories of abuse.

Specific behavioral reactions in children are often characteristic of that particular child's developmental level. The following outlines some abilities to be expected at specific levels:

Preschool Children

Preschool children demonstrate a variety of affective, cognitive, and behavioral symptoms in response to stress (Lusk & Waterman, 1986). Young children often respond to stress and/or trauma by exhibiting changes in eating and sleeping habits, chronic nightmares, regression, and an increase in fearful and clinging behaviors. Young children may also demonstrate changes in bowel and bladder control, with those who have been previously toilet trained beginning to wet and soil themselves. Preschool children may also demonstrate an increased activity level as well as aggressive behaviors in play activities and their interactions with others.

School-aged Children

School-aged children may demonstrate various emotional, cognitive, and behavioral changes that can be observed by parents and/or school personnel. These children may display notable moodiness, behaviors indicating a high level of anxiety and/or depression, and diminished academic functioning (Gomes-Schwartz et al., 1985). These affective and behavioral reactions may be accompanied by varied and repeated somatic complaints with no known physical cause.

Adolescents

Adolescents may come to the attention of mental health professionals in response to a crisis or an episode of acting out behavior such as a suicidal gesture, episodes of running away from home, or hostile, aggressive, and/or delinquent behaviors. Adolescents may also respond to personal and family stressors by withdrawing from family or friends, altering academic performance, or changing personal hygiene and appearance. It should be noted that due to the frequent delays in reporting incidents of child sexual abuse, adolescents may present with a history of chronic affective disturbances and behavioral problems. A comprehensive evaluation is indicated to fully assess the extent and origins of presenting problems.

Children may also come to the attention of professionals due to sexually reactive behaviors. While most stress-related behaviors are nonspecific for sexual abuse, Sgroi et al. (1988) have identified three sexually reactive behaviors likely to be seen in children who have been involved in direct or vicarious sexual experiences. Behaviors that have increased specificity for sexual abuse include excessive masturbation, sexual victimization of another child, and promiscuity. Developmentally inappropriate sexualized behaviors in children of all ages who have been sexually abused is one of the most consistent findings reported in the literature (Friedrich et al., 1986; Burns et al., 1988).

Children may also demonstrate sexualized behaviors that have not been identified as specific to sexual abuse but are suspicious for developmentally inappropriate sexual knowledge and/or experiences. If observed in a child or reported by a caregiver, such behaviors may warrant further evaluation.

These behaviors include but are not limited to the following:
— *Diminished personal boundaries, including indiscriminate kissing, hugging, and/or sexualized touching of other children or adults.*
— *Developmentally inappropriate "seductive" behavior to solicit attention, acceptance, and/or affection from significant others.*
— *Curiosity regarding genitalia or behavioral reactions to observed sexual material or situations that are atypical for that child's developmental level.*
— *Extreme reactions to bathing or toileting.*
— *Excessive fear or resistance to contact with the opposite sex.*
— *Strong resistance or refusal to participate in age-appropriate physical or social activities (i.e., physical education classes or sleeping over) where changing clothes or showering is involved.*

DIFFERENTIATING NORMAL FROM ABNORMAL SEXUAL BEHAVIOR

Since it has been well-documented that children who have a history of child sexual victimization often act out sexually and/or engage in sexual activity with other individuals, it is important that evaluators involved in evaluating allegations of abuse have an understanding of normal sexual behaviors in children. While information regarding developmental norms for sexual behaviors in children is limited, Sgroi et al. (1988) and Friedrich et al. (1991) have presented a developmental context for sexual behaviors observed within different age ranges for children. Normative data regarding sexual behavior of children at different developmental stages can guide an evaluator in differentiating normal sexual behaviors from those indicative of sexual abuse experiences.

Children who have a history of trauma, including sexual victimization, may present with symptoms associated with a diagnosis of post-traumatic stress disorder (PTSD). While post-traumatic phenomena have long been recognized in the literature, PTSD has only recently been examined as a possible consequence of child sexual abuse. Although now recognized as occurring in children, little is known about the course of PTSD in childhood. McLeer et al. (1988) cite evidence of PTSD symptom clusters in sexually abused children, including reexperiencing phenomena, avoidance behaviors, and autonomic hyperarousal. A follow-up study (Deblinger et al., 1989) of children hospitalized with psychiatric disorders with a history of sexual abuse reported that sexually abused children suffered significantly more re-experiencing phenomena than physically abused or nonabused subjects. McLeer and colleagues caution that children who develop PTSD may not only suffer from the direct trauma of their abuse, but may experience chronic symptoms that can interfere with a child's overall developmental progress.

♦ SCREENING AND REFERRAL PROCESS

Due to the complexity and the number of professionals who may be involved in evaluating alleged victims of child sexual abuse, it is necessary to organize initial screening and referral data. This can be accomplished using a standardized format *(see Telephone Referral/Screening Outline)*. The evaluators must exercise professional judgment when a request is received to interview an alleged victim of child sexual abuse, with an emphasis placed on meeting specific predetermined criteria before initiating any evaluation.

When it is determined that evaluation of an alleged victim of sexual abuse is appropriate, the standardized questionnaire can avoid duplicity of services and facilitate communication among professionals. Similarly, when other action is indicated and/or referral to another agency is made, the information can be easily documented.

Telephone Referral/Screening Outline

Date_____ Taken by _____

Patient Information:

Caller_____Relationship to Child _____

Child's Name_____BD_____Age_____Sex: M   F

Current Address_____Phone _____

Parent's Name _____

Living with: Parents___Mother___Father___Relative___Foster Care ___Other

Siblings (Names and Ages)_____

Current/Pending Legal Action: Divorce Y N   Custody Visitation Y N

    Other_____

Developmental Level of Child: Age Appropriate_____Delayed _____

Behavioral Indicators: Y N   Sexual Acting Out_____Stress-Related _____

Describe_____

Physical Symptoms: Y N   Describe _____

Referring Information:

Referred by_____ Agency _____

Address_____Phone _____

Reason for Referral _____

_____

_____

Hot Line Call Made: Y N   When_____Reported by _____

Other Agencies Involved: Y N   Name, Address, Telephone _____

_____

Is Child Currently Protected? Y N

Alleged Perpetrator(s) Name_____Relationship _____

Male_____Female_____Adult_____Child_____(Age)_____(Other)_____

Disclosure: None_____Purposeful_____Accidental_____Describe _____

Child Disclosed to: Mother___Father___Other Family___Peer___Other___

Reported Incidence: Single Multiple Last incident _____

Previous Interview(s): Y N By: DFS_____(Date)_____Police_____

        (Date)_____Other Professional_____(Date)_____

Results of Interview: Disclosed Sexual Abuse____Physical Abuse____Denied____

Previous P.E. Y N By:_____Date _____

Results of P.E. _____

Previous allegations of Sexual Abuse: Y N When _____

Disposition of those allegations _____

Previous Sexual Abuse Evaluation: Y N Location_____Date _____

Is child currently in counseling? Y N Provider _____

Plan:

Notified caller to make hotline report: Y N NA

Scheduled Appointment: Y N Interview_____P.E._____

        Parent consult_____Date_____

Referred child to DFS___Police___Therapist___Attorney___Medical Ser___

(Name)_____Other_____

Comments_____

_____

Additional Telephone Contacts: _____

_____

♦ EVALUATION PROCESS

The following interview protocols reflect guidelines for the evaluation of sexual abuse of children proposed by the American Professional Society on the Abuse of Children (1990), the American Academy of Child and Adolescent Psychiatry (1988), and the American Academy of Pediatrics (1991).

♦ CAREGIVER INTERVIEW

When abuse is suspected and it has been determined that a child will be interviewed, it is recommended that a minimum of one interview be conducted with the parent(s)/primary caregiver and/or other appropriate individual(s), in order to obtain applicable information in the following areas: family constellation and history, child's health history and current status, child's developmental level, behavioral indicators, psychosexual history including family's attitude and practices regarding privacy, nudity, sexual attitudes, and bath time and bedtime patterns, and allegations or suspicion of possible sexual abuse. Detailed information regarding the child's initial disclosure of the event is also obtained. This interview includes the parent or primary caregiver's interpretation of the child's statement and/or behavior regarding possible sexual abuse. It is recommended that this interview be conducted by the primary evaluator, prior to the initial child interview, and not with the child present. Information regarding sexual abuse allegations obtained from a caregiver in the presence of the child may contaminate any subsequent statements made by the child. A child may feel compelled to provide information to the evaluator which is consistent with the caregiver's statements. Statements made by caregivers should be documented specifically and in detail. Caregivers should be informed that information obtained may be shared with other professionals who are investigating allegations of abuse, as well as those making decisions regarding the appropriateness of legal action.

An information gathering interview may be conducted with the alleged perpetrator, if he or she is a member of the child's immediate family (parent), when this is deemed appropriate. The purpose of this interview is to gather pertinent data regarding the child's level of functioning and behaviors, the family situation, and the alleged or suspected perpetrator's knowledge of current allegations. The alleged or suspected perpetrator, as well as other family members, may also be referred for further evaluation by an independent assessor.

If information gathered during a parent interview reveals a current pending divorce or custody dispute and the allegations of sexual abuse were first disclosed during legal proceedings, it may be advisable to refer some or all parties (parent[s] and child/children) to an evaluator with the capabilities and expertise to evaluate all family members. Appropriate referral information should be provided to the family as indicated.

RELEASE OF INFORMATION
To facilitate review of all relevant information, parents are requested to sign release of information forms. This enables the evaluator to request information from other sources. Parents may also be requested to sign authorizations permitting the evaluation results to be shared with appropriate child protective, law enforcement, and/or treatment services.

Caregivers are informed that in the case of an open child abuse investigation, investigatory agencies (including child protective services, law enforcement agencies, and court officials) may have access to information gathered during an evaluation. They are also told that reports will be made as mandated by state law to child protective services. Information regarding evaluation procedures will be reviewed with parents at the initial interview.

ASSESSMENT OF FAMILY DYNAMICS
In conducting the parent/caregiver interview, the evaluator should carefully assess family dynamics and possible pathologies. It is important to identify stressors other than sexual abuse that may explain a child's statement or behaviors. Diagnostic information gathered at the time of the parent/caregiver interview is important, not only to the evaluation process, but also in the formulation of an appropriate treatment plan.

A behavior rating scale may also be used to gather specific information about the types and intensity of a child's problematic behaviors. The rating scale is completed by the child's parent(s) or primary caregiver.

The following is a sample of a parent/caregiver interview that organizes material gathered at the time of the initial contact with the parent or caregiver. This interview format may be modified to meet the needs of a particular agency and/or individual evaluator.

Parent/Caregiver Interview Outline

Date: _____
Primary Evaluator: _____

Parent/Caregiver Interview: (Not to be conducted in presence of the child).

Person(s) Interviewed_____Relationship to Child _____

Family Constellation: (Members in Household)

Adult _____Relationship to Child _____

Adult_____ Relationship to Child _____

Adult_____ Relationship to Child _____

Child_____ Relationship _____

Child_____ Relationship _____

Child_____ Relationship _____

Others_____ Relationship _____

Caretakers Outside of the Home _____

_____

_____

Family History:

Parents are: Married_____Divorced_____Separated_____Single _____

If parents divorced or never married, does child have visitation with noncustodial parent? Y N   Visitation Schedule _____

Date of last visit _____

Child lives with: Parents___Mother___Father___Foster Care___Other ___

Legal action pending: Y N Divorce___Custody/Visitation_____

History of Child Sexual Abuse in mother's family of origin: Y N

If Yes, Victim_____Alleged Perpetrator _____

History of Child Sexual Abuse in father's family of origin: Y N

If Yes, Victim_____ Alleged Perpetrator _____

History of Child Sexual Abuse of other siblings/children in household: Y N

If Yes, Victim _____

Alleged perpetrator _____

Has child had unsupervised contact with any above named alleged perpetrators? Y N If Yes, has child ever alleged child sexual abuse by person(s)? Y N Identify/Describe_____

History of psychiatric illnesses in family: Y N _____

History of drug/alcohol abuse in family: Y N_____

History of domestic violence in family: Y N_____

History of previous child sexual abuse in family: Y N _____

Physical abuse in family: Y N_____

Previous involvement of Child Protective Services: Y N Date _____

Describe_____

Police involvement: Y N Date_____Describe_____

Mother history of: Sexually Transmitted Disease_____Genital Warts_____

I.V. Drug Use_____ HIV+ _____

Father history of: Sexually Transmitted Disease_____Genital Warts_____

I.V. Drug Use_____ HIV+ _____

Has child been exposed to pornographic material?   Y N Describe_____

Background Information of Child:

Birth history: Unremarkable_____Remarkable _____Describe_____

Developmental level: Age Appropriate_____Delayed_____

Language development: Age Appropriate_____Delayed_____

Toilet trained: Y N Age: _____

Stress-related behaviors: Y N Describe _____

Onset and length of behaviors:_____

School/Daycare (Name):_____Grade _____

Academic performance: Average or Above_____Below Average_____

Special education services: Y N _____

History of chronic health problems: Y N _____

History of UTI/bladder infections: Y N Date: _____

History of chronic constipation: Y N _____

History of genital injuries, surgeries, diagnostic procedures: Y N _____

Current medication: Y N _____

Past or current physical symptoms: _____

Present sleeping arrangements in household: _____

Family stressors during past year?_____

Has child disclosed history of child sexual abuse? Y N _____

Describe _____

Child disclosed to: (Name) _____

Relationship_____Date _____

Disclosure: Purposeful_____Accidental_____Spontaneous_____

          Upon Questioning_____ By Whom_____

Has child displayed developmentally inappropriate sexual knowledge,
sexualized behaviors, and/or excessive masturbation? Y N Explain_____

Alleged perpetrator(s) (Name):_____

Relationship:_____Location:_____

Last known contact (Date): _____

Does child have current contact with named individual? Y N

Describe_____

Hot line Report made: Y N Date_____Reporter _____

Status of alleged perpetrator_____
Other agencies involved: *(See Referral Form)*

Previous interview(s), P.E.(s), and results *(See Referral Form)*

_____

Does parent/caregiver believe child sexual abuse allegations? Y N

Uncertain_____

Reason: _____

Collateral Information:

Child reports others present at time of abuse: Y N

Describe_____

Others state they observed incident(s) of abuse: Y N

Describe_____

Release of information signed to obtain/release information to:

Name/Address:

    Private Pediatrician Y N _____

    Hospital Y N_____

    Division of Family Services Y N_____

    Law enforcement Y N _____

    Therapist Y N _____

    Other Y N _____

◆ CHILD INTERVIEW GUIDELINES

The initial child interview is conducted after the caregiver interview has been completed. Ideally, a minimum of two interviews should be conducted with the child. A young child or a child identified as having special needs, such as developmental delay or language impairment, can require additional interviews. At some point in the evaluation process, the child will be questioned directly about sexual abuse. However, repeated questioning of a child regarding sexual abuse, when the child is not reporting or denying abuse, is contraindicated.

It is preferable that one evaluator conduct both caregiver(s) and child interviews to foster continuity and consistency. Following collection of parent, child, and collateral information, impressions regarding the credibility and reliability of a child's statements, the probability that sexual victimization has occurred, and the presence of alternative explanations may be formulated. Based on all available information, conclusions and recommendations can be provided to caregivers and appropriate investigative authorities. The evaluator should attempt to reconcile the content of the interview with other information.

It is important to focus on and be sensitive to the child's needs at the time of the interview. Children quickly assess the interest, investment, and ease of the evaluator.

The evaluator must create a safe and private atmosphere that fosters rapport and trust, diminishes feelings of anxiety, and enables the child to talk openly. This includes securing child-sized furniture and arranging the surroundings in a way that is child-friendly. Availability of materials such as paper, pencils, and crayons is suggested to put the child at ease, facilitate nonverbal communication, and help the child clarify verbal statements. Adequate time should be allotted so that neither the evaluator nor the child feels rushed. The evaluator must be sensitive to the child's pace and emotional responses. If a child is hungry, tired, or needing a bathroom break, the outcome of the interview may be compromised.

It is important to make the evaluation as predictable as possible for the child. Explain the purpose and format of the assessment, and address the child's expectations and/or fears. While appropriate reassurances can foster rapport and communication, the evaluator is cautioned not to make promises he or she will be unable to keep. Often a child will ask the evaluator, "If I tell you, will you tell my Mom/Dad?" or "If I tell you, will you promised not to tell anyone?" The evaluator needs to be honest and supportive regarding the need to ensure the child's safety. An evaluator can respond to a child's concern by saying, "After we talk, I'll do everything I can to help keep you safe and tell you what I know will happen next." If a child feels betrayed by the evaluator's use of information obtained, it can potentially have negative effects on the child's well-being and on the outcome of the evaluation.

THE DEVELOPMENTALLY APPROPRIATE INTERVIEW

The interviewing approach and the language used by the evaluator should be developmentally appropriate and match the child's age and level of functioning. It is necessary to establish the terminology the child uses for people, things, body parts, and sexual behaviors. The evaluator should ask the child to define words that may be ambiguous before using them in the interview. Words such as "case" and "counselor" may not mean the same thing to a child as they do to the evaluator and should be clearly defined.

Given the importance of communication between the evaluator and child during the interview process, close attention should be given to the language exchange. The evaluator should use language sensitive to a child's developmental level. Language should be adapted to fit the child's vocabulary and kept consistent throughout the interview.

Using developmentally sensitive language is particularly important when interviewing young children. Saywitz (1990) advocates using several short questions, such as "Who was there?" or "Where was your mom?" rather than long complex questions. Questions that are direct and use short words, simple verbs, and single negatives are also more likely to be understood by a young child. Miscommunication is likely to occur when children are asked long and complex questions. This is particularly the case with young children who typically respond only to the part of the question they understand, disregarding other information contained in the questions. Likewise, young children are unable to recognize their partial understanding or confusion in order to ask for clarification. The use of developmentally sensitive techniques can contribute significantly to the evaluator's confidence that the child has a good understanding of the questions asked, and has responded accordingly.

It is also helpful to clarify response options for the child before direct questioning. The child should know that he or she is not *required* to answer the question asked by the evaluator; the child has permission to refuse to answer. Explain to the child that saying "I don't want to talk about that now" in response to a direct question is preferable to giving inaccurate information or saying "I don't know" when he or she does in fact know. Also, if a child declines to respond to a specific inquiry, the evaluator may want to follow up with additional questions, such as "What do you think might happen if you talk about it?" This helps to clarify how the child is feeling and the source of any reluctance. Hopefully, more than one interview has been scheduled, so the evaluator will have the opportunity to return to sensitive questions that a child was unwilling to answer.

If following the initial interview with a child, the evaluator is uncertain of the child's cognitive functioning, has doubts about the child's level of language development, or suspects the presence of possibly severe emotional and/or psychiatric disturbance, further assessment by a mental health professional may be suggested as part of the evaluation. A psychological/psychiatric assessment is indicated in cases where the child's delayed development and/or disturbance could significantly interfere with the child's ability to participate in the evaluation. If the child was previously evaluated by a psychiatrist and/or psychologist, the evaluator should attempt to secure appropriate records before completing the sexual abuse evaluation.

As stated earlier, it is best to try to interview the child more than once. The following discussion outlines the stages of the process assuming that more than one interview is possible. If only one interview is feasible, the evaluator will need to be thorough and take sufficient time to obtain an accurate evaluation of the situation.

INITIAL INTERVIEW WITH THE CHILD

At the initial interview the evaluator's primary tasks are to establish a safe and comfortable environment, develop rapport, and assess the developmental level of the child. Young children may be fearful and resistant to separating from their parent(s). While a parent may accompany the child to the initial meeting to assist in giving the child a sense of security, the evaluator should advise the parent(s) that sexual abuse allegations will not be discussed with the parent(s) present.

At the initial interview, in the context of acclimating the child to the evaluation process, the evaluator is advised to ask the child "Do you know why you are here today?" or "How come you are here today?" or "What did your (Mom, Dad, Grandma, etc.) tell you about coming here today?" If the child indicates that his or her intent is to discuss allegations of sexual abuse by saying "To tell what happened" or "To talk about what my (uncle, etc.) did," the evaluator should follow a child's lead by saying "Tell me about that." At that time, the evaluator should encourage a narrative statement from the child with minimal questioning. Follow-up inquiries to clarify a child's initial report can then be asked. However, if a child claims no understanding of the purpose of the appointment and appears reluctant to discuss it further, the evaluator should provide a simple explanation, identifying the interview as an opportunity for the child and evaluator to talk about the child's everyday experiences and anything that might be troubling the child.

At the first session the evaluator can begin assessing the child's overall development (cognitive, language, social and interpersonal, and emotional) and relevant skills through structured dialogue, informal tasks, and play activities. Concepts such as size, number, location, and time should be assessed. Observation and interaction with the child can yield an estimation of the child's level of functioning. The establishment of developmental landmarks can assist the evaluator to interpret information obtained during child interviews. If significant delays are detected in a child's intelligence and/or verbal skills, the interviewer must modify the interview to fit the child's particular level of development and special needs. This is critical for the information gathered to be considered valid.

As part of developmental screening procedures, especially with young children, the evaluator can gather information by asking a child to:

1. Provide basic personal identifying information (i.e., name, age, place of residence, members of household, school placement, and caretakers). Other pertinent questions may be asked to gather information regarding custodial care and relationships. Children may be asked to outline a typical day at their parent's/caregiver's house. This can give information regarding family practices, including bath and bedtime patterns.

2. State gender of self and others.

3. Identify and label general body parts.

4. Identify and label genitalia and functions of identified body parts.

Dolls (with or without anatomic detail) or simple standard boy and girl drawings may be used to aid and clarify an child's identification of general body parts and genitalia.

Unless a child is deemed to be at immediate risk or spontaneously reports allegations of sexual abuse, direct questioning regarding possible sexual abuse is not recommended during the initial interview.

SUBSEQUENT INTERVIEWS WITH THE CHILD

The second (and subsequent) interview(s) begin with the evaluator reestablishing contact and rapport with the child. Conversation regarding the child's recent (since the first interview) family and school activities as well as play activities can put the child at ease. Reviewing activities and the content of the discussion of the initial interview can also help in reacclimating the child to the surroundings.

The primary purpose of the second and subsequent interviews is to directly question the child about possible occurrence of sexual abuse. The evaluator uses open-ended questions that facilitate the child's disclosure rather than questions that suggest particular responses. Initially the evaluator should attempt to obtain a narrative response that involves only minimal nondirective questioning. The child should be encouraged to relate information regarding possible inappropriate touch in his or her own words. Later questioning can be directed from general open-ended questions to more focused and specific inquiries, as is appropriate for each child. For young and/or special needs children, it may be necessary and appropriate to ask more specific or directive questions (Faller, 1990). As questioning moves from general open-ended inquiries to more directive questions, the confidence level in a child's responses diminishes, although evaluators should be aware that information obtained from directive questions can be accurate and reliable.

One technique to note is the "cognitive interview," which is useful in interviewing some children by aiding their recall of reported experiences (Saywitz, 1992). This technique, developed by R. Edward Geiselman, is a guided memory search which has recently been modified for use with children. Modifications provide specific instructions to children regarding the demands of the interview task, as well as revisions of general retrieval aids. Saywitz (1992) reports that results from recent studies utilizing these techniques indicate improvement in the quality of useful information gained from latency age children without creating increased inaccuracy.

Upon completion of the evaluation, it is important to acknowledge a child's participation, cooperation, and assistance in providing information regarding his or her experiences. The evaluator can express understanding that the evaluation may have been challenging and stressful, at times. The evaluator can be supportive by listening to and validating a child's feelings, although caution should be used not to suggest that a child should respond or feel a particular way. The child may be encouraged to ask the evaluator any questions, discuss any concerns or fears, or express current needs. As previously noted, one of the evaluator's responsibilities is to make the evaluation as predictable as possible for the child. Depending upon information known to the evaluator, the child should be informed in age appropriate language what is likely to happen next. A young child might be told, "We are done talking. You are going home with your mom now. Another man wants to talk to you about what you told me. He'll call your mom. Then you and your mom can go and see him at his office." If a child is referred for counseling, that may also be explained briefly. Lastly, the evaluator can help the child identify support people in his or her environment (i.e., "Who can you talk to if you have a question or feel worried, scared, etc.?") It is also reassuring for the child to know that the evaluator can be available if a child wants to talk further.

The following interview format or a modified version may be helpful in guiding and documenting child interviews.

Child Interview Outline

Child's name:_____Evaluator:_____

Date:_____Others present: _____

General identifying information obtained from child:

Name Y N ____Age Y N ____Birthdate Y N

Home address Y N ____School placement Y N ____

Identified members of household: _____

_____

Other: Caretakers/daycare:_____

_____

Developmental assessment (young children)

Identification of:

Primary colors Y N   Letters/numbers Y N

Drawings House Y N   Tree Y N   Person Y N   Other_____

Other measures:_____

_____

_____

Affect/mood: _____

Behavioral observations/activity level: _____

Information gathered during initial session (i.e., typical day): _____

_____

_____

Subsequent Child Interview(s):

Date:_____

Assessment of Possible Sexual Abuse:

Questioning presented to ascertain if child knows purpose of appointment on this date.

Do you know why you are here today? _____

Who brought (came with) you today? If child gives name(s) only, attempt to establish relationship to child. _____

_____

Ascertain if named person told child to relate any specific information to evaluator on this date.

Did (named person) tell you to say anything to me today? If yes, what? _____

_____

Use of dolls (anatomically detailed or nonspecific) for identification and clarification of general body parts Y N   Genitalia Y N

Demonstrates knowledge of general body parts Y N   Method of parts labeled (pointing/verbally labeled)

Identified private parts: Male Y N Female Y N

Method of parts labeled: (pointing/verbally labeled)

Labels male genitalia: Y N_____

Demonstrates knowledge of function: _____

Labels female genitalia: Y N _____

_____

Demonstrates knowledge of function: _____

Assessment of child's understanding of different kinds of touch.

Describe: _____

_____

_____

Adequate understanding demonstrated: Y N

Questioning to address possible sexual victimization of child:

If the child discloses sexual victimization, the evaluator should attempt to obtain a narrative of the sexual abuse allegation.

Tell me about that (what happened). Continue to gather information with similar statements.

_____

_____

_____

_____

If child gives a limited statement and/or is unable to give a narrative response, more direct questioning may be necessary to obtain additional identifying information and/or clarification.

If a statement of inappropriate touch is given, an attempt should be made to ascertain the following information: (If multiple perpetrators are identified, efforts should be made to gather information on a single individual or abusive experience at a time to avoid confusion.)

Identification of alleged perpetrator(s)

Relationship of alleged perpetrator(s) to child

Sex and age of alleged perpetrator(s)

Type(s) of inappropriate touch

Time, location(s), frequency, and context of alleged abuse

Presence or absence of element of secrecy

Circumstances of initial disclosure, including person, time, location, and context

Other children or adults directly or indirectly involved in present allegations of abuse

Physical and/or behavioral response(s) of child at time of abuse (i.e., physical discomfort, actions taken, etc.)

Any prior history or allegations of abuse

Any attempts by adults to instruct child to give inaccurate information

Dolls used in sexual abuse assessment for clarification of child's statements: Y N
Anatomically detailed: Y N Nonspecific: Y N

_____

_____

_____

_____

_____

_____

ANATOMICALLY DETAILED DOLLS

A word of caution should be added regarding the use of interview aids, such as anatomically detailed dolls and/or drawings. Although these may be useful for clarification and/or demonstration of a child's statement, the interpretation of a child's drawings or interactions with anatomically detailed dolls must be made cautiously. Information gathered from these techniques should be viewed as supplemental data, but never as conclusive evidence that sexual abuse has occurred. Doubt cast on the usefulness and reliability of the dolls was clearly illustrated by recent court decisions in California in which evidence obtained from use of anatomically detailed dolls was disallowed (*In re: Amber B. & Tella B., 191 Calif. 3rd 682, 1987; In re: Christine C & Michael C, Calif App. 3rd 676, 1987*). Critics alleged that anatomically detailed dolls are anatomically distorted and/or suggestive, and lead normal nonabused children to engage in sexually explicit play that may be misinterpreted by evaluators as evidence of abuse. Others charge that the use of anatomically detailed dolls during interviews of suspected victims teaches children responses favored and reinforced by the interviewer (Wakefield & Underwager, 1988).

Current research findings support the usefulness of anatomically detailed dolls in evaluating child sexual abuse, but professionals are cautioned to know accepted practice and limitations in their use. Examination of 17 different sets of anatomically detailed dolls revealed that when extrapolated to adult human proportions, the sizes of genitalia and breasts of the dolls were not found to be exaggerated (Bays, 1990). Furthermore, Sivan et al. (1988) assessed interactions of nonabused children with anatomically detailed dolls and concluded that doll play of children with no reported history of sexual abuse is unlikely to be characterized by aggressive or explicit sexual activity. Likewise, Everson and Boat (1990) examined sexualized doll play among young children and found that anatomically detailed dolls are not overly suggestive to young, sexually naive children. They found the dolls useful in assessing a child's sexual knowledge and exposure to developmentally inappropriate sexual behaviors. These findings also were supported by a study conducted by White et al. (1986) who reported that sexually abused children exhibit more sexually specific behaviors than do children who have no known reported history of sexual abuse.

To address the criticism that the use of anatomically detailed dolls impacts a child's subsequent sexual behaviors, Boat, Everson, and Holland (in press) conducted follow-up interviews of 30 mothers whose children had been exposed to anatomical dolls. While some children were reported as demonstrating a heightened awareness of sexual body parts, none of the children was identified as displaying behaviors that might be misconstrued as indicating that sexual abuse had occurred (Everson & Boat, 1990). Similarly, Aman & Goodman (1987) had previously indicated that the use of anatomical dolls, in and of itself, does not lead to false reports of abuse, even under conditions of suggestive questioning.

As with any assessment instrument, the use of anatomically detailed dolls should be only one aspect of a comprehensive evaluation. It appears that, at the present time, anatomically detailed dolls may be most useful as a supportive tool in a comprehensive evaluation to assist young or linguistically impaired children to clarify and/or demonstrate alleged inappropriate sexual contact. With regard to their admissibility as evidence into court proceedings, Myers & White (1989) advise interviewers to be prepared to describe the specific use and reason for using the dolls in a particular case; to be familiar with the research on anatomically detailed dolls and be certain that accepted practice in the field was followed; and to know the limits in the use of anatomically detailed dolls and recognize them for what they are—an interview tool.

DRAWINGS

As previously noted, drawings can be a useful interviewing aid. Drawing is a form of expression that is familiar even to young children. Often, through drawings, a child can communicate ideas and feelings to adults while achieving a sense of mastery and competence. The use of drawings may be especially helpful with young children, children who are hesitant, and/or those with immature verbal abilities.

For very young and/or highly traumatized children, drawings can provide a safe avenue for expression of both events and emotions (Burgess et al., 1981). A child may spontaneously depict an abusive experience that can be used to assist the child in disclosing a history of sexual victimization (**Figures 9-3 to 9-6**). Similarly, the evaluator can request that a child draw typical daily activities, family members, and/or interactions with significant others, which may illustrate areas in the child's life that warrant further evaluation. Drawings can also be used to clarify and validate a child's statement of sexual abuse (**Figure 9-2**). After a child completes a drawing, the evaluator should never assume understanding, but rather should ask the child to "Tell me about your picture." If the explanation is vague or incomplete, the evaluator can ask questions by beginning at the top of the figure(s) and progressively moving downward, asking "What is this?" or "Tell me about this part."

Clinical data in the literature suggest that sexually abused children are more likely to draw genitalia than those children who report no history of sexual victimization. Research findings on children 3 through 7 years of age reveal that young children with a history of sexual abuse are five to seven times more likely to draw genitalia than nonabused children (Hibbard et al., 1987; Hibbard & Hartman, 1990). However, it should be emphasized that although the presence of genitalia in a child's human figure drawing may be an indicator of possible sexual abuse, it is not conclusive. Likewise, the absence of genitalia does not exclude the possibility of sexual victimization (**Figures 9-4 and 9-7**).

♦ DOCUMENTATION

When an allegation of sexual abuse is assessed, the implications are profound for the child, alleged offender, and their respective families, as well as the evaluator. Accurate recording of information obtained is *critical*. It is common for court proceedings regarding sexual abuse allegations to take place months or even years after allegations were initially presented and evaluated. As a result, detailed written and/or taped documentation regarding evaluation procedures, including statements made by the child, caregiver, alleged offender, and collateral sources, is of utmost importance.

The ability of authorities to protect a child who is alleging sexual abuse frequently depends on the quality and comprehensiveness of the evaluator's records.

Pertinent information to be noted each time a child is seen includes the following:

1. Individual(s) who accompanied the child to evaluation sessions
2. Persons in the room at the time of the interview
3. The location of the interview
4. The date and time of day the interview took place
5. The length of the interview
6. The use of any interview tools

It is recommended that specific questions regarding possible sexual victimization as well as the exact responses (verbal and behavioral) made by a child are completely, accurately, and objectively documented. Myers (1991) has outlined factors in addition to interview questions and the content of a child's statement that have specific legal implications and should be carefully documented when obtained from a child or parent(s).

He stresses the need to document factors that immediately surrounded the disclosure statement, including:

1. The nature of the event(s) surrounding a child's disclosure
2. The lapse of time between the event(s) and the statement
3. The emotional condition of the child
4. The speech pattern displayed by the child (e.g., speech hurried)
5. The physical condition of the child at the time of the statement (e.g., injury and/or physical discomfort)
6. Spontaneity of child's statement
7. Child's statement in response to questions
8. Existence of first safe opportunity to make disclosure statement (e.g., child in prior custody of alleged offender with recent placement in safe setting).

As previously indicated, detailed documentation of all aspects of the evaluation, especially a child's statement, can have a significant impact on the protection of a child, as well as on the final disposition of the case. A primary responsibility of the evaluator is to accurately assess and document a child's competence to make a reliable statement. Factors surrounding a child's statement that should be documented include spontaneity in reporting an abuse experience, consistency of core details (over time and with prior statements), child's affective state, use of age-appropriate language and words to describe sexual contact(s), content of play behaviors or gestures that clarify or demonstrate a child's description of abuse, and evidence of developmentally inappropriate knowledge of sexual acts, anatomy, or vocabulary.

Myers (1991) also advises that information regarding a child's developmental competence and maturity, memory, and abilities to observe, communicate, and differentiate fact from fantasy should be noted in the record. Likewise, the evaluator should document any motive expressed by a child or adult to fabricate, deny, or postpone disclosure of sexual abuse. Drawings, handwritten statements, or other materials introduced by the child should be appropriately labeled and maintained as part of the permanent record.

Use of Audio and Videotaping

Audio and videotaping of child interviews continues to be controversial and lacking apparent consensus among professionals. It is suggested that evaluators who utilize audio and videotaping closely follow accepted practice for taping, storage, and release of information. Myers (1992) presents an overview of the advantages, disadvantages, and legal implications of videotaping.

♦Allegations of Sexual Abuse in Divorce and Child Custody Disputes

Sexual abuse allegations that arise during divorce and child custody proceedings, as noted earlier, present particular challenges to the evaluator. Such allegations are often viewed with immediate skepticism. This may, in part, be due to general public opinion that in the context of a divorce and/or custody dispute a parent or child may be motivated to deliberately give false information in an attempt to secure a favored legal decision.

Professionals disagree on the true incidence of false allegations of sexual abuse that emerge during court litigation involving child custody and visitation rights. Green (1986) reported the incidence of false allegations in such cases as "strikingly high," failing to confirm sexual abuse allegations in four of 11 children he evaluated for suspected sexual abuse during child custody disputes. Citing "an emerging national hysteria regarding the problem of sexual abuse," Blush and Ross (1987) identified a pattern (SAID syndrome) believed to be specific to sexual abuse allegations in present and past divorce situations. The SAID Syndrome (Sexual Allegations in Divorce) is defined as a particular phenomenon which occurs when sexual abuse allegations develop within a pre or post divorce context and when a family unit has become dysfunctional as a result of the divorce process.

While allegations of sexual abuse in divorce and child custody disputes may be regarded by some with suspicion, research findings do not consistently support the assumption that false allegations of sexual abuse in separated and divorcing families are common. Results of a study by Thoennes and Tjaden (1990) do not support previous clinical conclusions that suggest a disproportionately higher incidence of false allegations in custody and visitation disputes. Their findings indicate that allegations of sexual abuse made at the time of litigation regarding custody and/or visitation are no more likely to be determined false than are sexual abuse allegations in the general population.

In contrast to the dispute concerning false allegations, figures regarding the existence of sexual abuse allegations in families after separation or divorce do indeed indicate a higher incidence than in the general population (Corwin et al., 1987). Reasons cited for a higher incidence of allegations of sexual abuse in divorcing families include stress, familial dysfunction, and increased opportunities for sexual victimization due to parental separation or divorce. In addition, separation from the abuser may provide the first safe opportunity for a child to disclose that abuse has taken place. Corwin and associates suggest that separation weakens an abusive parent's ability to enforce secrecy, while increasing the willingness of the nonoffending parent to accept the disclosure and take protective action. It should also be noted that following a parental separation a child's risk for extrafamilial sexual abuse may be higher due to a change in caregivers, including the presence of a nonbiological parental figure in the home.

Allegations of sexual abuse made in the context of parental separation or divorce should not be readily dismissed due to situational factors, but rather given serious consideration and thoroughly evaluated. A complete evaluation of the parents, as well as the child, is indicated to ensure the child's safety and emotional well-being. Allegations of sexual abuse of a child by a parent indicate that a child is at emotional risk even when allegations are unsubstantiated (Bresee et al., 1986).

◆ EVALUATION OF INFORMATION OBTAINED IN INTERVIEWS

The interview with the child is often denoted as the "cornerstone" of a sexual abuse evaluation. Upon completion, the evaluator must assess the reliability and credibility of a child's statement(s) to determine the degree of probability that sexual victimization has occurred.

The use of predetermined criteria to assess a child's statements and behavior in allegations of sexual abuse can assist in minimizing evaluator bias. The following characteristics of a child's statement and behavior are associated with true allegations of sexual abuse (Faller, 1990):

Description and/or knowledge of sexual behavior:
— description of specific sexual acts
— description of sexual acts from a child's viewpoint
— sexual knowledge beyond that expected for the child's developmental stage

Emotional reaction of child to sexual abuse:
— child's state of mind and affective responses at the time of disclosure
— child's recollection of feelings at the time of the abuse

Details provided about the context of abusive situations:
— identity and relationship of alleged offender
— sex and estimated age of alleged offender
— when and where abuse occurred
— what the victim and alleged offender were wearing
— what clothing was removed and by whom
— whereabouts of other family members
— how alleged offender induced child to be involved
— elements of secrecy or coercion
— other idiosyncratic details/events

Note: Positive findings in the three major areas are not found routinely in every case of sexual victimization.

Schetky (1988) has also proposed factors that enhance a child's credibility. She notes numerous characteristics including (1) behavioral changes specific to sexual abuse and/or nonspecific stress-related changes; (2) the presence of sexual themes in a child's play and drawings; (3) progressive sexual activity over time; (4) secrecy; (5) delayed disclosure; (6) a description of psychological coercion; and (7) physical indicators.

In evaluating a child's statement for reliability and validity, close attention should be given to the child's language (words), ability to relate core events, and spontaneity. A child's interpretation and subsequent description of sexual victimization is dependent on the child's cognitive development, verbal abilities, and the extent of his or her life experiences.

Other factors that may corroborate a child's statement and should be considered include statements indicative of sexual victimization overheard by others, any eyewitness accounts, and the presence of multiple victims with consistent statements of sexual abuse (Myers, 1991).

◆CONCLUSIONS

Evaluators are faced with the dilemma that there are few absolutes in the area of child sexual abuse. Exceptions include pregnancy in a child under 12 years of age or medical evidence of specific sexually transmitted disease in young children *(see Chapter 8, Physical Examination in Sexual Abuse)*. However, after careful consideration of all available information, an evaluator can render one of the following possible findings (Swan, 1989). Conclusions are based on degrees of probability that sexual abuse has occurred.

Reliable history of sexual abuse
  Child gives clear, consistent statements of sexual abuse in age-appropriate
  language. There is no clear evidence of alternative explanations for a child's
  statement or behaviors, or motivation for a child or reporting adult to give false
  information. Corroborating factors may be present, including physical findings
  or behavioral indicators specific to sexual abuse.

Suspected sexual abuse
  The presence of physical or behavioral indicators that are consistent with
  sexual abuse although child does not make a clear statement or denies
  sexual victimization.

Appropriate concern/insufficient information
  A child may demonstrate stress-related behaviors or present vague statements of
  vulnerability. However, there is no statement or there is denial of inappropriate
  sexual contact, and supportive evidence is insufficient for findings.

No evidence of sexual abuse
  Information indicates child or reporting adult made false statement. Presence of
  alternative explanation for child's statement and/or behaviors, or
  misinterpretation of initial statement or behavior of child by significant adults.

◆RECOMMENDATIONS

Following evaluation of all available information and formulation of a conclusion, an interviewer may make recommendations regarding issues of protection, placement, custody and/or visitation, and the appropriateness of additional diagnostic or treatment services. The final deposition of cases regarding allegations of sexual abuse investigated by child protective services and/or law enforcement agencies is the responsibility of those agencies. However, conclusions and recommendations made by the evaluators may be valuable input in making placement and treatment decisions for children and their families.

Figures 9-3, 9-4, 9-5, and 9-6 are a series of drawings by one child.

Figure 9-1. *A 9-year-old victim of sexual abuse drew a picture of herself, at right, with her therapist. A rainbow protects them from the turmoil and chaos shown above. Drawings by sexually abused children often depict some type of shield from environmental stressors.*

Figure 9-2. *A 9-year-old depicts sexual abuse by adult. Picture shows type of abuse, location and time of abuse, as well as emotional responses of child and offender.*

Figure 9-3. *A 4-year-old victim depicts abusive mother, above, and father (Figure 9-4).*

Figure 9-4. Drawing by 4-year-old girl at initial interview when asked to draw a picture of her father. Presence of genitalia in drawing facilitated child's disclosure of sexual abuse.

Figure 9-5. Drawing by 4-year-old girl at initial interview when asked to draw a picture about her family. Child described fondling of her younger brother's genitalia at her father's instruction.

Figure 9-6. A 4-year-old draws nurturing caregiver in foster home. There is a striking difference between this drawing and the previous ones.

Figure 9-7. Drawing of human figure with genitalia by 3-year-old boy.

♦BIBLIOGRAPHY

Aman, C, and Goodman, G: Children's use of anatomically detailed dolls: An experimental study. Paper presented at the National Center on Child Abuse and Neglect's Symposium on Interviewing Children, Washington, DC, 1987.

Bays, J: Are the genitalia of anatomical dolls distorted? *Child Abuse Negl* 14:171-175, 1990.

Beitchman, J, Zucker, K, Hood, J, DaCosta, G, and Akman, D: A review of the short-term effects of child sexual abuse, *Child Abuse Negl* 15:537-556, 1991.

Berliner, L, and Conte, J: The process of victimization: the victim's perspective, *Child Abuse Negl* 14:29-40, 1990.

Blush, G, and Ross, K: Sexual allegations in divorce: The SAID syndrome, *Conciliation Court's Review* 25(1):1-11, 1987.

Boat, B, Everson, M, and Holland: Maternal perceptions of nonabused young children's exposure to anatomical dolls, *Child Welfare*, in press.

Bresee, P, Stearns, G, Bess, B, and Packer, L: Allegations of child sexual abuse in child custody disputes: A therapeutic assessment model, *Am J Orthopsychiatry* 56(4):560-569, 1986.

Burgess, A, McCausland, M, and Wolbert, W: Children's drawings as indicators of sexual trauma, *Perspect Psychiatr Care* 19(2):50-58, 1981.

Burns, N, Meyer-Williams, L, and Finkelhor, D: Victim impact. In *Nursery Crimes, Sexual Abuse in Day Care*, Sage Publications, Inc, Newbury Park, CA, 1988, pp. 114-123.

Conte, J, and Schuerman, J: Factors associated with an increased impact of child sex abuse, *Child Abuse Negl* 11:201-211, 1987.

Corwin, D, Berliner, L, Goodman, G., Goodwin, J, and White, S: Child sexual abuse and custody disputes: No easy answers, *J Interpersonal Violence* 2:91-105, 1987.

Deblinger, E, McLeer, S, Atkins, M, Ralphe, D, and Foa, E: Post-traumatic stress in sexually abused, physically abused and nonabused children, *Child Abuse Negl* 13:403-408, 1989.

DeJong, A: Sexual interactions among siblings and cousins: Experimentation or exploitation? *Child Abuse Negl* 13:271-279, 1989.

Everson, M, and Boat, B: Are anatomical dolls too suggestive? *The Advisor*, Newsletter of the American Professional Society on the Abuse of Children 3(2):6,14, 1990.

Everson, M, and Boat, B: Sexualized doll play among young children: Implications for the use of anatomical dolls in sexual abuse evaluations, *J Am Acad Child Adolescent Psychiatry* 29(5):736-742, 1990.

Faller, K: Types of questions for children alleged to have been sexually abused, *The Advisor*, Newsletter of the American Professional Society on the Abuse of Children, 3(2):3-5, 1990.

Faller, K: Criteria for judging the creditability of children's statements about their sexual abuse. Child Protective Investigative Team Training, UT Social Work/Office of Research and Public Service 1990.

Fay, J, Adams, C, Flerchinger, BJ, Loontjens, L, Rittenhouse, P, and Stone, ME: *He Told Me Not to Tell*, King County Sexaul Assault Resource Center, 1991.

Finkelhor, D: *A Sourcebook on Child Sexual Abuse*, Sage Publications, Inc, Beverly Hills, CA, 1986.

Finkelhor, D, and Browne, A: The traumatic impact of child sexual abuse: A conceptualization, *Am J Orthopsychiatry* 55(4):530-541, 1985.

Finkelhor, D, and Hotaling, G: Sexual abuse in the national incidence study of child abuse and neglect: An appraisal, *Child Abuse Negl* 8:23-33, 1984.

Finkelhor, D, Hotaling, G, Lewis, IA, and Smith, C: Sexual abuse in a national survey of adult men and women: Prevalence, characteristics, and risk factors, *Child Abuse Negl* 14:19-28, 1990.

Friedrich, W, Grambsch, P, Broughton, D, Kuiper, J, and Beilke, R: Normative sexual behavior in children, *Pediatrics* 88(3): 456-464, 1991.

Friedrich, W, Urquiza, A, and Beilke, R: Behavior problems in sexually abused young children, *J Pediatr Psychol* 11(1):47-57, 1986.

Gomes-Schwartz, B, Horowitz, J, and Sauzier, M: Severity of emotional distress among sexually abused preschool, school-age, and adolescent children, *Hosp Community Psychiatry* 36:503-508, 1985.

Green, A: True and false allegations of scxual abuse in child custody disputes, *J Am Acad Child Psychiatry* 25(4):449-456, 1986.

Guidelines for the clinical evaluation of child and adolescent sexual abuse: Position statement of The American Academy of Child and Adolescent Psychiatry, *J Am Acad Child Adolescent Psychiatry* 27:655-657, 1988.

Guidelines for the evaluation of sexual abuse of children. Committee on Child Abuse and Neglect: American Academy of Pediatrics, *Pediatrics* 87(2):254-260, 1991.

Guidelines for psychosocial evaluation of suspected sexual abuse in young children. Task Force chaired by Lucy Berliner, American Professional Society on the Abuse of Children, 1990.

Hechler, D: The battle for acceptance. In *The Battle and the Backlash, The Child Sexual Abuse War,* Lexington Books, Lexington, MA, 1988, pp. 1-12.

Hibbard, R, and Hartman, G: Genitalia in human figure drawings: Childrearing practices and child sexual abuse, *J Pediatr* 116(5):822-828, 1990.

Hibbard, R, Roghmann, K, and Hoekelman, R: Genitalia in children's drawings: An association with sexual abuse, *Pediatrics* 79(1):129-137, 1987.

Johnson, T: Child perpetrators: Children who molest other children: Preliminary findings, *Child Abuse Negl* 12:219-229, 1988.

Los Angeles Times poll, 1985.

Lusk, R, and Waterman, J: Effects of sexual abuse on children. In MacFarlane, K, and Waterman, J, eds: *Sexual Abuse of Young Children*, The Guilford Press, New York, 1986, pp. 101-118.

McLeer, S, Deblinger, E, Atkins, M, Foa, E, and Ralphe, D: Post-traumatic stress disorder in sexually abused children, *J Am Acad Child Adolescent Psychiatry* 27(5):650-654, 1988.

Myers, J: Legal implications of interviewing children, *Legal Issues in Child Abuse and Neglect*, Sage Publication, Newbury Park, 1992, pp. 80-83.

Myers, J: Legal implications of interviewing sexually abused children. Presentation: The Seventh National Symposium on Child Sexual Abuse, Huntsville, AL, 1991.

Myers, J, and White, S: Dolls in court? *The Advisor*, Newsletter of the American Professional Society on the Abuse of Children 3(2):5-6, 1989.

National Center on Child Abuse and Neglect, US Department of Health and Human Services, Washington, DC, 1981.

Pescosolido, F: Sexual abuse of boys by males: Theoretical and treatment implications. In *Vulnerable Populations: Volume II*, Lexington Books, Lexington, MA, 1989, pp. 85-109.

Saywitz, K: Developmental considerations for forensic interviewing, *The Advisor*, Newsletter of the American Professinal Society on the Abuse of Children 3(2):2,5,15, 1990.

Saywitz, K: Enhancing children's memory with the cognitive interview, *The Advisor* , Newsletter of the American Professional Society on the Abuse of Childern 5(3):9-10, 1992.

Schetky, D: The clinical evaluation of child sexual abuse. In *Child Sexual Abuse, A Handbook for Health Care and Legal Professionals*, Brunner/Mazel, Inc, 1988, pp. 57-78.

Sgroi, S, Bunk, B, and Wabrek, C: Children's sexual behaviors and their relationships to sexual abuse. In *Vulnerable Populations: Volume I*, Lexington Books, Lexington, MA, 1988, pp. 1-13.

Sgroi, S, Porter, F, and Blick, L: *Validation of Child Sexual Abuse. Handbook of Clinical Intervention in Child Sexual Abuse*, Lexington Books, Lexington, MA, 1983, pp. 39-41.

Sivan, A, Schor, D, Koeppl, G, and Noble, L: Interaction of normal children with anatomical dolls, *Child Abuse Negl* 12:295-304, 1988.

Smith, S: Children's Story: *Sexually Molested Children in Criminal Court*, Launch Press, Walnut Creek, CA, 1985.

Sorensen, T, and Snow, B: How children tell: The process of disclosure in child sexual abuse, *Child Welfare* 70:3-15, 1991.

Swan, H: Presentation: Sexual abuse and the law, St. Charles County Family Stress Council, Inc, and Sexual Abuse Task Force, St. Charles, MO.

Thoennes, N, and Tjaden, P: The extent, nature, and validity of sexual abuse allegations in custody/visitation disputes, *Child Abuse Negl* 14:151-163, 1990.

Tobin, P, and Farley, S: *Keeping Kids Safe: A Child Sexual Abuse Prevention Manual*, Learning Publications, Inc., Holmes Beach, 1990.

Wakefield, H, and Underwager, R: *Accusations of Child Sexual Abuse*, Charles C Thomas, Publishers, Springfield, IL, 1988.

White, S, Strom, G, Santilli, G, and Halpin, B: Interviewing young sexual abuse victims with anatomically correct dolls, *Child Abuse Negl* 10:519-529, 1986.

Chapter **10**

MULTIPLE PERSONALITY DISORDER

BARBARA Y. WHITMAN, PH.D.
PASQUALE J. ACCARDO, M.D.

Sheryl, a 12-year-old seventh grader, was referred to a multidisciplinary clinic for evaluation of continuing learning problems that had become more problematic after she entered a departmentalized learning situation with multiple teachers. She was noted to be behind in reading, had severe spelling and other sequential processing difficulties, and displayed attentional and reading comprehension problems. She was described as chronically withdrawn, asocial, and moody, and her parents would frequently find her sitting in the family room and staring for hours, particularly when upset. It was also reported that she exhibited occasional flashes of rage. However, it was noted that she seemed to display episodes of brilliance and talent. She occasionally wrote sophisticated and spellbinding poetry and sometimes produced astonishingly talented artwork. She was unable to explain what enabled her to perform so brilliantly or prevented her from regularly producing work of this caliber.

Although socially withdrawn and inept most of the time, it appeared that if Sheryl wanted to reach a goal she would single-mindedly pursue it. For example, she managed to get herself elected class president, and she succeeded at track and field events. She was described by both of her physician parents as a misfit in the family, unable to relate to or get along with her three highly successful siblings. After extensive psychoeducational and psychological testing, she was diagnosed as having a neurologically based specific learning disability, a dysthymic disorder, and an overanxious disorder of childhood. Appropriate therapies were recommended.

Sheryl made an emergency return to the clinic when she was a senior in high school.

She was talking of suicide, and her parents wanted additional evaluation. During this emergency visit, it was reported that psychotherapy had never been pursued because her parents felt her behavioral problems were related to stubbornness; they did not believe a child could be "depressed." This episode of suicidal ideation was actually her second. Her first episode had occurred two years previously, and Sheryl had been referred to her pastor for counseling. This second episode concluded with an immediate referral to a psychiatrist for medication and therapy.

The following September Sheryl enrolled as a freshman at a local private college. Within six weeks she was exhibiting major vegetative symptoms, so noticeable that college personnel contacted Sheryl's therapist. She was hospitalized for four weeks. After the first week she was allowed to leave the hospital during the day to attend classes. After being admitted to the hospital there was an instant stabilization of mood, occurring within 48 hours. During hospitalization it was noted that she had a shallow level of understanding of the need to explore how she got there, how to cope when leaving, and a generally oppositional demeanor toward any subject other than how she could "get out of here." After discharge she exhibited no engagement or effort during her weekly therapy sessions, a marked alteration in her demeanor. Before she left college for winter break, she reported being afraid to go home because "she didn't want the voices to start again."

After she returned from the school break, the subject of voices was vigorously pursued during therapy. Simultaneously, reports from a consulting psychiatrist noted that she was presenting an "entirely different" young

lady to him than was reported as being presented to the primary therapist. Confrontation of these discrepancies with Sheryl ultimately led to discussions of incidents such as memory loss, articles appearing that she didn't remember buying, and people telling her she had a good time at a movie she didn't remember attending. Ultimately the therapist invited the source of the "voices" to emerge. To date, 33 personalities have been identified. Etiology appears to have been chronic and sadistic sexual abuse from age 3 to age 10 by her maternal grandfather. Both Sheryl and her family indicated that "she was his special grandchild" and they further emphatically reported that "she was devastated when he died." She has, as yet, not divulged the facts of the abuse to her family.

Sheryl typifies the difficulty of diagnosing multiple personality disorder (MPD) in children. For her, there was never any indication or even an index of suspicion of any sort of abuse, which is the major etiologic factor for this disorder. Her "host" personality is indeed "learning disabled," although several of her other personalities are artisans. She was so scared of the "voices" that she never divulged their presence until moving to her college dorm. This move so greatly altered her external environment that she was unable to continue to function and hospitalization was required. Even with this episode, it was not until she was going home for a month and would be unable to see her therapist that she "let it slip" that she heard voices. Her age of presentation of this symptom, combined with her history, was compatible with a schizophrenic process. However, enough contradictory data were present that shortly thereafter, the MPD diagnosis was confirmed.

191

◆ DEFINITION

Multiple personality disorder (MPD) can be a devastating and refractory psychiatric disorder, the origins of which lie in the pre-latency period of childhood (Braun & Sachs, 1985; Kluft, 1985a; Frischholz, 1985; Putnam et al., 1986; Baldwin, 1990; Hornstein & Tyson, 1991). Since more than 90% of all cases are directly attributable to severe abuse in early childhood (Boor, 1982; Braun & Sachs, 1985; Greaves, 1980), current theories interpret MPD as one form of childhood post-traumatic stress disorder (Putnam, 1985; Spiegel, 1984, 1986).

MPD is characterized by the existence within an individual of two or more distinct personalities or personality states. In classic cases each personality is fully integrated, having his or her own unique memories, behavior patterns, and social relationships; in others there may be some sharing of memories and commonalities of behavior. When the personality is dominant, it determines the host individual's behavior (DSM-III-R, 1987). Transition from one personality to another is usually sudden (within seconds to minutes) and is most often precipitated by stress, reflecting a complex psychophysiologic process termed dissociation.

PREDISPOSING FACTORS

Two predisposing factors for MPD are currently recognized: (1) exposure to severe and overwhelming trauma, particularly during childhood, such as frequent and inconsistent alternating abuse and love, and (2) an innate and probably genetically determined psychophysiologic tendency to dissociate. Both factors—exposure and genetic tendency—are necessary; neither factor alone is sufficient to produce the disorder (Braun, 1984).

◆ EPIDEMIOLOGY AND HISTORY

Determining the incidence and prevalence of MPD has been hampered by two difficulties: (1) diagnosing the disorder and (2) dealing with the sociopolitical and professional context in which diagnoses are conceptualized. A brief understanding of the history of this disorder in psychiatric thinking is needed to understand the current state of knowledge regarding incidence and prevalence.

MPD is not a new psychiatric entity. Recognizable case histories of MPD in both adults and children were reported as early as 1817 (Taylor & Martin, 1944; Alvaredo, 1989). In the last major pre-Freudian psychology textbook, cases of MPD were given extensive coverage (James, 1890). The disorder was then lost in psychiatric controversy for a number of years and has only recently resurfaced as a "legitimate" psychiatric entity (Putnam, 1991a). Since 1980, a number of investigators have begun to clarify the epidemiology and consequences of this disorder.

In the earliest reports, MPD was described as the splitting of the total consciousness into complementary parts that coexist and mutually ignore each other, yet can share objects between or among themselves. The primary self often needs to invent "hallucinations" to mask and hide from itself the strange incidents and incongruous deeds of the secondary personalities. Each personality, nevertheless, has a conscious unity, continuous memory, habits, a name, and a sense of its own identity. This phenomenon was considered rare, associated with hysterical anesthesia, and discussed in conjunction with hypnotism, spiritualism, and the question of the location of the seat of the soul.

Although trauma similar to what might produce amnesia was considered a possible precipitating factor, the explanatory model used was post-hypnotic suggestion. Descriptions of the dissociative process were subjected to conflicting theoretical interpretations by Janet and Freud (Alexander & Selesnick, 1968). Unfortunately, the recommended use of a planchette to facilitate communication with these alter egos tended to link the entire MPD phenomenon with the interpretation of Charcot's hystero-epilepsy as a product of suggestion, if not fraud (Freud, 1948; Owen, 1971). Because of these linkages, Freud's theory of psychic repression prevailed over Janet's theory of dissociation (Masson, 1984) as the accepted description of unconscious functioning, resulting in a 60-year hiatus (circa 1920-1980) in the study of dissociative disorders. At the same time that interest in dissociation as a psychic concept was declining, Bleuler introduced the diagnostic entity "schizophrenia," which misinterpreted disorders of thought accompanied by hallucination as a psychic schism or two personalities. Subsequently, many MPD patients were misdiagnosed as schizophrenic (Rosenbaum, 1980).

Accurate statistical evaluation of MPD also relates to its etiologic relationship with severe abuse. Only recently have we recognized the widespread incidence of child abuse and child sexual abuse.

In 1980 in the brief section of the *Comprehensive Textbook of Psychiatry* dealing with incest, the only epidemiological comment is a reference to a 1955 paper estimating that incest affects one family out of a million in North America. This estimate was low by four orders of magnitude. . . . Child abuse underwent a 10,000 fold shift in prevalence in a very short time, and was transformed from a vanishingly rare curiosity to a major public health problem (Ross, 1991).

A parallel shift in the epidemiologic estimates of MPD is only now beginning to follow the earlier shift in its major etiologic determinant. Current prevalence estimates range from a very conservative 0.5% of the general population to a high of 10%. A recent prevalence study in the city of Winnipeg, Manitoba, Canada, yielded a 1% population prevalence rate (Ross et al., 1990); there is no reason to think American rates are substantially different. In a referred population (individuals who have come for counseling and been referred to psychologists and psychiatrists), prevalence rates may reach 25%.

♦ ETIOLOGY AND PATHOPHYSIOLOGY

MPD is most often associated with maltreatment beginning in early childhood and frequently extending through adolescence. The abuse, which can be sexual, physical, emotional, or often some combination of these, is usually "unprovoked" and often exhibits "marked deviance." "Unprovoked" implies that the abuse is not excessive discipline in response to child misbehavior, it is rather purposefully imposed, unusually severe, and often exhibiting both bizarre form and sadistic ambience. The extreme end of this abuse spectrum is exemplified by satanic cult practices, which can include witnessed child sacrifice (Young, 1988). Finally, the abuse is usually inflicted by the parent or another primary caregiver.

The last two decades have forced the recognition of the reality that sexual abuse of children is common. Simultaneously, mental health professionals have acquired a new and deeper understanding of the psychological impact of traumatic events. This knowledge is both derived from and focused by the post-traumatic stress disorders resulting from the Vietnam combat experience. Research has yielded better understandings of the nature of trauma and the trauma response mechanisms that define these disorders. Research has also highlighted the potential for long-term sequelae following traumatic events, particularly when appropriate psychological intervention is unavailable. Such knowledge has contributed to the evolution of procedures such as routine "crisis debriefing" and supportive therapy following major traumatic events, for example, earthquakes, hurricanes, riots, and other natural or man-made disasters.

While much of the progress in this area evolved from post-trauma work with adults, children have not escaped attention. Events such as The Chauchilla bus incident, firearm tragedies in schools, and similar events where children were the primary targeted victims have all broadened our understanding of both the immediate impact and the long-term sequelae of such trauma in children. While emotional health cannot be guaranteed through immediate and competent intervention, emotional devastation and long-term illness are inevitable when intervention is lacking. The prevalence of severe child abuse and child sexual abuse as well as the increased knowledge regarding the long-term consequences of such trauma allow the recognition and identification of MPD as the most severe form of post-trauma consequence.

DISSOCIATION

Since physical escape from abuse or trauma is often impossible for the victims, the only form of escape is psychological via dissociation route. Dissociation is a psychological separation from the current feeling or cognitive state. In MPD the dissociation is so complete that a discontinuity of "self" and "memory" results. In this situation, escape by dissociation, while psychologically creative, is also a psychologically devastating solution to an inescapable evil. The solution is creative in that the child maintains his or her love for the perpetrator in one personality, the memory of the painful experience and feelings in another, and frequently the angry and aggressive emotions and behaviors in yet another. Unfortunately, once that route of defense has been chosen, external stimuli unrelated to the original stress can precipitate dissociative episodes and the creation of additional personalities.

Not all victims of severe child abuse or child sexual abuse dissociate. Many authors note that some forms of dissociation are normal developmentally (Putnam, 1991b). Even among a severely abused population not all dissociation leads to MPD; many children and adults dissociate emotionally as a coping strategy. This dissociation, however, is limited to the emotional sphere with no loss of continuity of self or memory. Thus many victims will describe severe abuse in great detail, with no apparent demonstration of affect. They often note companion depersonalization and out-of-body phenomenon such as "there was a spot on the wall where I routinely went and watched as he raped me." For these victims, therapy involves a reintegration of the feelings and the experiences along with a working through of the feelings.

The ongoing puzzle of MPD is that the dissociation is so complete that the multiple personalities can continue to coexist. Each personality is either unaware of the others or there is an internal system of personalities who are aware of each other, but who operate outside the conscious awareness of the host personality. Frequently one or several of these personalities will emerge, engage in behavior not compatible with the host personality, and then retreat, leaving the host personality "holding the bag." Thus the prevailing personality, unaware of the existence of the others, must often manage the consequences of another personality's actions, such as meeting the demands of the promises made by these other selves. All the while the host personality remains unclear as to why he or she does not remember either the interactions described or the periods of time during which they occurred. People with MPD become masters at covering up these perceived deficiencies. Their lives are a constant balancing and disguising act for what each personality perceives as its "terrible memory," if not its "craziness," and which must be kept secret from other people.

◆DIFFERENTIAL DIAGNOSIS

Despite clear-cut and readily identifiable risk factors, the diagnosis of MPD in high–risk pediatric populations remains the exception rather than the rule. In addition to the factors already discussed, underdiagnosis is also due, in part, to the nature of the disorder itself.

DIAGNOSTIC CRITERIA

There are two diagnostic criteria for multiple personality disorder:

1. The existence within an individual of two or more distinct personalities or personality states, each with its own relatively enduring pattern of perceiving, relating to, and thinking about the self and the environment.

2. The recurrent assumption of full control of the person's behavior by at least two of these personalities.

These criteria are deceptively straightforward. Conceptually, confirming the diagnosis of MPD, particularly in children, is complex, as illustrated by the reported 6.8-year average interval between the first mental health contact and an accurate diagnosis made in adults (Putnam et al., 1984). Studies also indicate that the MPD child receives an average of 2.7 other psychiatric diagnoses before an accurate diagnosis of MPD is made (Hornstein & Putnam, 1992).

What is it about this disorder that makes diagnosis so difficult? Unlike the diagnosis of depression, where a clearly defined symptom list can be used to make systematic inquiry for critical findings, MPD presents the examiner with multiple personalities who frequently are not consciously aware of one another. Since dissociative processes occur, by definition, out of consciousness, one cannot merely ask "Do you dissociate?" In the majority of MPD adults, unless an episode of dissociation is witnessed and recognized, diagnostic data must be pursued through more indirect approaches.

Diagnosing childhood MPD is doubly difficult. The presenting plethora of affective symptoms, post-traumatic indicators, conduct disorders, hallucinatory signs, attention discrepancies, and school difficulties parallels the presentation of dissociative disorders in adults. The investigation of these symptoms in children, however, is more often performed through physical or developmental channels rather than psychiatric services. Thus, many MPD children are referred to neurologic services for possible seizure disorders presenting as "staring episodes," or to developmental clinics for evaluation of inconsistent attention and learning problems. Even when a child psychiatric evaluation is obtained, a number of developmental factors make it difficult to determine if a given child's dissociative behavior is normal or pathological. Even when clearly pathologic, some personalities can be nonverbal or preverbal. These personalities can exhibit marked acting out that is diagnostic, but they still could be unable to understand or respond to diagnostically useful questions.

For the diagnosis of children, the data collection must start from the diagnostic red flag of possible abuse and the examiner must obtain information from both the child and caregivers. A family history of MPD represents a significant and heavily weighted risk factor. To the extent that such a history is present, the clinical task is more to rule out MPD rather than to rule it in. The diagnostic process precisely parallels that of adult MPD but seeks signs that are exhibited within the child's developmental sphere of action (**Table 10-1**).

Table 10-1. Differences Between Adult and Child Dissociation	
Adult	**Child**
Forgetfulness and Amnesia	
Inexplainable and bothersome forgetfulness leading to a sense of always being on edge and needing to constantly conceal and check their behavior;	Amnesia for recent events such as abuse, schoolwork, tantrums, rage attacks;
Unexplained periods of lost time (both minutes and days) sometimes viewed by patient as "walking blackouts," but unrelated to alcohol use; *and/or* Waking up and not knowing how they got where they were or what they were doing in the recent past;	Perplexing forgetfulness such as time lost, tardiness with an inability to remember where they just were;
The appearance of items of clothing, jewelry, books or other personal goods in their possession that they cannot recall buying (or conversely the unexplained disappearance of such items);	The appearance of items of clothing, toys, school supplies that they have not been given by parents and cannot recall buying (or the unexplained disappearance of such items)
Long periods of lost time such as several childhood years in succession;	Adolescent MPDs may report this same phenomenon.
Flashbacks or broken threads of memory;	Adolescent MPDs may report this same phenomenon.
Forgetfulness Reflected in Interpersonal Relations	
People calling them other names and seeming to know them while they do not recognize these people; *and /or*	Confusion regarding the names of teachers or peers;
People telling them things they have done or said that they can't remember and the lack of memory is not explained by use of drugs or alcohol;	Denial of behavior witnessed by others—often accompanied by a fierce sense of injustice if punished or confronted for lying;
A childhood reputation for being called a liar that remains puzzling to the host personality.	Apparent inability to learn from experience such as discipline or punishment.
Affective Symptoms	
Unexplained severe mood swings;	Severe periodic depression sometimes including suicidal gestures but with no clear precipitating factor.

Table 10-1. Differences Between Adult and Child Dissociation —*Continued*	
Adult	Child
Multiple Psychiatric Diagnoses	
Behavior Symptoms	
Dichotomous behavior states and/or impulsive and dangerous risk taking as reported by friends.	Subtle alternating personality changes such as a basically shy child exhibiting depressed, angry, seductive, or regressive episodes.
	Extreme regressive episodes followed by amnesia such as thumbsucking in a pre-teen or sudden dramatic yet transient loss of language or motor skills.
An awareness of sometimes being unable to control their own behavior.	Frequent angry outbursts without apparent provocation and frequently with extreme physical strength.
Marked differences in handwriting from time to time.	Dramatic fluctuations in conduct and performance (especially in abilities relating to school work, games, and music.
	Continuously changing preferences in food, clothing, and social relationships.
Somatic Symptoms	
A history of many somatic complaints unexplained by a physical disorder or other psychiatric entities (e.g., panic disorder).	Physical complaints and injuries of vague origin, sometimes clearly self-inflicted.
Daydreaming, Sleepwalking, Depersonalization	
Frequent troublesome "dreamlike" states including sleepwalking.	Excessive daydreaming, sleepwalking, and trancelike and spacey behavior including concentration and attentional difficulties, not seizure disorder based.
Auditory "Hallucinations" and Imaginary Companions	
Occurrence of voices that argue in their heads but are not psychotic in character—that is, voices from inside (other personalities) perhaps speaking of "we" or "us."	Hallucinated voices either friendly or unfriendly, often attributed to imaginary companion.
History of imaginary companion beyond age 6.	Imaginary companion still real to a child 6 years or older.

♦CLINICAL PRESENTATION

MPD is depicted in the popular media as a flamboyant, rare female disorder. The cinematic presentations of *The Three Faces of Eve* (Thigpen & Checkley, 1957) and *Sybil* (Schreiber, 1973) compellingly depicted the complexity, devastation, and totality of this disorder. MPD, however, is neither rare nor, in most affected individuals, flamboyant (Kluft, 1985b, 1991). Unlike most psychiatric disorders, where the presenting problem usually indicates a specific differential diagnostic decision tree, the chief complaint in MPD rarely suggests an MPD diagnosis. The most frequently described presentation of MPD is depression in the host personality (Putnam, 1989). A typical MPD history will be vague and unclear. There are many "I can't remember for sure" answers or clever and subtle redefining of the questions by the MPD patient through oblique or tangential responses aimed at covering up half-realized memory gaps. Facts stated at one time may be "forgotten" or denied by another personality at another time. A useful diagnostic clue is presented when the therapist begins to wonder who is more forgetful—the professional or the patient. When this occurs it should raise the question of need for a major reorganization of the presenting data to account for this "forgetfulness." That perspective should lead to consideration of MPD in the differential diagnosis, particularly in the presence of a previous history of abuse.

Clinical diagnosis of MPD in both children and adults requires a different perceptual filter for the "third ear"; the usual clues and cues regarding truthfulness or defensiveness can be missing. A host personality asked about diagnostic behaviors could truthfully deny their presence because that personality can be completely unaware of events that were engaged in by another of the subject's personalities. The clinician's usual "lie detection" parameters such as eye gaze, body posture, nervous gestures, and defensive voice tones are of little use for the simple reason that the particular personality is not "lying." This phenomenon is of special importance to professionals investigating the possibility of multigenerational child sexual abuse. We will illustrate the diagnostic process from the perspective of diagnosing an adult. As complex as this process is, it must be remembered that this complexity is magnified in children due to their developmental level and language developmental issues.

TWO-LEVEL INVESTIGATION

Once adult MPD is suspected, confirmation requires a two-level diagnostic investigation. Since independent external validation of continuity and discontinuities of psychological functioning and behavioral contrasts is frequently sought from friends or relatives, a conclusive diagnosis will usually need to evolve over several sessions and involve sources of information other than the patient.

FIRST LEVEL

During the first level of investigation adult victims of child abuse are questioned about the presence of extreme, unexplainable, and bothersome forgetfulness that causes them to have a sense of always being on edge and needing to constantly conceal and check their behavior.

Other areas to be investigated are as follows:

1. Flashbacks or broken threads of memory

2. Unexplained periods of lost time, both minutes and days, sometimes viewed by the patient as "walking blackouts," but unrelated to alcohol use

3. Waking up and not knowing how they got where they were or what they were doing in the recent past

4. People they do not know frequently calling them by other names and seeming to know them

5. A childhood reputation for being a "liar" that remains puzzling to the host personality

6. The appearance of items of clothing, jewelry, books, or other personal goods in their possession that they cannot recall buying or, conversely, the unexplained disappearance of such items

7. Frequent and troublesome "dreamlike" states including sleepwalking

8. Marked differences in handwriting from time to time

SECOND LEVEL

When several of these symptoms have been documented, the clinician can then probe more deeply for the presence of second-level diagnostic markers: the occurrence of voices (other personalities) that argue in their heads but that are not psychotic in character; an awareness of sometimes being unable to control their own behavior; long periods of lost time such as several childhood years in succession; and unexplained severe mood swings and dichotomous behavior states (such as impulsive and dangerous risk-taking alternating with cautious or phobic states) as reported to them by friends.

When a diagnosis of MPD becomes almost certain and other personalities have not yet spontaneously revealed themselves, a direct invitation for them to come forward can be proffered. Thus the diagnosis proceeds from a suspicion to an investigation of possible external signs that, in turn, point the way to internal signs. Such signs sometimes are confirmed by the patient and lead to external validation of suspicious, and finally to the appearance of, alternate personalities.

◆ IS MPD REAL?

Despite substantial corroborative research, the persistent, overriding question surrounding MPD continues to be "Is it real?" This has remained unchanged for most of the professional community for the past century. As Putnam (1991a) notes, "The data supporting the validity of this diagnosis are quite robust, particularly when compared with some better-accepted disorders . . . . [There seems to be an] extra burden of proof on MPD that is not demanded of other psychiatric disorders." Recognition and acceptance of this disorder have been slow. For many, MPD is deemed an iatrogenic product of hypnotic suggestion recently termed False Memory Syndrome, hysteria or malingering, or a variant of other personality disorders. External validation of the abuse and of the functional status of many MPD victims provides clear evidence that this disorder is real and extraordinarily debilitating to those affected. In many case reports the therapist makes no use of hypnotism nor have the patients ever been subjected to hypnotism. Clearly then, the recognition of childhood MPD has lagged even further behind in acceptance than has adult MPD.

◆ PROGNOSIS

When these abused children are appropriately identified and adequately treated, outcomes and prognoses are positive (Fagan & McMahan, 1984; Kluft, 1986). When, however, children with MPD remain undiagnosed and untreated until adulthood, the therapeutic course is protracted, stormy, and prognostically uncertain. In contrast to many other psychiatric disorders, the etiologic factors of this disorder along with the psychological efficacy and cost effectiveness of early identification and treatment can be documented (Kluft, 1986).

The past decade has seen a reemergence in the study of this disorder and the stark realization that unless this disorder is recognized and treated at the point of its inception, early childhood, a public health problem of epidemic proportions can be created, potentially impacting succeeding generations.

Multiple personality disorder is currently recognized as a creative psychophysiologic defensive response to a specific set of inescapable and uncontrollable experiences occurring within a circumscribed developmental time frame. Effective treatment requires an understanding of the developmental antecedents and the initial adaption to cope with the overwhelming trauma while it is occurring. More importantly, both effective treatment and primary prevention require that professionals identify MPD in its incubation phase, those childhood years following identified abuse incidents.

ISSUES

Despite recent advances in the understanding of MPD and an increased ability to diagnose it in both children and adults, there remains resistance among professionals working with abused populations to screen for this disorder (Kluft, 1985c). One reason rests in an appropriate concern that an MPD diagnosis might invalidate an abused child's testimony; such a diagnosis should rather be considered prima facie evidence of abuse rather than negating the testimony. Thus the real answer to this objection lies in public and judicial education through pediatric and other professional advocacy.

More importantly, however, ignoring the possibility of this disorder in high-risk populations constitutes nothing less than continuing abuse of the child. One glimpse of the pain of these children, and that of those adults who have never been diagnosed or treated, can stun and momentarily immobilize the most sophisticated and experienced therapist. To recognize the energy it requires for any MPD victim to negotiate even one ordinary day is to gain a new understanding of coping and resilience. It is imperative that professionals working with abused children be able to recognize, diagnose, and obtain appropriate treatment for MPD. It should be routine that all such child victims receive therapy from a professional knowledgeable about MPD.

FORENSIC QUAGMIRE

MPD presents us with several forensic issues that are, as yet, unresolved. From the point of view of the person with MPD as a victim, recent court rulings have suggested that when one personality is seductive, promiscuous, and cooperative in getting into a compromising situation and another personality then emerges to stop, then continued forceful sexual interaction with this latter declining personality constitutes rape. This decision suggests that the person with MPD may be incapable of fully informed consent.

The more difficult ethical and legal conundrum occurs when one or more personalities has perpetrated abuse or murder. Incarceration or long-term institutionalization for these offenses accompanied by treatment for the "insanity or incompetency" may yield an integrated person who no longer has MPD. Does one then release this person, or does the person remain in care or custody based on the actions of a "person" who no longer exists? These and a number of other legal issues are just beginning to emerge as the diagnosis of MPD is more often a factor in litigation procedures.

MPD challenges our most basic beliefs and assumptions concerning the workings of the mind and leaves us with questions we are currently ill equipped to answer. Perhaps this gestalt also contributed to its loss of stature in the psychiatric literature for a number of years: What we don't see doesn't haunt us. Current evidence regarding the prevalence and destructiveness of this disorder strips us of the luxury of this blindness.

♦ BIBLIOGRAPHY

Alexander, FG, and Selesnick, ST: *The History of Psychiatry: An Evaluation of Psychiatric Thought and Practice from Prehistoric Times to the Present*, New American Library, New York, 1968, p. 223.

Alvaredo, C: Dissociation and state-specific psychophysiology during the nineteenth century, *Dissociation* 2:160-168, 1989.

Baldwin, L: Child abuse as an antecedent of multiple personality disorder, *Am J Occup Ther* 44:978-983, 1990.

Boor, M: The multiple personality epidemic: Additional cases and inferences regarding diagnosis, etiology, dynamics and treatment, *J Nerv Ment Dis* 2(170):302-304, 1982.

Braun, B: Towards a theory of multiple personality and other dissociative phenomena. In B Braun, ed: Symposium on multiple personality, *Psychiatr Clin North Am* 171-194, 1984.

Braun, B, and Sachs, R: The development of multiple personality disorder: Predisposing, precipitating, and perpetuating factors. In R Kluft, ed: *Childhood Antecedents of Multiple Personality*, American Psychiatric Press, Inc, Washington, DC, 1985, pp. 37-64.

Diagnostic and Statistical Manual of Mental Disorders, ed 3, revised, American Psychiatric Association, Washington, DC, 1987, pp. 269-277.

Fagan, J, and McMahan, P: Incipient multiple personality in children: Four cases, *J Nerv Ment Dis* 172:26-36, 1984.

Freud, S: *Hypnotism and Suggestion*, Collected Papers, Hogarth Press, London, 1948, pp. 16-22.

Frischholz, EJ: The relationship among dissociation, hypnosis, and child abuse in the development of multiple personality disorder. In R Kluft, ed: *Childhood Antecedents of Multiple Personality*, American Psychiatric Press, Inc, Washington, DC, 1985, pp. 99-126.

Greaves, GB: Multiple personality: 165 years after Mary Reynolds, *J Nerv Ment Dis* 164:385-393, 1980.

Hornstein, N, and Putnam, F: Clinical phenomenology of child and adolescent dissociative disorders, *J Am Acad Child Adolescent Psychiatry* 31:6, 1077-1085, 1992.

Hornstein, N, and Tyson, S: Inpatient treatment of children with multiple personality/dissociative disorders and their families, *Psychiatr Clin North Am* 14(3):631-648, 1991.

James, W: *Principles of Psychology*, Henry Holt, New York, 1890, 2 volumes.

Kluft, R: Childhood multiple personality: Predictors, clinical findings, and treatment results. In R Kluft, ed: *Childhood Antecedents of Multiple Personality*, American Psychiatric Press, Inc, Washington, DC, 1985a.

Kluft, R: The natural history of multiple personality disorder. In R Kluft, ed: *Childhood Antecedents of Multiple Personality*, American Psychiatric Press, Inc, Washington, DC, 1985b, pp. 197-238.

Kluft, R: Introduction: Multiple personality disorder in the 1980s. In R Kluft, ed: *Childhood Antecedents of Multiple Personality*, American Psychiatric Press, Inc, Washington, DC, 1985c, pp. viii-xiv.

Kluft, R: Treating children who have multiple personality disorder. In B Braun, ed: *Treatment of Multiple Personality Disorder,* American Psychiatric Press, Inc, Washington, DC, 1986, pp. 79-105.

Kluft, R: Clinical presentations of multiple personality disorder, *Psychiatr Clin North Am* 14(3):605-629, 1991.

Masson, JM: *The Assault on Truth: Freud's Suppression of the Seduction Theory,* Farrer, Strauss and Giroux, New York, 1984.

Owen, A: *Hysteria, Hypnosis and Healing: The Work of JM Charcot,* Garrett Publications, New York, 1971.

Putnam, F: Dissociation as a response to extreme trauma. In R Kluft, ed: *Childhood Antecedents of Multiple Personality*, American Psychiatric Press, Inc, Washington, DC, 1985, pp. 65-97.

Putnam, F: *Diagnosis and Treatment of Multiple Personality Disorder*, Guilford Press, New York, 1989.

Putnam, F: Recent research on multiple personality disorder, *Psychiatr Clin North Am* 14(3):489-502, 1991a.

Putnam, F: Dissociative disorders in children and adolescents, *Psychiatr Clin North Am* 14(3):519-531, 1991b.

Putnam, F, Guroff, J, Silberman, E, Barban, L, and Post, R: The clinical phenomenology of multiple personality disorder: Review of 100 recent cases, *J Clin Psychiatry* 47:285-293, 1986.

Putnam, FW, Lowenstein, RJ, and Silberman, EK: Multiple personality disorder in a hospital setting, *J Clin Psychiatry* 45:172-175, 1984.

Reagor, P, Kasten, J, and Morelli, N: A checklist for screening dissociative disorders in children and adolescents, *Dissociation* 5(1):4-19, 1992.

Rosenbaum, M: The role of the term schizophrenia in the decline of diagnoses of multiple personality, *Arch Gen Psychiatry* 37:1383-1385, 1980.

Ross, C: Twelve cognitive errors about multiple personality disorder, *Am J Psychother* 348-356, 1990.

Ross, C: Epidemiology of multiple personality disorder and dissociation, *Psychiatr Clin North Am* 14(3):503-517, 1991.

Ross, C, Joshi, S, and Currie, R: Dissociative experiences in the general population, *Am J Psychiatry* 147:1547-1552, 1990.

Schreiber, FR: *Sybil*, Regnery, Chicago, 1973.

Spiegel, D: Multiple personality as a post-traumatic stress disorder. In B Braun, ed: Symposium on multiple personality, *Psychiatr Clin North Am* 101-110, 1984.

Spiegel, D: Dissociation, double binds, and posttraumatic stress in multiple personality disorder. In B Braun, ed: *Treatment of Multiple Personality Disorder,* American Psychiatric Press, Inc, Washington, DC, 1986, pp. 61-78.

Taylor, W, and Martin, M: Multiple personality, *J Abnorm Psychol* 39:281-300, 1944.

Thigpen, C, and Checkley, H: *The Three Faces of Eve*, McGraw-Hill, New York, 1957.

Tyson, G: Childhood MPD/dissociative identity disorder: Applying and extending current diagnostic checklists, *Dissociation* 5(1):20-27, 1992.

Young, W: Issues in the treatment of cult abuse victims. Proceedings of the Fifth International Conference on Multiple Personality/Dissociative States, Chicago, 1988.

Sexually Transmitted Diseases in Abused Children

Allan D. Friedman, M.D., M.P.H.

A 2-year-old female was admitted to the emergency room for dysuria and a purulent bloody vaginal discharge. A vaginal smear was covered with polymorphonuclear leukocytes, many having gram-negative diplococci intracellularly. The vaginal mucosa was edematous and erythematous, with copious purulent discharge.

The hospital called Social Services and notified the Division of Family Services, via the hot line, of suspected sexual abuse.

The following day the vaginal cultures were reported positive for Neisseria gonorrhoeae and Chlamydia trachomatis. The child was taken into protective custody and placed in a foster home.

Because the child was preverbal, examiners could obtain no history. The mother and stepfather denied any possibility of sexual abuse. They postulated that the child had acquired the infection from either a towel or bedding, since she slept between the parents and shared a towel with them. The stepfather and a 12-year-old sibling tested positive for gonorrhea. The mother was negative. The sibling also denied abusing the child. The perpetrator was not discovered and the case went unresolved. The child was returned to the parents. She was seen again at 4 years of age with another gonococcal infection. At that time she was acting out sexually and disclosed that her brother had abused her. The sibling tested positive for gonorrhea.

Sexually transmitted diseases (STDs) are one of a few objective measures of sexual abuse in preadolescents (McIntyre, 1986). Until proven otherwise, an STD in a preadolescent means sexual abuse (Finkel, 1983; Felman & Nikitas, 1983). The spectrum of STDs that children acquire mimics that seen in adults. Therefore the practitioner must become familiar with the signs and symptoms of these infections, know how to properly establish the etiologic agent in these diseases, and know how to effectively treat the patient.

A thorough evaluation, including oral, rectal, and genital sites, is important if sexual abuse is suspected. The main infections for which children who are suspected victims of sexual abuse should be evaluated include gonorrhea, *Chlamydia*, syphilis, genital warts (human papillomavirus or HPV), herpes simplex, *Trichomonas*, and human immunodeficiency virus. **Not all children with an STD infection will be symptomatic; therefore, cultures should be obtained in all suspected cases of sexual abuse (De Jong, 1986).** Fifty percent of gonococcal infections in sexually abused children are asymptomatic. Thirty percent of these infections have been found in locations not reported by the children to have been involved in the abuse.

Table 11-1 lists the screening studies for sexually transmitted diseases, recommended by the Centers for Disease Control (CDC), in children suspected to be victims of sexual abuse. Ideally, all these studies should be obtained, although cost may dictate a more conservative approach.

General guidelines for the evaluation of children who are believed to be sexually abused include the following:

1. The interview and examination of children suspected to be sexually abused require special skills. Institutions providing health care for children should have a team of individuals who are trained to evaluate these children. If such a team is available, involve it in the workup.

2. For legal reasons, make certain all samples and cultures are labeled and logged carefully at all places where they are processed. Have them personally transported from the clinic or emergency room to the laboratory so as to ensure chain of custody.

3. If the child is believed to be sexually abused, contact Social Services immediately. Report the case via the hot line if it involves a caretaker or to the police sex crimes unit if it does not involve a caretaker. In the latter case, getting permission of the Division of Family Services or the parent is advisable before contacting the police. Do not discharge the child without first making sure he or she is going to a safe environment.

4. The majority of children (60% to 70%) have no physical findings of abuse. Do not let a negative examination influence your impression of sexual abuse or your decision to involve Social Services.

5. Do not begin therapy in symptomatic children before obtaining all appropriate samples. Therapy may be necessary in specific incidences before the organism and antibiotic sensitivities are known.

   Prophylactic antibiotics are not usually necessary in asymptomatic children suspected to be victims of sexual abuse. The infection rate is low in children, and prophylactic antibiotics are unlikely to prevent an infection. In addition the risk of STD complications is low in children, and the risk of pelvic inflammatory disease and peritonitis is very low in prepubertal children.

6. Use an experienced reference laboratory. On occasion, inexperienced laboratories have mistaken nonsexually transmitted gonorrhea organisms for *Neisseria gonorrhoeae.* Also, some laboratories that primarily deal with adults

have used rapid diagnostic tests such as the monoclonal antibodies in direct immunofluorescent stains or the enzyme-linked immunoassay test for *Chlamydia trachomatis* in children. These tests are neither sensitive nor specific enough, and have too many false positives, to be used in medical-legal cases. Too much is at stake to make these kinds of errors.

Table 11-1. Summary of Suggested Laboratory Tests for Sexual Abuse

AIDS and Hepatitis B
Test for HIV virus infection and hepatitis B if the perpetrator is in the high-risk group (drug user, homosexual, prostitute, multiple sex partners) for these infections or is known to be seropositive for these conditions. Some believe that with the high incidence of these infections in the population, all sexually abused children should be screened for these conditions. Perform follow-up test in 3 to 6 months.

Neisseria gonorrhoeae
Obtain rectal, throat, vaginal/urethral cultures.

Chlamydia trachomatis
Obtain vulvovaginal, urethral, rectal, pharyngeal cultures.

Gardnerella vaginalis
Wet preparation of vaginal secretions for clue cells and amine odor with 10% KOH solution.

Herpes simplex
Obtain lesion culture or vulva/cervix culture, if no lesions are present.

Human papillomavirus
Confirm clinical examination with biopsy and histologic examination. Acetic acid (10%) solution can aid in detecting subclinical cases.

Neisseria gonorrhoeae
In males, checking the first 10 cc of freshly voided urine for white blood cells can be an effective screening procedure. Obtain blood, joint fluid, and conjunctival cultures if clinically indicated.

Treponema pallidum, **syphilis**
Perform VDRL, with follow-up test at 6 to 12 weeks.

Trichomonas vaginalis
Examine urine for organisms and culture vaginal secretions.

In cases of acute assault, obtain follow-up cultures after 2 weeks and repeat serology testing after 6 weeks. Perform a pregnancy test in pubertal children and repeat this test in 2 weeks in cases of acute assault.

♦GONORRHEA

Gonorrhea is caused by the gram-negative intracellular diplococcal organism *Neisseria gonorrhoeae.* The organism is fragile and will not grow without proper culturing procedures. Although precise numbers are difficult to find, it has been estimated that between 3% and 26% of sexually abused children are infected with gonorrhea (Frau & Alexander, 1985). In the author's institution the incidence is about 1% in sexually abused children. The infection occurs only in humans. In the United States the infection is reported in about 1 million patients of all ages each year, but the actual number of cases is probably significantly greater (Friedman, 1987).

CLINICAL PRESENTATION

Gonorrhea may be asymptomatic or may present as urethritis, cervicitis, vulvovaginitis, proctitis, conjunctivitis, pharyngitis, epididymitis, bartholinitis, or pelvic inflammatory disease (American Academy of Pediatrics, 1988).

In prepubertal females gonococcal infections most frequently present as vulvovaginitis and urethritis. In postpubertal girls the presentation is usually cervicitis or pelvic inflammatory disease. In males the primary site of infection is the urethra, but urethritis is infrequent in prepubertal males. Bacteremic spread can result in arthritis, dermatitis, perihepatitis, meningitis, or endocarditis (American Academy of Pediatrics, 1988).

Incubation periods for gonorrhea vary with the infection site. Urethritis in males can occur as early as 2 to 5 days after infection. In females symptoms may not occur until 2 weeks after exposure or later (Parish & Gschnait, 1989). This longer incubation period increases the risk of unknowingly spreading the infection to sexual partners.

Symptoms in females include vaginal discharge, frequency of micturition, dysuria, backache, lower abdominal pain, pelvic pain, and rectal discharge and bleeding. Local complications include skenitis. In males, uncomplicated gonorrhea presents as purulent urethral discharge with dysuria. Frequency may also be a symptom. The urethral discharge is often yellow or yellowish green and the external urethral meatus may be swollen and red. Untreated, a posterior urethral infection may occur, which may result in pain, burning, urgency, and frequency with a few drops of blood at the end of micturition. Ultimately, this can lead to prostatitis, epididymitis, vesiculitis, and cystitis.

Less common symptoms of gonorrhea result from the involvement of the rectal mucosa, the pharynx, and the conjunctiva. Symptoms of anorectal gonorrhea may be mild and cause anal pruritus, a mucopurulent discharge, and scant rectal bleeding. If severe, gonorrhea can cause an acute proctitis that presents as rectal pain, tenesmus, and constipation. The mucosa is often red, friable, edematous, and mucopurulent. Most anorectal infections are symptomatic.

Pharyngeal gonorrhea is usually symptomatic. Common findings are fever, sore throat, and cervical adenopathy.

After the neonatal period, gonococcal conjunctivitis is uncommon. It results from direct contamination of the eye, often from fomites or fingers (Parish & Gschnait, 1989).

Children appear to be more susceptible to gonococcal infection than adults. The vaginal mucosa in prepubertal girls is thin with an alkaline pH and a poor glycogen content, making vulvovaginitis more likely. The discharge may be profuse. The vulva may be swollen, red, and sore (Parish & Gschnait, 1989).

LABORATORY DIAGNOSIS

Culture of the gonococcal organism is necessary to confirm the clinical diagnosis of gonococcal disease. In males, swabs from the urethra should be obtained for Gram stain and culture. In females, when possible, cervical and urethral specimens should be obtained. Because sexual abuse may involve other orifices, swabs should also be obtained from the anus and pharynx. The specimen should be directly plated onto appropriate media and placed in an optimal environment for growth. Modified Thayer-Martin media are commonly used and are effective in preventing overgrowth of other organisms and facilitating the growth of most *N. gonorrhoeae*.

Positive cultures for *N. gonorrhoeae* should be confirmed by a reference laboratory. As stated earlier, nonpathogenic *Neisseria* organisms can be mistaken for *N. gonorrhoeae*. Nonculture techniques for diagnosing gonorrhea are not appropriate in children because they lack the requisite sensitivity and specificity.

THERAPY

Current recommendations for the treatment of gonorrhea are based on the following considerations: the spread of infections due to organisms resistant to older therapies, the strong association of gonorrhea with chlamydial infections, the risk of serious complications of untreated gonorrhea or chlamydial infection, and the lack of accurate, fast, inexpensive diagnostic tests for chlamydial infection. In addition, sexually abused children may also have pharyngeal and anal infections. Infections at these sites are less susceptible to traditional therapies.

Children less than 45 kg body weight who have gonococcal vulvovaginitis, cervicitis, urethritis, pharyngitis, or proctitis should receive 125 mg intramuscularly of ceftriaxone once. If the patient is unable to tolerate ceftriaxone therapy, he or she can receive 40 mg/kg of spectinomycin intramuscularly once (not effective for pharyngeal infection). Children 45 kg or greater should follow the adult regimen which is 250 mg of ceftriaxone intramuscularly once or, if the patient cannot tolerate ceftriaxone, 2 gm of spectinomycin intramuscularly once. **Table 11-2** summarizes treatment of STDs in children. Other acceptable regimens include oral cefuroxime axetil with probenecid (1 gm of each); cefixime, 400 mg orally once; cefotaxime, 1 gm intramuscularly and ceftizoxime, 500 mg intramuscularly, once.

In patients proven to have infection not resistant to penicillin, 3 gm of amoxicillin may be given orally with 1 gm of probenecid. All patients 8 years of age and older should also receive doxycycline, 100 mg orally, twice daily for 7 days.

Table 11-2. Treatment of STDs in Children*

Chlamydia trachomatis
Erythromycin base 40-50 mg/kg/day x 7 days po *or* sulfisoxazole 120-150 mg/kg/day x 14 days po *or* tetracycline 500 mg g6h x 7 days po (> 8 yrs old) *or* doxycyline 100 mg bid x 7 days po (> 8 yrs old)

Gardnerella vaginalis
Metronidazole 15 mg/kg/day x 7 days po *or* clindamycin 300 mg bid x 7 days po (older children)

Herpes simplex
Acyclovir oral 200 mg 5 times daily for 10 days (older children); topical (5%) 5 times daily x 7 days

Human papillomavirus
Podophyllin (10%-20%), apply for 2-4 hours then wash off

Neisseria gonorrhoeae
<45 kg body weight: ceftriaxone 125 mg IM x 1 *or* spectinomycin 40 mg/kg IM x 1 (may fail to eradicate pharyngeal disease); ≥ 45 kg body weight: ceftriaxone 250 mg 1M x 1 *or* spectinomycin 2 gm 1M x 1

Treponema pallidum
Penicillin G (benzathine) 50 x 10 u/kg (up to 2.4 x 10 u) IM x 1 (early disease) *or* penicillin G (benzathine) 2.4 x 10 u IM q week x 3 (>1 yr duration of disease) *or* penicillin G (aqueous crystalline) 20 x 10 - 30 x 10 u/kg/d (up to 2-4 x 10 u q 4 hr) IV x 10-14 days (CNS disease)

Trichomonas vaginalis
Metronidazole 15 mg/kg/day x 7- 12 days po *or* metronidazole 2 gm po x 1 (adolescents) *or* metronidazole 500 mg po bid x 7 days (adolescents)

* Alternative treatment may exist.

With disseminated disease, children less than 45 kg should receive 50 mg/kg/day of ceftriaxone (maximum of 1 gm/day) for 7 days for bacteremia or arthritis, and 10 to 14 days of therapy for meningitis (maximum of 2 gm/day). After treatment is completed, cultures should be obtained to ensure that therapy was effective (Centers for Disease Control, 1989).

◆CHLAMYDIAL INFECTIONS

Chlamydia trachomatis is the most common cause of sexually transmitted disease and is believed to account for as many as 3 million new infections each year (Holmes, 1981). As many as 20,000 adolescent females become sterile from their chlamydial infection each year (Schachter et al., 1975). Whenever a child has a chlamydial infection in the vagina or rectum, abuse must be considered. The infection reportedly can be contracted at birth; however, it is not known how long the infection can be carried asymptomatically and therefore at what age neonatal infection need no longer be considered (Ingram et al., 1986).

CLINICAL PRESENTATION

The most common clinical presentation of chlamydial infection in females is cervicitis. However, asymptomatic infections are common. If the patient is symptomatic, a mucopurulent discharge is present initially. A purulent yellow discharge on a cervical swab introduced into the cervical canal indicates leukorrhea. Urethritis may also occur in female patients, often in association with cervicitis.

Symptoms often include dysuria and increased frequency of micturition (Stamm et al., 1980). In teenage and adult female patients, salpingitis may result from chlamydial infection and may lead to infertility. Symptoms of salpingitis, such as mild to moderate abdominal pain, may be absent. Other complications of chlamydial infection include perihepatitis which often presents with acute, right upper quadrant abdominal pain and endometritis (Muller-Schoop et al., 1978).

In males, urethritis is the most common symptomatic presentation of chlamydial infection which is believed to be the most common cause of nongonococcal urethritis. Discharge, when present, is mucoid or mucopurulent. Symptoms develop 1 to 3 weeks after infection. Untreated, these patients may progress to epididymitis and infertility. Simultaneous infection with both *N. gonorrhoeae* and *C. trachomatis* may result in recurrence of symptoms after appropriate gonococcal therapy, due to the longer incubation time for the chlamydial infection. Proctitis and Reiter's syndrome may also occur as a result of chlamydial infection (Holmes et al., 1975).

LABORATORY DIAGNOSIS

Both serologic and cell culture methods are available for the diagnosis of chlamydial infection. Serologic methods, however, are of limited value because of the high prevalence of chlamydial antibodies in the population. Cultures are highly specific, but the sensitivity depends on obtaining an adequate specimen. Appropriate cultures are obtained by vigorously swabbing the site so that cells attach to the swab. Either cotton wool or calcium alginate-tipped swabs can be used to collect the specimen (Schachter et al., 1979).

Using chlamydial antigen detection tests to evaluate suspected sexual abuse in children has been largely unsuccessful. Both false positive and false negative results have been reported. Because of the profound implications for both the victim and the accused, accurate diagnosis is essential. Therefore adequate cultures must be obtained (Hammerschlag et al., 1988; Fuster & Neinstein, 1987).

THERAPY

Children 8 years of age or older can be treated according to adult regimen. Treatment is doxycycline, 100 mg orally, twice daily for 7 days, or tetracycline,

500 mg orally, four times a day for 7 days. Alternative therapy for simple cervicitis or urethritis is azithromycin, 1 gm orally, once. Younger children, or children who are unable to take the tetracyclines, can receive erythromycin base in a dose of 40 to 50 mg/kg/day, by mouth, four times a day for 7 days or erythromycin ethylsuccinate, 40 to 50 mg/kg/day orally, four times a day for 7 days. Children unable to tolerate erythromycin receive sulfisoxazole or amoxicillin, although little clinical data are available regarding the efficacy of the alternative regimens (Centers for Disease Control, 1989).

◆ BACTERIAL VAGINOSIS

Previously called nonspecific vaginitis, bacterial vaginosis is a result of overgrowth of *Gardnerella vaginalis* and anaerobes. This condition is thought to affect children infrequently, as the organisms prefer an estrogenic vagina; nevertheless, the organism can occasionally be recovered from prepubertal girls. Although the organism can be recovered from the male urethra, it is not clear either what role male colonization with the organism has in female infection or if there is a symptomatic condition associated with this infection in males (Spagna & Prior, 1985; Bartley et al., 1987).

The organism is more prevalent in sexually active adolescent males and females. It is also more common in sexually abused children than in controls. Though the organism is not pathognomonic for sexual abuse, its presence should raise suspicion about possible sexual abuse.

CLINICAL PRESENTATION

Adults with bacterial vaginosis may be asymptomatic. The classic symptoms are foul smelling, fishy vaginal odor that in postpubertal females may increase with menses and after intercourse (Spagna & Prior, 1985). The patient may have a discharge that is thin, gray, and homogeneous. The pH of the discharge is greater than 4.5, and the fishy odor becomes obvious after mixing KOH with the discharge.

Children may be asymptomatic. Symptoms may include pruritus and the classic discharge described for adults. Occasionally the discharge is more white than gray (Parish & Gschnait, 1989).

LABORATORY DIAGNOSIS

The presence of a discharge with a foul, fishy smell upon adding 10% KOH is helpful in making the diagnosis of bacterial vaginosis. Further evidence of infection is the presence of clue cells on Gram stain or Papanicolaou stain. Usually few white blood cells are found (Parish & Gschnait, 1989). Culture of the discharge or of a vaginal swab for *G. vaginalis* is of controversial value because at least in postpubertal females, the organism may be present as nonpathogenic flora (Spagna & Prior, 1985). Nevertheless, its presence in children should always raise concern about possible sexual abuse.

THERAPY

The treatment of *Gardnerella vaginalis* is 15 mg/kg/day of metronidazole given orally in three divided doses for 7 days. In older children and adults the infection can be treated with 500 mg orally twice a day for 7 days. Patients unable to take metronidazole can be treated with clindamycin 300 mg by mouth twice a day for 7 days (Centers for Disease Control, 1989).

◆ SYPHILIS

In children, syphilis is almost always sexually transmitted. The causative organism is *Treponema pallidum*, a spirochetal organism with an incubation period of about 3 weeks. In children syphilis undergoes a primary and a secondary stage. In adults a tertiary stage can also occur. In one series, about 6% of sexually abused children were infected with *T. pallidum* (Frau & Alexander, 1985). In the author's institution, however, the incidence of syphilis in postnatal sexually abused children has been essentially zero. This is consistent with other centers. A survey of 80 physicians showed that only 25 children had syphilis in a population of 49,000 sexually abused children. All these tested children were infected with other sexually transmitted diseases. Though the incidence of syphilis is believed to be low in these children, with the recent rise in syphilis in the adult population it is prudent to screen all children who have been sexually abused.

CLINICAL PRESENTATION

Primary syphilis presents with a macule that evolves into a papule. The surface of the lesion then erodes with a sharply defined border. The lesion contains serous material. Usually only one primary lesion develops. This chancre is painless and is associated with nonsuppurative regional lymphadenopathy. It heals without therapy in 3 to 8 weeks.

The second stage occurs about 6 to 8 weeks after the chancre appears. A nonpruritic rash may develop that is maculopapular and generalized and involves the palms and soles.

Mucosal lesions, called mucous patches, and enlarged nontender lymph nodes may be present also. Skin lesions contain the organism and are a source of spread of the infection (Chapel, 1980). Less commonly, alopecia, periostitis, hepatomegaly, and acute glomerulonephritis may occur (Crissey & Denenholz, 1984).

LABORATORY DIAGNOSIS

Spirochetes can be identified by dark-field microscopic examination of specimens taken from moist areas. False negative results are common. Reliable nontreponemal tests for syphilis include the Venereal Disease Reference Laboratory slide test (VDRL), the rapid reagin card test (RPR), and the automated reagin test (ART). These tests are convenient rapid screens that are useful in indicating disease activity. False positive nontreponemal tests can occur in patients with connective tissue disease, tuberculosis, and endocarditis. False negatives occur in early primary syphilis and in late disease.

Specific treponemal tests should be performed to confirm results. These tests include the fluorescent treponemal antibody absorption test (FTA-ABS), the microhemagglutination test (MHA-TP), and the immobilization test (TPI). FTA and MHA remain positive for life even after successful treatment. The TPI is rarely used today.

THERAPY

The recommended treatment for early acquired syphilis, which includes primary, secondary, and latent disease of less than 1 year duration, is penicillin G (benzathine), intramuscularly, 50,000 units/kg, but not to exceed 2.4 million units. If patients are allergic to penicillin, they can receive tetracycline, 2 gm/day, by mouth, divided into four doses for at least 15 days. If the child is 8 years or younger, treatment may be either hospitalization and desensitization of the child to penicillin or the use of erythromycin for 15 days with good follow-up, since erythromycin is not believed to be as effective as penicillin or tetracycline (Centers for Disease Control, 1989).

♦ HERPES SIMPLEX

Approximately 10% of the adult population has symptomatic genital herpes (Friedman, 1987). Although herpes simplex type 2 is more commonly associated with genital infection, type 1 can also be found. After the neonatal period the presence of herpes lesions, especially in the genital region, strongly suggests sexual abuse.

Fomite transmission of the disease is unlikely. Transmission requires direct contact of live virus with a mucous membrane or an abraded skin area of the person becoming infected.

Other viruses and bacteria that cause lesions in the genital area of children can resemble herpes simplex. Viral cultures should, therefore, be obtained from all suspect lesions.

CLINICAL PRESENTATION

Symptoms of herpes simplex vary from mild to severe. Soreness, itching, and dysuria along with inguinal or femoral lymphadenopathy are common. Systemic symptoms such as headache and fever may also occur. Female patients with primary herpes may experience erosive cervicitis and vaginal discharge. Males may have urethritis with dysuria. There may be little or no discharge. Lesions, if present, start as vesicles or vesiculopustules and are often found on the shaft of the penis or the vulva. These lesions ulcerate and are painful. Healing begins during the second week and is complete by the end of the third week. Recurrent infections are milder. Contact with lesions spreads the disease, but infection may be present without obvious lesions (Friedman, 1987).

LABORATORY DIAGNOSIS

Lesions can be scraped and stained with Giemsa or Papanicolaou stains for multinucleated giant cells. This test is highly suggestive but not diagnostic, as other herpes viruses may also stain positively. A more specific test is immunofluorescent staining against herpes simplex antigen. Both tests require a good specimen from an unroofed lesion. Diagnostic confirmation is by viral culture for herpes simplex. Cultures are positive in 40 to 72 hours.

THERAPY

Acyclovir is effective in treating primary herpes infections. The drug is available in topical, oral, and intravenous forms. Topical therapy can be applied six times a day for 7 days. Oral therapy (200 mg capsules) given five times a day for 7 to 10 days is available for older children.

For serious infection, intravenous therapy is available (Nelson, 1989). Recurrences of genital herpes infection are common. Although usually symptomatic, recurrences can be asymptomatic. In patients with frequent recurrences, long-term oral acyclovir can decrease the frequency of infection as long as the patient continues to take the medicine.

♦ HUMAN PAPILLOMAVIRUS

Condyloma acuminatum is an infection caused by human papillomavirus (HPV). The incidence of these infections reportedly has increased more than 450% since 1954. Most patients are between 15 and 29 years of age, but infections have been reported in children and when present must lead to a suspicion of sexual abuse (Norins et al., 1984). Neonates, however, may acquire the infection while passing through the birth canal. Condyloma infection in the first two years of life is likely the result of contact during delivery, although sexual abuse is still a possibility. Since these children are preverbal, if there are no other physical or historical findings consistent with sexual abuse, it must be assumed the infection is not due to sexual abuse. Other members of the family should be examined for possible lesions, even if they are asymptomatic.

The incubation period for HPV is 3 to 20 months. Among the consequences of infection in children are the concerns about the oncogenicity of certain strains of the virus (HPV-16, HPV-18) and the possibility of transmission (Schachner & Hankin, 1985). Spread is by direct contact with the lesions.

CLINICAL PRESENTATION

Genital and anorectal lesions are flesh colored, focal, and verrucous tumors. Lesions on the cervix are flat and wart-like. These lesions may be missed by the naked eye but can show up in colposcopy. In males the lesions are typically skin colored, slightly pink, or white verrucous papules. They may be solitary lesions or confluent, forming the typical cauliflower appearance. They may appear anywhere along the penile shaft or on the glans. Anal and perianal lesions also may occur. Lesions in both sexes range from small and painless to large, ulcerated lesions that are secondarily infected. These lesions may be pruritic and burn.

Infection can be subclinical. An application of acetic acid (10%) turns nonapparent lesions white. The solution should be allowed to remain in contact with the suspected area for 5 to 10 minutes before determining that this test is negative for HPV lesions. The solution is painful when applied to mucous membranes. Care must be taken when deciding to use it on children.

LABORATORY DIAGNOSIS

Histological examination is diagnostic. Characteristic findings include acanthosis, papillomatosis, and parakeratosis of the epithelial projections. Koilocytotic cells are visible in the upper stratum malpighii.

THERAPY

Condyloma acuminatum is treated topically. Infected areas should be kept cool and dry. Podophyllin, 10% to 20%, should be administered and then washed off after about 2 to 4 hours. Alternative therapies include trichloroacetic acid, electrocautery, and cryotherapy. Human lymphoblastoid interferon has also been used successfully (Centers for Disease Control, 1989).

◆ TRICHOMONIASIS

Trichomonas vaginalis is the protozoon responsible for trichomoniasis. It is uncommon in prepubescent patients and can be transmitted both sexually and nonsexually. In adults the prevalence varies from 5% to 75% depending on the population studied (White et al., 1983).

CLINICAL PRESENTATION

T. vaginalis is often asymptomatic. Infected females are more likely to be symptomatic than males. Erythema and edema of the external genitalia are often present. A frothy, gray discharge may occur. The patient may have vaginitis along with symptoms of cervicitis and punctate hemorrhages (White et al., 1983). Untreated, the infection may progress to prostatitis and salpingitis.

LABORATORY DIAGNOSIS

The parasite is a motile protozoan that can appear under microscopy. A specimen of vaginal discharge should be placed on a wet mount slide preparation with a drop of saline. The swimming motion of the organism is visible. Alternative means of identification are culture and Papanicolaou smear. Because the wet mount test for diagnosing *T. vaginalis* infections has been shown to miss 40% of those proven by culture, in children suspected to be infected with *T. vaginalis*, cultures and wet mount should be done.

THERAPY

The drug of choice is oral metronidazole, 15 mg/kg/day, divided into three doses, for 7 to 10 days. In older children and adults 2 gm of metronidazole may be given once or 500 mg twice a day for 7 days.

♦ ACQUIRED IMMUNODEFICIENCY SYNDROME (AIDS)

The human immunodeficiency virus (HIV) is the causative agent of AIDS. Fortunately, few reported cases of AIDS have been attributable to sexual abuse. The risk of transmitting the disease during sexual contact is well-documented, however, and the consequence of infection can be devastating.

HIV is particularly tropic for CD4 (T-helper) lymphocytes and macrophages. Humans are the only reservoir of HIV. The incubation period for this infection is variable, and infection acquired in adolescence may not result in clinical disease until adulthood.

CLINICAL PRESENTATION

The spectrum of disease due to HIV infection ranges from asymptomatic to full-blown, devastating, opportunistic infection in a severely debilitated, immunocompromised host. Common clinical findings include lymphadenopathy, hepatosplenomegaly, parotitis, recurrent diarrhea, failure to thrive, progressive neurologic disease, recurrent invasive bacterial infections and opportunistic infections, malignancies, and lymphoid interstitial pneumonia. Opportunistic organisms commonly occurring in children with HIV infection include *Pneumocystis carinii, Candida, Mycobacterium, Avium-intracellularae*, and *Cryptosporidium.*

LABORATORY DIAGNOSIS

HIV infection can be detected by serological testing. Enzyme-linked immunosorbent assays (ELISA) with confirmatory Western blot and immunofluorescent antibody testing are used. Serological tests may not become positive for months after infection has occurred, so retesting is indicated. Because symptoms resulting from infection may be delayed months to years, children suspected of sexual abuse should be evaluated for HIV infection along with the other infections. If the perpetrator is known, he or she should be tested for HIV infection. The victim should also be tested for baseline HIV status and retested at least one more time, 3 to 6 months later, during which period most infected people develop antibody.

THERAPY

Currently, HIV infection has no cure. Drugs reported to have a beneficial effect on the progression of the disease include azidothymidine (AZT), also called zidovudine; dideoxyinosine (ddI); and dideoxycytidine (ddC). Management also involves the treatment and prevention of secondary infections (Centers for Disease Control, 1989).

♦ MOLLUSCUM CONTAGIOSUM

While molluscum contagiosum is often sexually transmitted in adults, in children it is easily spread by casual contact. Without a reliable history of sexual abuse, molluscum in children should be considered nonsexually transmitted. When genital lesions are present in children, a careful history usually reveals that the lesions began on other parts of the body.

♦ MISCELLANEOUS INFECTIONS

Many other infections can be spread through sexual contact but have a relatively low incidence in the United States.

Although examiners do not routinely screen for them, chancroid (*Hemophilus ducreyi*), lymphogranuloma venereum (*C. trachomatis,* LGV serovars), viral hepatitis (mostly hepatitis B), and ectoparasites (pediculosis pubis, scabies) are other diseases that should be considered in abused children.

♦ SUMMARY

While not all of the illnesses discussed in this chapter are exclusively transmitted sexually, it would be inappropriate to assume nonsexual transmission before doing a full evaluation of the child. Many of these infections can be asymptomatic. A child suspected of being sexually abused requires a full workup to identify both symptomatic and asymptomatic infections. *Table 11-2* summarizes treatment for the infections discussed in this chapter.

When evaluating children for sexually transmitted diseases, the practitioner should keep in mind that it is common for more than one disease to be transmitted at the same time. It is therefore essential to do a comprehensive evaluation. The presence of one infection makes the presence of another more, not less, likely.

♦ BIBLIOGRAPHY

American Academy of Pediatrics, Committee on Infectious Diseases: *Report of the Committee on Infectious Diseases*, Elk Grove Village, IL, 1988, pp. 193-203.

Bartley, DL, Morgan, L, et al: *Gardnerella vaginalis* in prepubertal girls, *Am J Dis Child* 141:1014-1017, 1987.

Centers for Disease Control: 1989 Sexually Transmitted Diseases Treatment Guidelines, US Department of Health and Human Services, 1989, pp. 21-26.

Chapel, TA: The signs and symptoms of secondary syphilis, *Sex Transm Dis* 7:161-164, 1980.

Crissey, JT, and Denenholz, DA: Syphilis, *Clin Dermatol* 2:1-166, 1984.

DeJong, AR: Sexually transmitted diseases in sexually abused children, *Sex Transm Dis* 13:123-126, 1986.

Feigin, R, and Cherry, J: *Textbook of Pediatric Infectious Diseases*, ed 3, WB Saunders Co, Philadelphia, 1992.

Felman, YM, and Nikitas, JA: Sexually transmitted diseases and child sexual abuse, Part 1, *NY State J Med* 83:341-343, 1983.

Finkel, KC: *Recognition and Assessment of the Sexually Abused Child*, Ontario Medical Association, Toronto, 1983.

Frau, LM, and Alexander, ER: Public health implications of sexually transmitted diseases in pediatric practice, *Pediatr Infect Dis* 4:453-467, 1985.

Friedman, AD: *Handbook of Pediatric Infectious Diseases*, Ishiyaku EuroAmerica Inc, St. Louis, 1987, pp. 109-111.

Fuster, CD, and Neinstein, LS: *Vaginal Chlamydia trachomatis* prevalence in sexually abused prepubertal girls, *Pediatrics* 79:235-238, 1987.

Hammerschlag, M, and Rawstron, S: Sexually transmitted diseases. In S Krugman, S Katz, A Gershon, and C Wilfert, eds: *Infectious Diseases of Children*, ed 9, Mosby-Year Book, St. Louis, 1992, pp. 419-456.

Hammerschlag, MR, Rettig, PJ, and Shields, ME: False positive results with the rise of chlamydial antigen detection tests in the evaluation of suspected sexual abuse in children, *Pediatr Infect Dis* 7:11-12, 1988.

Holmes, KK: The chlamydia epidemic, *JAMA* 245:428-435, 1981.

Holmes, KK, Handsfield, HH, Wang, SP, et al: Etiology of non-gonococcal urethritis, *N Engl J Med* 292:1109-1205, 1975.

Ingram, DL, White, ST, Occhiuti, AR, et al: Childhood vaginal infections: Association of Chlamydia trachomatis with sexual contact, *Pediatr Infect Dis* 5:226-229, 1986.

McIntyre, L: Sexual abuse and sexually transmitted diseases in children, *CMAJ* 134:1272-1273, 1986.

Muller-Schoop, JW, Wang, SP, Munzinger, J, et al: C. trachomatis as a possible cause of peritonitis and perihepatitis in young women, *Br Med J* 1:1022-1024, 1978.

Nelson, JD: *Pocketbook of Pediatric Antimicrobial Therapy*, ed 8, The Williams & Wilkins Co, Baltimore, 1989, p. 36.

Norins, AL, et al: Genital warts and sexual abuse, *J Am Acad Dermatol* 11:529-530, 1984.

Parish, LC, and Gschnait, F: *Sexually Transmitted Diseases, A Guide for Clinicians*, Springer-Verlag, New York, 1989, pp. 59-76.

Schachner, L, and Hankin, DE: Assessing child abuse in childhood condyloma acuminatum, *J Am Acad Dermatol* 12:157-160, 1985.

Schachter, J, Cles, L, Ray, R, et al: Failure of serology in diagnosing chlamydial infections of the female genital tract, *J Clin Microbiol* 10:647-649, 1979.

Schachter, J, Hanna, L, Hill, EC, et al: Are chlamydial infections the most prevalent venereal disease? *JAMA* 231:1252-1255, 1975.

Spagna, VA, and Prior, RB: *Sexually Transmitted Diseases, A Clinical Syndrome Approach*, Marcel Dekker, Inc, New York, 1985, pp. 147-152.

Stamm, WE, Wagner, KF, Amsel, R, et al: Causes of the acute urethral syndrome in women, *N Engl J Med* 303:409-415, 1980.

White, ST, Loda, FA, Ingnam, DL, et al: Sexually transmitted diseases in sexually abused children, *Pediatrics* 72:16-21, 1983.

POISONING

KEVIN COULTER, M.D.
ANTHONY J. SCALZO, M.D.

A 13-month-old boy was seen in the emergency room because of convulsions. The mother and boyfriend both smelled of alcohol and social services was notified.

The child was found to have a blood glucose level of 15 mg%; the etiology of the convulsion was determined to be hypoglycemia, with alcohol-induced hypoglycemia suspected. A blood alcohol level was obtained and the child reported to the Division of Family Services via the abuse hot line for suspected abuse, specifically alcohol poisoning. The blood alcohol level was determined to be significantly elevated. The mother initially denied any possibility of the child ingesting alcohol but later acknowledged that the boyfriend had convinced her to give the child vodka to "help him sleep."

Poisoning is one of the most common medical emergencies faced by health practitioners caring for children. It accounts for numerous emergency room visits and is a significant cause of pediatric morbidity and mortality. The Centers for Disease Control in 1986 reported 4,740 unintentional poisoning deaths. Of these deaths, 93 were children under 5 years, 24 were between 5 and 9 years, and 249 were adolescents (Olsen & Banner, 1991). A review of calls to 63 poison control centers participating in a national data collection program during 1987 disclosed 1.2 million ingestion cases. In this study, 60% of the ingestion cases involved children under the age of 5 years, 22 children died, and 107,844 had symptoms of poisoning. In another study the median age of the victims, 2 years, was similar to that in physical abuse, and indeed, evidence of coincident battering was present in 20% of the children (Dine, 1982). The most common agents used were found to be salt (eight cases), water (six cases), tranquilizers (six cases), and barbiturates (five cases). In his landmark discussion of the battered child syndrome in 1962, Kempe was the first to propose poisoning as part of the spectrum of injury in child abuse. As he stated, "In an occasional case the parent, or parent-substitute, may also have assaulted the child by administering an overdose of a drug or by exposing the child to natural gas or other toxic substances" (Kempe et al., 1962).

Poisoning as it relates to child abuse can occur in two major contexts: as an intentional act or as the result of neglect. Each has its own implications and complexities. Over the past 30 years intentional poisoning has remained an uncommon form of reported child abuse. Similarities in the epidemiology of abuse and poisoning point to two overlapping and possibly frequently related problems. Both of these "environmental dangers" are commonly seen in children under 5 years of age and in social settings marked by similar stresses. Marital discord, unemployment, parental psychiatric disturbances, inadequate housing, and geographic mobility are common factors in both child abuse and poisoning. The similarities are not surprising when considering the relationship between neglect and the child with repeated ingestions. While many pediatric ingestions may represent a failure to provide adequate protection in chaotic, stress-burdened homes (acts of omission), health practitioners must remember that some ingestions, the exact proportion being unknown, result from intentional poisoning (acts of commission) (Kresel & Lovejoy, 1981).

◆INTENTIONAL POISONING
Since Kempe first suggested that poisoning could be nonaccidental, scattered reports of this type of abuse have appeared in the literature. The intentional poisoning of children seems to occur by two general mechanisms: the acute assault of a child by forced ingestion or aspiration of a drug or other substance as a method of discipline. Case reports of these types of abuse in the literature include the forced ingestion of water through a garden hose in a 4-year-old boy who developed hyponatremic seizures (Mortimer, 1980) and homicidal pepper aspiration (Cohle et al., 1988).

CHARACTERISTICS OF THE PERPETRATOR
Cases of abuse are usually perpetrated by an individual with poor impulse control, a low tolerance for a child's upsetting behavior, and a tendency to act out violently against the child using a poison. While some of these cases undoubtedly represent a deranged individual attempting to directly harm a child, other cases can be viewed as a spectrum of parental dysfunction in attempting to cope with the stresses of caring for children. At one end of the spectrum are the young parents distressed by their fussy, colicky infant. They may try at times, with the direction of their physician, to sedate their infant with an antihistamine or paregoric. Usually this does not prove to be injurious. There is the danger that the parents will continuously increase the dose to accomplish sedation without awareness of the potential ill effects that can be associated with these agents. In addition, with

highly stressed, impulsive parents the situation may escalate to physical abuse, often by shaking, or possibly to chemical abuse with doses of potent sedatives such as alcohol or narcotics. At the far end of this spectrum are adults or older children who intentionally introduce children to the effects of illicit drugs. A recent survey was conducted of adolescent females in a drug treatment program who had been baby sitters. Nine girls (11%) stated they had blown marijuana smoke into the faces or mouths of the children being cared for in an attempt to make them "high" (Schwartz et al., 1986). In a far more malicious setting, pedophiles may attempt to chemically sedate children before molesting them.

MUNCHAUSEN SYNDROME BY PROXY

A mechanism for intentional poisoning that occurs only rarely is Munchausen Syndrome by Proxy (MSBP). Briefly, this syndrome is defined as an illness in a child that is simulated or produced by a parent, usually the mother. The illness is frequently dramatic and results in repeated visits to physicians, leading to multiple diagnostic and therapeutic procedures. The perpetrator of this medical hoax denies any knowledge of the cause of the illness. Physical signs of illness usually promptly resolve when the child is separated from the perpetrator. In cases of MSBP where disease is actually produced, surreptitious poisoning of the child is a common mechanism. In a review of published cases of MSBP (Rosenberg, 1987), seven of the eight most common presentations of MSBP were poisoning (**Table 12-1**); the lone common presentation not involving poisoning was fever. In the majority of cases where actual illness was produced, including that produced by poisoning, the abuse continued after the child was admitted to the hospital. The placement of intravenous lines or gastrostomy tubes while in the hospital in some cases afforded other routes of poisoning (Saulsbury et al., 1984).

For a more complete review of MSBP, refer to Chapter 13.

NEGLECT

While all childhood poisonings represent some degree of lack of proper supervision, it can be difficult to decide when a poisoning has resulted from true neglect. In an important study on the epidemiology of caustic ingestions, no difference was found in the number of safety hazards or safety precautions between homes where the ingestions occurred and control homes (Sobel, 1970). Similar factors appear in studies of homes of children who have experienced multiple ingestions. Sobel's and other studies consistently show that the common denominator in homes with accidental ingestions is not neglect but significant family stress. Marital conflicts, mental or physical illness, transiency, and other factors combined with poor coping mechanisms for stress seem to set the stage for poisonings. The resultant poisoning brings to the attention of the health care provider the child whose basic needs are unmet. The child may appear dirty, malnourished, and lack immunizations. There may be a delay in seeking medical care for the ingestion because the child is left unattended for long periods of time or the parents have been in a prolonged alcohol- or drug-induced stupor. When neglect is suspected, child protective services must be contacted to save the child from further harm (Fischler, 1983).

As noted, neglect may be a factor in some poisonings involving families with parental drug and alcohol abuse. As the extent and variety of drug use has proliferated over the latter portion of this century, the risk of ingestion of these drugs by children has similarly increased. Case reports of phencyclidine ingestion began to appear in the 1970s. Poisonings were presumed to have occurred from passive inhalation in a smoke-filled car. Younger children especially may be at increased risk of passive exposure to the smoke of crack cocaine due to their decreased mobility, although this remains an unproven theory. Accidental ingestion of PCP crystals left from a party was cited in one report (Schwartz & Einhorn, 1986). Benzodiazepines, opiates, and methamphetamines have been detected in children poisoned in drug-abusing environments (Bays, 1990).

Table 12-1. Munchausen Syndrome by Proxy
Presentations Produced by Poisoning
Bleeding
Seizures
CNS Depression
Apnea
Diarrhea
Vomiting
Fever

ILLICIT DRUG USE

The danger to a child living in the presence of illicit drug use includes not only the prenatal effects of drug exposure and the increased risks of neglect and physical abuse postnatally (Leventhal et al., 1989), but also the risk of the child actually ingesting an illicit drug. Close proximity to recreational drugs can result in the poisoning of a child through four possible routes: passive inhalation, accidental ingestion of drugs left around the home, accepting drugs from an older child or other nonparent adult, or deliberate poisoning (Schwartz et al., 1986).

The phrase "morning after syndrome" was first used to describe children poisoned by ethanol after sampling alcohol left out in the home, frequently from a party the night before. Typically these children presented to an emergency room obviously intoxicated and then progressed to seizures and coma secondary to alcohol-induced hypoglycemia (Tolis, 1965).

COCAINE INTOXICATION

As the epidemic of cocaine use has spread, reports of cocaine intoxication in young children have appeared. Apnea and seizures have been reported in infants exposed to cocaine in breast milk (Chasnoff et al., 1987) and in a breast-fed infant whose mother placed topical cocaine on her painful nipples (Chaney, 1988). Much of the epidemic of cocaine use has been fueled by the ready availability of the relatively cheap form of freebase cocaine referred to as "crack," which is easily vaporized by heat and then smoked. Passive inhalation of these cocaine vapors was the presumed route of ingestion of four children presenting to Harlem Hospital, two of whom had seizures and two of whom were lethargic. Toxicologic screens of the urine identified the presence of cocaine in all four children (Bateman & Heagerty, 1989). One of these children, who also presented with burns of uncertain etiology, also had an opiate found in the urine. In this case, deliberate poisoning seems a more likely mechanism. Oral ingestion of cocaine was believed to have caused seizures reported in four children under 3 years old who were unexpectedly found to have cocaine on routine urine toxicologic screening (Ernst & Sanders, 1989). On further evaluation by social services, all the children were found to have been in the company of cocaine-abusing adults. One infant, a 4-month-old, was believed to have been intentionally fed cocaine in an attempt to quiet her.

In addition to the ingestion of cocaine, the chemicals used in the conversion of cocaine hydrochloric acid to freebase cocaine ("crack") can be a serious hazard. A 20-month-old child who sustained severe caustic esophageal burns requiring gastrostomy feedings and central hyperalimentation has been reported. The injury occurred following the ingestion of a lye solution, which was used in making freebase cocaine. The lye had been left in her home following a party. This child's urine was also positive for cocaine metabolites (Kharasch et al., 1990).

Children who present with clinical evidence of acute cocaine poisoning are likely to be only a small portion of all children who actively or passively ingest cocaine. This was demonstrated in a survey of children between 2 weeks and 5 years of age presenting to the emergency room at Boston City Hospital (Kharasch et al., 1991). In those children who did not have life-threatening emergencies or any history suggestive of cocaine exposure, the urine was screened for cocaine metabolites. Of 250 children whose urine was collected before discharge from the emergency room, six (2.4%) tested positive for cocaine. All of the children testing positive were less than 2 years old and four of the six were less than 1 year old. Only one of these children was being breast-fed at the time of the study.

Regardless of the mechanism by which cocaine gains access to children's bodies, it seems clear that children in close proximity to this drug are at significant risk. They may not show obvious clinical signs of exposure, but can be at risk of behavioral, intellectual, and physical damage from repeated exposure. Although it may be difficult to determine the mechanism of ingestion in any given case of a child poisoned by an illicit drug, child protective services should be routinely involved in evaluating the home situation. Whether it is the purposeful intoxication of children by parents or babysitters (Schwartz et al., 1986) or an accidental ingestion, one must presume the child is a victim of abuse or neglect and act accordingly.

◆ MANAGEMENT

HISTORY

In most incidents involving accidental poisoning the ingestion is either witnessed or is discovered soon after ingestion. The child still has the container in hand, with the pills or solution in the mouth or nearby. Usually little has been ingested and the child has no symptoms, or very mild, transient symptoms. Death is an uncommon occurrence following accidental ingestion. Accidental poisoning can also occur in homes that have not been child-proofed, for example, at a friend's or relative's home where there are no children.

The child who has been poisoned by intent or neglect presents with a confusing or misleading history. *One of four presentations commonly occurs (Meadow, 1989):*

1. A parent brings the child to the hospital for treatment of an acute poisoning under the guise of an accidental ingestion.

2. A child presents with signs and symptoms of unknown etiology.

3. The child presents with recurrent unexplained illnesses (MSBP).

4. The child is found dead or near death because of significant time lapse since ingestion.

Given the confusing history, the physician must be alert to the myriad signs and symptoms children can manifest following an ingestion. **Table 12-2** lists common presenting signs and symptoms reported in intentionally poisoned children with their respective etiologies.

Table 12-2. Symptoms and Signs Following Intentional Poisoning

Symptoms and Signs	Drug	Reference
Seizures	Phenothiazine	Dine, 1965
	Hydrocarbons	Saulsbury et al., 1984
	Salt	Rogers et al., 1976
	Water	Mortimer, 1980
	Cocaine	Rivkin & Gilmore, 1989
Drowsiness, Coma	Tricyclic Antidepressants	Simon, 1980
	Chloral Hydrate	Lansing, 1974
	Insulin	Bauman & Yalow, 1981
	Acetaminophen	Hickson et al., 1983
	Salicylates	Pickering, 1976
	Phenothiazines	Schnaps et al., 1981
	Barbiturates	Rogers et al., 1976; Lorber, 1978
	Opiates	Rogers et al., 1976
	Valium	Dine, 1982
	Alcohol	Dine, 1982
	Glutethimide	Dine, 1982
Apnea	Tricyclic Antidepressants	Watson et al., 1979
	Salt	Rogers et al., 1976
	Pepper	Cohle et al., 1988
Vomiting	Ipecac	Sutphen & Saulsbury, 1986
Diarrhea	Phenolphthalein	Fleisher & Ament, 1977
	Epsom Salts	Fenton et al., 1988

PHYSICAL EXAMINATION

Various drug ingestions in children can rapidly lead to severe depression of the central nervous system and coma. The physical examination can differentiate drug-induced encephalopathy from the other common causes of coma in children such as mass lesions and seizures. Intact pupillary reflexes to light in the comatose patient indicate a functional midbrain. In most forms of metabolic coma, including drug-induced, pupillary reflexes remain intact.

The physical examination can also enable the physician to identify a specific toxicologic syndrome accounting for the patient's unexplained symptoms (**Table 12-3**).

Table 12-3. Identifying Specific Toxicologic Syndrome		
Poison Syndrome	**Signs and Symptoms**	**Drugs**
Sympathomimetic	Increased pulse and blood pressure, fever, pupillary dilatation, sweating, agitation, psychosis	Cocaine, barbiturates, phencyclidine
Sympatholytic	Decreased pulse and blood pressure, hypothermia, small pupils, decreased peristalsis, obtundation, coma	Ethanol, barbiturates, sedative hypnotics, opiates
Cholinergic	Bradycardia, miosis, sweating, hyperperistalsis, salivation, bronchorrhea, urinary incontinence	Organophosphates, carbamates, nicotine
Anticholinergic	Tachycardia, hypertension, fever, pupillary dilation, hot dry skin, decreased peristalsis, urinary retention	Tricyclic antidepressants, antihistamines, phenothiazines, atropine, scopolamine

(Adapted from: Olsen K., Banner W. Emergency Management of Childhood Poisoning. In Grossman M., Dieckmann R. Eds. Pediatric Emergency Medicine. Philadelphia, JB Lippincott, 1991, pp. 332-339.)

LABORATORY DATA

Laboratory data that can help in arriving at a diagnosis include serum osmolality, electrolytes, glucose, BUN, and creatinine.

SERUM OSMOLALITY

The serum osmolality is normally about 290 mOsm/l. Serum osmolality should be directly measured with a freezing point depression osmometer and can be estimated by calculation using the following equation:

Osmolality = 2 (Na) [mEq/l] + Glucose [mg/dl] / 18 + BUN [mg/dl] / 2.8

The difference between the measured and calculated osmolality is known as the osmolar gap. Ethanol ingestion is a common cause of elevated osmolar gap.

ELECTROLYTES

Serum electrolytes are helpful in determining the presence of a metabolic acidosis associated with an anion gap. **Table 12-4** identifies drugs that can cause an elevated anion gap metabolic acidosis.

The anion gap can be calculated as follows:

Anion gap = Na - (Cl + HCO3) = 8 - 16 mEq/l in children

ADDITIONAL LABORATORY TESTS

Serum glucose, BUN, creatinine, and urinalysis should also routinely be measured in the poisoned patient.

Table 12-4. Drugs Associated with an Elevated Anion Gap Acidosis
Methanol
Ethylene Glycol
Phenformin
Isoniazid
Iron
Salicylates
Cyanide
Carbon Monoxide

RADIOLOGIC STUDIES

Abdominal radiographs can demonsrrate radiopaque tablets in the gastrointestinal tract. Although iron- and enteric-coated tablets can be seen by X-ray, a negative film does not rule out their ingestion. In infants and toddlers, additional radiographs in the form of a skeletal survey (humanogram) should be considered to detect other signs of abuse as indicated. This may be especially helpful in children with certain stigmata of abuse, for example, inflicted burns *(see Chapter 6)*.

TOXICOLOGY SCREENING

The routine toxicology screen employed by most hospitals can be valuable in the identification of the poisoning agent, if the child has been poisoned with a drug included in the screen. In many recorded cases of intentional poisoning, however, the drug was not part of the standard toxicology screen. It is important for the physician to consider which particular drugs may be responsible and ask the laboratory to perform specific assays for them. If the clinical presentation of the child is particularly confusing, it is wise to preserve samples of blood, urine, and gastric aspirate until a more specific request can be made of the toxicology laboratory. These samples and any samples sent for specific toxicologic assays should be prepared in a chain of custody protocol. Urine and blood should be collected in special containers and sealed with tamper-evident seals. Most hospitals and reference laboratories have lists available and policy and procedure manuals for collecting specimens under the chain of custody, which is a system where personnel collecting, transferring, or analyzing biological specimens or controlled substances retrieved from patients (for example, rocks of crack cocaine retrieved in gastric lavage) must sign a legal log for each step in the handling of the specimen. This affords the legal system evidence that is admissible in a court system. The timing of samples is critical and must be noted in the medical record.

Certain substances may require a second analytical method for confirmation. Toxins detected by screening methods such as thin layer chromatography (TLC) or gas chromatography (GC) may need to be confirmed by gas chromatography–mass spectrophotometry (GC-MS). A Regional Poison Center and toxicologist should be consulted for advice in individual cases on the recommended assays for laboratory testing. It is also helpful to discuss the case with the analytical or forensic toxicologist involved with the clinical laboratory that will be analyzing the patient's specimens.

When attempting to identify the potentially offending agent, it could be helpful to contact that parent's physician to determine which drugs have been prescribed for each of the parents. Also, the parent's occupation may give a clue as to which drugs may be present in the home. It should be noted that a negative screen may be the result of obtaining the sample too late to identify a drug with a short half-life.

◆ EXAMPLES OF POISONING AGENTS

A few specific poisonings will be discussed to highlight particular aspects of this phenomenon.

SALT

The literature contains several instances of infants intentionally poisoned with salt (Meadow, 1977; Rogers et al., 1976). These infants presented with multiple episodes of hypernatremia. They exhibited a variety of findings, including seizures, lethargy, ataxia, coma, and dehydration. All had extreme elevations of serum and urine sodium. Normal renal function was demonstrated on recovery. Several authors have postulated that these infants would have been able to excrete the excess salt in the urine efficiently, but this mechanism failed probably because they were likely also deprived of water. The clinical and biological findings in these salt-poisoned children are very similar to findings in children with hypernatremic dehydration secondary to intentional withholding of water (Pickel et al., 1970). Mothers were the perpetrators in all cases of salt poisoning and all had histories of severe psychiatric problems.

PEPPER ASPIRATION

Eight children dying of pepper aspiration have been reported (Cohle et al., 1988). In each case the child was asphyxiated by forced pepper ingestion as a punishment for some perceived wrongdoing. The children all died due to airway obstruction. Typically, the airways were totally occluded by pepper and mucosal edema. All but one of the victims was under 5 years old and the perpetrators were all caretakers of various types. Four of the children showed signs of chronic abuse.

COCAINE

Children clinically intoxicated with cocaine usually present with a combination of central nervous system and cardiovascular findings. Seizures are common and frequently difficult to control. Since cocaine can cause fever in children, one might reasonably presume the fever to be the etiology of the seizure. Cardiovascular findings can provide the clue to the true cause of the child's condition. Hypertension, tachycardia, cardiac arrhythmias, and poor peripheral perfusion often are present. As part of the sympathomimetic syndrome induced by cocaine, the pupils may be dilated. It is important to stress that any combination of these findings can be present. The study by Kharasch and associates reminds us that cocaine exposure can be clinically undetectable. In areas where cocaine use is common, its presence in children presenting with unexplained neurologic or cardiovascular findings should be explored.

ALCOHOLS, GLYCOLS, AND HYDROCARBONS

Children intoxicated with ethanol may present to emergency departments with altered mental status, metabolic acidosis, and often hypoglycemia. The source may be half-consumed containers of alcohol (beer or wine coolers) or mixed drinks left after an adult party. Toddlers may access these beverages when there is inadequate supervision or neglect. Furthermore, parents have offered children alcohol to quiet them when the adults are frustrated by the child's "excessive" crying.

Alcohols, glycols, and hydrocarbons are three compounds that should be given special attention when investigating potential child abuse. These three agents are a unique group because they are common to most households and because their dangerous properties are not always realized. In addition, abusive forced ingestion can readily be passed off as accidental injury if the investigator does not probe into this possibility. This is particularly true during "holiday" seasons.

There are cases of intentional ethylene glycol (antifreeze) poisoning in small infants (Woolf et al., 1992; Saladino & Shannon, 1991). Ethylene glycol is sweet tasting and only a small amount is toxic, factors that may contribute to its ease of administration. In fact, cases of animal abuse or accidental poisoning have occurred secondary to these physical characteristics. Infants presenting with anion gap metabolic acidosis of unexplained etiology should be evaluated for infection, toxic overdose from agents such as ethylene glycol, ethanol, methanol, salicylates, and iron, and metabolic conditions such as diabetic ketoacidosis, uremia, and inborn errors of metabolism.

Hydrocarbons in various forms have been associated with intentional poisoning from practices such as lighter fluid administration in an intravenous line (Saulsbury et al., 1984) and recurrent pine oil intoxication in an infant (Hill et al., 1975). An unusual hydrocarbon-type odor and unexplained respiratory failure with pulmonary edema may be a clue to this form of abuse.

◆ SUMMARY

The intentional poisoning of children is an uncommon but highly dangerous form of child abuse. It can occur in the context of extreme neglect, bizarre means of discipline, or Munchausen Syndrome by Proxy. The physician must approach the family with as much understanding and compassion as possible. In some instances what appears to be an attempt to harm a child may instead be the injudicious but well-intentioned use of a folk remedy the family felt too embarrassed to discuss. On the other hand, perpetrators of MSBP may be extremely sophisticated in their ability to conceal their intent.

As always, the duty of the physician is to approach the ill child with a sensitivity to the history and close attention to the physical findings and laboratory studies. When the latter is not explained by the former, child abuse must always be considered. The persistent search for an explanation of those findings, particularly in the intentionally poisoned child, may save that child from future harm and even death.

◆ BIBLIOGRAPHY

Bateman, D, and Heagerty, M: Passive freebase cocaine ("crack") inhalation by infants and toddlers, *Am J Dis Child* 143:25, 1989.

Bauman, W, and Yalow, R: Child abuse: Parenteral insulin administration, *J Pediatr* 99:588, 1981.

Bays, J: Substance abuse and child abuse, *Pediatr Clin North Am* 37:881, 1990.

Chaney, NE: Cocaine convulsions in a breast-feeding baby, *J Pediatr* 112:134, 1988.

Chasnoff, IF, Lewis, DE, and Squires, L: Cocaine intoxication in a breast-fed infant, *Pediatrics* 80:836, 1987.

Cohle, S, Trestail, J, and Graham, M: Fatal pepper aspiration, *Am J Dis Child* 142:633, 1988.

Dine, M: Tranquilizer poisoning: An example of child abuse, *Pediatrics* 36:782, 1965.

Dine, M: Intentional poisoning of children: An overlooked category of child abuse: report of seven cases and review of the literature, *Pediatrics* 70:32, 1982.

Ernst, A, and Sanders, W: Unexpected cocaine intoxication presenting as seizures in children, *Ann Emerg Med* 18:774, 1989.

Fenton, AC, Wailoo, MP, and Tanner, MS: Severe failure to thrive and diarrhea caused by laxative abuse, *Arch Dis Child* 63:978, 1988.

Fischler, R: Poisoning: A syndrome of child abuse, *Am Fam Physician* 28:104, 1983.

Fleisher, D, and Ament, M: Diarrhea, red diapers, and child abuse, *Clin Pediatr* 17:820, 1977.

Friedman, E: Caustic ingestions and foreign body aspirations: An overlooked form of child abuse, *Ann Otol Rhinol Laryngol* 96:709, 1987.

Green, J, Craft, L, and Ghishan, F: Acetaminophen poisoning in infancy, *Am J Dis Child* 137:386, 1983.

Hickson, GB, Greene, J, Ghishan, FK, et al: Apparent intentional poisoning of an infant with acetaminophen, *Am J Dis Child* 137:917, 1983.

Hill, RM, Barer, J, and Leighton, H: An investigation of recurrent pine oil poisoning in an infant by the use of gas chromatographic-mass spectrometric methods, *J Pediatr* 87:115, 1975.

Kempe, CH, Silverman, FN, Steele, BF, et al: The battered child syndrome, *JAMA* 181:17, 1962.

Kharasch, S, Glotzer, D, Vinci, R, et al: Unsuspected cocaine exposure in young children, *Am J Dis Child* 145:204, 1991.

Kharasch, S, Vinci, R, and Reece, R: Esophagitis, epiglottitis, and cocaine alkaloid ("crack"): "Accidental" poisoning or child abuse, *Pediatrics* 86:117, 1990.

Kresel, JJ, and Lovejoy, FH: Poisonings and child abuse. In N Ellerstein, ed: *Child Abuse and Neglect*, Churchill Livingstone, New York, 1981, pp. 307-313.

Lansky, L: An unusual case of childhood chloral hydrate poisoning, *Am J Dis Child* 127:275, 1974.

Levanthal, JM, Garber, RB, and Brady, CA: Identification during the postpartum period of infants who are at high risk of child maltreatment, *J Pediatr* 114:48l, 1989.

Lorber, J: Unexplained coma in a two-year-old, *Lancet* 2:680, 1978.

Mahesch, V, Stern, P, and Kearns, G: Application of pharmokinetics in the diagnosis of chemical abuse in Munchausen Syndrome by Proxy, *Clin Pediatr* 27:243, 1988.

McClung, HJ, Murray, R, and Braden, NJ: Intentional ipecac poisoning in children, *Am J Dis Child* 142:637, 1988.

Meadow, R: Munchausen Syndrome by Proxy: The hinterland of child abuse, *Lancet* 2:343, 1977.

Meadow, R: Munchausen Syndrome by Proxy, *Arch Dis Child* 57:92, 1982.

Meadow, R: ABC of child abuse: Poisoning, *Br Med J* 298:1445, 1989.

Mortimer, JG: Acute water intoxication as another manifestation of child abuse, *Arch Dis Child* 55:401, 1980.

Olsen, K, and Banner, W: Emergency management of childhood poisoning. In M Grossman and R Dieckmann, eds: *Pediatric Emergency Medicine*, JB Lippincott, Philadelphia, 1991, pp. 332-339.

Pickel, S, Anderson, C, and Holliday, M: Thirsting and hypernatremic dehydration: A form of child abuse, *Pediatrics* 45:54, 1970.

Pickering, D: Salicylate poisoning as a manifestation of the battered child syndrome, *Am J Dis Child* 130:675, 1976.

Rendle-Short, J: Non-accidental barbiturate poisoning of children, *Lancet* 2:1212, 1978.

Rivkin, M, and Gilmore, H: Generalized seizures in an infant due to environmentally acquired cocaine, *Pediatrics* 84:1100, 1989.

Rogers, D, Tripp, J, and Bentovim, A: Non-accidental poisoning: An extended syndrome of child abuse, *Br Med J* 1:793, 1976.

Rosenberg, D: Web of deceit: A literature review of Munchausen Syndrome by Proxy, *Child Abuse Negl* 11:547, 1987.

Saladino, R, and Shannon, M: Accidental and intentional poisonings with ethylene glycol in infancy: Diagnostic clues and management, *Pediatr Emerg Care* 7:93, 1991.

Saulsbury, FT, Chobanian, MC, and Wilson, WG: Child abuse: Parenteral hydrocarbon administration, *Pediatrics* 73:719, 1984.

Schnaps, Y, Frand, M, Rotem, Y, et al: The chemically abused child, *Pediatrics* 68:119, 1981.

Schwartz, HR, Peary, P, and Mistretta, D: Intoxication of young children with marijuana: A form of amusement for "pot"-smoking teenage girls, *Am J Dis Child* 140:326, 1986.

Schwartz, RH, and Einhorn, A: PCP intoxication in seven young children, *Pediatr Emerg Care* 2:238, 1986.

Simon, F: Uncommon type of child abuse (letter), *J Pediatr* 96:785, 1980.

Sobel, R: The psychiatric implications of accidental poisoning in childhood, *Pediatr Clin North Am* 17:653, 1970.

Sutphen, J, and Saulsbury, FT: Intentional ipecac poisoning: Munchausen Syndrome by Proxy, *Pediatrics* 82:453, 1986.

Tolis, A: Hypoglycemic convulsions in children after alcohol ingestion, *Pediatr Clin North Am* 12:423, 1965.

Watson, JB, Davies, JM, and Hunter, JL: Non-accidental poisoning in childhood, *Arch Dis Child* 54:143, 1979.

Woolf, AD, Wynshaw-Boris, A, Rinaldo, P, et al: Intentional infantile ethylene glycol poisoning presenting as an inherited metabolic disorder, *J Pediatr* 120:421, 1992.

Chapter 13

MUNCHAUSEN SYNDROME BY PROXY

JAMES A. MONTELEONE, M.D.

John was followed from birth in the hemophiliac clinic. His mother was a known carrier. She had two brothers with a bleeding disorder. John was found to be a mild bleeder, having only two episodes of bleeds requiring special attention in the emergency room in his first two years. The bleeding was controlled easily and required short hospitalization. When he was 2 his mother asked to be taught home care to manage his future bleeds. She was an eager and excellent student. Soon she was calling every day, stating that he had sustained a fall or that she noted blood in

his stool. This was followed by her appearing in the clinic on a daily basis stating that John had fallen or that she found blood in this stool. No one had ever witnessed the falls. He was hospitalized 37 times and while in the hospital was found to have unexplained drops in his hemoglobin levels. The child was placed in foster care and experienced no bleeds over an extended period of time. The mother was ordered by the court to see a counselor. The child was returned to his mother's care with supervision. He continued to do well.

♦OVERVIEW

Baron von Munchausen was a teller of outrageous tales who lived in the 18th century. Some of his tales, authored by one of his friends, Rudolph Raspe, were published in a children's book entitled *Baron von Munchausen's Narrative of His Marvelous Travels and Campaigns in Russia* (1936).

In 1951, Asher described an unusual group of patients who went from physician to physician fabricating stories of illness; they were willing to subject themselves to numerous tests and needless surgery. He called this the von Munchausen's (or Munchausen) syndrome. Later, Roy Meadow (1977) described a variant of the Munchausen syndrome in a case report of two hospitalized children. Unlike the original Munchausen syndrome, in this case, the parent fabricated the illness in the child and presented the child to a physician for treatment. Meadow called this phenomenon the *Munchausen Syndrome by Proxy (MSBP)*. Since then, the syndrome has become more widely recognized, although before Meadow coined the name, others (Rogers et al., 1976) had reported incidents in which several mothers had deliberately poisoned their children and then tried to convince their physicians that their children were ill, by either simulating or actually inducing illness in their children.

Naturally, such falsification of medical illness can cause emotional harm by propagating a self-image in the child as chronically ill and causes physical injury with unnecessary medical testing and possible pointless use of medications to treat false symptoms. In some cases, it has led to the child's death.

♦CLINICAL PRESENTATION

SIGNS AND SYMPTOMS

Munchausen Syndrome by Proxy affects children of widely variable ages. Children have presented with factitious illness by proxy from as young as neonates (Rogers et al., 1976) to as old as 21 years (Rosenberg, 1987). Perpetrators of MSBP are found in all socioeconomic groups; some deceptions are unsophisticated while others are complex requiring complicated investigative techniques to unravel. In general, the child appears to have a persistent or recurrent condition or illness that cannot be explained. There may be abnormal laboratory studies without strong evidence of underlying disease or, conversely, there may be normal lab results which do not support the illness reported. Treatments are not well-tolerated or else seem ineffective. For example, a child may develop a rash but is unable to tolerate prescribed drug treatments because of reported vomiting or other untoward reactions. The parent, most often the mother, is willing to have her child undergo diagnostic procedures and medical treatments even when they are invasive. If the child is hospitalized the situation may go from bad to worse, with the child becoming febrile or lapsing into a coma; on the other hand, with hospitalization the severity of illness simulated or described by the parent may not continue, and the child may appear well. Experienced specialists often remark that they have never seen a case like this before.

Presenting complaints can vary widely, with the parent complaining that the child is tired all the time, that the child stops breathing and becomes cyanotic, or that the child convulses. Deliberate poisoning may be seen, sometimes involving medications prescribed by a physician. Children have also been injected with medications such as insulin to produce coma and with foreign substances, such as feces, to produce infection.

MEDICAL RECORD REVIEW

Typically, when reviewing the history and the medical record, it is noted that there have been numerous visits to the doctor and numerous hospitalizations. The child has undergone many diagnostic procedures, often involving several hospitals and physicians. The perpetrator, again most often the mother, usually denies knowledge of the etiology of the child's illness. The mother may report that she or another child have complained of symptoms similar to the ones she says are being experienced by the child. A rare disease is often diagnosed or strongly considered.

OCCURRENCE

The frequency of Munchausen Syndrome by Proxy is difficult to estimate. Most published articles on this syndrome are single case studies that focus on the type of medical deception used by the parent. Meaningful research has been difficult to conduct and is therefore limited in the literature. Still, it may not be as rare as previously thought. For instance, Warner and Hathaway (1984) estimated that 5% of cases evaluated for food allergies were consistent with Munchausen Syndrome by Proxy.

◆ETIOLOGY

The first significant review of the literature on MSBP was by Roy Meadow. He was the first to recognize and describe MSBP occurring in children. Others had described MSBP symptoms in children, but Meadow made the connection between the symptoms and the syndrome. Meadow reviewed the cases of 19 children from 17 families, 10 boys and 9 girls. The children ranged in age from 4 months to 7 years, with a mean age of 3 years, 2 months. The children had a wide range of signs and symptoms usually suggesting a multisystem disorder. The false symptoms and signs had occurred for 1 1/2 months to 4 years prior to diagnosis, the average being 13 months. The most common fabricated sign in Meadow's review was bleeding, which was reported in 12 of the 19 children. Neurological signs were also common (**Table 13-1**). Most of the children had been seen by many different doctors and had many referrals to various specialists. Even though the initial reported symptoms and signs were false, most of the children incurred secondary symptoms and signs as a result of medical investigations, operations, and medications. During their illness, many different diagnoses were considered. Meadow concluded that the doctors, who were treating the false illness, did the most harm to the child, unknowingly.

In addition to Meadow's study, Rosenberg's review is significant because all the cases known at the time (1987) were assembled for his study. This review was of greater significance than Meadow's because the number of cases studied was larger.

Table 13-1. Summary of Meadow's Results: Fabricated Signs	
Number of Cases: 19	
Bleeding:	12
Hematuria	7
Hematemesis	5
Hemoptyses	3
Blood in feces	3
Neurological Signs:	7
Drowsiness with coma	5
Seizures	3
Unsteadiness	2
Other Fabricated Signs	
Rashes	6
Glycosuria	5
Fevers	4
Biochemical abnormalities	4
Feculent vomitus	2

Rosenberg (1987) summarized the findings in 117 cases, comprising essentially all the known literature. Patient population was identified as 46% males, 45% females; in 9% of the cases no sex was indicated. The mean age (67 cases) was 39.8 months ± 32.1 months. Mean time of onset of symptoms and signs to the time of diagnosis was 14.9 months ± 14 months. The range of age at diagnosis was 1 month to 21 years. The range from time of onset of symptoms and signs to time of diagnosis was from several days to 20 years.

Presenting symptoms and signs covered a wide range. The most common presentations were: bleeding from various sites (44%), seizures (42%), central nervous system depression (19%), apnea (15%), diarrhea (11%), vomiting (10%), fever (10%), and rash (9%). Many children had more than one presenting problem.

SIMULATED VERSUS PRODUCED ILLNESS

Rosenberg identified two categories of presentation, simulated illness and produced illness. Simulated illness is defined as illness that is faked by the mother. An example of a simulated illness would be the mother's contamination of the child's urine specimen with her own blood and her subsequent claim that the child had been urinating blood. Produced illness is defined as illness that the mother actually inflicted on the child. An example of a produced illness would be the injection by the mother of a foreign material such as feces or a drug into the child's intravenous line or formula.

In 72 cases in which the presentation was known, 25% involved simulation of illness; in 72% of these cases the simulation took place while the child was in the hospital. Production of illness was found in 50% of the 72 cases; in 95% of this group, the production of illness took place while the child was in the hospital. In 25% of the cases, both simulation and production of illness were involved and in 84% of these cases both the simulation and the production of illness took place while the child was in the hospital.

PRESENTATION DECEPTIONS

The child's mother was the perpetrator in each of the cases Meadow and Rosenberg reviewed. Meadow found that the mothers in his study were able to accomplish the deception in a number of ways. Bleeding was generally the result of the mother adding her own blood to the child's vomit, urine, or feces. Sometimes blood was smeared on the child's face or perineum. The blood was usually obtained by the mother pricking herself. One mother used blood from an open thigh wound; another stirred a vaginal tampon in the child's urine specimen. A few mothers simulated blood in a specimen from the child by adding paint, cocoa, or phenolphthalein. One mother produced feculent vomitus by adding soft feces, which she stored in a container in her room, to the child's vomit. Fevers were produced by rubbing thermometers or immersing them in hot liquid. Biochemical abnormalities were simulated by adding chemicals, such as salt, to a specimen. In order to accomplish the deception, a variety of tricks distracted the person who had taken the specimen.

Rashes were fabricated by rubbing the skin repetitively with a fingernail or a sharp object to obtain a bullous lesion, by applying caustic solutions to areas of skin, or by painting with a dye such as phenolphthalein.

The neurological symptoms were the result of the mother giving the child a sedative or tranquilizer that had been prescribed for herself. The mother gave the medications in doses greater than those prescribed for herself. One mother applied pressure to the child's neck to induce seizures.

Seizures are a common presenting complaint in MSBP. Meadow noted that the best way to rule out a convulsive disorder was by taking a careful history. Often, the children were said to have had a seizure at school or similar place, in the presence of a third party or parties; questioning the party or others present at the time of the reported seizure usually revealed that no seizure had happened.

There is a high prevalence of MSBP in the subgroup of apnea patients. These patients have had two or more episodes of apnea that terminated after mouth-to-mouth resuscitation. The episodes have their onset only in the presence of the parent, but are witnessed secondarily by other persons after they have been called for assistance. When these infants die, the presumptive cause of death may be sudden infant death syndrome (SIDS). It may be impossible to distinguish between SIDS and other causes of death even with an autopsy. However, it is essential that all infants with unexplained deaths have an autopsy.

MULTISPECIALTY INVOLVEMENT

Rosenberg in particular found that many of the children had symptoms involving more than one organ system and saw more than one pediatric subspecialist. The overall problem in such cases is that the subspecialists see only their part of the elephant. Rosenberg felt that the pediatric subspecialists should consider factitious illness in their differential diagnosis and that they could make the correct diagnosis quicker if they reviewed the child's medical record thoroughly and carefully.

♦ DEMOGRAPHICS

PARENTAL CHARACTERISTICS

Certain characteristics seem to be held in common in these families. Most of the mothers, according to Meadow's study, seem loving and caring. They do not appear cruel, negligent, or uncaring. The father is usually distant and minimally involved. If the mother has other children, they are rarely discussed. All her energy is focused on the sick child. The mother spends an excessive amount of time on the hospital ward with the child and refuses to leave the child alone in the hospital even for one hour. She often insists that she is the only one to whom the child can relate and from whom the child will accept food, drink, and medication. The mother, despite her child's problems, does not seem as concerned about her child as are the medical and nursing staff. She may actually be conciliatory about the child's condition with the hospital staff.

The mother is typically familiar with medical terminology and procedures. Many of them have had some nursing education or have worked in a medical setting and may become overly friendly with the hospital staff. The occupations of 40% of the 97 mothers was unknown (**Table 13-2**). There is often conflict among medical professionals in the case, each taking a side as to whether or not the child is ill, or, if suspected, a victim of MSBP. The child usually improves when separated from the parent. With parental confrontations, the symptoms may stop and the child may improve, or the child may be in greater danger.

Seven of 12 mothers in the Meadow study who were questioned on the subject had a history with some features of Munchausen's Syndrome. Five of 10 mothers had a history within the previous 3 years of symptoms and signs similar to those which she fabricated for the child. Munchausen Syndrome or features of the syndrome were noted in 24% of the mothers in Rosenberg's study.

Table 13-2. Occupational Distribution Among Mothers in Rosenberg's Study	
Nurse or training for nursing	27%
Housewife	20%
Unemployed	4%
Medical office worker	3%
Social worker	2%
Schoolteacher	1%
Home helper	1%
Baby food demonstrator	1%
Orderly	1%

FAMILY DYNAMICS

At the time the fabrication was discovered, 15 of the 17 pairs of parents in the Meadow study were living together. Their mean age was 29 years, ranging from 24 to 37 years of age. Most of the mothers lived in the hospital with the child or visited the child for long periods each day. The fathers kept a low profile; 10 of 15 rarely visited the child in the hospital, which was particularly noteworthy in view of the severity of the child's illness. Six of 11 had jobs that required them to be away from home for long periods or in the evenings, and two others were considered extremely unsupportive of their wives. The fathers did not appear to know of the fabrication and had difficulty in believing it when told. In 10 of 15 families, there was a discrepancy between the social and the intellectual level of the parents. In each instance, the wife either came from a higher social background or seemed much more intelligent than her husband. In 15 of 17 families there were other children. In five families a second child incurred the syndrome or died of suspicious circumstances. In 10 families there was nothing to suggest involvement of older or younger siblings.

In describing the 97 perpetrators in her 117 cases, Rosenberg assessed that 98% were biological mothers and 2% were adoptive mothers. Many of the mothers were described as friendly and socially adept. Once the deception by the mother was discovered, evidence of secondary paternal collusion occurred in only 1.5% of all cases. In 15% of the cases the mother admitted completely to the deception; an additional 7% partially admitted; and 18% of the mothers denied the deception. The mother's reaction to confrontation was unknown in 60% of the cases.

Mother's Occupation of 16 of the 19 Mothers in Meadow's study

Nurses:	8
Registered	1
Partial training	7
Pediatrician's receptionist	1
Home health worker	1
Primary school teacher	1
Baby food demonstrator	1
No regular paid employment	4

Meadow's Prognoses for Victims of Munchausen Syndrome by Proxy

Meadow (1989) listed the following consequences for children who are falsely labelled as ill:

1. *They will receive needless and possibly harmful treatments.*
2. *They may develop a genuine disease.*
3. *They may die.*
4. *They may develop chronic invalidism.*
5. *They may develop Munchausen Syndrome as an adult.*

When a psychiatric diagnosis was described, depression was cited most often, and some personality disorders were noted. Many authors made a point of indicating that the perpetrator was not psychotic. Only one mother was described as a hysterical psychopath and one as probably psychotic. Loneliness and isolation were prominent in these women's lives.

♦ OUTCOMES

In Meadow's report, 17 of the 19 children survived. One died from presumed poisoning and one from uncertain circumstances. Of the survivors, eight were taken away from the family, nine remained at home after confrontation with the parents and involvement of social services with arrangements for continued supervision. Seven of these nine children were well and free of all symptoms at follow-up one to four years later. Two mothers continued to take their children to a variety of doctors with minor complaints, but no harmful fabrication took place.

Ten of the 117 children in Rosenberg's review died, giving a mortality rate of at least 9%. The age at the time of death was known for eight. All were younger than 3 years of age. The causes of death were from suffocation (4), salt poisoning (3), other poisoning (2), and uncertain (1). All the children died in the custody of their mothers. No mother admitted to homicide. In two of the children who died, the parents had been confronted with the diagnosis of MSBP and the children had been sent home with them, subsequently to die. Rosenberg warns that the fact that the parents had been confronted does not preclude the possibility of subsequent murder of the child.

Among the 117 victims reviewed by Rosenberg, 10 siblings had died under unusual circumstances. Those 10 siblings were not included in the original case reports.

SHORT-TERM MORBIDITY

Rosenberg defined short-term morbidity as pain and/or illness that did not leave permanent disfigurement or permanent impairment of function. One hundred percent of the children studied suffered short-term morbidity. In 75% of the cases, the morbidity was caused by both medical staff and the perpetrator. In 25% of the cases, the morbidity was caused most directly by the medical staff. The morbidity caused by the medical staff was related to investigations and procedures.

LONG-TERM MORBIDITY

Rosenberg defined long-term morbidity as pain or illness that caused permanent disfigurement. Of the 107 survivors, 8% had long-term morbidity, including impairment of gastrointestinal function following multiple esophageal surgeries, serious psychiatric problems, destructive joint changes, a limp, and mental retardation with cerebral palsy and cortical blindness. Several had multiple abdominal surgeries for laparotomy, colectomy, or ileostomy. Rosenberg felt the incidence of long-term morbidity was an underestimate since few of the cases had long-term follow-up.

Twelve of the perpetrators on whom information was available were suicidal. Of these, seven attempted suicide before the disclosure and five after the disclosure; 38 did not attempt suicide. No information was available on 47 of the perpetrators.

♦ CATEGORIES OF MSBP

Before examining guidelines for approaching suspected MSBP, it may be helpful to the examiner to be aware of various categories of the syndrome established by researchers. This can sometimes aid in diagnosis of both the syndrome and its degree of severity, which in turn aids in the choice of intervention.

Meadow (1989) and Libow and Schreier (1986) suggest a spectrum of categories for MSBP, including the following. Meadow identifies such categories as Perceived Illness, Doctor Shopping, Enforced Invalidism, and Fabricated Illness. Libow and Schreier classify perpetrators as Help Seeker, Active Inducer, and Doctor Addict. As with all forms of child abuse, it is the degree of abuse that matters. This will influence actions taken by social agencies.

PERCEIVED ILLNESS

Perceived illness describes the anxious mother, inexperienced, under stress and lonely, who needlessly worries that her healthy child is ill. She perceives symptoms in her child that others do not observe. The child is taken to the doctor on many occasions because the mother cannot be reassured, resulting in unpleasant investigations and treatments for the child. This process would not be classified as child abuse, unless the mother's persistence and refusal to accept normal results were excessive and the quality of the child's life was seriously impaired.

DOCTOR SHOPPING

Meadow uses the term doctor shopping to describe the parent who seeks help from a succession of different doctors claiming that a healthy child is ill. As each doctor in turn refuses further investigation, she consults yet another doctor. She tells none, in a chain of doctors, that she has seen anyone else for diagnosis or treatment. The result for the child is a series of repetitive investigations. When the parent's convictions about illness reach these proportions, it is child abuse.

ENFORCED INVALIDISM

Enforced invalidism develops when a parent with an ill or disabled child seeks to keep the child ill or increases the degree of disability. If the child has no disability, the parent ensures that the child is regarded as incapacitated and in need of special attention or assistance.

FABRICATED ILLNESS

Fabricated illness results when the parent lies to the doctor about a child's health, giving a convincing history of illness, and fabricates physical signs or alters health records that cause the doctor to perform detailed investigations and prescribe treatment. The parent invents the illness while the child is young and continues and intensifies the story as the years pass. When they are older some children will participate in the deception. Some have become independent illness addicts and have grown up to have the Munchausen Syndrome.

HELP SEEKER

The help seeker, which would be comparable to Meadow's Perceived Illness category, fabricates illness in a child on a limited basis, but the desperate request for help with parenting is the clear motivation. These mothers may respond to psychiatric intervention.

ACTIVE INDUCER

At the other extreme of the Munchausen Syndrome by Proxy is the active inducer —the prototype who will make life-threatening assaults on very young children. This type of parent, again usually the mother, is a very dangerous person. This person will go to extreme lengths to actively induce injury or illness.

DOCTOR ADDICT

The category of doctor addict, comparable with Meadow's Doctor Shopping group, represents the other major class of cases. Neither as dramatic as Active Inducers in symptomatology and danger, nor as blatant as the Help Seekers in their request for intervention, the Doctor Addict mothers may frequently be written off as cranks or overanxious and their children as psychosomatic or depressed. They are less likely to be identified than the prototypical cases since doctor addiction can evade resolution for longer than the prototypical cases in which the victim is hospitalized with an acute condition.

◆ GUIDELINES WHEN MSBP IS SUSPECTED

If the diagnosis of Munchausen Syndrome by Proxy is to be made, the physician must remember that sometimes a story is false. A small degree of suspicion should be maintained at all times, especially when the course of a child's condition does not make sense.

If the attending physician suspects MSBP, he or she should take the following steps:

1. The child's safety is the primary concern. These children are at risk. Approximately 10% of them will die, and the majority will have long-term morbidity. The physician should continue to behave as if the mother's story of her child's illness is accurate; it may be. Perform whatever diagnostic tests are necessary to confirm the diagnosis, using other professionals, crime labs, veterinarians, or others who might be useful in aiding with the diagnosis. Veterinarians are included in the diagnostic process because they are familiar with animal blood and tissue, which some parents have attempted to pass off as coming from the child. It is often not possible, or necessary, to obtain laboratory evidence to prove MSBP.

2. The child should be separated from the parents for a sufficient length of time to determine if the symptoms and signs occur in their absence. Try to get the parents to leave voluntarily. If not, this action may require legal enforcement and a court order.

3. If the child is verbal, interview him or her alone. An experienced counselor is recommended.

4. Check with other physicians, other hospitals, employers, and schools for details of the history relating to the child and family. Check out the social and work histories as well. It is common for the parent to fabricate details such as schooling, employment, illnesses, and hospitalizations. Check out the parent's history of witnesses to illness in the child and interview them about the facts they have allegedly witnessed. Check past medical records. Do not allow the parent to talk you out of the search. Look for unusual illnesses in siblings of the patient or unusual illnesses in the parents.

5. Pay careful attention to documentation in the medical record. Follow chain of evidence procedures in handling specimens.

6. The possibilities of simulating or producing illness are endless and as diverse as the human imagination. Nothing is farfetched, especially when one suspects poisoning. Decide which poisons are suspected and obtain specific assays on the appropriate body fluids and exogenously administered fluids. Consider all sources, food, syringes, and intravenous bottles as possible evidence. Save all specimens for toxicological assay. It may be necessary to have more than one reference laboratory assay the specimen. Check the reliability of the signs, that the rash does not wash off with water or alcohol, that the blood is blood and that it is the child's.

7. An experienced nurse who has been carefully instructed about the problem should be stationed in the room at all times. All specimens must be carefully collected and guarded. No food, drink, or medicines may be brought in by the family. The child should never be left alone with a parent, and the person in attendance should be aware that the parent may try to harm the child; the nurse must watch carefully at all times while the parent is with the child.

8. The child should have a psychiatric and/or psychologic evaluation. As with the parents, the purpose of these evaluations is not to confirm the diagnosis (which cannot be done by testing) but to aid with the impact of the situations and to identify other potential problems.

9. Local social service and child protective services must be involved immediately.

10. The medical team, social service, and protective agencies must work out a plan of action. It is wise for the child protection team to have a protocol outlining the procedures to follow. Remember, the child is not free of risk because he is in the hospital. If the parent is producing illness, there is a 70% chance that he or she will produce it in the hospital. The protective plan may include video monitoring of the child. As in any other child abuse case, the plan should include whether the child should be removed from the home or can remain there under supervision.

11. Be supportive, not accusing when presenting the diagnosis to the family. State the case clearly and simply. Tell the parents that the case has been reported to child protective services. Be prepared to immediately protect the child. Child protective services and the court should be on notice so that a court holding order on the child may be obtained if necessary. The object of presenting the diagnosis to the parents is not to persuade them that it is true or to obtain a confession, it is to inform them that such a diagnosis has been made and that steps will be taken to protect the child and confirm the diagnosis.

12. The parent may be suicidal. Psychiatric care should be made immediately available to the mother and father after disclosure of the diagnosis.

COMPLICATIONS IN EVALUATION

Sometimes the evaluation is complicated because a genuine organic disease is present in addition to the fabricated illness. The child may actually have a legitimate illness, such as hemophilia, asthma, or convulsive disorder which the parent uses as a basis for complaints. For example, the parent of a hemophilia patient may precipitate problems by causing a bleed; another might withhold or increase the prescribed medications in the child with an asthmatic or convulsive disorder.

CHILD SURVEILLANCE

Video surveillance has been effective as a means of confirming the diagnosis of Munchausen Syndrome by Proxy (Epstein et al., 1987). In answer to the critics of video surveillance who state that it is not ethical, Frost and Glaze (1988) respond that the critics of videotaping forget that it is the patient, the child, who is being watched secretly by the camera, not the mother. Videotaping is performed for the child's protection and is therefore ethical. There is no entrapment since the presence of the surveillance apparatus does not increase the likelihood that the illegal act will be committed. The method is legal and the information obtained has been used as evidence in legal proceedings.

◆ CONFRONTATION

Meadow suggested that these parents be confronted by the physician immediately after he or she suspects the charade. In his experience the fabrication usually ended following confrontation. He warned that those he did not confront continued the abuse and in one case he believed it resulted in the death of the child. He further stated that, when confronted, most perpetrators do not acknowledge the abuse but they do stop the actions.

If MSBP is not recognized, the child is at higher risk for morbidity. When the diagnosis is being considered, the hospital is the best place to confirm the diagnosis, if necessary. The child's involvement in the pretense can result in his or her death.

♦BIBLIOGRAPHY

Amegavie, L, Marzouk, O, Mullen, J, Sills, J, and Gauthier Le Tendre, JBM: Munchausen's Syndrome by Proxy: A warning for health professionals, *Br Med J* 293:855-856, 1986.

Asher, R: Munchausen Syndrome, *Lancet* 1:339-341, 1951.

Blix, S, and Brack, G: The effects of a suspected case of Munchausen's Syndrome by Proxy on a pediatric nursing staff, *Gen Hosp Psychiatry* 10:402-409, 1988.

Clark, GD, Key, JD, Rutherford, P, and Bithoney, WG: Munchausen's Syndrome by Proxy (child abuse) presenting as apparent autoerythrocyte sensitization syndrome: An unusual presentation of Polle syndrome, *Pediatrics* 74:1100-1102, 1984.

Drell, MJ: More on Munchausen by Proxy, *J Am Acad Child Adolescent Psychiatry* 27:140, 1988.

Epstein, MA, Markowitz, RL, Gallo, DM, Holmes, JW, and Gryboski, JD: Munchausen Syndrome by Proxy: Considerations in diagnosis and confirmation by video surveillance, *Pediatrics* 80:220-224, 1987.

Frederick, V, Luedtke, GS, Barrett, FF, Hixson, D, and Burch, K: Munchausen Syndrome by Proxy: recurrent central catheter sepsis, *Pediatr Infect Dis J* 9:440-442, 1990.

Frost, JD, and Glaze, DG: Munchausen's Syndrome by Proxy and video surveillance, *Am J Dis Child* 142:917-918, 1988.

Griffith, JL, and Slovik, LS: Munchausen Syndrome by Proxy and sleep disorders medicine, *Sleep* 12:178-183, 1989.

Guandolo, VL: Munchausen Syndrome by Proxy: An outpatient challenge, *Pediatrics* 75:526-530, 1985.

Herzberg, JH, and Wolff, SM: Chronic factitious fever in puberty and adolescence: A diagnostic challenge to the family physician, *Psychiatr Med* 3:205-212, 1972.

Holborow, PL: A variant of Munchausen's Syndrome by Proxy, *J Am Acad Child Psychiatry* 24:238, 1985.

Hosch, IA: Munchausen Syndrome by Proxy, *Am J Maternal Child Nurs* 12:48-52, 1987.

Jones, JG, Butler, HL, Hamilton, B, Perdue, JD, Stern, P, and Woody, RC: Munchausen Syndrome by Proxy, *Child Abuse Negl* 10:33-40, 1986.

Kahan, BB, and Yorker, BC: Munchausen Syndrome by Proxy, *J Sch Health* 60:108-110, 1990.

Kurlandsky, L, Lukoff, JY, Zinkham, WH, Brody, JP, and Kessler, RW: Munchausen Syndrome by Proxy: Definition of factitious bleeding in an infant by 51Cr labeling of erythrocytes, *Pediatrics* 63:228-231, 1979.

Lazoritz, S: Munchausen Syndrome by Proxy or Meadow's syndrome, *Lancet* 2(8559):631, 1987.

Libow, JA, and Schreier, HA: Three forms of factitious illness in children: When is it Munchausen Syndrome by Proxy? *Am J Orthopsychiatry* 56:602-611, 1986.

Light, MJ, and Sheridan, MS: Munchausen Syndrome by Proxy and apnea (MBPA), *Clin Pediatr* 29:162-168, 1990.

Liston, TE, Levine, PL, and Anderson, C: Polymicrobial bacteremia due to Polle syndrome: The child abuse variant of Munchausen by Proxy, *Pediatrics* 72:211-213, 1983.

MacDonald, TM: Myalgic encephalomyelitis by proxy, *Br Med J* 299:1030-1031, 1989.

Makar, AF, and Squier, PJ: Munchausen Syndrome by Proxy: Father as a perpetrator, *Pediatrics* 85:370-373, 1990.

Malatack, JJ, Wiener, ES, Gartner, JC, Zitelli, BJ, and Brunetti, E: Munchausen Syndrome by Proxy: A new complication of central venous catheterization, *Pediatrics* 75:523-525, 1985.

Masterson, J, Dunworth, R, and Williams, N: Extreme illness exaggeration in pediatric patients: A variant of Munchausen's by Proxy? *Am J Orthopsychiatry* 58:188-195, 1988.

McGuire, TL, and Feldman, KW: Psychologic morbidity of children subjected to Munchausen Syndrome by Proxy, *Pediatrics* 83:289-292, 1989.

McKinlay, I: Munchausen's Syndrome by Proxy, *Br Med J* 293:1308, 1986.

Meadow, R: Munchausen Syndrome by Proxy: The hinterland of child abuse, *Lancet* 2:343-345, 1977.

Meadow, R: Munchausen Syndrome by Proxy, *Arch Dis Child* 57:92-98, 1982.

Meadow, R: Munchausen Syndrome by Proxy and pseudo-epilepsy, *Arch Dis Child* 57:811-812, 1982.

Meadow, R: Munchausen by Proxy and brain damage, *Dev Med Child Neurol* 26:672-674, 1984.

Meadow, R: Management of Munchausen Syndrome by Proxy, *Arch Dis Child* 60:385-393, 1985.

Meadow, R: Munchausen Syndrome by Proxy, *Br Med J* 299:248-250, 1989.

Meadow, R, and Lennert, T: Munchausen by Proxy or Polle syndrome: Which term is correct? *Pediatrics* 74:554-556, 1984.

Money, J: Paleodigms and paleodigmatics: A new theoretical construct applicable to Munchausen's Syndrome by Proxy, child-abuse dwarfism, paraphilias, anorexia nervosa and other syndromes, *Am J Psychother* 43:15-24, 1989.

Nicol, AR, and Eccles, M: Psychotherapy for Munchausen Syndrome by Proxy, *Arch Dis Child* 60:344-348, 1985.

Orenstein, DM, and Wasserman, AL: Munchausen Syndrome by Proxy simulating cystic fibrosis, *Pediatrics* 78:621-624, 1986.

Palmer, AJ, and Yoshimura, GJ: Munchausen Syndrome by Proxy, *J Am Acad Child Psychiatry* 23:503-508, 1984.

Pickford, E, Buchanan, N, and McLaughlan, S: Munchausen Syndrome by Proxy: A family anthology, *Med J Aust* 148:646-650, 1988.

Raspe, RE: *The Adventures of Baron Munchausen*, Grosset & Dunlap, New York, 1936.

Richardon, GF: Munchausen Syndrome by Proxy, *Am Fam Physician* 36:119-123, 1987.

Rogers, D, Tripp, J, Bentovim, A, Robinson, A, Berry, D, and Goulding, R: Non-accidental poisoning: An extended syndrome of child abuse, *Br Med J* 1:793-796, 1976.

Rosen, CL, Frost, JD, Bricker, T, Tarnow, JD, Gillette, PC, and Dunlavy, S: Two siblings with recurrent cardiorespiratory arrest: Munchausen Syndrome by Proxy or child abuse? *Pediatrics* 71:715-720, 1983.

Rosenberg, DA: Web of deceit: A literature review of Munchausen Syndrome by Proxy, *Child Abuse Negl* 11:547-563, 1987.

Senner, A, and Ott, MJ: Munchausen Syndrome by Proxy, *Issues Compr Pediatr Nurs* 12:345-357, 1989.

Sheldon, SH: Munchausen Syndrome by Proxy, *Pediatrics* 76:855-856, 1985.

Sheridan, MS: Munchausen Syndrome by Proxy, *Health Soc Work* 14:53-58, 1989.

Sigal, M, Gelkopf, M, and Meadow, RS: Munchausen by Proxy Syndrome: The triad of abuse, self-abuse, and deception, *Comp Psychiatry* 30:527-533, 1989.

Sigal, MD, Altmark, D, and Carmel, I: Munchausen Syndrome by adult proxy: A perpetrator abusing two adults, *J Nerv Ment Dis* 174:696-698, 1986.

Sutphen, JL, and Saulsbury, FT: Intentional ipecac poisoning: Munchausen Syndrome by Proxy, *Pediatrics* 82:453-456, 1988.

Waller, DA: Obstacles to the treatment of Munchausen by Proxy Syndrome, *J Am Acad Child Psychiatry* 22:80-85, 1983.

Warner, JO, and Hathaway, MJ: Allergic form of Meadow's syndrome (Munchausen by Proxy), *Arch Dis Child* 59:151-156, 1984.

Wood, PR, Fowlkes, J, Holden, P, and Casto, D: Fever of unknown origin for six years: Munchausen Syndrome by Proxy, *J Fam Pract* 28:391-395, 1989.

Woody, RC, and Jones, JG: Neurologic Munchausen-by-Proxy Syndrome, *South Med J* 80:247-248, 1987.

Zitelli, BJ, Seltman, MF, and Shannon, RM: Munchausen's Syndrome by Proxy and its professional participants, *Am J Dis Child* 141:1099-1103, 1987.

NEGLECT AND ABANDONMENT

WAYNE I. MUNKEL, M.S.W., L.C.S.W.

This chapter cannot begin to explain the complex issue of neglect but can only look at the outcomes. Usually, if there is no unfortunate outcome, neglect goes undetected and unreported. It takes a death or shocking evidence before many cases of neglect are brought to light.

A severely malnourished 7-year-old boy was taken to the emergency room by ambulance. The child's mother found him unresponsive in bed and not breathing. The mother stated that the child had had a cold for the past few days and appeared to be recovering.

He was emaciated and dirty, he had bed sores on his buttocks and hips, and the soles of his feet were crusted with dirt that had to be scraped off. Under the dirt were several infected wounds, one looking like a cigarette burn. Attempts at resuscitation were successful and he was intubated and given fluids and antibiotics. He had severe bilateral pneumonia. After several hours in the hospital he suffered cardiac arrest. Attempts at resuscitation were futile.

There were three other children in the family. All, although poorly clothed, were well nourished and healthy. The mother was single, and none of the children had the same father. The mother was receiving public aid and had been reported for abuse and neglect several times in the past. She was regularly visited by state child protection services, the last visit the week before the child's admission. The worker did not see the child during the visit, although he was supposedly sick and in bed at that time.

The school was contacted. The three siblings had been to school regularly. The dead child had missed a number of days in the past and had been absent for the previous two weeks. One of the teachers stated that on several occasions the child had come to school in obvious distress. He was dirty, malnourished, and unable to work on his school assignments. On one occasion, the child was so weak he had to crawl up the stairs. His teacher had suggested they report the child to the Division of Family Services. The school principal decided that since the other children seemed to be doing well, he would just send the child home.

The media caught wind of the story and took pictures of the home, which should have been condemned. But as we review the case it is clear that the media had chosen this family as a scapegoat for the child protection system itself. In truest perspective, the system was the cause of the child's death. Had the mother received better services, the child would have survived and thrived. The school's role in the tragedy, although understandable, compounded the situation.

Given this history, typical of so many cases, it is easy to see that neglect resulted in death. But too often the causative responsibility is shared among several factors that can be difficult to define. Furthermore, neglect is often difficult to prevent. This chapter will attempt to identify the various forms of neglect and abandonment as they present in the medical setting, just touching on the *"who"* and the *"why,"* which constitute a social problem beyond the scope of this chapter.

As is true with most problems, there is a spectrum of neglect that ranges from mild to severe. It is easy to agree on what constitutes severe neglect and what should be done about it. Beyond that, unless an obviously bad outcome is brought to light, nothing is done or, in most cases, can be done.

The following case illustrates this point:

A 2-month-old child was found dead in his crib by his mother. The cause of death was suffocation. The child shared the crib with a 2-year-old and a 4-year-old sibling. The medical examiner decided the cause of death was accidental. One of the siblings, while sleeping, probably laid on the child to cause the suffocation.

Was neglect involved here? Who was neglectful? The mother? No one told her the child would be in danger if he slept with others. If the mother had had more money, she could have afforded beds for each child. If she had been better educated, she might have known better.

A mother leaves seven children in the home while she goes on a date. The eldest is 8 years old. He has been told not to play with matches and had been reprimanded for this very thing. While the mother is gone, there is a fire and all of the children are killed. It is declared an accident caused by a child playing with matches. The neighbors and firemen had trouble reaching the children because the windows were barred and the door had a "deadman" board against it. The family was known to the state protective services.

This case certainly illustrates neglect and shows that the neglect must be shared among the mother, the landlord, the neighbors who were aware that the mother would often leave the children alone, the fire inspector, and the state protective system.

Some feel that the consideration of neglect should be simplified. Missouri law defines neglect as "**reckless** failure to provide, by those responsible for the care, custody, and control of the child, the proper or necessary support, education as required by law, nutrition or medical, surgical, or any other care necessary for his well-being; and **food, clothing or shelter sufficient for life or essential medical and surgical care.**" This definition in the law clearly allows for broad interpretation by the courts.

♦ INCIDENCE AND DEFINITIONS

In 1980, neglect reports accounted for 48% of all child maltreatment reports (NIS-1, 1981). A change in definition expanded the percentage to 63% in 1986 (NIS-2, 1988). With an increased percentage of reports defined as neglect, one could assume that an increased focus on this problem would appear in the professional literature. However, there is a conspicuous lack of research on neglect as compared to other forms of abuse. Neglect is often noted as a component in some studies of other forms of abuse, but the concept of neglect as a separate entity for study is poorly defined. This is still true as we see the challenge of preventing neglect growing even greater in a climate of uncertain economic conditions and changing political realities.

Simply stated, neglect is the failure of caretakers to provide for the basic needs of their children. Failure to meet these needs may vary in degree from mild to severe and can be acute or chronic. No workable definition that quantifies the degree of neglect has yet been found. While there is general agreement on what constitutes extreme neglect, little agreement has been reached concerning what constitutes milder forms of neglect and the harm caused by neglect.

DEVELOPING CRITERIA TO DEFINE NEGLECT OBJECTIVELY

The degree of harm suffered by the child was the impetus for the first national study on the incidence of child neglect. The National Study of the Incidence and Severity of Child Abuse and Neglect (NIS-1, 1981) defined neglect as a situation in which it could be shown that, as a result of caretaker inattention to the child's basic needs for care, protection, or control, the child experienced predictable injury or impairment of serious or greater severity.

In addition, an affirmative answer had to be obtained for the following questions:

1. Had the caretaker been informed of the child's need or problem by a competent professional, or under the circumstances of the situation, would the child's need have been apparent to most reasonably caring and attentive adults?

2. Was the caretaker physically and financially able to obtain or provide the needed care, protection, or supervision? (Mayhall & Norgard, 1983)

Using an expanded definition, the Department of Health and Human Services (NIS-2, 1988) added a category titled "endangered." This new category allowed for reporting children who had no present evidence of abuse through neglect but for whom it was reasonable to suspect there was the risk of injury due to neglect. This change added a substantial number of children who were considered to be neglected. While the risk of harm or endangerment is a category of neglected children that may need intervention to prevent future neglect, the lack of sufficient resources available to child protective services (CPS) and other human services leaves this category of neglect unserved in many states. The dramatic 55% increase in child abuse and neglect reports between 1980 and 1986 was accompanied by a meager 4% increase in funding (Krugman, 1990). During the same period the substantiation rates for child protective services declined (Kessler & New, 1989; Eckenrode et al., 1988; Besharov, 1985). The NIS-2 (1988) concluded that child protective services were more selective in the reports investigated.

Overreporting, which is defined as reported cases that are investigated and closed without services being provided (Berger et al., 1989), has led some parent groups to advocate for changes in laws to redefine abuse and neglect and to protect parental rights. Others feel that rather than redefine abuse and neglect, children and parents would be better served by expanding the support and resources of the child protection system and the training of child protection workers.

The following discussion uses the NIS-1 definition of "demonstrable harm," which provides the physician with a workable definition. This facilitates reporting of children who are endangered by neglect, in the judgement of the reporter, in accordance with reporting statutes.

◆ TYPES OF NEGLECT

When a child presents with an injury or other signs that potentially result from neglect, it is the responsibility of the physician to find a mechanism to explain the physical signs. For example, a child who falls and is seriously injured may reasonably present as having suffered an accident. When the physician has suspicions about the cause, a good social history is necessary to determine if it was, in fact, an accident or if neglect or intent played a role in the event.

Neglect can be due to inadequate physical environment, presence of environmental hazards, inadequate care standards, or developmental neglect.

PHYSICAL ENVIRONMENT

INADEQUATE SHELTER

Frequently, a house where neglect exists is overcrowded with people, furnishings, trash, or garbage; for example, 25 persons may live in a four-bedroom house. The children simply get lost in the house because of the adults' inattention. They are not supervised because each adult assumes someone else is managing the child's care.

INADEQUATE SLEEPING ARRANGEMENTS

When a child does not get adequate sleep, he or she may appear as chronically fatigued or listless, particularly as noted by schoolteachers or neighbors. The child's need for sleep may not be met because there are too many people living in the house, too much noise, too many people sleeping in one bed, or no beds available. The practice of allowing or forcing children to sleep with adults can contribute to sexual abuse of the child. This is frequently exacerbated by the lack of consideration for personal boundaries and/or poor self-control (often as a result of drug or alcohol use). Another problem involves bedding that is inadequate for cold weather or soiled with feces or urine. Furthermore, the child may be denied privacy from opposite-sex children or adults, contributing to a sense of shame that can lead to a lack of sleep. Another source of anxiety results from fear when different people are free to roam the premises, posing a threat to the child's security.

UNSANITARY CONDITIONS

As noted, frequently in neglect cases the house is filled with an accumulation of garbage and trash. Toilets are unusable, and there may be animal and/or human feces on the floors. Often, uncontrolled vermin—rats, spiders, cockroaches—are present. Food preparation under these circumstances is unhealthy and can cause ongoing illness in the child as well as others in the house.

STRUCTURAL HAZARDS

Not uncommonly, the house or dwelling has partially collapsed. Stairs may have broken steps and railings are missing, as are protective barriers on porches or balconies. Windows and doors are in poor repair, with broken or jagged glass. The doors and windows are without screens, and floors and ceilings have holes. Badly worn floors may be covered with large splinters.

HOUSEKEEPING PROBLEMS

The condition of the house and furniture indicates the lack of even minimal care. Dirt and filth cover the surfaces, especially in the kitchen and bathroom. Clutter and trash are everywhere, obviously having accumulated over a long period of time.

ENVIRONMENTAL HAZARDS

FIRE HAZARDS

Exposed or frayed wiring is frequently found in the home. Fuel containers are stored in living areas, and combustible materials are placed near heat sources. Beds are too close to heat sources, which could result in burns of unaware children, as well as fires. Metal bars on windows and "deadman" props against doors impede evacuation should a fire occur in the house.

SUBSTANCE ACCESSIBILITY AND USE

Chemicals or drugs may be within reach or easy accessibility of children who can climb up to storage areas. Illicit drugs in the house or the use of the house in drug traffic are particularly hazardous to children and often accompany neglect.

EXCESSIVE HOT WATER TEMPERATURE

In houses where neglect is practiced, the hot water available at the tap may be greater than 130° Fahrenheit. The time required to burn skin with water at this temperature is less than 30 seconds; if the water is at 140°F a burn can occur in 3 seconds; at 147°F it only takes 1 second for a burn to be inflicted (Johnson, 1990). Thus, if an unsupervised child accidentally turns on the hot water tap, a serious burn can result in 1 second.

INADEQUATE CARE STANDARDS
NUTRITION
The food may be of poor quality and lacking in nutritional value. The diet is inadequate with regard to the basic food groups and does not offer any variety, indicating a lack of meal planning or haphazard planning. Often no adult caretaker prepares meals on a consistent basis. The food provided may also be inappropriate for the child's age and developmental abilities. Food found stored in either a cupboard or in a refrigerator may be spoiled. Unfortunately, in many cases no food is available. The mealtime itself may be marked by chaos or unpleasant routines for the child, further adversely affecting his or her nutritional status.

CLOTHING
Clothing for neglected children is inadequate and inappropriate for the weather and season. It may also be dirty, ill-fitting, or in a poor state of repair. The child's footwear can be inadequate for the season, too small, too large, or in poor repair.

PERSONAL HYGIENE
Neglected children often show evidence of not having bathed for a lengthy period of time, smelling of urine, feces, or sweat, covered with crusted dirt, and hair unkempt. The child often states that he or she has not bathed. Poor dental hygiene is evident by severe dental caries and mouth odor. When asked, the child may state that he or she does not brush his or her teeth. Furthermore, neglect is evident when there is the persistent presence of lice.

HEALTH CARE
Neglect implies that even minimal health care is not obtained and the child lacks immunizations. The adult either overuses emergency services, going to the hospital for even slight problems, or does not use them at all, even with severe injury and illness. When medicine or rehabilitative equipment is prescribed, the prescription goes unfilled. Dental caries and other dental needs remain untreated. Regimens recommended for the treatment of chronic illness are not followed or compliance is poor. Prescribed psychological help is not obtained.

SUPERVISION
The lack of supervision by the parent and/or caretaker can lead to injuries that could have been avoided and to repeated injuries. The key question to be answered is whether the behavior of the parent and/or caretaker contributed significantly to the child's injury.

DEVELOPMENTAL NEGLECT
EDUCATION
Neglected children are often not enrolled in school after the state-required age. The adult caretaker permits chronic truancy and fails to provide encouragement for the educational process. The adult caretaker also fails to provide the necessary control, discipline, or role model for learning, socialization, and responsible behavior.

EMOTIONAL GROWTH
When there is emotional neglect, the child's needs for emotional support and encouragement are not provided by the adult caretaker. The adult caretaker is unavailable emotionally, is indifferent, or rejects the child. Because there is inadequate supervision, the child engages in dangerous behaviors for long periods of time. The child's need for emotional security is not met.

◆ ATTACHMENT DISORDERS

Attachment disorders are defined as the caregiver's rejection of the child and the parental role. Abandonment can occur because attachment to the child, or bonding, which normally develops during the prenatal or immediate antenatal period, fails to occur. The parent has no feelings of attachment to the child and no sense of responsibility for providing for the child's basic needs.

ABANDONMENT

In general, abandonment is a legal term with legal implications that refers to the physical aspects of neglect and fulfills certain rigid criteria. However, in addition to physical abandonment, which frequently results from attachment disorders, there is emotional abandonment, which, in the long run, is potentially more devastating. In emotional abandonment the parent, usually the mother, in one way or another completely withdraws from nurturing and meeting the child's needs for security. This parallels the general aspects of abandonment, where the caregiver does not meet the child's needs for physical security. The child's needs are either not met or are provided for by others.

Parental characteristics, rather than those associated with the child, and environmental factors are the best predictors of the potential for abandonment. Among the predisposing characteristics are sexual promiscuity with or without alcoholism, financial problems, and relatively poor state of health. Depression, especially when severe, can be a factor in causing abandonment (Martin & Walters, 1982).

The circumstances and conditions associated with abandonment can be categorized by the following six types:

1. Fatal or near-fatal abandonment

2. Abandonment with physical needs provided by others

3. Throwaways

4. Parental custody refusal

5. Lack of supervision

6. Emotional abandonment

FATAL OR NEAR-FATAL ABANDONMENT

Children abandoned with the intent to kill either die or are saved by fortuitous circumstances. Children can be abandoned in places where they are likely to be found and subsequently cared for. Sometimes, however, they are not found in time to prevent serious health problems or death. A set of twins was put in trash bags and placed in a dumpster by the mother, who then called the father and told him where they were. A young mother placed her child in a gangway in subzero weather where the baby would be found by a passerby. A 2-year-old was found, bound hand and foot, in a suitcase under a hospital dumpster by a security guard. The child's gag had been slipped off her mouth and the zipper of the suitcase was left open so the child's cries could be heard. A newborn infant was found by an alert security guard in a gym bag on an icy street in a public park. Abandonment at its worst is abandonment infanticide. In these instances the child is left to die or is left in conditions likely to result in his or her death.

These children and their parent(s) obviously had great need of protective services. Fortunately, most children are found in time to prevent serious health problems or death.

ABANDONMENT WITH PHYSICAL NEEDS PROVIDED BY OTHERS

Children can be abandoned under conditions that result in the child's physical needs being met by others (Heger & Yungman, 1989). These children are left at hospitals, sitters, relatives, friends, neighbors, licensed providers, or extended care facilities. Children who are not picked up two days after the agreed upon or arranged pickup are considered abandoned. *(NOTE: This time may vary from state to state.)* In other cases, hospitals and extended care facilities care for children for various periods of time and the caregiver has little responsibility, if any, for providing basic needs. These interludes of absence initiate separations between parent and child and provide an opportunity for parents to abandon the child. Handicapped children are especially susceptible. Prematurely born children often have serious health problems that require lengthy hospitalizations in high technology environments. In some cases, no attachment is formed between the parent and child. Temporary abandonments by parents because of incarceration or emergency hospitalization without care plans are not considered legal abandonment unless there is a previous history of physical abandonment.

THROWAWAYS

Some children, particularly adolescents, are thrown out of their homes by their parents or caregivers. They may be physically thrown out, locked out, or refused admittance to the home upon their return after having run away or after delinquent behavior or becoming pregnant. Some children choose to leave the home and parental care. In some cases the parents or caregivers relinquish parenting and turn legal custody of the child over to juvenile authorities. The child's delinquent or incorrigible behavior is often cited as the reason for this action rather than the parents' inability to parent. These children are emancipated prematurely and abandoned to others for care. They are vulnerable to exploitation, often wander the streets, and are totally left to their own resources to provide for their care and survival.

PARENTAL CUSTODY REFUSAL

Some parents are unable or unwilling to accept custody responsibilities for their children. The children in these circumstances live an uncertain existence. They spend days or weeks with different relatives, parents' friends, or even total strangers. The shuffling of children from one caregiver to another is a chronic situation and is usually based on the parents' unwillingness to parent rather than an acute financial or housing problem. The child's need for a stable environment is not met. Financial and housing difficulties, however, do occur among these families and can play a significant role. Each case must be investigated individually.

LACK OF SUPERVISION

Children who are unsupervised for long periods of time, who engage in dangerous activities, who stay away from home overnight—and the caregiver does not know where they are and makes no attempt to locate them—are in a sense abandoned. They may become throwaways later in life or their parents or caregivers may refuse custody when these children get into predelinquent or delinquent activities.

EMOTIONAL ABANDONMENT

Emotional abandonment has been described in the backgrounds of many adults. As children, they did not form secure attachments (Armsworth, 1990). The parent may have been physically present but emotionally absent or unavailable to the child. Often these were severely dysfunctional families in which these individuals describe periods of emotional abandonment and overcontrol. Some experienced physical abandonment in conjunction with the emotional absence. Often these adults were sexually victimized as children and later by others. The dynamics present in these emotionally scarred adults can be found in members of other severely dysfunctional families where physical abuse and neglect occur.

The effects of the parents' behavior, through abandonment, leave the child in a confused, emotionally stressed state. The child's sense of trust in an adult's availability to meet his or her needs is severely shaken. This lack of trust may have lifelong consequences in relationships with others. As adults these victims may exhibit no understanding of what is right and what is wrong. They often experience difficulty bonding to their own offspring and may have marital problems. If their youth included juvenile delinquency, this can be carried into adulthood as antisocial behavior. Unless they receive treatment, a cycle of emotional and/or physical abandonment can continue.

◆ FAILURE TO THRIVE

Nonorganic failure to thrive is an interactional disorder in which parental expectations, parental skills, and the resulting home environment are intertwined with the child's developmental capabilities. Spinner and Siegel (1987) have found that an effective approach to this syndrome must consider the multiple etiologic factors involved.

Nonorganic failure to thrive in some instances relates to child abuse or neglect. This syndrome can be associated with maternal deprivation or emotional abuse and for that reason has also been referred to as psychosocial dwarfism. Nonorganic failure to thrive is characterized by physical and developmental retardation associated with a disturbed mother-infant relationship.

Berkowitz and Senter (1987) published a study that quantified the differences noted in interactions between a mother and her failure-to-thrive infant whose condition was not induced by organic causes. These mother-infant pairs were videotaped and evaluated in comparison to a control group of mother-thriving infant pairs. Twenty-one different behavioral categories were assessed, and statistically significant differences were noted in five.

A high percentage of failure-to-thrive cases, where children are slow to develop or learn, involve victims of deprivation and neglect. Cooper (1978) highlighted the importance of underdiagnosing the incidence of failure to thrive without organic cause. She emphasized that growth retardation is more readily demonstrated in the first three years of life when the growth period is most rapid (Lacey & Parkin, 1974). Pediatricians must evaluate the psychosocial environment of children who are not growing properly. Often the reason given is that the parents were also small, but in many instances the parents were small for the same psychosocial reasons. In evaluating children with failure to thrive without organic cause, Lacey and Parkin mentioned that the typical child's height is below the third percentile for his age and birth weight. He is thin and even emaciated. Pot belly, hypotonia, episodes of diarrhea, tension, misery, and cold, dull, pale, and mottled skin are characteristic. These children are apathetic and withdrawn, avoid personal contact, and are emotionally and verbally unresponsive, often avoiding eye contact. They may have short temper tantrums. Many appear to be insensitive to pain and have self-inflicted injuries. Some are encopretic and enuretic. Insomnia and disrupted sleep are common, with the result that they often roam the house at night, probably searching for food. Some eat and drink inappropriate substances from the garbage can, toilet bowl, or a dog's or cat's dish. Questions regarding their behavior in the home must be evaluated cautiously, because families usually hide any psychological harassment and physical abuse of children. Lacey and Parkin summarize the definition of "deprivation dwarfism" in **Table 14-1**.

Table14-1. Findings in Deprivation Dwarfism

The Child's Appearance
   Short stature
   Usually thin
   Infantile proportions
   Pot belly (with episodes of diarrhea)
   Skin dull, pale, and cold
   Limbs pink or purple, cold and mottled
   Edema of the feet, legs, hands, and forearms
   Poor skin care, excoriations, abrasions, and ulcers
   Sparse, dry hair with patches of alopecia
   Dejection and apathy
   May have bruises, small cuts, burns, or scars

The Child's Behavior
   Passive with or without catatonia
   Rocking or head banging
   Retarded speech and language
   Delayed development
   Solitary and unable to play
   Easily bullied
   Gorging food and scavenging from wastebaskets, etc.
   Particularly notable—during their convalescent stay in a hospital they
      have marked growth spurts that relapse as soon as they return to their
      home environment.

The Child's Progress in the Hospital
   Rapid recovery of growth and liveliness
   Slower progress with speech and language
   Affection seeking, but may be shallow or even promiscuous
   Attention seeking
   Severe tantrums at the slightest frustration
   Rocking and head banging when upset
   Remain greedy and scavenge food

The Child's Later Behavior
   Speech and language immaturity
   Gorging of food that may last six months or more
   Restlessness with short attention span
   Rocking and head banging if stressed
   Difficulties with peer group and learning in school
   Soiling and wetting
   Stealing and lying
   Tantrums and aggression

The characteristic endocrine abnormality of these children is a deficient growth hormone response to insulin-induced hypoglycemia. Most have a deficient growth hormone response to arginine infusion and to exercise. Apparently a deficit also exists in slow-wave sleep associated with the deficiency in growth hormone secretion (Guilhaume et al., 1982). Although failure to thrive can be caused by a number of organic conditions, failure to thrive caused by parental behavior is clearly defined. With nutritional neglect or deprivation, the child does not consume enough calories and other nutrients to grow and develop at the expected rates (Helfer, 1984). In failure to thrive the child is found to be below the third percentile on standardized growth grids and is not growing at the expected rate; he may, in fact, lose weight and show no change in length or height. In some cases the child may receive sufficient calories, but because of emotional deprivation he still does not thrive. This phenomenon has been called maternal deprivation or psychosocial dwarfism.

FAMILY DYNAMICS

Nonorganic failure to thrive is an interactional disorder in which parental expectations, parental skills, and the resulting home environment are intertwined with the child's developmental capabilities. An effective approach to this syndrome must consider the multiple etiologic factors involved (Spinner & Siegel, 1987).

Family dynamics have been researched in an attempt to understand failure to thrive. Although stress, parental skill and education, and personality each play a role in failure to thrive, parental interaction with the child, the family support system, and parental relationships are more basic to the problem (Heger & Yungman, 1989).

Since the mother is the primary caretaker in most families, many studies have focused on the maternal role. The concept of parental deprivation was used by Gagan to explain the dynamics in his study (Gagan et al., 1984). He concluded, "It is parental deprivation and deficient social support networks for the mother, rather than maternal deprivations, which are central to the etiology of non-organic FTT."

Alderette and deGraffenried (1986) found nonorganic failure to thrive in families whose interactional style was described as disengagement. These families had poor communication between all members, and there was minimal interaction among family members. The preexisting disengaged style is responsible for the lack of parental bonding. The pervasive lack of nurturing and attachment by the parents causes the child to respond similarly. The child responds with a feeding and behavioral problem. Infants in these families adopt the disengaged style by becoming withdrawn, undemanding, and unresponsive. Thus the failure-to-thrive infant is viewed as the symptom of a breakdown in the family system.

Parental denial of the physical and behavior problems in failure-to-thrive children was found to be significant (Ayoub & Milner, 1985); "the absence of attachment pervaded the parent-child encounters." The more severe the family dynamics problem, the more likely the child will have a reactive attachment disorder.

CHILDREN AT RISK

Children begin an interactive role at age 4 months. The mother-child interactional roles are defined when the child is between 5 and 12 months of age. During this first year of life most children are initially admitted to hospitals for nonorganic failure to thrive, with 25% admitted during the first month of the child's life (Gagan et al., 1984). These children are most vulnerable at this time, at the highest risk for morbidity and mortality.

Failure-to-thrive children can also be targeted for abuse if the family situation is left untreated. Koel (1969) reported several failure-to-thrive children who were victims of violent deaths when they were sent back to parents who had not been treated or counseled.

◆ FETAL NEGLECT

Included in good prenatal care are instruction in nutrition management, medical check-ups to monitor fetal development and the mother's health, and education regarding the avoidance of toxins harmful to the developing fetus. Poor nutrition and cigarette smoking are well known to cause lower birth weights. In addition, fetal alcohol syndrome is a recognized result of alcohol abuse by the mother during her pregnancy. Heavy metal intoxication causes brain damage and adversely involves other systems of the developing fetus. Rubella is known to cause birth defects. The effects of illicit drugs (e.g., heroin, marijuana, amphetamines, cocaine) and crack cocaine have been documented for harm caused to the developing fetus as well as for contributing to inadequate parenting skills and interest on the part of the mother. Cocaine use during pregnancy specifically results in newborn infants with growth retardation and microcephaly (Hadeed & Siegel, 1989; Doberczak et al., 1987); increased rates of anomalies of the genitourinary, cardiac, and central nervous system (Bays, 1990); renal malformation; and cerebral cortical atrophy (Cregler & Mark, 1986), among numerous other harmful effects.

Two issues emerge regarding neglect in the prenatal period of development. First, what level of responsibility does a mother have toward her developing fetus? Second, what should society do about mothers who ingest harmful toxins and injure their developing child? Opinions differ as to the rights of the fetus (Risenberg, 1989) and the rights of the pregnant woman (Fleisher, 1987, 1988). The debate over this topic is unlikely to conclude soon.

The significance of fetal neglect becomes clear after examining the growing body of knowledge about preventive and prenatal predictors of child maltreatment. Lally (1984) pointed out that the emotional relationship between parent and child begins before the child is born and is particularly malleable throughout pregnancy and during the first year of life. Research has shown that prevention efforts are effective at these early stages. Murphy et al. (1985) found that prenatal testing of pregnant women could predict which women were at risk for neglecting their yet unborn child. Main and Goldwyn (1984) observed child-mother relationships. They found that mothers whose children avoided them gave descriptions of their own childhood experiences that had cognitive distortions of their relations with their mothers. These researchers inferred that mothers who have been rejected by their mothers, in turn, reject their own children.

◆ Drugs and Alcohol

Aside from the physical effects produced in fetuses, drug and alcohol use is a significant contributing factor in the maltreatment of children. Parents and/or caretakers under the influence of these toxins commit thousands of neglectful and abusive acts each year. Drugs and alcohol facilitate the sexual abuse of children by lowering inhibitions in both the adult and the child. Their contribution to the problem of neglect is considerable. The purchase of drugs and alcohol by a parent or caretaker diverts financial resources, often a scarce commodity, from providing for the basic needs of the family—food, shelter, and warmth. Under the influence of these substances, the parent or caretaker cannot provide optimum care for the children. The level of care declines; for infants, the lack of care can be catastrophic.

The presence of illicit drugs in a child's environment produces the risk of serious harm. Children and infants may become intoxicated themselves through deliberate poisoning, passive inhalation, accidental ingestion of drugs or alcohol, or accepting drugs proffered by an adult or older child (Schwartz & Einhorn, 1986). Cases involving children who have been healthy but who come seeking medical attention with unexplained neurologic symptoms or seizures, children who apparently fall victim to SIDS, or those who die unexpectedly in other situations should be screened for the presence of alcohol or drug intoxication (Bays, 1990).

◆ The Effects and Outcomes of Child Neglect

Neglected children suffer hurts in their bodies, their minds, their emotions, and their spirits. The hurts in their bodies mend and heal, but the hurts in their minds, emotions, and spirits have far-reaching ramifications. Neglect of their bodies can be recognized through delayed intellectual development that affects performance in preschool and school. Emotional hurts can be exhibited by aggression and depression. When the spirit is hurt, the child no longer tries to succeed, instead withdrawing from life. The joy of childhood is lost.

DEVELOPMENTAL EFFECTS

The early years of life are critical periods of development for the child. Neglect during this time can cause development to stop, freeze permanently, or even fail to occur (Helfer et al., 1976). The body, mind, and emotions of children operate on a developmental timetable that is individually determined. These developments cannot be put in an emotional deep freeze or placed on hold while parents work through problems sufficiently to make it safe for the child to live in the home (Kempe, 1976). Some families are untreatable or cannot be treated in time to meet the developmental needs of the child (Jones, 1987).

Each neglected or maltreated child needs an individual treatment plan to meet his or her needs. Often the treatment services provided by child protective services are parent oriented rather than child oriented. Services are dropped when the crisis appears to have resolved (Alfaro, 1984). But some children need help from the day they are born (Brazelton, 1990) and still others may need a lifetime of treatment services.

LONG-TERM EFFECTS OF NEGLECT

The long-term effects of neglect reveal extreme variations in the child's behavior or illness. Extreme neglect can result in child fatalities. One-fifth of unexpected child deaths (defined as those occurring before arrival at the hospital or within 10 days of being hospitalized) were suspicious for abuse or neglect (Christoffel et al., 1985). Children who do not die from abuse or neglect may suffer long-term sequelae. The effects of malnutrition, for example, include lower intelligence, slowed growth, poor teeth, deformities, and life-long poor health.

Children who have been neglected have an increased incidence of psychopathology. They tend to be slow and cognitively impaired (Vondra, 1990), have difficulty relating to others, and have an increased frequency of unsocialized conduct disorders (Rogeness et al., 1986). Adults who were neglected as children may be unable to trust others, develop problems with anger, suffer feelings of low self-esteem, have a decreased ability to form enduring, satisfying relationships, and exhibit impaired social skills (Tower, 1989). Mothers who neglect their children seem unable or unwilling to provide for the health, safety, or well-being of their children. In turn, their children have difficulty mustering the energy or resources to deal with various tasks. As preschoolers they are dependent, have poor ego controls, are negativistic, and frequently are noncompliant (Egeland et al., 1983).

Another widely studied effect of physical abuse and neglect is the link to delinquency and adult criminality. Most studies link abuse and neglect in some combination. One study, however, separates neglect and its outcomes (McCord, 1983). In her findings, 45% of abused and neglected boys had been convicted of serious crimes, become alcoholics or mentally ill, or died before age 35. If there was a history of abuse or neglect, juvenile delinquency tended to result. This finding is similar to the bidirectional relationship between child abuse and delinquency (Howing et al., 1990).

Victimization in childhood has demonstrable consequences in adult criminal behavior. In one study individuals who were abused or neglected as children had higher arrest rates as adults than control subjects (Widom, 1989). While there is a clear relationship between childhood victimization and later adult criminal behavior, the majority of subjects in both the McCord (53%) and Widom (71%) studies did not demonstrate extreme behavioral problems or damage. Widom points out the need to look for more subtle forms of damage in evaluating these cases.

Among the outcomes in those with subtle forms of damage, we see the developmentally frozen child or the untreated, neglected child becoming the neglecting parent in the next generation of the cycle of neglect. Whether extreme or subtle, the effects of neglect create unhappy, unproductive, and sometimes violent adults. The cycle can be broken through the treatment of neglected children and neglecting families as well as the prevention of neglect.

♦PREVENTION

Though it may not always be possible to break the intergeneration cycle of neglect, an effort should be made. Primary prevention of neglect involves finding those at risk and connecting them with resources that provide supportive programs aimed at preventive measures. However, most current efforts in preventing neglect involve secondary prevention. Thus, the system waits until a neglected child is recognized before efforts are made to prevent further neglect and to treat the harm already done to the child. Prenatal and perinatal predictors of neglect that have been identified could form the basis of primary prevention programs. Early diagnosis of attachment disorders (Harris et al., 1989; Call, 1984; Caffo et al., 1982), problem parenting, family stress, failure to thrive, and parental rejection of the current parent point to areas where preventive efforts may be directed to help both the infant and the family (Avison et al., 1986; Murphy et al., 1985; Edwards et al., 1990; Ayoub & Milner, 1985; Gagan et al., 1984; Main & Goldwyn, 1984).

Truly effective programs addressing primary prevention of neglect are generations away even if we start now. However, if we treat the victims of neglect today we can be accomplishing primary prevention for a future generation. Treatment of the neglecting parent or caretaker can also decrease the damage at the present time.

Families are only one context in which neglect occurs. These families live in a society that neglects children. The social welfare infrastructure developed to offer support for families has been reduced or dismantled by budget cuts over the last decade. Many of these services reduced stress factors known to be associated with neglect, such as insufficient income, inadequate housing, social isolation, family discord, and use of drugs and alcohol. The loss of these supportive services has stressed families even more. Cuts in funding for education, mental health, public medical care, and limited access to this medical care have exacerbated the neglect of children. As stated earlier, the drug problem and associated crime have led to the deaths of children and extreme physical neglect. In addition, the economic changes noted have led to neglect in families involved with traditionally secure professions, such as farming and manufacturing.

The child protection system was designed to evaluate families and to provide services to aid in correcting conditions known to produce neglect and abuse (Krugman, 1990). Yet it has not met the increasing demands for investigation, treatment, and prevention services that we have seen over the past decade. The result has been the loss of trained, clinically oriented workers, decreased treatment capabilities, and poor general ability to perform the functions mandated by statutes. The impact of the cocaine and crack epidemic has overwhelmed child protection services as well as the foster care system. There is a crisis in the child protection system that now represents a national emergency (U.S. Advisory Board on Child Abuse and Neglect, 1990).

During the last decade the issue of prevention gained legislative attention. Forty-nine states now have trust funds for prevention programs. In 1988 the funds for prevention programs totaled $32 million (Krugman, 1990). These monies are earmarked for programs aimed at prevention of abuse.

Treating and preventing chronic neglect consumes both time and resources. It is frustrating to work with neglectful families, and success comes slowly, if at all. As stated earlier, some families are untreatable (Jones, 1987). Focusing prevention or treatment on the individual neglected child or neglecting parent will not guarantee that neglect will not occur.

Physician Roles

The prevention of child neglect must be addressed at the level of the individual, family, society, and culture. The prevention of neglect requires a concentrated effort at each of these levels and a long-term commitment to accomplish its goals. Leadership is needed in this effort, and the physician can play a key role in preventing and treating neglect.

The physician recognizing neglect is legally responsible for reporting it to child protective services. The physician's evaluation of the child provides direct evidence of neglect as well as signs that point to neglectful conditions in the child's environment. The American Medical Association issued guidelines to assist physicians in evaluating and reporting child abuse and neglect (Council on Scientific Affairs, 1985). Immunity has been granted to physician reporters and penalties provided for failure to report.

Physicians still fail to recognize and report child maltreatment. Some physicians do not report it because experience has caused them to question the ability of child protective services to protect children or to follow through with appropriate intervention for neglected children (Helfer, 1990; Krugman, 1990). Their reluctance to report abuse and neglect may also be due to lack of training and fear of potential loss of patients. Pollack and Levy (1989) state that countertransference (also referred to as vicarious traumatization (McCann & Pearlman, 1990), where the therapist takes on the symptoms of trauma of the child and reacts to them adversely), is an inevitable part of work with child abuse and neglect cases and recommend education and training so that all persons employed in this field better understand these reactions.

Child Advocate

By virtue of their knowledge and expertise, physicians are in a unique position to impact outcomes for abused and neglected children. The role of child advocate accompanies the recognition and reporting roles. Most physicians are reluctant to be involved in the court system, viewing it as a possibly unpleasant experience. Yet the physician's testimony in court can be the determining factor in helping the court decide whether abuse or neglect occurred, what degree of harm the child has suffered, and future problems the child could face related to this harm. The physician can and should make recommendations regarding the child's safety and protection.

Physicians can also impact the legislative process on behalf of children. They can speak to the needs of children, the effects of abuse and neglect, and the effects of specific public policies on children. In this period of declining resources, children need articulate spokespersons who are willing to represent them at all levels of government.

◆Regional Centers

Programs or regional centers have been developed to address the unique needs posed by premature infants, genetic disorders, hemophilia, and learning disabilities. Many child protection workers feel that regional child abuse centers could concentrate resources and expertise to manage and treat child abuse and neglect more effectively. These centers can gather research data and information for prevention and treatment programs (Kessler & New, 1989; Heger & Stewart, 1988). Regional centers could be located in medical facilities or be freestanding. A multidisciplinary center can bring together all the agencies involved in the investigation, coordination, treatment, and prevention of child abuse and neglect. In view of the current lack of funding in numerous fields, the regional center concept may be the most cost-effective means to manage the existing problem of child abuse and neglect and to further advance the knowledge base related to the problem.

♦BIBLIOGRAPHY

Alderette, P, and deGraffenried, DF: Non-organic failure-to-thrive syndrome and the family system, *Soc Work*, May-June: 207, 1986.

Alfaro, J: Helping children overcome the effects of abuse and neglect, *Pediatr Ann* 13:778, 1984.

Armsworth, M: A qualitative analysis of adult incest survivors' response to sexual involvement with therapists, *Child Abuse Negl* 14:541, 1990.

Avison, W, Turner, RJ, and Nolt, S: Screening for problem parenting: Preliminary evidence on a promising instrument, *Child Abuse Negl* 10:157, 1986.

Ayoub, C, and Milner, JS: Failure to thrive: Parental indicators, types and outcomes, *Child Abuse Negl* 9:491, 1985.

Bays, J: Substance abuse and child abuse: Impact of addiction on the child, *Pediatr Clin North Am* 37:881, 1990.

Berger, D, et al: Child abuse and neglect: An instrument to assist case referral decision making, *Health Soc Work* 14:60, 1989.

Berkowitz, CD, and Senter, SA: Characteristiscs of mother-infant interactions in nonorganice failure to thrive, *J Fam Practice* 25(4): 377-381, 1987.

Besharov, DJ: Doing something about child abuse: The need to narrow the grounds for state intervention, *Harvard J Law Pub Pol* 8:539, 1985.

Brazelton, T: Why is America failing its children? *NY Times Magazine* Sept 9, 1990.

Caffo, E, et al: Prevention of child abuse and neglect through early diagnosis of serious disturbances in the mother-child relationship in Italy, *Child Abuse Negl* 6:453, 1982.

Call, JD: Child abuse and neglect in infancy: Sources of hostility within the parent/infant dyad and disorders of attachment in infancy, *Child Abuse Negl* 8:185, 1984.

Christoffel, KK, Zieserl, EJ, and Chiaramonte, J: Should child abuse and neglect be considered when a child dies unexpectedly? *Am J Dis Child* 139:876, 1985.

Cooper, CE: Child abuse and neglect: Medical aspects. In SM Smith: *The Maltreatment of Children*, University Park Press, Baltimore, 1978.

Council on Scientific Affairs: AMA diagnostic and treatment guidelines concerning child abuse and neglect, *JAMA* 254:796, 1985.

Cregler, LL, and Mark, H: Medical complications of cocaine abuse, *N Engl J Med* 315:1495, 1986.

Doberczak, DM, Thornton, JC, Bernstein, J, et al: Maternal drug dependency and growth impact, *Am J Dis Child* 141:1163, 1987.

Eckenrode, J, et al: Substantiation of child abuse and neglect reports, *J Consult Clin Psychol* 56:9, 1988.

Edwards, A, et al: Recognizing failure to thrive in early childhood, *Arch Dis Child* 65:1263, 1990.

Egeland, B, Stroufe, LA, and Erickson, MA: The developmental consequences of different patterns of maltreatment, *Child Abuse Negl* 7:459, 1983.

Fleisher, LD: Wrongful birth: When is there liability for prenatal injury? *Am J Dis Child* 141:1260, 1987.

Fleisher, LD: Fatal neglect as child abuse, *Am J Dis Child* 142:914, 1988.

Gagan, R, Cupoli, JM, and Watkins, AH: The families of children who fail to thrive: Preliminary investigation of parental deprivation among organic and non-organic cases, *Child Abuse Negl* 8:93, 1984.

Guilhaume, A, Benoit, O, and Gourmelen, M: Relationship between sleep IV deficit and reversible HGH deficiency in psychosocial dwarfism, *Pediatr Res* 16:299-303, 1982.

Hadeed, AJ, and Siegel, SR: Maternal cocaine use during pregnancy: Effect on the newborn infant, *Pediatrics* 84:205, 1989.

Harris, ES, Weston, DR, and Lieberman, A: Quality of mother-infant attachment and pediatric health care use, *Pediatrics* 84:248, 1989.

Hathaway, P: Failure to thrive: Knowledge for social workers, *Health Soc Work* May:122, 1989.

Heger, A, and Stewart, D: Sexual abuse: The pediatrician's role. Paper presented at the American Academy of Pediatrics, Spring Session, 1988, New York.

Heger, RL, and Yungman, JJ: Toward a causal typology of child neglect, *Child Youth Services Rev* 11:203, 1989.

Helfer, RE: The epidemiology of child abuse and neglect, *Pediatr Ann* 13:745, 1984.

Helfer, RE: Where to now, Henry? A commentary on the battered child syndrome, *Pediatrics* 76:993, 1985.

Helfer, RE: The neglect of our children, *Pediatr Clin North Am* 37:923, 1990.

Helfer, RE, McKinney, JP, and Kemper, R: Arresting or freezing the developmental process. In Child Abuse and Neglect: *The Family and the Community,* Ballinger Publishing Co, Cambridge, MA, 1976.

Howing, P, et al: Child abuse and delinquency: The empirical and theoretical links, *Soc Work* May:244, 1990.

Howze, DC, and Kotch, JB: Disentangling life events, stress and social support: Implications for the primary prevention of child abuse and neglect, *Child Abuse Negl* 8:401, 1984.

Johnson, CF: Inflicted injury versus accidental injury, *Pediatr Clin North Am* 37:791, 1990.

Jones, DPH: The untreatable family, *Child Abuse Negl* 11:409, 1987.

Justice, B, Calvert, A, and Justice, R: Factors mediating child abuse as a response to stress, *Child Abuse Negl* 9:359, 1985.

Kempe, CH. In H Martin and CH Kempe, eds: *The Abused Child: Multidisciplinary Approach to Developmental Issues and Treatment,* Ballinger Publishing Co, Cambridge, MA, 1976, pp. xi-xiii.

Kessler, DB, and New, M: Emerging trends in child abuse and neglect, *Pediatr Ann* 18:471, 1989.

Koel, BS: Failure to thrive and fatal injury as a continuum, *Am J Dis Child* 118:565, 1969.

Krugman, RD: Future role of the pediatrician in child abuse and neglect, *Pediatr Clin North Am* 37:1003, 1990.

Lacey, KA, and Parkin, JM: The normal short child, *Arch Dis Child* 49:417, 1974.

Lally, JR: Three views of child neglect: Expanding visions of preventive intervention, *Child Abuse Negl* 8:243, 1984.

Main, M, and Goldwyn, R: Predicting rejecting of her infant from representations of her own experience: Implications for the abused-abusing intergenerational cycle, *Child Abuse Negl* 8:203, 1984.

Martin, MJ, and Walters, J: Familial correlates of selected types of child abuse and neglect, *J Marriage Fam* 44:267-276, 1982.

Mayhall, PD, and Norgard, KE: *Child Abuse and Neglect: Sharing Responsibility*, John Wiley and Sons, New York, 1983.

McCann and Pearlman, LA: Vicarious traumatization: A framework for understanding the psychological effects of working with victims, *J Trauma Stress* 3:133, 1990.

McCord, J: A forty-year perspective on effects of child abuse and neglect, *Child Abuse Negl* 7:265, 1983.

Murphy, S, Orkow, B, and Nicola, RM: Prenatal prediction of child abuse and neglect: A prospective study, *Child Abuse Negl* 9:225, 1985.

Pollack, J, and Levy, S: Countertransference and failure to report child abuse and neglect, *Child Abuse Negl* 13:515, 1989.

Rekowitz, CD, and Senter, SA: Characteristics of mother infant interactions in nonorganic failure to thrive, *J Fam Pract* 25(4):377-381, 1987.

Risenberg, HM: Fetal neglect and abuse, *NY State J Med* March:148, 1989.

Rogeness, GA, et al: Psychopathology in abused and neglected children, *J Am Acad Child Psychiatry* 25:659, 1986.

Schwartz, RH, and Einhorn, A: PCP intoxication in seven young children, *Pediatr Emerg Care* 2:238, 1986.

Spinner, MR, and Siegel, L: Nonorganic failure to thrive, *J Prevent Psychiatry* 3:279-287, 1987.

Study Findings (NIS-1): National study of the incidence and severity of child abuse and neglect, US Department of Health and Human Services, 1981.

Study Findings (NIS-2): Study of the national incidence and prevalence of child abuse and neglect, US Department of Health and Human Services, 1988.

Tower, CC: The neglect of children. In *Understanding Child Abuse and Neglect*, Allyn and Bacon, 1989.

US Advisory Board on Child Abuse and Neglect: Child abuse and neglect: Critical first steps in response to a national emergency, US Department of Health and Human Services, 1990.

Vondra, JI: Self-concept, motivation, and competence among preschoolers from maltreating and comparison families, *Child Abuse Negl* 14:525, 1990.

Widom, CS: Child abuse, neglect, and adult behavior: Research design findings on criminality, violence, and child abuse, *Am J Orthopsychiatry* 59:355, 1989.

Chapter

15

EMOTIONAL ABUSE

PEGGY S. PEARL, ED.D.

As far back as anyone can remember, Carol has regularly told Mary how lazy and stupid she is. Everywhere they go, Carol is heard telling Mary what she is doing wrong. Carol routinely tells Mary, as well as anyone else who will listen, that all of Carol's problems began when Mary was born. Carol has long complained that she couldn't keep a job because Mary was so demanding. When Mary entered school, she was behind her age-mates, wouldn't attempt new assignments, and did not appear to enjoy any activity. At the first parent conference, Carol told the teacher that she had always recognized that Mary was lazy, stupid, and a troublemaker. Mary had a very short attention span. In third grade, Mary was referred to the school psychologist for depression. Later that year she was found sitting on the playground in below-zero-degree temperatures without a coat, gloves, or hat. When asked what was wrong she said, "Nothing...," without looking at the teacher. Although Mary never complained to anyone, another student called the teacher's attention to the fact that Mary's hands "looked weird." The school nurse referred Mary to a pediatrician. Mary had frostbite.

259

Emotional abuse is the core issue in the broader topic of child maltreatment and therefore exists in all types of neglect, physical abuse, and sexual abuse (Dean, 1979; Straus & Kantor, 1987). Emotional abuse is a concerted attack on a child's development of self and social competence. It may or may not be a conscious act by the parents or other caregivers. Regardless of the intent, the consequences to the child are the same. Its pattern of psychologically destructive behavior by an adult can take the form of an act of omission, such as ignoring the child, or an act of commission, such as repeatedly telling the child that he or she is stupid. It is the most elusive and damaging of the types of maltreatment (Fortin & Reed, 1984; Yates, 1982; Green, 1978; Garbarino et al., 1986; Dean, 1979; Burgess et al., 1990; Hickox & Furnell, 1989). Emotional abuse interrupts the process of attachment, affective development, and the evolution of empathetic capacities. As a result of the child's failure to develop empathy, the child is impaired in his or her ability to appropriately receive and transmit emotional information. Some researchers think that lack of attachment, continual attack on the child's sense of worth, and failing to provide emotional nurturance, coupled with neglect and perhaps early physical abuse, impair the child's total capacity to respond emotionally (Brothers, 1989). An inability to consciously experience and communicate feelings has been linked to primate studies in deprivation (Sackette, 1966) and appears to be linked to human maternal deprivation. Since affective development must precede cognitive and physical development, early diagnosis and treatment of emotional abuse are important to minimize an individual's developmental damage and maturational impairment. Early diagnosis and treatment are the most effective means of reducing societal costs of emotional abuse and increasing the likelihood that the victim will live a fuller and more productive life.

◆ FORMS OF EMOTIONAL ABUSE

Emotional abuse can take many forms. It is always involved in the adult's struggle for absolute control of the child. The younger the child and the less developed the child's sense of self and identity, the more serious the physical, social, and emotional consequences. Emotional abuse of older children with a well-established sense of self may have less impact than the same action on a younger child or a previously maltreated child.

Emotional abuse varies in intensity from occasional to mild to extreme over a sustained period of time. Categories of emotional abuse include ignoring, rejecting, isolating, terrorizing, corrupting, verbally assaulting, and overpressuring (**Table 15-1**).

In most dysfunctional families children experience many types of maltreatment. In some families all children are treated or mistreated similarly, while in others each child is treated uniquely and is individually affected. The child's developmental stage influences both the parent-child interaction and the impact of the interaction on the child. The more nurturing the child has had prior to the maltreatment and the more secure the child's attachment to his or her caregiver(s) early in life, the less impact the maltreatment will have on the child.

Table 15-1. Categories of Emotional Abuse

1. *Ignoring* the child and failing to provide necessary stimulation, responsiveness, and validation of the child's worth in normal family routine.
2. *Rejecting* the child's value, needs, and requests for adult validation and nurturance.
3. *Isolating* the child from the family and community; denying the child normal human contact.
4. *Terrorizing* the child with continual verbal assaults, creating a climate of fear, hostility, and anxiety, thus preventing the child from gaining feelings of safety and security.
5. *Corrupting* the child by encouraging and reinforcing destructive, antisocial behavior until the child is so impaired in socioemotional development that interaction in normal social environments is not possible.
6. *Verbally assaulting* the child with constant name-calling, harsh threats, and sarcastic put-downs that continually "beat down" the child's self-esteem with humiliation.
7. *Overpressuring* the child with subtle but consistent pressure to grow up fast and to achieve too early in the areas of academics, physical/motor skills, and social interaction, which leaves the child feeling that he or she is never quite good enough.

◆IGNORING

Ignoring parents or other caregivers fail to acknowledge the child's presence or needs (**Table 15-2**). The ignoring parent is neither physically nor psychologically available for the child, either consistently or on an unpredictable basis. Ignoring is often part of serious physical neglect where the child is not fed, clothed, sheltered, bathed, supervised, or acknowledged as being in need of these basics.

CASE EXAMPLE

Martha seldom if ever calls any of her children by name. She neither talks to them nor looks at them. Martha's house is spotlessly clean, but meals are rarely prepared and seldom is there food that the children can readily prepare for themselves. Following a visit with her daughter, Martha's mother brought the youngest child to the emergency room, concerned about the child's lack of appetite. He was diagnosed as nonorganic failure to thrive. On examination of the other children, each child was found to be in the lowest percentile on growth charts, with abnormally short limbs, poor skin coloring, and extreme delays in muscle development. A visit to the school found the oldest child was barely passing, had poor social skills, and was withdrawn and passive. Discussion with Martha revealed that her husband, Tom, is a workaholic, a very successful lawyer who spends long hours at the office. His income is one of the highest in the community, from which he generously provides for his family. However, he spends little time at home and little of that time with his children. Even from cursory observation of Martha, she appears depressed and merely says that she misses her husband's company.

Studies of ignored children in institutions describe socioemotional deprivation severe enough to cause infant mortality of more than 33% (Spitz, 1945; Spitz, 1946). Because of medical intervention, however, each year the number of failure-to-thrive cases is growing.

CASE EXAMPLE

Jane is a 21-year-old single mother of three children. She has had normal pregnancies and each child was observed as normal at birth. However, each child now appears developmentally delayed and malnourished. Their skin is dry with little resiliency and a pale color. Their hair is dull, dry, and brittle. Their scalp is very dry. The children appear lethargic, as if drugged. The oldest child, 3 years 6 months old, lacks language. In the doctor's waiting room, nurses observed the eldest child feeding the 6-month-old infant. The mother sat nearby, ignoring the children and their activities.

RESULTING CHARACTERISTICS

Once treated, failure-to-thrive infants remain apathetic and lethargic. They are developmentally delayed, both physically and behaviorally. After they begin to look normal physically, behavioral problems remain for children who were failure-to-thrive infants. They experience a higher frequency of temper tantrums at all ages, isolation, and socioemotional delay, and they commit more petty theft (Bullard et al., 1967; Gardner, 1972). MacCarthy (1979) described these children as engaging in attention-seeking behavior, superficial displays of affection, selfishness, and spiteful actions.

Other physical conditions are linked to severe emotional neglect during childhood. The conditions include psychosocial and deprivation dwarfism, sleep and eating disorders, and motor abnormalities (Powell et al., 1967; Gardner, 1972). Egeland and associates' study (1983) of psychologically unavailable parents found that the children failed to thrive and develop normally. These children were both emotionally and cognitively delayed. One extreme form of parental ignoring is Munchausen Syndrome by Proxy (**Table 15-3 and Chapter 13**). The child's needs are ignored as the parent attempts to meet her own needs. In this syndrome, a parent, usually the mother, fabricates symptoms for the child, or actually causes illnesses, that result in unnecessary medical procedures (**Table 15-4**).

Table 15-2. Parental Ignoring Behaviors
Does not respond to child's needs
Fails to stimulate child in appropriate manner
Does not look at child
Does not call child by name
Does not attach or bond to child
Fails to recognize child's presence
Shows no affection for child
Is psychologically unavailable for child on consistent basis
Fails to allow child normal and appropriate privacy

Table 15-3. Signs of Munchausen Syndrome by Proxy

1. Persistent symptoms and/or illnesses for which a cause cannot be found.

2. Unusual symptoms, signs, and/or laboratory findings that do not make sense.

3. A diagnosis of disorders that are less common than MSBP.

4. Symptoms and signs that go away when the child is not with the mother or appear when only the mother is present.

5. Overly attentive parent. Parent becomes attached to medical staff, seems less concerned about child's condition than medical staff, and is highly involved in the care of other patients.

6. Affect of parent inconsistent with the apparent seriousness of the child's condition.

7. In a two-parent functional home, father absent or uninvolved in making medical decisions for what appears to be a seriously ill child.

8. Parental suggestions for or welcoming of medical tests even when painful for the child.

Table 15-4. Substances and Maneuvers Creating or Simulating Illness in Victims of Munchausen Syndrome by Proxy

Psychoactive Drugs

Phenothiazines	Chloral hydrate
Imipramine	Methaqualone
Amitriptyline	Amphetamines
Codeine	Barbiturates

Drugs/Substances Altering Fluid and Electrolyte Balance

Excessive table salt	Phenformin
Excessive water	Salicylates
Insulin	Theophylline
Furosemide	Chlorthalidone

Miscellaneous Toxins

Pepper	Laxatives
Naphtha	Lye
Warfarin	

Other Mechanisms

Starvation
Suffocation
Fabricated history of previous diagnosis of serious illness, e.g., operable cardiac disease, epilepsy, various conditions
Inflicted vaginal/rectal injury to produce bleeding
Altered laboratory studies, e.g., simulation of cystic fibrosis by altering sputum samples, putting salt in collection for sweat test, adding fat to stool collection
Injection of contaminated material into intravenous lines
Putting parent's blood into urine
Removal of blood from child's central venous line

(From Wissow, 1991.)

In addition to the physical harm, the child learns to live under absolute control with adults who cannot be trusted (McGuire & Feldman, 1989). Children of depressed mothers who were emotionally unavailable to their children on a consistent basis showed both emotional and cognitive developmental delay (Polanky et al., 1981). The schizophrenic parent or character disorder parent also is in such need emotionally that she or he is consistently unavailable to the child. Ignoring is an act of omission, passive and neglectful, as compared to rejecting, which is an act of commission, active and abusing.

♦ REJECTING

Rejecting parents refuse to touch or show affection to their child and/or do not acknowledge this child's presence or accomplishments as well as constantly "rejecting and demeaning" age-appropriate behaviors. **Table 15-5** lists parental rejecting behaviors.

With an infant, the parent refuses to form an attachment. The parent does not respond to the child's behaviors to have basic needs met, such as when the child cries for food or with a wet diaper. Nor does the parent respond to the child's smiles and vocalizations of pleasure. As the child grows the parent does not talk with the child or get involved in the preschooler's activities. The child is not included in family activities. The child may spend long periods of time in solitary play often in another room with the door closed. As the child develops, the parent consistently communicates a negative definition of self to the child. The parent belittles the child and his or her accomplishments, both privately and publicly calling the child "dummy, clumsy, dunce, nerd," and/or "freak." The parent has very low expectations of the child in school, telling the child that he or she can't expect to pass or do well in school because he or she is too dumb.

Table 15-5. Parental Rejecting Behaviors

Refusing to allow child to get needed psychological or medical treatment or educational services

Belittling and ridiculing child

Purposefully and continually embarrassing child

Singling child out for criticism and punishment

Failing to allow child to develop autonomy or independence

Confusing child's sexual identity

Undermining attachment of child with others

Routinely rejecting child's ideas

Ridiculing or punishing age-appropriate behaviors as too immature

Routinely calling child dumb, stupid, freak, nerd

Privately and publicly routinely putting child down

Inappropriately attributing undesirable characteristic(s) to child

Continuing to treat adolescent as young child

Denying child's needs and making child meet adult needs

Making child perform household tasks because the parent finds the task undesirable

---

The school-aged child or adolescent is treated like a small child and not allowed to act in age-appropriate ways. The parent does not acknowledge, or openly rejects, the changes associated with adolescence, including social roles, physical size, sexual development, or increased cognitive ability. The child is told of his failures and seldom if ever included as a valued individual within the family. The parent commonly fails to have empathy for the child's needs (Trowell, 1983; Rohner & Rohner, 1980).

Rejecting parents generally appear overwhelmed by the convergence of social and economic hardships. Commonly, rejecting parents are reacting to large families, limited material resources, limited education and job skills, and few emotional and social supports, all of which stress the parents and limit their ability to nurture their children (**Table 15-6**). These parents feel materially and psychologically unable to move beyond concern for themselves to concern about their role as caregivers, teachers, and providers of emotional support for their children (Garbarino et al., 1986; Pemberton & Benady, 1973; Trowell, 1983).

CASE EXAMPLE

Jane feeds her son regularly on schedule but seldom if ever holds him while she feeds the child his bottle. She lays him on the sofa and props the bottle, telling him and others how much of her time he takes and what better things she could be doing than taking care of him. When she feeds him baby food she fails to make eye contact or talk to him. When she changes his diaper the only comments she makes are in disgust at how terrible it smells and what a mess he has made that she must clean up. She is seldom in the same room as the child and does not talk to him or play with him when they are physically near each other. She describes him as a "troublesome baby." However, other family members comment that he is a good baby since they never hear him cry.

Table 15-6. Family Circumstances Associated with Increased Risk for Rejection

Unwanted pregnancies

No opportunity for caregiver to spend time alone

Lack of involvement by father in child rearing

Marital discord

Social and instrumental isolation of family from the community

---

RESULTING CHARACTERISTICS

Children who have been psychologically and/or physically rejected by parents or other primary caregivers are hostile and aggressive, have impaired self-esteem, and show either excessive dependency on parents and/or other adults or "defensive independence" (Rohner & Rohner, 1980). These children and teens appear emotionally unstable and unresponsive, eventually perceiving the world in negativistic terms (Pemberton & Benady, 1973). They see themselves as having few strengths and skills. They view the world as being hostile and unwilling to assist them. They feel isolated and in turn reject others, including their own children.

◆ISOLATING

Isolation of children can come from a variety of parental motivations, but the resulting behavior prevents children from having normal opportunities for social relations with both adults and peers. **Table 15-7** lists parental isolating behaviors. Some isolating parents are themselves fearful of the outside world and want to protect their children from the dangers they believe exist from contact with others. These families usually have a very limited amount of social contact, which deprives the children of learning social skills with a variety of individuals. Isolation is also present in sexually abusive families and in families where ritualistic abuse occurs. The isolation is to keep what happens in the family a secret and to keep the children from learning that there is any other way of life. Other isolating parents are themselves without social skills and merely lack social contacts and/or supports and do not provide the opportunity for their children.

Table 15-7. Parental Isolating Behaviors
Not allowing child to participate in normal family routine
Not allowing child normal contact with peers
Physically separating child from family unit
Failing to allow child to participate in the social aspects of school
Avoiding physical contact with child, e.g. hugging, touching, holding
Routinely teaching child to avoid and distrust peers
Locking child in room, basement, attic
Punishing requests for interaction with family or others
Binding or gagging child to prevent interaction
Refusing, without justifiable reason, to allow child contact with noncustodial parent, grandparent, or siblings
Hiding child from outside world

CASE EXAMPLE

Neither Maria, 14, nor Christine, 10, are allowed to have friends over to play or go to other homes to play. Their mother believes that other children will introduce her girls to drugs and other "evils of the world." The girls were home-schooled until recently when their mother had to go to work to help pay off some medical and home repair bills. Since entering the public schools the girls have not made friends. Christine has had problems doing group social studies and language arts. Both girls are excessively anxious about trying new experiences at school. They worry about someone taking advantage of them, and as a result peers tease them.

RESULTING CHARACTERISTICS

Isolating families often directly teach their children that contact outside the family is undesirable. School-aged children are not allowed to participate in co-curricular school activities, youth activities, or neighborhood play groups. Adolescent children are given home responsibilities and are prohibited from participation in school activities. Some families even remove children from school or do not encourage school attendance. Frequently, children who have been isolated for long periods of time lack the social competence to experience success or enjoyment at school and therefore do not like to attend (Garbarino et al., 1986; Rohner & Rohner, 1980).

♦ TERRORIZING

Terrorizing involves threatening the child with extreme or frightening punishment. **Table 15-8** lists parental terrorizing behaviors. The parent intentionally stimulates intense fear, creates a climate of unpredictable threat, or sets unattainable expectations and punishes the child for not attaining them. The discipline techniques are often arbitrary or beyond the child's ability to understand. The parent may tease or scare a young child in the name of humor, but the results terrorize and confuse the child. The parent disciplines the child by playing on fears that are normal for that age, such as loud noises or the dark. The terrorizing parent uses the feared situation "to scare the child into behaving." Parents may tell preschool-aged children that if they don't behave the "monsters will drag them away in the night," or the night-light is "watching and if you're not good, the night-light will zap you." One of the normal fears of adolescents is that their peers will see them as different or that they will not fit into social settings. The terrorizing parent threatens the adolescent with "public humiliation" (Garbarino et al., 1986).

CASE EXAMPLE

Sam repeatedly has had his dad threaten him and other family members with a gun, a bullwhip, and a switchblade. He has never seen them used on a family member but regularly hides so he cannot be found in case his dad comes home mad.

RESULTING CHARACTERISTICS

Terrorizing parents play mind games with older children. These games are designed to be no-win where the child becomes very anxious fearing the consequences. When parents place the child in the middle of arguments, as often happens in divorces, the child also becomes terrorized by the no-win situations. A child may be blamed for everything that goes wrong in the family, regardless of whose behavior is inappropriate. Constant criticism often leaves children so traumatized that they will not act because they fear they will be criticized.

Table 15-8. Parental Terrorizing Behaviors
Excessive threats and psychological punishment
Threatening and frightening child with guns, knives, whips, etc.
Bizarre means of discipline
Excessive use of guilt-producing activity
Chaotic behavior to frighten child
Laughing at or ridiculing child when frightened, or putting child down for expressing normal fears
Punishing child by playing on normal childhood fears
Refusing to comfort infant in distress
Inconsistent and capricious disciplining of child
Continually threatening suicide or to leave child
Threatening to harm others in child's presence
Knowingly permitting child to view or be involved in violent behavior
Routinely engaging in fights and frightening behavior in front of child
Binding and/or gagging child
Permitting others to terrorize child
Failing to provide shelter, consistency, and safety for child

♦ RITUALISTIC ABUSE

Ritualistic or multiple-victim, multiple-perpetrator abuse is one of the most damaging forms of abuse (Burgess et al., 1990; Snow & Sorensen, 1990). It is the systematic, bizarre misuse of the child physically, socially, sexually, and emotionally that includes some supernatural and/or religious activities by a group of adults. Ritualistic abuse is " carefully integrated and linked with a symbol of overriding power, authority, and purpose," such as a religion or pseudo-religion (Burgess et al., 1990). In this type of abuse, children are routinely involved in ceremonial sexual activity with adults, other children, and to a lesser extent with animals. Use of bondage, excessive threats, and force can be present. This activity is usually performed in front of other adults and children. Children are physically tortured, drugged, and forced to ingest drugs, human and/or animal feces, urine, blood, and flesh. They are buried alive in boxes and bound to crosses, and some stories are told of sacrificing children to the devil (**Table 15-9**).

The children, as well as the adults involved in this activity, are removed from normal social interaction and activity and are taught a very antisocial value system. The "family" environment is one of absolute control by one individual. The children are told that what is happening to them is because of their bad behavior or sin and that they must be punished or they must cleanse themselves during the ceremonies. Children are systematically told they are of no value except for how they can be used by the "all-powerful one," the group leader (Young et al., 1991; Snow & Sorensen, 1990; Burgess et al., 1990; Kelley, 1988).

In ritualistic abuse cases, children are systematically terrorized into participation and silence. Initially the victim appears normal and denies any ritualistic involvement or multiple-perpetrator activity. Over time when the child feels safe, the child is able to recall memories and begins to describe experiences to a therapist or other trusted individual. The following are commonly used methods of terrorizing children to silence in ritualistic abuse:

Preschool-aged children are given a "mock operation." The child is laid blind-folded and nude on a table. The stomach is brushed with either a local antiseptic or a very cold liquid. Then a sharp pointed object is used to draw an outline on the child's stomach. The child is told that an animal is being placed in his stomach, and if he tells anything that has happened to him the animal or demon will eat the child up to protect the secret. The child may be drugged to drowsiness before the "operation" and then given additional drugs to induce sleep. On waking, the child is asked what has just happened to check for effectiveness and to begin the terrorizing.

Children of any age can be systematically programmed so that when they see a specific thing or hear a specific word they will "forget everything" they know or they will remember specific bizarre threats of what can happen to them if they tell. The word or object is usually something that the child frequently hears, or sees, such as a postal truck or the word "light."

Table 15-9. Common Behaviors and Interests of Ritualistically Abused Children
Excessive masturbation
Preoccupation with feces and urine
Detailed, age-inappropriate sexual knowledge
Spontaneous sexual offers to adults
Somatic complaints
Night terrors
Frequent sexual interplay between children
Preoccupation with death and burial
Extreme fears of death, confinement, and abduction
Stories of being buried
References to the devil and magic
Bizarre treatment of animals or talking of the bizarre treatment
Fear of rituals, candles, chants
Multiple personalities
Lack of traditional belief system
Delinquent behavior, often bizarre

Children are taught to believe that others can "read" their minds to always know what they are thinking. They are also taught to believe that "good is bad and bad is good, hate is smart and love is dumb."

◆ SEXUAL ABUSE

Sexual abuse of children involves different types of emotional abuse. Commonly, children are terrorized with extreme threats and the excessive use of power and control. The adult uses extreme methods to both gain and maintain control over the child's mind. The child is told if he or she tells anyone about the abusive events, the parent or perpetrator will go to jail, the child will be taken away and never be allowed to see family members again, the child will become very ill and die, or some family member or beloved pet will die. Victims experience emotional trauma from shame, guilt, uncertainty, and fear of breaking up the family. The role changes in the incestuous family do not conform with societal norms. The common use of sexual exploitation within the family teaches the child socially inappropriate interpersonal communication skills. Corrupting also occurs in incestuous families as the child is taught inappropriate adult and child behaviors that do not conform with the community standards (Snow & Sorensen, 1990; Burgess et al., 1990; Kelley, 1988).

♦ CORRUPTING

Corrupting parental behaviors (**Table 15-10**) teach and reinforce antisocial or deviant patterns that tend to make the child unable to function in a normal social setting. In milder forms, the parents convey approval of or encourage the child's precocious interest and/or behavior in the area of sexuality, aggression, violence, or substance abuse. In the more serious forms, the parents continue to encourage and reinforce as the child's antisocial behavior grows more intense and destructive to self, others, or property. Reinforcing or ignoring delinquent behavior is parental corrupting behavior.

Corrupting can begin with rewarding the infant for oral sexual contact, creating drug dependence, encouraging violence toward peers, laughing at antisocial behaviors, and continuing to encourage these behaviors as they grow more habitual and serious. Common parental corrupting behaviors include allowing adults to use their children for sexual activity including prostitution and child pornography, allowing children to sell and deliver drugs, and encouraging drug use. In ritualistic abuse cases, often children reveal, after they feel very safe, that they were encouraged to have sex with younger children.

Table 15-10. Parental Corrupting Behaviors
Allowing and/or forcing child to watch pornographic materials
Teaching child sexually exploitative behaviors
Teaching child illegal activity
Knowingly allowing others to teach illegal activity to child
Praising child for antisocial/delinquent behavior
Positively responding to child's antisocial behavior
Instructing child in antisocial/illegal activity
Assisting child in delinquent behavior
Failing to discipline child for delinquent behavior
Teaching child that "bad is good and good is bad"
Giving drugs or other contraband to child
Exposing child to harmful influences or situations
Using child as a spy, ally, or confidante in parent's romantic relationships or marital or divorce problems

Parents who knowingly allow children to engage in any illegal activity are corrupting those children. Corruption is also occurring, however, when parents merely fail to teach their children the social skills necessary for successful interaction in the world around them and leave them vulnerable to learn inappropriate behaviors from those who would take advantage of them (Garbarino et al., 1986; Burgess et al., 1990).

In families where parents are corrupting their children, the parents could be repeating the parenting cycle. They pass on the type of parenting they received. Parents who themselves have antisocial behaviors commonly transmit those values, actions, and attitudes to their children. These parental behaviors result from some events or series of events in their own lives. Research suggests that most antisocial and criminal behavior is a consequence of child maltreatment (Cerce et al., 1988).

CASE EXAMPLE

Katrina's mother has had a series of boyfriends living in the home for many years, most of whom have had substance abuse problems. Both alcohol and drugs are common in the home. Katrina, 16, tells her friends that she can supply them with almost any drug they want anytime they want them. She has her own car and no curfew. This year her school attendance record has been poor, but she has notes from her pediatrician, who is her grandfather, to "excuse" each absence.

RESULTING CHARACTERISTICS

Children who are mistreated during the first year of life fail to develop a basic sense of trust and, therefore, see the world around them as negative. They believe that people are not to be trusted or valued. These children frequently are taught that you have to take care of yourself, "take or get taken." This lack of respect for others leads them to have no respect for themselves. The consequence of corrupting children is that from an early age the children demonstrate antisocial behavior. These children have a pseudo-mature behavior unlike normal behavior of age-mates. They are "street-smart kids." From a very young age, they demonstrate few positive emotions and an inability to play in an age-appropriate manner. They are often rewarded for stealing and assaulting peers. As a result they are unaware that their behavior is inappropriate. Commonly these families devalue formal public education and fail to send their children to school on a regular basis or fail to discourage school absences, further isolating the children from learning appropriate social skills, values, and attitudes.

◆VERBAL ASSAULTING

Verbally assaulting the child with constant name-calling, harsh threats, and sarcastic put-downs that continually "beat down" the child's sense of worth with humiliation is a type of emotional abuse. **Table 15-11** lists parental verbally assaulting behaviors. In the verbally assaultive family, words are used to humiliate and control. Repeatedly, the child is told of the things that he is doing wrong without regard for what he does well. The child is often unfavorably compared with other family members or with downcast individuals. The child is regularly called derogatory names. The verbal put-downs and attacks can occur in the privacy of the home. Frequently, however, the child is publicly told what she has failed to do and how worthless she is. The verbally assaultive behavior is so pervasive in the family's functioning that child care professionals routinely hear the verbal assaults. These verbal assaults are usually delivered in a loud voice which further accents their negativeness (Vissing et al., 1991; Trowell, 1983; Rohner & Rohner, 1980).

Table 15-11. Parental Verbally Assaulting Behaviors

Continuous verbal attacks, especially in loud voice

Failing to protect child from verbal attacks of others

Constant belittling

Excessive criticism

Routinely humiliating the child

Openly telling the child he or she is worthless and no good

Excessive name-calling

Scapegoating the child

Calling child derogatory or demeaning names

Cursing child

Continually yelling at child

Attributing to child behaviors or characteristics that are totally unacceptable to child

CASE EXAMPLE

Phil is 3 years old. He had been developing normal language but a radical change has occurred. The neighbor is worried; she hears Phil's dad continually telling Phil to shut up all of that chattering and not to talk when the television is on. "No one wants to hear you talk, we want to listen to the television." Phil's mom is telling all her friends, in front of Phil and whomever else is around, that he's "just retarded, can't talk, and the most awkward child she has ever seen."

RESULTING CHARACTERISTICS

As a consequence of verbal battering, children have a flat or negative affect, low self-esteem, and often self-mutilating behavior. These children are withdrawn and shy and have no sense of initiative. The children feel they are incapable of any achievements. They are unable to recognize positive social feedback when it is given to them. In some families, one child is scapegoated and routinely verbally assaulted or the brunt of routine family sarcasm while other children receive no emotional abuse. The scapegoated children are a high risk for failure to thrive, psychological dwarfism, childhood depression, and suicide. Usually, the child's physical appearance is one of poor posture and flat affect or excessive acting behavior (Egeland et al., 1983; Pemberton & Benady, 1973; Burgess et al., 1990; Baily & Baily, 1983).

♦ OVERPRESSURING

Primarily a middle-class phenomenon, overpressuring parents consistently have inappropriately high expectations for their children. As David Elkind described in *The Hurried Child: Growing Up Too Fast Too Soon* (1982), many parents today tend to be more concerned about a child's intellectual achievements than his or her emotional well-being. Children are expected to perform intellectual tasks early to prevent being "normal or average" as compared to peers. **Table 15-12** lists parental overpressuring behaviors. Overpressuring begins when parents toilet train too early or attempt to teach 3- and 4-year-old children to read, count, and work on computers, and continues with inappropriate "pressuring and hurrying" throughout the child's life.

Graduating tenth rather than first in the high school class or obtaining an ACT score of 25 is seen as failure by the parent. The parent views the child's consistently coming in second in a swimming meet or a golf tournament as not really trying rather than having done a "good job." The overpressured child is praised and valued for what is accomplished but not for just being.

Table 15-12. Parental Overpressuring Behaviors
Excessively advanced expectations of child
Excessively critical of age-appropriate behaviors as inadequate
Punishes child for acting in age-appropriate manner, calls child "immature"
Ostracizes child for not achieving far above normal abilities
Does not provide assistance with remedial work, refusing to acknowledge that child would need assistance with such "simple" materials
Refuses to provide age-appropriate experiences, insisting on providing experiences that are advanced
Begins toilet training very early and insists that child control body functions
Makes comparisons of child to those who are very advanced, consistently leaving child "poor by comparison"
Routinely buys toys that are far too advanced for child with clear expectations that the toy will be used appropriately, setting the child up for almost certain failure

CASE EXAMPLE

Sara's parents expected her to be "Harvard material." She was expected to do well in everything, playing the piano, sports, and academics. But she was average. Her parents regularly expressed their expectations and disappointment with her level of achievement, her appearance, and choice of friends. At 15, she was convinced that she was a failure and attempted suicide "to save her parents the embarrassment," the note said.

RESULTING CHARACTERISTICS

Parents can set high standards for their children and still demonstrate acceptance and love. Nurturing parents demonstrate positive feelings to their children, recognize their achievements, and convey pride. Overpressuring parents, however, fail to demonstrate that they feel acceptance, love, and pride toward their children. As a result, the overpressured child feels worthless, discouraged, lazy, unreliable, unacceptable, and inferior. The child feels inadequate or unacceptable as she (or he) is since parents are always trying to change her. The child's identity is in terms of accomplishments rather than herself.

Stress-related illnesses are common in these children. Because they lack parental support and good self-esteem, they are more vulnerable to negative experiences. These children commonly suffer from depression and are at high risk for eating disorders, suicide, and poor peer relationships throughout their lives.

♦ TOILET TRAINING

Beginning to toilet train too early (clearly before 18 months of age, but may be later in some children) says to the child "you are not acceptable as you are and need to change." Often parents combine the age-inappropriate toilet training with terrorizing and threats of what will happen to the child if she (or he) does not gain control of her (or his) bowels and bladder. These children may later be seen in the physician's office with extreme constipation and/or urinary tract infections as the child continues to try to gain control of his or her "environment" by control of body functions. When children repeatedly hear parents or grandparents say, "Your dad or mother was potty trained at 9 months," they feel the pressure to be toilet trained but lack the muscle control. The children feel inferior because they are unable to perform as wanted by these significant adults. To the child this is a subtle but consistent put-down for not performing at the same level as the parent. When this put-down is combined with other forms of overpressuring, the results are frequently stress-related illnesses and excessive anxiety.

◆CAUSES OF EMOTIONAL ABUSE

Many theories exist regarding the causes and correlates of child abuse. The four theories discussed here are 1) the psychiatric approach, 2) the social approach, 3) the developmental approach, and 4) the ecological approach.

PSYCHIATRIC APPROACH

The psychiatric approach to emotional abuse of children assumes that the perpetrating parent suffers from some mental illness. Kempe and Kempe (1978) estimated that 10% of all maltreating parents are psychopathic or sociopathic. Studies of mentally ill patients show they are at high risk for failing to meet a child's psychological needs because of the amount of effort they must expend to meet their own emotional needs. As compared to a control group, emotionally abusive parents showed significantly more psychosocial problems, more difficulty coping with stress, more difficulty building relationships, and more social isolation (Pemberton & Benady, 1973). According to one study, emotionally abusive parents described themselves as having poor child management techniques and being victims of maltreatment in their childhoods (Hickox & Furnell, 1989). The mother who is overwhelmed with her own depression and psychologically stressed after childbirth lacks the physical or emotional energies to give the child what is needed. The parent preoccupied with the death of a parent, sibling, or spouse may also be unable to meet a child's needs. Although postpartum depression and grief tend to be short-term and reversible, they negatively impact the parent-child relationship and can adversely affect the developing child. Mothers who are psychologically unavailable to their children appear to impair both socioemotional and cognitive development of the children (Erickson et al., 1986; Polanky et al., 1981). Emotional abuse stemming from the mental illness of parents is one possible explanation but explains only a small number of emotional abuse cases.

SOCIAL APPROACH

Social approach theory places emphasis on the role of stress as a force impacting the family dynamics and causing emotional abuse. Fifty-nine percent of all abuse cases were associated with stress (Gil, 1970). Social stress interacting with other variables leads to aggression in the form of emotional abuse. The stressors for all families include limited resources, problems at work, death of the significant other, unemployment, health problems, overcrowding, isolation, substance abuse, high levels of mobility, poverty, and marital problems (Newberger & Newberger, 1982).

Individuals respond differently to stress. Women as a group demonstrate a tendency toward depression rather than violence as a response. Men as a group respond to stress with violence. Stressed women usually are psychologically unavailable to their children, thus ignoring, rejecting, or isolating them. Men, on the other hand, have a tendency to physically or verbally assault their children. The family's socialization to violence determines if the father is physically or verbally assaultive (Straus & Kantor, 1987). *Since all parents experience stress, the following mediating variables can assist in identifying which parents will abuse their children and which will not:*

1. Presence or lack of appropriate coping mechanisms

2. Degree of family integration or isolation

3. Presence or absence of positive social networks

These mediating variables and the underlying causes of the stress determine the length and degree of the emotional abuse and, consequently, the amount of damage to the child's development (Casanova et al., 1992; Hickox & Furnell, 1989; Newberger & Newberger, 1982; Straus & Kantor, 1987).

DEVELOPMENTAL APPROACH

The developmental approach to emotional abuse is based on a theory that parenting attitudes and behaviors parallel Piaget's stages of cognitive development and Kolberg's stages of moral development. The stages require increasing cognitive sophistication and moral reasoning. At the lower developmental level, behavior is marked by immediate, direct, and unmodulated responses to external stimuli and internal need states. At higher levels of maturation, behavior is characterized by the appearance of indirect, ideational, conceptual, and symbolic or verbal behavior. Parents at the higher levels are more apt to use words and reasoning as part of parenting. Parents at the higher levels look at each child as an individual and at what is best for that individual. Parents at the lower levels are more impulsive, directive, and physical in their parenting. Parents at the lower levels parent from their own point of view and to make themselves feel good (Newberger & Cook, 1983). Abusive parents, therefore, are parenting at their developmental level (Zigler & Hall, 1989).

The orientations toward the parent-child relationship as identified by Newberger and Cook (1983) are egoistic, conventional, individualistic, and analytic orientations. **Table 15-13** describes the characteristics of parental reasoning at each of these cognitive-developmental stages.

Table 15-13. Cognitive-Developmental Stages of Parental Reasoning

Egoistic (Self) Orientation

The basis for parental activity and for understanding of the child is the child's actions in relation to the parent's needs. Child care tasks and parenting are seen as being carried out in response to external cues that affect the parent's emotional and physical comfort, or which offer approval to the parent. Intentions of the child are recognized, but as a projection of parental feelings, and are not separate from actions. The organizing principle is achieving what the parent wants, and the object of socialization of the child is to maximize parental comfort.

Examples:

> *What do you feel children need most from their parents?*
> Love and attention
>
> *When you say love, what do you mean?*
> Holding them, telling them you love them, making them behave so they won't get on that dope and stuff when they get older. I want my kids to feel proud of me. I know eventually when they get older maybe I'll fail, but I'm gonna try my darndest when they're younger and just hope they don't turn out that way.

Conventional (Norms) Orientation

The basis for parental activity and for understanding of the child is the child's actions and inferred intentions in relation to preconceived, externally derived expectations. The child is conceived as having internal states and needs that must be acknowledged, but the parent conceives of the child's subjective reality in a stereotypical way. The child is not seen as unique, but as a member of the class of "children" and the parent draws upon tradition, "authority," or conventional wisdom, rather than solely upon the self, to inform expectations and practices. The parent and child are understood to have well-defined roles which are their responsibility to fulfill. The parent-child relationship is conceived as mutual fulfillment of role obligations.

Examples:

> *What do you feel children need most from their parents?*
> Love

Table 15-13. Cognitive Developmental Stages of Parental Reasoning—*Continued*

Explain.
Just letting them know you love them. Letting them know you care, that you are concerned about what they do, and just trying to be the best parent you can.

Why do you think that is most important, conveying that love?
Because if children know they have love, then they are secure.

Individualistic (Child) Orientation
Each child is recognized to have unique as well as universally shared qualities and is understood in terms of his or her own subjective reality. The parent tries to understand the child's world from the child's particular point of view, and conceptualizes the parent-child relationship as an exchange of feelings and sharing of perspectives, rather than only fulfillment of role obligations.

Examples:

What do you think children need most from their parents?
Love and time, they need to have their needs considered, that they aren't always happy with things that we do and with the things that we want to make them do and with the things we want to make them happy. You have to look at them and if they don't tell, you have to ask them. You have to really try to find out what each child wants and what is going on in their heads.

Analytic (Systems) Orientation
The parent can view the relationship between parent and child as a mutual and reciprocal system and understand that the child has a complex psychological self-system. The parent can understand that the motives underlying a child's actions may reflect simultaneous and conflicted feelings. The parent can also recognize that there may be ambivalence in his or her own feelings and actions as a parent, and still love and care for the child. Individuals and relationships are understood not only in terms of their stable elements, but also as a continual process of growth and change. The parent-child relationship is built not only on shared feelings, but also on shared acceptance of each other's faults and frailties as well as virtues, and each other's separateness as well as closeness.

Examples:

What do you feel children need most from their parents? I will say love and you will say to me; "What do you mean by love?" and I will say, "I think it is an acceptance, unqualified, for what that person is in time...." It has nothing to do with grades or cleanliness. I would like her to be clean and tidy, but it has nothing to do with love and feeling that someplace in this world you are loved for what you are by the people who know you best and nevertheless love you. I think that it is something that will help the children begin to love themselves.

What do you mean to begin to love itself? Well, I think that people can be so cruel to themselves, "Oh, I'm dumb, I'm stupid." Words which tear down instead of build up. And I think one way to serenity about the way you are and the way you see the world, even if life is difficult, is if you can be gentle with your errors and failures and see them as part of a process. Then I think you will have a kind of stability and mental health that is a legacy from parents who love you unqualified (Newberger & Cook, 1983).

ECOLOGICAL APPROACH

The ecological approach to emotional abuse of children includes all of the various aspects of the family's life including what the parents bring to the relationship, the child, the social context of the family and its support system, and the total societal influences and values. The parents bring to the parent-child relationship a variety of influences including how they were parented, their parental developmental level, their feelings toward the child, their knowledge of child development, their marital relationship, and their individual mental health. The child influences how (he or she) will be parented. The child's health, temperament, ordinal position in the family, and other family relationships all influence how a child will be parented. Additionally, the support systems of the family and the total societal expectations are influencing factors. The interaction of all the influencing factors determine the type of parenting (Polanky et al., 1981; Zigler & Hall, 1989; Hickox & Furnell, 1989).

♦Identifying Emotional Abuse

Emotional abuse, although the core of all types of maltreatment, is very difficult to specifically identify and diagnose. With careful multidisciplinary documentation, each professional can provide a valuable part of the total picture (Fortin & Reed, 1984). Many young emotional abuse victims, especially ritualistically abused victims, may initially have few overt indicators. The complete picture becomes evident as the child feels safe with more professionals. The assessment of the child's situation begins with a professional seeing some minor abnormalities and then becoming more concerned as he or she obtains additional information. **Table 15-14** summarizes indicators of emotional abuse in children.

Table 15-14. Indicators of Emotional Abuse

Socioemotional Indicators
Impaired capacity to enjoy life
Refuses to defend self
Pseudo-mature behavior
Sexually precocious behavior
Lies notably when it is not to protect self but often in circumstances when there is nothing to lose by telling the truth
Cheats, steals
Refuses to accept responsibility for actions; blames others
Psychiatric symptoms
Tantrums
Bizarre behavior
Low self-esteem
Withdrawal
Opposition
Compulsivity

Aggressive, defiant, domineering
Controlling but lacks self-control
Extreme behaviors
Seeking love, acceptance, and affection outside of home
Pregnant adolescent wanting her baby to love her
Apathy

Cognitive Indicators
School learning problems
Short attention span
Hypervigilance
Hyperactivity, attention deficit
Language delayed
Motor delayed
Lack of exploration and curiosity

Physical Indicators
Nonorganic failure to thrive

Slowed growth in trunk and distinctly short limbs, dwarfism
Circulatory problems
Accident prone
Awkwardness
Small abrasions that heal slowly on limbs
Coarse, dry, brittle hair and dry scalp
Self-destructive both physically and socially
Eating disorders, anorexia nervosa, bulimia, obesity
Gastrointestinal and bowel problems including chronically loose stools, refusal to void
Poor posture
Reduced energy level, lethargy
Catatonia
Sleep disorders

Behavioral Indicators

The emotionally abused infant's behavior is characterized by a wide range of behaviors including apathy, crying and irritability, refusal to be calmed, and avoidance of eye contact with adults, especially parents.

Negative Affect

Emotionally maltreated infants commonly show a negative affect to anyone in the environment. They also fail to grimace or show pain when appropriate, such as not crying after a fall or a shot. They don't respond as other children would when things such as toys or food are taken away from them. In situations in which a normal child would cry or seek comfort, these children have no affect, appearing indifferent.

Failure to Thrive

In extreme cases of emotional abuse, the infant can undergo the process of nonorganic failure to thrive characterized by insufficient weight gain, impaired health, slow physical growth, retarded language development, distorted social responses, irritability, an anxious attachment, apathetic solitariness, and catatonia.

Passivity

Abused children appear numb to either negative or positive environmental stimuli.

If left alone with familiar objects, they do not have normal age-appropriate play skills and do not demonstrate normal pleasure and satisfaction from either solitary play or play with adults. They are excessively passive and obedient (MacCarthy, 1979; Trowell, 1983).

NEGATIVE SELF-IMAGE

Young children who have experienced emotional abuse demonstrate a negative view of their world and themselves. They see themselves as unworthy and view the world as a hostile place. They are fearful, angry, anxious, aggressive, and sometimes violent. They may engage in both physically and socially self-destructive behavior. They are often depressed, withdrawn, passive, and shy, exhibiting poor interpersonal communication skills. These children are often suicidal. They may frequently complain of headaches and sleep disturbances.

Children who externalize their feelings tend to be disobedient, impulsive, and overactive. They lack self-control and often are violent toward other people and their environment. Maltreated children who are aggressive exhibit a continuous and generalized aggression. The aggression is a state of being rather than a response to a specific action or individual. They behave according to impulses rather than social norms (Fontana, 1973; Rohner & Rohner, 1980). Children who internalize their feelings are withdrawn, indifferent, submissive, and hostile (Egeland et al., 1983).

ABNORMAL RESPONSES

Some emotionally maltreated children have low levels of social responsiveness or hesitant response patterns. They approach unfamiliar adults indiscriminately, seeking attention while avoiding physical contact with them (Balla & Zigler, 1975; Harter & Zigler, 1974). Other emotionally maltreated children cling to adults other than their parents and remain distant from peers (MacCarthy, 1979). In both instances, the child's social behavior can be situationally inappropriate. In most instances the child is unable to respond to environmental rewards such as children asking them to join in group activities, smiles, and verbal praise (Watkins & Bradbard, 1982). The child is often indifferent to positive feedback about his or her own success and responds negatively with social challenges or peer rejection.

Maltreated children respond negatively to parents and/or merely attempt to avoid the parent to avoid more maltreatment. The child may also try to take care of the parent's needs to reduce the instance and degree of maltreatment in the future. In the home, as in other social environments, the child may rebel and aggressively act out or may withdraw and attempt to escape physically or emotionally.

BEHAVIOR EXTREMES

Child abuse victims characteristically exhibit behavior at the extremes of the normal spectrum (**Table 15-15**).

CHILD AND FAMILY ASSESSMENT

The early indicators of emotional maltreatment should alert child care professionals to possible problems, prompting early intervention and treatment. Assessment tools combined with observational data from all professionals who work with a child and his or her family can give an accurate evaluation of family functioning. Most cases of emotional abuse are mild and will not enter the protective services system; instead, the family in trouble will seek assistance with its own problems. If protective services and the courts become involved, the case should include professional summaries from a variety of professionals and an assessment by a psychologist with at least three of the assessment tools listed in **Table 15-16**.

Table 15-15. Extreme Behaviors of Victims of Child Abuse

Compulsively neat and meticulously clean, or destructive and extremely messy

Very polite, compliant, or very noncompliant and belligerent

Overly obedient, willing to do anything to please, or overly controlling, resistant

Socially very polite, kind, overly generous, or egocentric, revengeful, self-centered, antisocial behavior

Passive, or openly hostile and angry

Indiscriminately friendly, "shows affection" to or hugs anyone, or cold, indifferent, avoids peers, family, strangers

Overly obedient, helpful, "loving," or extremely disagreeable, angry, "purposefully hurts others"

These children have no moderation in their behavior. One child can be at both extremes on the spectrum in different areas of behavior, but is more likely to be consistently on one end of the spectrum in all areas of development

Although many different professionals can observe behavioral indicators of emotional abuse, assessment for state involvement either by the protective services agency or the courts commonly requires that the case records include assessment by a licensed psychologist (Furnell, 1986; Garbarino, 1978; Yates, 1982). The multidisciplinary assessment of child maltreatment involves a psychologist who has specialized training in administering developmental tests to evaluate (1) the child's cognitive developmental level, (2) the child's personality characteristics, and (3) the quality of the parent-child interaction. Most commonly used instruments for personality assessment include Minnesota Multiphasic Personality Inventory (MMPI), Rorschach test, Thematic Apperception Test, and Draw-a-Person Test. A variety of instruments can be used for assessing infant, child, and adolescent psychological maltreatment and parent-child interaction.

PARENTAL AND ENVIRONMENTAL INDICATORS

Most researchers and practitioners caution against overemphasis on identifying potential child abusers. Professionals, however, should be aware of parental behaviors and family dynamics that foster the child's behaviors indicating that emotional abuse could be occurring. Emotionally abusive parents as a group share some common characteristics (**Table 15-17**), although nonabusing parents can also have some of these same characteristics. Because parents have some of the identified characteristics does not mean that they are or will become abusing parents, but it denotes the potential for abuse.

PARENTS MALTREATED AS CHILDREN

Not all maltreated children grow up to maltreat their children. Parents who were maltreated as children, however, lack the role model of appropriate parenting and can suffer from lowered self-esteem, higher anxiety levels, and a more negative view of the world, all conditions that may have a negative impact on their child-rearing practices (Claussen & Crittenden, 1991; Caffo et al., 1982; Burgess & Conger, 1978; Straus & Kantor, 1987; Baily & Baily, 1983; Pemberton & Benady, 1973).

MENTAL ILLNESS AND CRIMINAL BEHAVIOR

Parents with a history of mental illness or criminal behavior, especially violent criminal behavior, should alert protective service workers and other professionals to the possibility of child maltreatment. Many individuals involved in criminal activity corrupt and/or terrorize their own children (Caffo et al., 1982; Burgess & Conger, 1978; Garbarino, 1977).

PARENT-CHILD INTERACTION PATTERNS

A recent study identified the following pattern of parent-child interaction that consistently appeared in emotional abuse cases:

1. Verbal communication between mother and child was virtually one-way, with the mother using words as commands rather than initiating or allowing dialogue.

2. The mother repeatedly gave confused messages to the child about what was wanted; contradictions sometimes occurred within seconds.

3. The mother carried out activities for the child (for example, putting clothes on a doll) at the child's instigation. This was done without involving the child in the task and consequently did not lead to play or the teaching of skills.

Table 15-16. Instruments Used to Assess Psychological Maltreatment and Child-Parent Interaction

Bayley Scales of Infant Development (Bayley, 1969)

Tennessee Self-Concept Scale (Fitts, 1965)

State-Trait Anxiety Inventory (Spielberger, 1971; Spielberger et al., 1970; Rohner et al., 1978)

Child Behavior Checklist (Achenbach, 1978; Achenbach & Edelbrock, 1979)

Child Assessment Schedule (Hodges, 1982)

Table 15-17. Characteristics Common to Emotionally Abusive Parents

Emotionally abused as children

Stressed

Lack of appropriate coping skills

Mental illness, e.g. schizophrenia, character disorder, depression

Angry

Hostile

Ambivalence toward parenthood

Few resources, financial, social, etc.

Inappropriate expectations of children

Lack of knowledge of normal child development

Marital problems

Lack of impulse control

Chemically abusive

4. The child was not involved in "doing things together with baby." The situation provided numerous (missed) opportunities for activities likely to provide environmental benefit for the child and also to facilitate interaction between the child and her younger brother (Furnell, 1986, p. 182).

Emotionally abusive parents, as all maltreating parents, have a negative view of their children and their children's behavior. This negative view of their children will be obvious to professionals working with the family. Some of the characteristic responses of abusive parents to their infants are listed in **Table 15-18**. The negative attitudes toward infants will persist as the child grows and develops if conditions remain the same. Professionals can observe similar parent-child interaction with children of any age. As compared to control groups of parents, the abusive parent sees the infant as purposefully acting in ways to "get even with" or "annoy" the parent (Hickox & Furnell, 1989). This may be due to the parent's lack of knowledge about child growth and development, as well as the parent's alexithymia and lack of trust of others.

Table 15-18. Characteristic Responses of Abusive Parent to Infant
Considered abortion or giving child up for adoption
Excessively irritated by baby's crying
Repulsed and irritated at having to change diapers
Describes the child in negative terms—ugly, deformed, makes repulsive sounds
Passive, unconcerned about child's needs
Disciplines—spanks, slaps, yells at—infant under 6 months for "bad" behaviors
Does not talk to the child
Tells others of disappointments with appearance, sex of infant
States that the infant does "things on purpose to irritate or to get even with parent(s)"
Not involved with child
Plays very little with child
Very concerned about how soon infant will have control of bowels and bladder
Calls the child derogatory names, e.g., little bastard, fart-head, freak

Table 15-19 summarizes the parental behaviors that may indicate emotional abuse (Baily & Baily, 1983; Giovannoni & Becerra, 1979; Rohner & Rohner, 1980; Burgess et al., 1990).

♦CONSEQUENCES OF EMOTIONAL ABUSE

Consequences of emotional abuse vary with the child's age and the level of development of self at the time the abuse occurs. **Table 15-20** lists some of the common consequences of emotional abuse. The consequences of the maltreatment will become evident by differing behaviors as the child progresses through different developmental stages. When emotional abuse is combined with sexual maltreatment, the psychopathology appears to be most evident prior to puberty. Disturbances in body functions as a result of maltreatment are most evident in children under the age of 4 years, whereas psychoneurotic conflicts mostly manifest during preadolescence. Behavior disorders and psychomotor delays appear at all ages (Martinez-Roig et al., 1983; Cerce et al., 1988; Hartman & Burgess, 1989).

Ignoring and rejecting a child's basic needs appears to result in children who are destructive, impulsive, low in ego control, passive, low in impulse control, less

> **Table 15-19. Summary of Parental Behaviors that Indicate Potential for Emotional Abuse**
>
> Seldom shows emotions; when present, emotions tend to be negative
>
> Routinely ignores or denies child's basic needs
>
> Belittles child or calls child derogatory names in public
>
> Consistently yells at child rather than talking in normal tone
>
> Isolates child from normal contact with peers and community
>
> Routinely ignores child behaving inappropriately
>
> Fails to define appropriate behavior for child; instead punishes
>
> Routinely verbally assaultive in public
>
> Consistently demonstrates inappropriate expectations from child
>
> Demonstrates a lack of basic knowledge of normal child development
>
> Demonstrates sadistic behavior toward child
>
> Threatens child with guns, knives, bondage, abandonment
>
> Routinely humiliates child in public or in front of peers
>
> Scapegoats the child
>
> Consistently demonstrates impulsive behavior
>
> Routinely places own needs before child's to child's detriment
>
> Consistently uses bizarre or frightening form of punishment
>
> Teaches child antisocial or criminal activity
>
> Knowingly allows child to engage in antisocial or criminal activity
>
> Sexualizes activities with child
>
> Consistently criticizes or calls child a "baby" when child behaves in age-appropriate manner
>
> Begins toilet training very early and harshly disciplines child for "accidents"
>
> Demonstrates jealous behavior toward child
>
> Has diminished capacity due to mental retardation, psychopathology, substance abuse
>
> Feels his or her life is out of control
>
> Has history of violent behavior
>
> Lives in poverty
>
> Describes self as "no good"
>
> Lacks parental warmth toward child

flexible, less creative, less persistent and those who avoid mothers. The young children lack the self-esteem and trust necessary to explore the environment or attend to cognitively oriented tasks (Egeland et al., 1983). Since individuals view themselves as they believe "significant others" view them, and parents are the most "significant others" of young children, rejected children view themselves as unworthy of love and inadequate as individuals. Negative self-esteem and negative self-adequacy lead children to be less tolerant of stress, less emotionally stable, emotionally insulated, more dependent (clingy, intensely possessive), more defensive, more emotionally detached, and more angry. Rejected children in all cultures view God, the gods, or whatever form the supernatural takes, as being malevolent. They believe that God is hostile and punitive and inflicts death, sickness, and misfortune (Rohner & Rohner, 1980).

Table 15-20. Consequences of Emotional Abuse
Psychiatric disorders—depression, character disorder, borderline personality disorder, multiple personality disorder, attention deficit
Self-destructive behaviors
Antisocial and delinquent behaviors, often violent
Increased vulnerability
Language delayed
Cognitive delayed
Fine and gross motor delayed
Decreased exploratory activity
Relationship problems
Low self-esteem
Negative view of self and others
Sleep disorders
Eating disorders
Maternal deprivation syndrome
Deprivation dwarfism
Nonorganic failure to thrive
Circulatory problems
Munchausen Syndrome by Proxy

INCREASED VULNERABILITY

Threats, trauma, or deprivation in a child's life increase vulnerability to other maltreatment. For instance, the emotionally deprived child is more vulnerable to negative experiences in day care than are children from enriched home environments (Gamble & Zigler, 1985). Children can overcome the experiences of physical assault or sexual abuse provided they have been nurtured and valued by psychologically supportive parents (Finkelhor, 1984).

EATING DISORDERS

Anorexia nervosa, bulimia, obesity, and other eating disorders in individuals at all ages are common consequences of emotional abuse. The food behaviors of an abuse victim can range from refusing to eat or holding food in the mouth but refusing to swallow, to gulping food down, scavenging, stealing, and hoarding. These children are enuretic and encopretic; loose stools are common. Victims of emotional abuse commonly attach more emotional than physical significance to food.

MUNCHAUSEN SYNDROME BY PROXY

Munchausen Syndrome by Proxy victims manifest psychologically impaired development. These infants fail to develop a basic sense of trust in infancy and therefore are developmentally impaired throughout life. The children develop eating disorders, become withdrawn or hyperactive, and develop oppositional behaviors. They are passive and tolerate medical procedures. The older children and adolescents grow to cooperate with their parents' deceptions and begin to fabricate their own history of symptoms. The child victims of Munchausen Syndrome by Proxy become Munchausen Syndrome patients. It is very difficult to stop this cycle of learned behavior because of the extreme denial and manipulation that occurs in both generations (McGuire & Feldman, 1989).

LANGUAGE DELAY

Most maltreated children demonstrate some degree of language delay. The more securely attached infants with better infant-mother attachment, however, consistently demonstrate better linguistic output and general language development (Cicchetti, 1989; Martinez-Roig et al., 1983).

DELAYED COGNITIVE FUNCTIONING

Maltreated children are to be delayed in their cognitive functioning. Children who have been verbally assaulted are less persistent in exploring their environment and have increased difficulty with problem solving and task completion. These skills are necessary in order for learning to occur (Egeland et al., 1983). The abusive environment appears to encourage the development of aggressive behavior as an adaptive coping strategy. Cognitive-affective imbalance in maltreated children can cause them to interpret ambiguous stimuli as being threatening and aggressive. Maltreated children are more likely than normal children to interpret behavior as aggressive and respond in a like manner. This results in difficulty when interacting with their peers. Perhaps this can explain why maltreated children have more negative expectations of interpersonal relations (Cicchetti, 1989).

ATTACHMENT DISORDERS

Bowlby (1977) believed that parental threats to abandon the child and commit suicide are forms of emotional abuse by rejection and would have pathogenic effects on the child's attachment mechanism. These pathological conditions can emerge as early as the preschool years and are manifested as childhood borderline disorders, attention deficit disorders, dissociative disorders, and childhood depression (American Psychiatric Association, 1987; Bemporad et al., 1982). Children of psychologically unavailable mothers, as compared to a control group of children 4 to 6 years old, were more aggressive, less involved with peers, unpopular

278

with peers, nervous, overactive, and lower overall in academic performance. Emotional abuse to children as a result of mothers being psychologically unavailable appears to impair both socioemotional and cognitive development of the children (Erickson et al., 1986). Interaction with their mothers was characterized by negativity, noncompliance, lack of affection, and a high degree of avoidance.

◆ SUMMARY

Following all types of emotional abuse, children experience impairment in all areas of development. The impairment can be minimized when the child is securely attached, when the abuse is not combined with other forms of maltreatment, and when the abuse is mild or over a short period of time. Howerver, in all cases, some impairment occurs in all areas of development. The child's self-esteem is lowered. The child enjoys life less and either becomes withdrawn and passive or aggressive and hostile. Cognitive and language ability are also delayed. Physically the child's growth and motor abilities may be delayed. Ritualistic or multiple-victim multiple-perpetrator abuse leaves the most profound impairment because it is systematically planned, is continuous, and involves multiple types of maltreatment including "brain-washing" of the child.

◆ BIBLIOGRAPHY

Achenbach, TM: The child behavior profiles. I: Boys aged 6-11, *J Consult Clin Psychol* 46:478-488, 1978.

Achenbach, TM, and Edelbrock, CS: The child behavior profiles. II: Boys aged 12-16 and girls aged 6-11 and 12-16, *J Consult Clin Psychol* 47:223-233, 1979.

American Psychiatric Association Committee on Nomenclature: *Diagnostic and Statistical Manual of Mental Disorders III (Revised)*, American Psychiatric Association, Washington, DC, 1987.

Baily, TF, and Baily, WH: *Operational Definitions of Child Emotional Maltreatment*, Maine Department of Human Services, Augusta, ME, 1983.

Balla, DA, and Zigler, E: Preinstitutional social deprivation, responsiveness to social reinforcement, and IQ change in institutionalized retarded individuals: A 6 year follow-up study, *Am J Ment Defic* 80:228-230, 1975.

Bayley, N: *Manual for the Bayley Scales of Infant Development*, Psychological Corporation, New York, 1969, pp. 201-210.

Bemporad, J, Smith, H, Hanson, C, and Cicchetti, D: Borderline syndromes in childhood: Criteria for diagnosis, *Am J Psychiatry* 139:596-602, 1982.

Bowlby, J: The making and breaking of affectional bonds, *Br J Psychiatry* 130:201-210, 1977.

Brothers, L: A biological perspective on empathy, *Am J Psychiatry* 146(1):10-19, 1989.

Bullard, DM, Glaser, HH, Hagarty, MC, and Pivchik, EC: Failure-to-thrive in the "neglected" child, *Am J Orthopsychiatry* 37(1):680-690, 1967.

Burgess, AW, Hartman, CR, and Kelly, SJ: Assessing child abuse: The TRIADS Checklist, *J Psychosoc Nurs* 28(4):7-14, 1990.

Burgess, R, and Conger, R: Family interaction in abusive, neglectful, and normal families, *Child Dev* 49:1163-1173, 1978.

Caffo, E, Guaraldi, GP, Magnani, G, and Tassi, R: Prevention of child abuse and neglect through early diagnosis and serious disturbances in the mother-child relationship in Italy, *Child Abuse Negl* 6(4)453-463, 1982.

Casanova, GM, Domanic, J, McCanne, TR, and Milner, JS: Physiological responses to non-child-related stressors in mothers at risk for child abuse, *Child Abuse Negl* 16(1):31-44, 1992.

Cerce, D, Rokouus, F, Diamond, D, Knight, R, and Prentky, R: Predicting criminal outcome from early developmental history. A paper presented at the National Symposium on Child Victimization, Anaheim, CA, April 27-30, 1988.

Cicchetti, D: How research on child maltreatment has informed the study of child development: Perspectives from developmental psycho pathology. In D Cicchetti and V Carlson, eds: *Child Maltreatment: Theory and Research on the Causes and Consequences of Child Abuse and Neglect*, Jossey-Bass Publishers, San Francisco, 1989.

Claussen, AH, and Crittenden, PM: Physical and psychological maltreatment: Relations among types of maltreatment, *Child Abuse Negl* 15(3):5-18, 1991.

Dean, D: Emotional abuse of children, *Child Today* 8(4):18-20, 1979.

Devereux, EC, Bronfenbrenner, U, and Suci, GJ: Patterns of parent behavior in the USA and the Federal Republic of Germany: A cross national comparison, *Int Soc Sci J* 14:488-506, 1962.

Egeland, B, Stroufe, A, and Erickson, M: The developmental consequences of different patterns of maltreatment, *Child Abuse Negl* 7:459-469, 1983.

Elkind, D: *The Hurried Child: Growing Up Too Fast Too Soon*, Addison-Wesley Publishing Co, Reading, MA, 1982.

Erickson, MF, Egeland, B, and Pianta, R: Effects of maltreatment on the development of young children. In D Cicchetti and V Carlson, eds: *Child Maltreatment: Theory and Research on the Causes and Consequences of Child Abuse and Neglect*, Jossey-Bass Publishers, San Francisco, 1986.

Finkelhor, D: *Child Sexual Abuse*, Free Press, New York, 1984.

Fitts, WH: Manual: *Tennessee Self-Concept Scale*, Counselor Recording and Tests, Nashville, 1965.

Fontana, VJ: *Somewhere a Child is Crying: Maltreatment-Causes and Prevention*, Macmillan, New York, 1973.

Fortin, PJ, and Reed, SR: Diagnosing and responding to emotional abuse within the helping system, *Child Abuse Negl* 8:117-119, 1984.

Furnell, JRG: Emotional abuse of children: A psychologist's contribution to legal establishment, *Med Sci Law* 26(2):179-184, 1986.

Gamble, T, and Zigler, E: The effects of infant day-care, *The Network* 6(4):4, 1985.

Garbarino, J: The human ecology of child maltreatment, *J Marriage Fam* 39: 721-736, 1977.

Garbarino, J: The elusive 'crime' of emotional abuse, *Child Abuse Negl* 2:89-99, 1978.

Garbarino, J, Guttmann, E, and Seeley, JW: *The Psychologically Battered Child*, Jossey-Bass Publishers, San Francisco, 1986.

Gardner, LI: Deprivation dwarfism, *Sci Am* 227(1):76-82, 1972.

Gil, D: *Violence Against Children: Physical Child Abuse in the United States*, Harvard University Press, Cambridge, MA, 1970.

Giovannoni, JM, and Becerra, RM: *Defining Child Abuse*, Free Press, New York, 1979.

Green, A: Psychopathology of abused children, *J Am Acad Child Psychiatry* 17:92-103, 1978.

Harter, S, and Zigler, E: The assessment of effectance motivation in normal and retarded children, *Dev Psychol* 10:169-180, 1974.

Hartman, CR, and Burgess, AW: Sexual abuse of children. In D Cicchetti and V Carlson, eds: *Child Maltreatment: Theory and Research on the Causes and Consequences of Child Abuse and Neglect*, Jossey-Bass Publishers, San Francisco, 1989.

Helfer, RE, Schneider, CJ, and Hoffmeister, JK: *Report on Research on Using the Michigan Screening Profile of Parenting (MSPP): A 12-Year Study to Develop and Test a Predictive Questionnaire*, Office of Child Development, Department of Education, Washington, DC, 1978.

Hickox, A, and Furnell, JR: Psychosocial and background factors in emotional abuse of children, *Child Care Health Dev* 15(4):227-240, 1989.

Hodges, KK: The Child Assessment Schedule (CAS) diagnostic interview: A report on reliability and validity, *J Am Acad Child Psychiatry* 21:468-473, 1982.

James, B: The dissociatively disordered child, *The Advisor* 3(4):8-10, 1990.

Kelley, SJ: Ritualistic abuse of children: dynamics and impact, *Cult Studies J* 5(2):228-236, 1988.

Kempe, CH, and Kempe, R: *Child Abuse*, Harvard University Press, Cambridge, MA, 1978.

MacCarthy, D: Recognition of signs of emotional deprivation: A form of child abuse, *Child Abuse Negl* 3:423-428, 1979.

Martinez-Roig, A, Domingo-Salvany, F, Llorens-Terol, J, and Ibanez-Cacho, JM: Psychologic implications of the maltreated-child syndrome, *Child Abuse Negl* 7(3):261-263, 1983.

McGuire, TT, and Feldman, KW: Psychological morbidity of children subjected to Munchausen Syndrome by Proxy, *Pediatrics* 82(2):289-292, 1989.

Moos, RH: *Evaluating Correctional and Community Settings*, John Wiley and Sons, New York, 1975.

Newberger, CM, and Cook, S: Parental awareness and child abuse: A cognitive-developmental analysis of urban and rural samples, *Am J Orthopsychiatry* 53:512-524, 1983.

Newberger, CM, and Newberger, E: Prevention of child abuse: Theory, myth and practice, *J Prevent Psychiatry* 1:443-451, 1982.

Olson, DH, Russell, DH, and Sprenkle, CS: Circumplex model of marital and family system. VI: Theoretical update, *Fam Process* 22:69-83, 1979.

Pemberton, DA, and Benady, DR: Consciously rejected children, *Br J Psychiatry* 123:575-578, 1973.

Polanky, N, Chalmers, M, Butterweiser, E, and Williams, D: *Damaged Parents*, University of Chicago Press, Chicago, 1981.

Polanky, NA, Borgman, RD, and De Saix, C: *Roots of Futility*, Jossey-Bass Publishers, San Francisco, 1972.

Powell, GF, Brasel, JA, and Blizzard, RM: Emotional abuse deprivation and growth retardation simulating idiopathic hypopituitarism, *N Engl J Med* 276(23):1271-1278, 1967.

Rohner, RP: Worldwide test of parental acceptance-rejection theory: An overview, *Beh Sci Res* 15:1-21, 1980.

Rohner, RP, and Rohner, EC: Antecedents and consequences of parental rejection: A theory of emotional abuse, *Child Abuse Negl* 4(3):189-198, 1980.

Rohner, RH, Saavedra, JM, and Granum, EO: *Development and Validation of the Personality Assessment Questionnaire*: Test Manual , ERIC Clearinghouse on Counseling and Personnel Services, Ann Arbor, MI, 1978.

Sackette, GP: Monkeys reared in isolation with pictures of visual input: Evidence for an innate reasoning, 5(4):1468-1473, 1966.

Schaefer, ES: Children's reports of parental behavior: An inventory, *Child Dev* 36(2):412-424, 1965.

Schwartz, JC, and Zuroff, DC: Family structure and depression in female college students: Effects of parental conflict, decision making power, and inconsistency of love, *J Abnorm Psychol* 88:398-406, 1979.

Snow, B, and Sorensen, T: Ritualistic child abuse in a neighborhood setting, *J Interpersonal Violence* 5(4):474-487, 1990.

Spielberger, CD: Trait-state anxiety and motor behavior, *J Motor Beh* 3:265-279, 1971.

Spielberger, CD, Gorsuch, RL, and Wishene, RE: *The Trait Anxiety Inventory*, Consulting Psychologists' Press, Palo Alto, CA, 1970.

Spitz, RA: Hospitalism: An inquiry into the genesis of psychiatric conditions in early childhood, *Psychoanal Study Child* 1:53-74, 1945.

Spitz, RA: Hospitalism: A follow-up report, *Psychoanal Study Child* 2:113-117, 1946.

Straus, MA, and Kantor, GK: Stress and child abuse. In RE Helfer and RS Kempe, eds: *The Battered Child*, ed 4, University of Chicago Press, Chicago, 1987.

Trowell, J: Emotional abuse of children, *Home Visito*r 56(7):252-255, 1983.

Vissing, YM, Straus, MA, Gelles, RJ, and Harrop, JW: Verbal aggression by parents and psychosocial problems of children, *Child Abuse Negl* 15(3)223-238, 1991.

Watkins, HD, and Bradbard, MR: Child maltreatment: An overview with suggestions for intervention and research, *Fam Relations* 31:323-333, 1982.

Yates, A: Legal issues in psychological abuse of children, *Clin Pediatr* 21(10)587-590, 1982.

Young, WC, Sachs, RC, Bruan, BG, and Watkins, RT: Patients reporting ritual abuse in childhood: A clinical syndrome. Report of 37 cases, *Child Abuse Negl* 15(3):181-189, 1991.

Zigler, E, and Hall, NW: Child abuse in America. In D Cicchetti and V Carlson, eds: *Child Maltreatment: Theory and Research on the Causes and Consequences of Child Abuse and Neglect*, Jossey-Bass, San Fransicisco, 1989.

Appendix: Instruments for Assessing Characteristics of the Maltreating Family and Parents and the Maltreated Child

	Instrument	Purpose	Theoretical Basis	Examples of What Is Measured	Filled Out By
Family Context	Family Environment Scale	Assess social climate in family	Ecological approach to human systems	Interpersonal relationships Personal growth Family structure	Each family member
	Family Adaptability and Cohesion Scale	Assess family's level of cohesion and adaptability	Systems framework of family relationships	Emotional bonds Sharing Roles Feedback	Each family member
	Interparental Conflict and Influence Scales	Assess content and frequency of arguments, relative power in decision making	Parental conflict and decision-making power	Finance Spouse characteristics Child-rearing practices Joint family activities	Each family member
Parental Factors and Parent-Child Interactions	Parental Acceptance-Rejection Questionnaire	Assess degree of parental acceptance or rejection	Parental acceptance-rejection theory	Warmth/affection Hostility Indifference Undifferentiated rejection	Each family member
	Children's Reports of Parental Behavior Inventory	Assess degree of parental love/hostility, autonomy/control, firm control/lax control	Relation of child's adjustment level to perception of parents	Sharing Affection Ignoring Intrusiveness Strictness	Each family member; mainly the child
	Bronfenbrenner's Parental Behavior Questionnaire	Assess parental loving, punishing, demanding	Relation of child's adjustment level to perception of parents	Nurturance Companionship Power Indulgence	Each family member; mainly the child
	Michigan Screening Profile of Parenting	Assess degree of existing maltreatment and predict further maltreatment	Child maltreatment is related to parental maltreatment as a child	Relationship with parents Expectations of children Coping skills	Parents
	Maternal Characteristics Scale	Assess how mother's personality affects maternal competence	Polansky's studies of neglectful mothers	Apathy-futility Childlike impulsivity	Practitioner
	Childhood Level of Living Scale	Assess quality of mother's child-rearing practices	Polansky's studies of neglectful mothers	Physical care of child Emotional-cognitive care of child	Practitioner
Children's Behavior and Personality	Bayley Scales of Infant Development	Assess infant's development of motor, mental, and social skills	Infant development and the interrelatedness of motor, mental, and social abilities	Verbal communication Coordination of muscles Tendency to approach stimulation	Trained practitioner, rating the child
	Tennessee Self-Concept Scale	Assess self-concept, self-acceptance, perception of own behavior	Theories of self-concept as influence on behavioral patterns	Self-criticism Positive self-perception Integrity across topics	Each family member; mainly the child
	State-Trait Anxiety Inventory	Assess extent to which child is tensed overall and at specific situations	State and trait theory of anxiety	Calmness Unhappiness Worry Fright	Each family member; mainly the child
	Personality Assessment Questionnaire	Assess personality and behavioral dispositions	Rohner's acceptance-rejection theory	Hostility Dependence Self-esteem Emotional stability	Each family member
	Child Behavior Checklist	Evaluate behavioral problems and competencies of child	General classifications of behavior problems	Participation in sports or activities Membership in organizations Grades in school Somatic complaints Hyperactivity	Each family member
	Child Assessment Schedule	Assess child's personality and personality disorders	Standard psychiatric diagnostic criteria and general classifications of behavior problems	Fears Moods Thought disorders Self-understanding	Practitioner

Garbarino, J., Guttmann, E. and Seeley, J.W. (1986). Assessing the Causes and Effects of Maltreatment, in The Psychologically Battered Child: Strategies for Identification, Assessment, and Intervention. 101-102. San Francisco: Jossey-Bass.

THE CYCLE OF ABUSE

JAMES J. WILLIAMS, M.D.

Relatively scant societal attention and resources have been directed to the study of human violence. While societal awareness of interpersonal violence has been raised by various groups who have come forward and identified it in their own lives, children are largely a silent group. To this list of sufferers must be added children who are themselves abusers. Our ideas about human violence are flawed when they ignore child maltreatment and its links to human violence. Abusive children have probably always existed, and they are a manifestation of a number of tragic circumstances. Family violence and neglect should be among the most preventable of situations. This chapter will deal with that particular cause, describing the cycle of abuse.

◆ FAMILY VIOLENCE

Family violence is not entirely mysterious. To a large degree, it is predictable and understandable. When unchecked, its costs reach far beyond the tragedy of individual families. To the immediate costs of therapy are added the social costs of school failure, substance abuse, impaired parenting, psychiatric hospitalization, and criminal violence. These costs are more substantial for the victims but ultimately affect us all. Child protection has always varied with the value society has placed on the lives of its children. Successful intervention first requires recognition that abusive children exist and then a social commitment to respond to their suffering.

Though victims of family violence now receive increased public attention, the medical, legal, and social professions are still largely unaware of children who abuse other children. Revelations that children are battered or denied the necessities of life evoke contradictory and complex mixtures of denial and horror, disgust and fascination from the professions, media, and the public. It is even more incredible and unpleasant to contemplate that small children are the aggressors in situations of physical and sexual abuse. The response of the protective service system to young child perpetrators has been nearly nonexistent. The children remain essentially invisible, and society has great difficulty acknowledging them.

Historically, the widespread recognition of violence between family intimates is a modern phenomenon. Certain family functions, such as how children are disciplined and how spouses react to anger and frustration, have been addressed in western societies, exposing problems that have probably always existed. Paradoxically, the increased recognition has come in the same social context that minimizes spouse abuse. Child abuse exploded into public awareness in the 1960s (Caffey, 1946; Silverman, 1953; Kempe et al., 1962) and was championed by the child protection movement. In the 1970s, society became more aware of spouse abuse (e.g., Martin, 1976). Apart from the obvious physical differences between the sexes, social inequality explains why women and children remain the most vulnerable targets for men in family violence. Women and children continue to be viewed as *owned* by the male head of the household.

Sexual abuse was brought into the open as incest survivors told their stories of unacknowledged pain. With the additional recognition of elder abuse, violence is now seen to span the generations, making the family itself the center of concern. Despite the progress in recognizing these problems, major concerns remain. We need to consider the violence instigated by children as a marker for assessing family violence. Ignoring the violence impedes efforts to protect children and to understand family functioning.

The home retains its aura of privacy for citizens in our society, making well-designed studies of family violence difficult to pursue. Yet the home is where aggressive interactions begin.

Reliable information on the levels of violence by children is particularly difficult to find. Nationwide surveys suggest that several factors allow this violence to be overlooked (Straus et al., 1980). Many parents in the survey by Steinmetz (1977) exhibited poor recall of their children's violence. When social norms minimize rivalry and sibling abuse, parents often regard sibling conflicts as a routine part of family relations, not as particularly violent. Many parents expect their children to engage in minor acts of violence as an inevitable part of growing up, and only intervene to discourage more serious conflicts. Parents may believe that rivalry and aggression prepare the child for the competitive world outside the home and enhance self-image and social competence (Stark & McEvoy, 1970; Bank & Kahn, 1982).

Corporal punishment is another overlooked factor in children's violence. Parents who strongly believe in the utility of corporal punishment often do not recognize their children's violence as such or tend to dismiss it as normal and routine. In homes characterized by spouse abuse and high levels of corporal punishment, young males may receive a double message that their bodies are not safe from stronger males' violence and that it is part of their identity to be aggressive toward more vulnerable family members.

♦ PHYSICALLY ABUSIVE CHILDREN

Despite the limited literature on abusive children, research has shown that they have a common background of family violence and/or neglect. Many have experienced coercive parenting, witnessed spouse abuse, suffered severe abuse or neglect, or seen other family members being abused or neglected.

At the core of child maltreatment is a breakdown in the parent-child interaction (Dietrich et al., 1983). Parents may promote childhood antisocial behavior through poor monitoring of the child's activities; little or no parental empathy with the child; and harsh and inconsistent discipline (Bahr, 1979; Patterson et al.,

1989). No variable alone can be traced to the development of abusive behavior, but each factor influences the course of the parent-child relationship (Belsky, 1980), which the child considers as normative in applying to interactions with other people.

Victimization is a leading pathway to human violence. The child's experiences may develop into a persistent and dynamic state of post-traumatic pain, which is central to the pursuit of aggressive behaviors. This is internalized "victimization." The rules of violence learned by the victim become crucial to the perpetuation of violence from one generation to the next (**Table 16-1**). At the time of the abuse, confusion, fear, anger, and sometimes arousal are too intense for the child to feel safely. Victimization becomes a part of the child's self-image. To survive the repeated episodes of abuse, the child gives up any expression of distress and learns how not to feel. The child learns to alter thoughts and feelings about the abuse (Rieker & Carmen, 1986) and to accept the judgment of care providers concerning the experience of abuse. "My mother told me that nothing was really happening," one incest victim said, "so I remembered that my older brother teased me but I forgot the terrible things he did to me." Other survivors minimize the abuse they experienced. "My father hit me a few times, but I deserved it," a physical abuse victim said, "and I'm grateful that I was never allowed to get away with being bad." The thought patterns of the child survivor remain stable and firmly embedded in the personality long after the abuse has ceased.

Brutalized by experiences with family members, the severely abused child incorporates these personal interactions into a deranged schema of the self and the world. An adult who learned as a child to blame herself for abusive treatment said, "Even after years of therapy, there's a part of me that still blames myself for what happened." This forgetfulness or blocking of the events, denial of one's true feelings, and acceptance of the intrusion of others' judgments is called "victimization."

With increasing repetition and severity of abuse, the child's emotional numbness develops into habitual cognitive and behavioral patterns that some have described as "soul murder" (Shengold, 1979). Harmful care providers are then reinterpreted, delusionally, as good. The delusions protect the child and allow him or her to survive the abuse and the loss of self-image. The delusion can persist and lead to destructive behaviors directed at self and others later. The family system perpetuates and reinforces the child's negative self-image, leading to possibly higher levels of violence.

Table 16-1. Social and Family Factors Involved with an Increased Likelihood of Child Abuse
History of abusive experience
Corporal punishment in the home
Being a witness to family violence
Lower educational status
Poor quality primary attachment with the parent
Poor parental supervision
Single parenthood and unwanted pregnancy

Other sources of family disruption:
    Spouse abuse
    Drug/alcohol addiction
    Child neglect

◆ DEFINITIONS
Like abuse by adults, which has been studied for more than a generation, there is no adequate definition of what constitutes abuse by children (Giovanni, 1989). Despite the lack of precision, child abuse has been addressed from various directions—medicine, law, education, social work, sociology, and research—which greatly contributes to its recognition and treatment (Newberger & Bourne, 1978).

◆ PREVALENCE AND EARLY STUDIES
The Biblical story of Cain slaying his brother Abel (Genesis, Chapter 4) has been cited as the earliest recorded instance of sibling abuse. Throughout the ages, many children have died as the result of adult brutality or neglect (Langer, 1973; DeMause, 1974; English, 1984; Radbill, 1987). However, little attention has yet been paid to sibling abuse. Many jurisdictions in the United States do not even recognize sibling abuse as grounds for an investigation.

Several national surveys illustrate the problem, showing that children have many opportunities to learn and practice aggressive behaviors within the privacy of the home. Straus and Gelles (Straus et al., 1980; Straus & Gelles, 1986) found that conflict between children is the most prevalent single form of family violence. While 80% of the children engaged in some form of violence against their siblings, more than 50% employed at least one act of "severe violence" during the year studied. Nearly 5% of the children had, at some time in their lives, used or threatened to use a knife or gun against a sibling. Additionally, 1% of the children were beaten by their parents and 1% of parents beat each other, but 16% of the children had beaten a sibling. Males were only slightly more violent than females. This retrospective study depended on parents' ability to recall information and thus is limited in its predictive power and description. The actual extent of violence may have been much greater if single-parent households had been included and the data gathered directly from the children themselves.

Developmentally, all but the most severe violence decreases as children age, but aggression by older children may be more purposeful and severe than that among younger children. Studies of primary school children found that conflicts occur most frequently when the only children in the home are male who are less than four years apart in age (Furman & Buhrmester, 1985). Despite the bias of retrospective studies, the high rate of sibling conflict leads to the conclusion that childhood aggression is learned within the family and may be a characteristic of *normal* children, not only those referred for behavior problems.

◆CHILD MALTREATMENT AND AGGRESSION

Various concepts in child development and psychology provide a background from which to review childhood aggression. Perspectives on human aggression range from biologically based psychoanalytic theory (Freud, 1920/1955), ethological theory (Lorenz, 1966), drive theory (Berkowitz, 1962), and ego psychology (Horney, 1950), to social learning theory (Bandura, 1973, 1978), attachment theory (Bowlby, 1969/1982), and social network theory (Lewis, 1982). Fundamental to most formulations is the conviction that a person's early experiences are foundational and become internalized to influence later life experiences.

ATTACHMENT

The attachment model of human development (Bowlby, 1969/1982) is particularly germane to this study, since failure to recognize behavioral cues and personal boundaries are commonly found in physically and sexually abusive persons. Humans depend strongly on social supports for continued growth and development, which begins with the initiation of an affective bond with a parent (Ainsworth et al., 1978). By the end of the first year of life, the child uses the parent as a base from which to explore the environment and to return during need; later, the parent is the child's base for developing social skills (Sroufe & Waters, 1977). Children who receive consistent and positive nurturing from the parent internalize these dimensions and will act similarly in future caregiving roles. During periods of stress and frustration, secure children can then remember empathetic attachment figures to regulate and label their emotional states (Matas et al., 1978; Bretherton et al., 1986). Conversely, research suggests that insecurely attached children have an impaired sense of self and are vulnerable to recurrent failure in relationships (Olweus, 1980; Egeland & Sroufe, 1981). Such a child may become an insecure adult parent who believes that the physical protection of his or her children is impossible. To protect this insecurity, the parent may prefer to withdraw from perceived threats rather than face them.

SOCIAL LEARNING

Learning by modeling the self on others is crucial in human development. The social learning concept posits a link between cognition and aggression (Bandura, 1978). The abuser's modeling, reinforcement, punishment, and threats mediate a great deal of what the child learns from maltreatment or neglect. Accordingly, children resort to violence after they have witnessed or experienced abuse or neglect and internalized its negative messages (Mischel, 1973; Parke & Slaby, 1983). A schema of retaliatory norms and strategies develops before they are able to reject what they have learned.

The basis for children's relationships is through attachment and interaction with the parent (Bowlby, 1969/1982) and later with persons they associate with who model and reinforce behaviors (Bandura, 1973). In a sense, sibling aggression reflects what children see parents doing or neglecting to do for them and what they see parents doing to each other. Children at a pre-operational level of cognition perceive aggression and punishment to be the same. Parents, who may seek to curtail misbehaviors by severe corporal punishment one time and by ignoring them at another time, only add to the child's confusion about when aggressive behavior may be proper. Parental inconsistency and intrusiveness have disorganizing effects on children. In an observational and prospective study, Jacobvitz and Sroufe (1987) found, for example, that inconsistent maternal styles made it difficult for children to internalize self-control. The aggressive child evokes punitive behavior from the parent who, in turn, elicits a negative and frustrated emotional state in the child, further contributing to his high level of assertiveness. The pathology in the parent-child relationship must be discovered long before the child begins to abuse other children.

Neglectful parents can be unaware of what is happening between siblings. Children have felt murderous rage at younger siblings who displace them in the mother's affections. Unable to grasp the permanence of death, children have even killed younger siblings. Neglectful parents tend to disbelieve their child when he or she complains of being hurt or dismiss it as sibling rivalry, saying in effect, "you must have deserved it." Parental interventions, even in severe situations, are often ineffectual or nonexistent if their attention is diverted, for example, by an unwanted pregnancy, mental illness, substance abuse, or spouse abuse. Parents can be immature, disinterested in raising children, or feel trapped in their current situation.

Modern family life presents a less protective environment for children than has been previously assumed. The changing composition of the American family, with increasing numbers of nonrelated children living in the same household, gives new meaning to sibling rivalry and child protection. The vulnerability of children is increased when the parents expect the child to take over some or all of the care of younger children in the home during the parent's absence. Tragic instances have occurred when children, acting as caregivers, are too immature to understand how to parent. The older children may refer to their own experiences of violence and engage in destructive behavior.

Children's attachments and modeling progress during school age into peer group relationships. These contribute to the child's learning about empathy and social cooperation (Lewis, 1982). Children in the third year of life typically begin to describe their negative feeling states through increasingly complex language. They are more and more able to discern another's inner psychological state concurrent with their maturing ability to read social cues (Eisenberg & Mussen, 1989). However, abusive children have an inadequate basis on which to develop empathy, since they have learned not to label and share their distress (Wheeler & Berliner,

1988). Instead, their distressing experiences have been kept out of conscious awareness. The victimization remains alive, however, possibly to erupt inexplicably in future situations of stress. Eventually, aggressive children's behaviors increase the likelihood of rejection by less aggressive peers, association with antisocial peers, and academic failure in school (Patterson et al., 1989).

Aggressiveness is a stable personality trait over time. Critical contributions to the development of empathy and interpersonal cooperation are not made in an environment of parental and peer rejection. Aggression becomes a more likely outcome. Rejected male children tend to try to lessen their painful feelings by identifying with the aggressor. As victims who have become victimizers, the children are even less able to express feeling for the victim's distress.

The commonsense belief that "violence breeds violence" has been used by professionals to explain the origins of child abuse. Child abuse and adult violence are said to form an intergenerational continuum. Child victims carry their inner- or outer-directed distress into relationships with other children and, as adults, into the lives of their own children. There is conceptual support for this in several studies. Steinmetz (1977) found striking parallels between the methods used by parents and those used by their children to resolve conflicts. Adults who resolve disputes by verbal or physical methods tend to use these methods in disciplining their children. Their children tend to use similar behaviors in relationships with siblings and peers. Straus et al. (1980) found that parents who were punished severely as children were more than twice as likely to be violent with their own children. Male gender, being poorly socialized, and coming from a physically punitive family are factors associated with a higher likelihood of child violent action after witnessing or experiencing victimization. Yet recent reviewers have found the violence breeds violence hypothesis to be limited in its predictive power. Possibly its conclusion has been overgeneralized from retrospective and uncontrolled data.

♦EFFECTS OF PHYSICAL ABUSE

The age and developmental level of the child at the time of the abuse have an important bearing on its lasting effects. The child's response is determined by how the experience is perceived (Finkelhor & Browne, 1985). Equally important is how the abuse affects family functioning and the parent-child interaction. Violent intrusions challenge the child's most basic assumptions about personal safety and the world as a predictable place. Emotional exploitation, the background of all child maltreatment and neglect, attacks the child's basic sense of self as lovable and worthy of care. Abuse at an early level of cognitive development is more likely to be internalized to mean that the child is *bad* (Piaget, 1965; Kohlberg, 1981), a feeling that is carried into future relationships. From current clinical research, severe maltreatment leads to impaired emotional development, poor social competence, and deviations in cognitive development and character formation (Dietrich et al., 1983). Gelles and Straus (1988) report that children from violent homes are more than twice as likely to experience personal troubles. These include having few friends, receiving failing grades in school, and engaging in aggressive fights with family members and persons outside the home. As they grow older, aggressive male children tend to report that their negative behaviors are often directed toward restoring a low self-image (Perry et al., 1986). As adolescents, severely abused children may be institutionalized for psychiatric illnesses or have antisocial, delinquent, or self-destructive behaviors. As adults, abuse victims are at risk for abusing their own children, being abused by others, or having emotional disorders, criminal records, and substance abuse problems.

The early case literature on abusive children reported only the most violent examples. A prior history of victimization and family disorganization were common denominators in most of the reports. The children were negativistic, lacked impulse control (Elmer, 1967), angry (Fontana, 1973), and exhibited overly hostile behavior (Morse et al., 1970). Some committed homicide (Bender, 1940; Adelson, 1972; Tooley, 1977). In their study, Easson and Steinhilber (1961) found confirmed or suggestive past histories of parental maltreatment in five of eight boys who had committed murder. Some were encouraged by their care provider to be violent (Easson & Steinhilber, 1961; Sargent, 1972; Tooley, 1975; Rosenthal & Doherty, 1984) or were identified as *dangerous* by the parent because they took the place of a hated ex-spouse or boyfriend (Rosenthal & Doherty, 1984). Other studies speculated that poor primary bonding and negative role modeling were factors in children's murderous assaults (Bender, 1953). Adelson's study (1972) of five children, all of whom were under 8 years of age at the time they committed homicide, postulated that many felt jealousy and rage at the infant sibling's presence in the home.

Later studies on maltreatment outcomes support the social learning and attachment perspectives on aggression. As violent behavior becomes accepted as "normal" by the victimized child, it is more available to him to employ against siblings and peers. When he gains greater physical strength, such violence is more readily available in confrontations with parents and other adults. The level of violence between children seems directly related to the amount of violence between their care providers. Straus et al. (1980), for example, found that severe sibling violence occurred in 100% of the 2,143 homes where parents frequently attacked each other and their children, compared to 20% of nonviolent homes.

Controlled empirical studies have increased our understanding of victimization's effects. Thus, abused infants, 14 months old, were more likely to turn away from their parent's attentions than controls (Wasserman et al., 1983). Abused toddlers, 1 to 3 years of age, avoided peers four times more often than controls. They hit peers, verbally or physically assaulted care providers, and were less likely to approach care providers in response to friendly gestures (George & Main, 1979) than nonabused children. Abused children, 4 years old, were more likely than controls to engage in aggressive behaviors with peers (Hoffman-Plotkin & Twentyman, 1984). Abused children, 6 to 7 years old, were more aggressive than controls in fantasy, free play, and the school environment (Reidy, 1977). Abused children, 5 to 12 years old, were more likely to depict themselves as sad, unpopular, poorly behaved, and outwardly aggressive toward others than nonabused controls (Kinard, 1980).

Available data concerning the effects on children who witness violent spouse abuse also suggest a similar development (Hershorn & Rosenbaum, 1985; Wolfe et al., 1985; Jaffe et al., 1990). This work consistently shows the lasting negative effects of domestic violence as evidenced by the emergence of increased aggression in children who witness such instances.

SELF-DESTRUCTIVENESS
Studies show that child abuse also leads to withdrawal and self-destructive behaviors. Martin and Beezley (1977) noted the development of these behaviors in 12 of the 50 abused children they studied. Carmen et al. (1984) and Mills et al. (1984) studied children who were both sexually and physically abused and noted that they were more likely to be physically harmful to themselves compared to subjects who were only physically abused. Hendin (1969) found a history of physical abuse in many case histories of suicidal black adults.

The Centrality of Violence

Prospective controlled studies have established the central place of violence and neglect in the maldevelopment of the child. Earlier studies were unable to predict which children who had been maltreated subsequently became abusive or violent. Prospective studies surpassed the earlier ones and developed baseline data on violent behavior in various demographic groups. Widom (1989a), in well-designed research on a group of 319 abused children, matched and controlled for age, sex, and race, found that maltreatment increased the risk of delinquency and subsequent violent criminal behavior by as much as 42% over controls.

Dodge et al. (1990), in a study of 309 children age 4 to kindergarten, concluded that early abuse increased the risk of developing deviantly aggressive behavior by nearly threefold. This increase was unexplained by the relative contributions made by poverty, divorce, marital violence, and the child's health and temperament. Abused children comprised 15% of the sample and were identified through interviews with mothers, visible bruises, and a medical history. Behaviors were assessed by teacher evaluations, peer ratings, and direct observation. Dodge's study has benefitted others by establishing a baseline rate for abuse in children who do not come to official attention.

Aggression develops at a cognitive-emotional as well as a behavioral level. Research has been interested in not only specific behaviors, but also in psychological processes that underlie, proceed, and follow aggression. Dodge and Somberg (1987), for example, found that young aggressive children, compared to their peers, have biased and deficient patterns of processing social cues. They overattribute hostile intent to their playmates, even when it is unwarranted, and they become less accurate in their attributions when they are under stress. They display far more aggression than they receive. Their bias leads peers to expect greater hostility from them. Given the series of inevitable negative interactions, their perceptions perpetuate a cycle of hostile attributions, aggressive behavior, school failure, and peer rejection.

Nevertheless, cognitive biases only partially explain the origin of aggressive behavior. It has been suggested that abused and aggressive children's deficits are conceptually similar to the inhibition deficit found in impulsive children (Dodge & Frame, 1982), who fail to inhibit inappropriate behaviors that are more readily available (Camp, 1977; Dodge & Neuman, 1981). Abused and aggressive children cannot only be cognitively delayed, but also develop along a deranged path resulting from early relationships and socialization.

◆Sexually Abusive Children

Sexually abusive prepubertal children have been greatly understudied and are poorly recognized in the constellation of family violence. Yet the increasing numbers of reports of severe outcomes of sexual assault have forced clinicians to reconsider the nature of sexual activity between children (e.g., Johnson, 1988, 1989). The position taken here is that children's abusive behaviors arise from severe prior sexual or physical victimization. Sexual abuse by children is the sexual expression of aggression, not the aggressive expression of sexuality. When these problem behaviors are present, they are among the few specific indicators that sexual abuse has occurred (Corwin, 1988; Friedrich et al., 1987; Friedrich & Luecke, 1988). Younger children who manifest extreme sexual aggression were likely to have been victimized in a preexisting abusive family context.

There are several reasons why sexual abuse by children has remained unnoticed. In western culture, sexuality is not usually ascribed to children. There is little empirical knowledge of what is typical sexual behavior between children despite clinical impressions by many that it is common. Society has assumed that sexually abusive behaviors are perpetrated by adults so that what occurs between children is often dismissed as "just a phase." When adolescent perpetrators were identified in high numbers in the 1980s (e.g., Scherzer & Lala, 1980; Ryan et al., 1987), clinicians came to realize that children may also be sexual abusers. Sexually abused children have similar adverse outcomes despite the age level of the perpetrator. Also, "sex play" has been misused as a cover for behaviors as diverse as "you show me yours and I'll show you mine" to forced oral, genital, or rectal penetration. Next, it has been assumed that sexual activity between children in the home is less serious than with contacts outside the home. Increasing numbers of sexual abuse have been reported in which biologically and nonbiologically related children living in the same home have been the identified perpetrators. The former distinction between inside and outside the home cannot be made a discriminator for abuse.

♦EXPERIMENTATION OR ABUSE?

The clinician is often called upon to distinguish between consensual sexual play of nonabused children and reenactment behavior of sexually abused children. Children's typical sexual behaviors are age, activity, and culturally dependent. Sexual behaviors may appear shortly after birth. Genital self-stimulation occurs in the first year of life as infants develop motor coordination and awareness of the penis or clitoris (Litt & Martin, 1981). By 3 years of age, most children have identified themselves as either boys or girls. Between 3 and 6 years of age, children become increasingly aware of anatomical genital differences, and genital play is common during this time (Rutter, 1971). Usually, the play involves age-mates in some degree of undressing and touching in games, such as "doctor" or "house." This has sometimes been misinterpreted as a sign of earlier sexual abuse. The current understanding, however, is that typical childhood behavior is mutual and noncoercive in nature and in keeping with the child's developmental level (**Table 16-2**). Simulated intercourse will sometimes occur after viewing overt sexuality in motion pictures or in the home. More invasive acts, such as penetration of the genitalia or rectum, with or without coercion, are not typical and require investigation. During latency, sexual exploration continues to increase, although more covertly, within the peer group. With the onset of puberty, peer and family-related exploration diminishes and interest in sexual roles and sexual identity is added to curiosity and pleasure in motivating sexual contacts. In doubtful cases, an interview with the child may be most helpful in distinguishing the motivation.

Table 16-2. Consequences of Sexual Abuse
Age-inappropriate sexual behavior
Adult sexual adjustment problems
Being at increased risk for sexual victimization
Sexually victimizing others
Physical aggressiveness
Acting out
Conduct disorders
Self-destructive behaviors
Marked anxiety, fear, withdrawal, depression
Guilt, low self-esteem
Overly compliant, anxious to please
Dissociative disorders, split personality

♦PREVALENCE

While the data on the prevalence of child sexual abuse by adults are sparce and unreliable, there are no data on the extent of child sexual offenders. Rates of child sexual victimization vary greatly in surveys. Finkelhor (1979) found that 9% of the men and 19% of the women, in a survey of 796 college students, had experienced either contact or noncontact sexual abuse during childhood. Fritz et al. (1981) found that 5% of the males and 8% of the females, in a sample of 952 students, had been sexually abused. Russell (1983, 1984) reported that 28% of 903 women had experienced some form of unwanted sexual contact before 14 years of age. Wyatt (1985) reported that 45% of the 248 women surveyed had experienced some form of sexually abusive contact. Kinsey et al. (1953), in the earliest U.S. estimate, found that 9% of 4,441 nonrandomly selected women had sexual contacts with an adult before the age of 14. Variations in the samples make the results difficult to compare, but the figures establish that sexual abuse occurs in the lives of many children.

Abusive sexual activity among siblings, cousins, and nonrelated children, who are age-mates, is considered to be common but is infrequently documented. In a sample of 831 abused children referred to a university hospital, De Jong (1989) found that 10% of the sexual abuse was by siblings or cousins, in which a majority described attempted vaginal or rectal penetration. Finkelhor's (1979, 1980b) student survey found that sibling incest occurred among 15% of the abused females and 10% of the abused males. Russell (1983) found that 2.5% of the women had been victimized by a sibling and that 15% of all incest was by siblings. Wyatt (1985) found that 3% of 248 randomly selected women reported sibling incest, or 12% of all incest. Cousin incest, which is at least as common as sibling incest, accounted for 15% (De Jong, 1989) to 28% (Finkelhor, 1979, 1984) of incest in various surveys. While most perpetrators in these surveys were adolescents, we have no idea of the frequency of incestuous sexual abuse by children under 12 years of age.

◆ THE IMPACT OF SEXUAL ABUSE

To understand children with sexual behavior problems, we must first try to conceptualize the negative impact of sexual abuse itself. Sexual victimization can be understood as a combination of posttraumatic stress responses and socially learned cognitive and behavioral adaptations.

TRAUMATIZING FAMILY PRECURSORS

Sexual abuse often results from complex, pathological family interactions. Children become involved in sexual activity for a variety of reasons. Many children acquiesce to the abuser's sexual advances because the love, care, and approval they need are otherwise lacking in their lives. Their care providers may be physically or emotionally absent, neglectful, distracted by other needs and/or substance abuse, or sexually punitive; they offer little protection to the child and may have a history of being victimized themselves.

TRAUMATIZING ABUSE

The impact of abuse varies with the child's perceptions of it as stigmatizing, sexualizing, and whether it is marked by powerlessness and betrayal (Finkelhor & Browne, 1985). Traumatic powerlessness occurs when the child perceives that his or her personal boundaries have been invaded and damaged. This can lead to severe posttraumatic pain and to later significant impairment of the ability to modulate aggressive behavior. Feeling in control of oneself is a foundational element of social development that is missing from the abused child's self-image. Male victims of abuse are more likely to turn outward in anger with antisocial and aggressive behaviors. They may define themselves as the abuser. "I wanted it," one male child victim said, "and I seduced him, not the other way around." Stigmatization is experienced when the child feels internally disfigured and shamed by the abuse. Betrayal is experienced when an emotionally significant person, on whom the child depended for his or her identity, care, and safety, is perceived to have caused harm. Traumatic sexualization occurs when the child's emotional growth is thwarted by the introduction of developmentally inappropriate behaviors. These factors result in an acceleration of sexual knowledge but at the cost of distorting the child's sense of intimate friendship. The victim can feel that the abuser owns his or her body. Male victims may become confused over sexual identity or attempt to master their pain by repeating the victimization on younger children (Finkelhor, 1981). Finkelhor's *traumagenesis model* explains the multiplicity of symptoms found in sexual abuse. It points out that more severe symptoms occur in situations (1) where the perpetrator is closely related or emotionally significant to the child, (2) where the abuse is repetitive or of long duration, (3) when physical force is used, (4) when the victim is older and can understand what happened, and (5) when the experience involves oral, genital, or rectal penetration.

TRAUMATIZING FAMILY RESPONSES

The coping abilities of the child and the family have a great influence on recovery. Greater damage occurs to the child who lives in a family environment that is itself abusive. Such families are characterized by exploitation, coerciveness, invasiveness of physical and emotional boundaries, and betrayal of trust. Care providers can engage in coercive sexual or physical behavior toward each other, the child, or others, and they often lack empathy and functional interpersonal skills. Maintaining family secrecy is central to this family's value system (Rush, 1980). It is not surprising, therefore, that if the child discloses abuse, his or her revelations are likely to be delayed, unconvincing, and often followed by their retraction and denial (Summit, 1983).

◆THE EFFECTS OF SEXUAL ABUSE

Children who sexually abuse other children are likely to have suffered prior sexual or physical victimization. Empirical studies find sexual abuse to be associated with a wide range of psychological and behavioral effects (Table 16-3). Some abused children are described as "wild" and "out of control," with their distress channeled outward into aggressiveness and inappropriate sexual activity. As with physical abuse, child sexual abuse victims are at risk for compulsive repetition of the abuse and loss of conscious memory of the trauma (Terr, 1988). Symptoms may also be directed inwardly and include somatic complaints, sleep problems, academic failure, running away, substance abuse, self-hatred, disturbed relationships with others, and inability to trust others and protect oneself. With severe victimization, self-destructive behaviors can occur (Wyatt & Powell, 1988). In studying the traumatic precursors of borderline personality, van der Kolk et al. (1988) found significant associations between child sexual abuse and later development of self-harm, particularly starving and cutting oneself.

Table 16-3. Criteria for Defining Sexual Abuse Between Children
Sexual contact between children may be considered inappropriate or abusive in the presence of any of these conditions:
1. Sexual activity between children who are not of a similar age (within 5 years) or developmental level.
2. Sexual activity that is not consistent with the developmental level of the child.
3. Sexual activity in which force or threats are used.
4. Sexual activity between children in which there is outside coercive influence from another, older individual.
5. Sexual activity that results in documented injury or predominantly negative feelings in the victim.

SEXUAL BEHAVIOR PROBLEMS

Researchers have attempted to distinguish sexually abused from nonsexually abused children based on problematic sexualized behaviors (Friedrich et al., 1987; Mannarino & Cohen, 1986; Mian et al., 1986; Corwin, 1988; Gale et al., 1988; Friedrich & Luecke, 1988; Kolko et al., 1988). It is not clear whether these behaviors represent reenactment of the victimization or premature and distorted activation of sexual capacities. Still, there are no reliably predictive profiles of who will become a sexual abuser. Not all sexually abused children will develop problem behaviors. However, it should be assumed that the abusive experience is so potentially toxic to developing sexuality that therapeutic measures should be taken accordingly.

SEXUALLY REACTIVE CHILDREN

Children with sexual behavior problems have been tentatively described as either sexually reactive or sexually aggressive (Friedrich, 1990). The sexually reactive child exhibits physically or sexually inappropriate behaviors reflecting the acute issues of recent abuse. The symptoms may result from confusion about self-boundaries. He may be a toddler, for example, who engages in increased masturbation, sexual exploration, exposure of genitals, sexualized play, or inviting others to become inappropriately sexually involved. These behaviors may have elements of aggressiveness but they are noncoercive in nature. Generally, they reflect a sexualization of activities only, and do not imply an underlying psychopathology. The frequency of these behaviors is not known because care providers may minimize them as transitory or "sex play."

SEXUALLY ABUSIVE CHILDREN

Other children are referred to therapy because of behaviors that far exceed those typical of sex play. These behaviors involve overt and often coercive sexual activity. The child's aggressiveness has been firmly entrenched for some time. It has been maintained by ongoing abuse, by caregivers who treat the child like a scapegoat, and by a neglectful family environment. Children whose sexual behavior is driven by anger, depression, and anxiety are often male and their history of sexual abuse is severe and prolonged. Typically, they have been victimized repeatedly, often by multiple perpetrators. Often they also have a preexisting physical abuse history. Less severe behavior problems, rejection by peers, and failure in school may occur before the sexually coercive behaviors toward other children become obvious.

The psychotherapeutic literature detailing the condition of these children is very sparse. Data come from case reports and small groups of children who are referred for treatment after their problem behavior problems were discovered. Feherenbach et al. (1986) report that 22% of the sample of youthful sex offenders were between 11 and 13 years old. Poor academic achievement, behavior problems, social isolation, and a background of sexual or physical abuse were common. In two studies, Johnson described 47 boys (1988) and 13 girls (1989), 4 to 13 years old, who overtly and coercively molested other children. Nearly half of the molested children were siblings. The behaviors included fondling and oral copulation with anal and/or vaginal penetration. Nearly 50% of the boys were victims of prior sexual abuse and 19% had been physically abused. All of the girls had been previously sexually abused, and 31% had been physically abused. A family history of substance abuse was also found in many cases.

The proportion of male to female sexually abusive children parallels that of adult sex abusers. Most of the reported offenders are boys. Girls, however, seem to suffer more abuse or neglect before becoming sexually abusive themselves. However, girls are less likely to follow the path toward abusing other children.

Friedrich and Luecke (1988) studied 16 sexually aggressive children (12 were males), 4 to 11 years old, and compared them to a group of sexually abused children who did not have problem behaviors. All the problem behavior children had prior sexual abuse of greater severity and duration than was found in earlier surveys (e.g., Finkelhor, 1979, 1984; Gomes-Schwartz et al., 1986). Most of the problem children were sexually preoccupied, and their behaviors paralleled their abuse experiences. All experienced oral, anal, or vaginal penetration, and many were also exposed to physical violence. In the study by Fehrenbach et al. (1986), in contrast, only 23% of the sexually offending children were involved in the sexual coercion of other children, but a majority were so involved in Friedrich's sample.

A high degree of personal and parental psychopathology, predating their abuse of other children, was found in Friedrich's group. All the children had a concurrent DSM-III (APA, 1980) diagnosis of a conduct or oppositional disorder, indicating extreme aggression. Their nonabusive parents had a high rate of depression and substance abuse and often covertly reinforced the children's aggressive behavior by labeling them as *bad*, categorizing them as being the same as offending adults. Family issues centered on inconsistent and neglectful parenting and lack of empathy.

♦ ABUSED-TO-ABUSER CYCLE

Research is leading clinicians to speculate on the possibility that there exists a cycle of violence for victims of physical and sexual abuse. Although limited in scope and predictive power, available studies suggest that sexual abuse in childhood appears to increase the risk for later sexual aggression, probably for the more severely traumatized children (Longo, 1982; Gaffney et al., 1984; Becker, 1988). The greater the trauma of the abuse, the more likely the experience will be deflected from awareness, perhaps to reappear as abusive activity in the future. Studies of sex offenders have revealed that many began their activities in mid-childhood after being sexually molested. Sexual abuse as a child and the later development of juvenile delinquency and/or adult criminality have been associated in several studies. Lewis et al. (1988), in a study of 14 juveniles condemned to death for murder in 1987, showed that 12 young people had been brutally physically abused and five had been severely sexually abused by relatives. Burgess et al. (1987), in a prospective study of 34 sexually abused boys, found an association between drug abuse, delinquency, and criminality six to eight years later. Boys who were physically and sexually abused, unsupported in disclosing the abuse, and socially rejected were more likely to become delinquent or criminal than boys from supportive families.

Information has also come from adolescent sex offenders. In a review of the literature, Peters et al. (1986) discovered prior child sexual abuse in 3% to 30% of male and in 8% to 38% of female offenders interviewed. Adolescent sex offender treatment programs have reported prior sexual abuse in 19% to 47% of their clients (Longo, 1982; Becker, 1988). Many adult sex offenders may have been sexually abused in adolescence even before puberty.

Although the limited research cannot reliably predict who will become abusive, there is ample evidence of the damaging influence of abuse. While little direct evidence exists for an intergenerational transmission of sexual abuse, the complex traumatic components of child maltreatment are clearly associated with the behavioral symptoms, especially the physical and sexual aggressiveness of abused children (Finkelhor & Browne, 1985; Dodge et al., 1990).

♦ FACTORS IN ALTERING THE CYCLE OF ABUSE

Maltreated or neglected children are not necessarily predestined to develop into sexually or physically offending adults. In 1987, Kaufman and Zigler reviewed the extant literature and estimated that the actual transmission rate of physical abuse was 30% to 50%. Subsequent reviews (Widom, 1988, 1989a,b) have generally supported this conclusion. Although 30% is six times the rate of abuse in the general population (Parke & Collmer, 1975; Gelles & Straus, 1988a,b), the implication is that most abused children escape at least the severe outcomes of the cycle and do not come to official attention.

Clinical research is not so naive as to attempt to prove direct causality in the cycle of violence. The child copes not only with the effects of victimization or witnessing family violence, but violence also results from the multiple family changes it sets in motion. These effects include (1) reduced maternal parenting effectiveness, (2) increased family dysfunction, and (3) increased (male) child aggressiveness as a result of modeling an abusive parent's behavior. As the child's efforts to cope with the violence place greater strain on the parents' relationship, a vicious cycle is set in motion. Similarly, mental health professionals' efforts at therapeutic interventions to correct a child's deviant aggressive behavior have often been undermined by continuing spouse abuse.

The relation between trauma and an aggressive outcome is not linear, for clinical experience has shown that variables serve to modify and buffer its impact. These variables have been found within individuals, the family, and the social environment. They include good cognitive abilities, absence of major psychopathology, and available nonabusing adults and peers.

A negative self-image, derived from early abusive relationships, is carried forward as the persistence of abusive behaviors in the abuse cycle unless it is interrupted. Children who are given a chance to make sense of their abuse with a nonabusing adult are less likely to repeat the patterns of victimization in their later lives. The same is true in abuse prevention for adults who have a high risk of abusing their children (Kempe, 1976; Olds et al., 1986; Olds & Kitzman, 1990). Egeland et al. (1988), in a controlled sample of 44 mothers who had been abused as children, found that those who did not maltreat or neglect their children had either a supportive adult available during childhood or extensive psychological counseling at some time in their lives. Parents who became abusive had neither. Therefore, the availability of alternate relationships is important in interrupting the cycle of abuse.

♦ TREATMENT PERSPECTIVES

The family's response to the physically or sexually aggressive child is critical for the success of treatment. Parent training in how to respond to the child's sexual behaviors and a peer support group may be all that is needed for the child who is reactive to abuse. Parents who deal in a consistent and caring manner with the recently molested child, who is acting with increased masturbation, for example, will go far in eliminating the behavior by helping him to understand the proper boundaries regarding touching. On the other hand, parents who view the child as a scapegoat or as *damaged goods* add to his or her trauma.

Sexually or physically abusive children present far greater challenges. Their behaviors are more firmly established than those who have been abused but do not act aggressively. Typically, their families possess few, if any, mitigating resources. While therapy may start with small and easily achievable goals, there are larger patterns of failure requiring attention, including parent training, social competence and peer relations, and academic performance. Both parents and child need intense behavioral, cognitive, and affective therapy (Azar & Siegel, 1990). Therapy must be based on such factors as the child's developmental age at the onset of the abuse, the age at which the child's aggressions began, the duration of the behaviors, and prior efforts at intervention. It is also necessary to evaluate all siblings for collateral abuse and their need for treatment.

Foster home placement, while sometimes necessary, is insufficient to treat the emotional damage of abusive children. In Reidy's study (1977), abused children in foster placement displayed as much physical aggression as abused children in their natural homes. Foster care was inadequate to reduce their level of aggression and problems at school.

Family system failure must also be addressed. The families of sexually aggressive children often have a long history of coercive interactions and inconsistent parenting. Their response to the child's aggressive behaviors has often been inappropriate or even encouraging. Greater assistance from local protective service agencies is needed to involve the parents in the treatment of their abusive children. Many are wary of or indifferent to professional involvement. Without an official agency's firm support, the parents often do not follow through and bring the child to treatment. Therapy will take a long period of time. Parents do not realize the length of the commitment nor do they have the energy or interest to invest in it.

Therapeutic intervention involves alternate adult and peer models of social interaction for the children and their parents. Integrating abused children into programs with normal peers and parents into support groups aids with more appropriate behavior models. Research is greatly needed in this area.

◆ BIBLIOGRAPHY

Abel, GG, Mittelman, MS, and Becker, JV: Sexual offenders: Results of assessment and recommendations for treatment. In MH Ben-Aron, SJ Hucker, and CD Webster, eds: *Clinical Criminology: Current Concepts*, M&M Graphics, Toronto, 1985, pp. 191-205.

Abramaovitch, R, Corter, C, and Landro, B: Sibling interaction in the home, *Child Dev* 50:997-1003, 1979.

Abramovitch, R, Corter, C, and Pepler, D: Observations of mixed-sex sibling dyads, *Child Dev* 51:1268-1271, 1980.

Abramovitch, R, Corter, C, Pepler, JF, and Stanhope, L: Sibling and peer interaction: A final follow-up and a comparison, *Child Dev* 57:217-229, 1986.

Adelson, L: The battering child, *JAMA* 222:159-161, 1972.

Ainsworth, MDS, Blehar, M, Waters, E, and Wall, S: *Patterns of Attachment: Observations in the Strange Situation at Home*, Erlbaum, Hillsdale, NY, 1978.

Azar, ST, and Siegel, BR: Behavioral treatment of child abuse: A developmental perspective, *Beh Mod* 14:279-300, 1990.

Bahr, SJ: Family determinants and effects of deviance. In WR Burr, R Hill, FI Nye, and IL Reiss, eds: *Contemporary Theories About the Family, Volume 1*, Free Press, New York, 1979, pp. 615-643.

Bandura, A: *Aggression: A Social Learning Analysis*, Prentice Hall, Englewood Cliffs, NJ, 1973.

Bandura, A: Social learning theory of aggression, *J Commun* 28:12-29, 1978.

Bank, SP, and Kahn, MD: *The Sibling Bond*, Basic Books, New York, 1982.

Bays, J: Substance abuse and child abuse: Impact of addiction on the child, *Pediatr Clin North Am* 37:881-904, 1990.

Becker, JV: The effects of child sexual abuse on adolescent sexual offenders. In GE Wyatt and GJ Powell, eds: *The Lasting Effects of Child Sexual Abuse*, Sage Publications, Newbury Park, CA, 1988, pp. 193-207.

Belsky, J: Child maltreatment: An ecological integration, *Am Psychol* 35:320-355, 1980.

Bender, L: Children and adolescents who kill, *J Crim Psychopathol* 1:297-322, 1940.

Bender, L: Children with homicidal aggression. In L Bender, ed: *Aggression, Hostility, and Anxiety in Children*, Charles C Thomas, Springfield, IL, 1953, pp. 91-115.

Bender, L: Children and adolescents who have killed, *Am J Psychiatry* 116:510-513, 1959.

Berkowitz, L: *Aggression: A Social Psychological Analysis*, McGraw-Hill, New York, 1962.

Black, R, and Mayer, J: Parents with special problems: Alcoholism and opiate addiction, *Child Abuse Negl* 4:45-54, 1980.

Blumberg, ML: Psychopathology of the abusing parent, *Am J Psychother* 28:21-29, 1974.

Bowlby, J: *Attachment and Loss: Volume 1. Attachment*, Basic Books, New York, 1969/1982.

Bowlby, J: *Attachment and Loss: Volume 3. Loss, Sadness, and Depression*, Basic Books, New York, 1980.

Bretherton, I, Fritz, J, Zahn-Waxler, C, and Ridgeway, D: Learning to talk about emotions: A functionalist perspective, *Child Dev* 57:530-548, 1986.

Burgess, AW, ed: *Child Pornography and Sex Rings*, Lexington Books, Lexington, MA, 1984.

Burgess, AW, Hartman, CR, and McCormack, A: Abused to abuser: Antecedents of socially deviant behavior, *Am J Psychiatry* 144:1431-1436, 1987.

Caffey, J: Multiple fractures in the long bones of infants suffering from chronic subdural hematoma, *AJR* 56:163-173, 1946.

Camp, B: Verbal mediation in young aggressive boys, *J Abnorm Psychol* 86:145-153, 1977.

Carmen, E, Reiker, PP, and Mills, T: Victims of violence and psychiatric illness, *Am J Psychiatry* 141:378-383, 1984.

Chasnoff, IJ, Burns, WJ, Schnoll, SH, Burns, SH, et al: Maternal-neonatal incest, *Am J Orthopsychiatry* 56:577-580, 1986.

Conte, JR, and Schuerman, JR: The effects of sexual abuse on children: A multidimensional view. In GE Wyatt and GJ Powell, eds: *Lasting Effects of Child Sexual Abuse*, Sage Publications, Newbury Park, CA, 1988, pp. 157-170.

Coons, PM, Bowman, ES, Pellow, TA, and Schneider, P: Post-traumatic aspects of the treatment of victims of sexual abuse and incest, *Psychiatr Clin North Am* 12:325-335, 1990.

Corwin, D: Early diagnosis of child sexual abuse: Diminishing the lasting effects. In GE Wyatt and GJ Powell, eds: *Lasting Effects of Child Sexual Abuse*, Sage Publications, Newbury Park, CA, 1988, pp. 251-269.

Curtis, GC: Violence breeds violence-perhaps? *Am J Psychiatry* 120:386-387, 1963.

Cummings, EM, Iannotti, RJ, and Zahn-Waxler, C: Aggression between peers in early childhood: Individual continuity and developmental change, *Child Dev* 60:887-895, 1989.

De Jong, AR: Sexual interactions among siblings and cousins: Experimentation or exploitation? *Child Abuse Negl* 13:271-279, 1989.

DeMause, L: *The History of Childhood*, Harper & Row, Publishers, New York, 1974.

Dietrich, KN, Starr, RH, and Wiesfeld, GE: Infant maltreatment: Caretaker-infant interaction and developmental consequences at differing levels of parenting failure, *Pediatrics* 72:532-540, 1983.

Dodge, KA, Bates, JE, and Pettit, GS: Mechanisms in the cycle of violence, *Science* 250:1678-1683, 1990.

Dodge, KA, and Frame, CL: Social cognitive biases and deficits in aggressive boys, *Child Dev* 53:620-635, 1982.

Dodge, KA, and Neuman, JP: Biased decision making processes in aggressive boys, *J Abnorm Psychol* 90:375-379, 1981.

Dodge, KA, and Somberg, DR: Hostile attributional biases among aggressive boys are exacerbated under conditions of threats to the self, *Child Dev* 58:213-224, 1987.

Dubowitz, H: Prevention of child maltreatment: What is known, *Pediatrics* 83:570-577, 1989.

Easson, WM, and Steinhilber, RM: Murderous aggression by children and adolescents, *Arch Gen Psychiatry* 4:27-35, 1961.

Egeland, B, Jacobvitz, D, and Sroufe, LA: Breaking the cycle of abuse, *Child Dev* 59:1080-1088, 1988.

Egeland, B, and Sroufe, LA: Attachment and early maltreatment, *Child Dev* 52:44-52, 1981.

Eisenberg, N, and Mussen, P: *The Roots of Prosocial Behavior in Children*, Cambridge University Press, Cambridge, 1989.

Elmer, E: *Children in Jeopardy*, University of Pittsburg Press, Pittsburg, PA, 1967.

English, PC: Pediatrics and the unwanted child in history: Foundling homes, disease, and the origins of foster care in New York City, 1860-1920, *Pediatrics* 73:699-711, 1984.

Famularo, R, Kinscherff, R, Fenton, T, and Bolduc, SM: Child maltreatment among runaway and delinquent children, *Clin Pediatr* 29:713-718, 1990.

Famularo, R, Stone, K, Barnum, R, and Wharton, R: Alcoholism and severe child maltreatment, *Am J Orthopsychiatry* 56:481-485, 1986.

Fehrenbach, PA, Smith, W, Monastersky, C, and Deisher, RW: Adolescent sexual offenders, *Am J Orthopsychiatry* 56:225-233, 1986.

Finkelhor, D: Psychological, cultural and family factors in incest and sexual abuse, *J Marriage Fam Counseling* 4:41-49, 1978.

Finkelhor, D: *Sexually Victimized Children*, Free Press, New York, 1979.

Finkelhor, D: Risk factors in the sexual victimization of children, *Child Abuse Negl* 4:265-273, 1980a.

Finkelhor, D: Sex among siblings: A survey of prevalence, variety, and effects, *Arch Sex Beh* 9:171-194, 1980b.

Finkelhor, D: The sexual abuse of boys, *Victimization* 6:76-84, 1981.

Finkelhor, D: *Child Sexual Abuse: New Theory and Research*, Free Press, New York, 1984.

Finkelhor, D: The trauma of child sexual abuse: Two models. In GE Wyatt and GJ Powell, eds: *The Lasting Effects of Child Sexual Abuse*, Sage Publications, Newbury Park, 1988, pp. 61-82.

Finkelhor, D, and Browne, A: The traumatic impact of child sexual abuse: A conceptualization, *Am J Orthopsychiatry* 55:530-541, 1985.

Finkelhor, D, Williams, L, and Burns, N: *Nursery Crimes: Sexual Abuse in Day Care*, Sage Publications, Newbury Park, CA, 1988.

Fisher, M: Adolescent adjustment after incest, *Sch Psychol Int* 4:217-222, 1983.

Fontana, V: *Somewhere a Child is Crying*, Macmillan, New York, 1973.

Freud, S: *Beyond the Pleasure Principle*, Volume 18 (Strachey, J, ed and translator), Hogarth, London, 1920/1955.

Friedrich, WN: Behavior problems in sexually abused children: An adaptational perspective. In GE Wyatt and GJ Powell, eds: *The Lasting Effects of Child Sexual Abuse*, Sage Publications, Newbury Park, CA, 1988, pp. 171-191.

Friedrich, WN: *Psychotherapy of Sexually Abused Children and Their Families*, WW Norton, New York, 1990.

Friedrich, WN, Beilke, RL, and Urquiza, AJ: Sexually abusive families: A behavioral comparison, *J Interpersonal Violence* 2:391-402, 1987.

Friedrich, WN, Beilke, RL, and Urquiza, AJ: Behavior problems in young sexually abused boys, *J Interpersonal Violence* 3:21-28, 1988.

Friedrich, WN, and Luecke, WJ: Young school-age sexually aggressive children, *Prof Psychol Res Pract* 19:155-164, 1988.

Friedrich, WN, Urquiza, A, and Beilkie, R: Behavior problems in sexually abused young children, *J Pediatr Psychol* 11:47-57, 1986.

Fritz, G, Stoll, K, and Wagner, A: A comparison of males and females who were sexually molested as children, *J Sex Marital Ther* 7:54-59, 1981.

Furman, W, and Buhrmester, D: Children's perceptions of the qualities of sibling relationships, *Child Dev* 56:448-461, 1985.

Gabarino, J: What kind of society permits child abuse? *Infant Ment Health J* 1:270-280, 1980.

Gabarino, J: An ecological approach to child maltreatment. In LH Pelton, ed: *The Social Context of Child Abuse and Neglect*, Human Sciences Press, New York, 1981, pp. 228-267.

Gaffney, GR, Laurie, SF, and Berlin, FS: Is there familial transmission of pedophilia? *J Nerv Ment Dis* 172:546-548, 1984.

Gale, J, Thompson, RJ, Moran, T, and Sack, WH: Sexual abuse in young children: Its clinical presentation and characteristic patterns, *Child Abuse Negl* 12:163-170, 1988.

Gelinas, D: The persisting negative effects of incest, *Psychiatry* 46:312-332, 1983.

Gelles, RJ: Violence in the family: A review of research in the seventies, *J Marriage Fam* 42:873-885, 1980.

Gelles, RJ, and Straus, MA: How violent are American families? In GT Hotaling, D Finkelhor, JT Kirkpatrick, and MA Straus, eds: *Family Abuse and Its Consequences*, Sage Publications, Newbury Park, CA, 1988a, pp. 14-36.

Gelles, RJ, and Straus, MA: *Intimate Violence*, Simon and Schuster, New York, 1988b.

George, C, and Main, M: Social interactions of young abused children: Approach, avoidance, and aggression, *Child Dev* 50:306-318, 1979.

Gil, D: *Violence Against Children: Physical Child Abuse in the United States*, Harvard University Press, Cambridge, MA, 1973.

Giovanni, J: Definitional issues in child maltreatment. In D Cicchetti and V Carlson, eds: *Child Maltreatment: Theory and Research on the Causes and Consequences of Child Abuse and Neglect*, Cambridge University Press, Cambridge, UK, 1989, pp. 3-37.

Gold, ER: Long-term effects of sexual victimization in childhood: An attributional approach, *J Consult Clin Psychol* 54:471-475, 1986.

Gomes-Schwartz, B, Horowitz, J, and Sauzier, M: Severity of emotional distress among sexually abused preschool, school age, and adolescent children, *Hosp Community Psychiatry* 36:503-508, 1986.

Hendin, H: Black suicide, *Arch Gen Psychiatry* 21:407-422, 1969.

Hershorn, M, and Rosenbaum, A: Children of marital violence: A closer look at the unintended victims, *Am J Orthopsychiatry* 55:260-266, 1985.

Hoffman-Plotkin, D, and Twentyman, C: A multimodal assessment of behavioral and cognitive deficits in abused and neglected preschoolers, *Child Dev* 55: 794-802, 1984.

Horney, K: *Neurosis and Human Growth*, WW Norton, New York, 1950.

Hotaling, G, and Sugarman, D: An analysis of risk markers in husband to wife violence: The current state of knowledge, *Violence Victims* 1:101-124, 1986.

Hunter, RS, and Kilstrom, N: Breaking the cycle in abusive families, *Am J Psychiatry* 136:1320-1322, 1979.

Jacobvitz, D, and Sroufe, LA: The early caregiver-child relationship and attention-deficit disorder with hyperactivity in kindergarten: A prospective study, *Child Dev* 58:1496-1504, 1987.

Jaffe, PG, Wolfe, DA, and Wilson, SK: *Children of Battered Women*, Sage Publications, Newbury Park, CA, 1990.

Johnson, TC: Child perpetrators: Children who molest other children: Preliminary findings, *Child Abuse Negl* 12:219-229, 1988.

Johnson, TC: Female child perpetrators: Children who molest other children, *Child Abuse Negl* 13:571-585, 1989.

Johnson, CF, and Showers, J: Injury variables in child abuse, *Child Abuse Negl* 9:205-215, 1985.

Kaplan, PJ, Waters, J, and White, G, et al: Toronto multi-agency research project: The abused and the abuser, *Child Abuse Negl* 8:343-351, 1984.

Kaufman, J, and Zigler, E: Do abused children become abusive parents? *Am J Orthopsychiatry* 57:186-192, 1987.

Kempe, CH: Approaches to preventing child abuse: The health visitor's concept, *Am J Dis Child* 130:941-947, 1976.

Kempe, CH, Silverman, FN, Steele, BF, Drogemueller, W, and Silver, HK: The battered child syndrome, *JAMA* 181:17-24, 1962.

Kinard, EM: Emotional development in physically abused children, *Am J Orthopsychiatry* 50:686-696, 1980.

Kinsey, AC, Pomeroy, WB, Martin, CE, and Gebhard, PH: *Sexual Behavior in the Human Female*, WB Saunders Co, Philadelphia, 1953.

Kohan, MJ, Pothier, P, and Norbeck, JS: Hospitalized children with history of sexual abuse: Incidence and care issues, *Am J Orthopsychiatry* 67:258-264, 1987.

Kohlberg, L: *The Philosophy of Moral Development, Volume 1*, Harper & Row, Publishers, San Francisco, 1981.

Kolko, DJ, Moser, TM, and Weldy, SR: Behavioral/emotional indicators of sexual abuse in child psychiatric inpatients: A controlled comparison with physical abuse, *Child Abuse Negl* 12:529-541, 1988.

Langer, WL: Infanticide: An historical survey, *History Child Q* 1:353-365, 1973.

Lewis, D, Pincus, J, Bard, B, et al: Neuropsychiatric, psychoeducational and family characteristics of 14 juveniles condemned to death in the United States, *Am J Psychiatry* 145:584-589, 1988.

Lewis, JO, Shanok, SS, Grant, M, and Ritvo, E: Homicidally aggressive young children: Neuropsychiatric and experiential correlates, *Am J Psychiatry* 140:148-153, 1983.

Lewis, M: The social networks systems model. In T Field, ed: *Review of Human Development*, Plenum Press, New York, 1982.

Litt, IF, and Martin, JA: Development of sexuality and its problems. In M Levine, WD Carey, AC Crocker, and RT Gross, eds: *Developmental-Behavioral Pediatrics*, WB Saunders, Philadelphia, 1981, pp. 633-649.

Longo, RE: Sexual learning and experiences among adolescent sexual offenders, *Int J Offender Ther Comparative Criminology* 26:235-241, 1982.

Lorenz, K (Wilson, MK, translator): *On Aggression*, Harcourt, Brace & World, New York, 1966.

Mannarino, AP, and Cohen, JA: A clinical-demographic study of sexually abused children, *Child Abuse Negl* 10:17-23, 1986.

Martin, D: *Battered Wives*, Simon and Schuster, New York, 1976.

Martin, HP, Beezley, P, Conway, E, and Kempe, CH: The development of abused children, *Adv Pediatr* 21:25-73, 1974.

Martin, HP, and Beezley, P: Behavioral observations in abused children, *Dev Med Child Neurol* 19:373-387, 1977.

Matas, L, Arend, R, and Sroufe, L: Continuity of adaptation in the second year: The relationship between the quality of attachment and later competence, *Child Dev* 49:547-556, 1978.

Mian, M, Wehrspann, W, Klanjner-Diamond, H, et al: Review of 125 children 6 years of age and under who were sexually abused, *Child Abuse Negl* 10:223-229, 1986.

Mills, T, Reiker, PP, and Carmen, E: Hospitalization experiences of victims of abuse, *Victimology* 9:436-449, 1984.

Mischel, W: Toward a cognitive social learning reconceptualization of personality, *Psychol Rev* 80:252-283, 1973.

Morse, C, Sahleer, O, and Friedman, S: A three-year follow-up study of abused and neglected children, *Am J Ment Defic* 79:327-330, 1981.

Morse, CW, Sahleer, OJZ, and Friedman, SB: A follow-up study of abused and neglected children, *Am J Dis Child* 120:439-446, 1970.

Murphy, S, Orkow, B, and Niola, RN: Prenatal prediction of child abuse and neglect: A prospective study, *Child Abuse Negl* 9:225-235, 1985.

Newberger, EH, and Bourne, R: The medicalization and legalization of child abuse, *Am J Orthopsychiatry* 48:593-607, 1978.

Nielsen, T: Sexual abuse of boys: Current perspectives, *Personnel Guidance J* 62:139-142, 1983.

Olds, DL, Henderson, CR, Chamberlin, R, and Tatelbaum, R: Preventing child abuse and neglect: A randomized trial of nurse home visitation, *Pediatrics* 78:65-78, 1986.

Olds, DL, and Kitzman, H: Can home visitation improve the health of women and children at environmental risk? *Pediatrics* 86:108-116, 1990.

Olweus, D: Familial and temperamental determinants of aggressive behavior in adolescent boys: A causal analysis, *Dev Psychol* 16:644-660, 1980.

Parke, R, and Collmer, C: Child abuse: An interdisciplinary analysis. In EM Hetherington, ed: *Review of Child Development Research*, Volume 5, University of Chicago Press, Chicago, 1975.

Parke, RD, and Slaby, RG: The development of aggression. In PH Mussen and EM Hetherington, eds: *Handbook of Child Psychology*, Volume IV, John Wiley and Sons, New York, 1983, pp. 547-641.

Patterson, GR: Performance models for antisocial boys, *Am Psychol* 41:432-444, 1986.

Patterson, GR, DeBarysche, BD, and Ramsey, E: A developmental perspective on antisocial behavior, *Am Psychol* 44:329-335, 1989.

Perry, DG, Perry, LC, and Rasmussen, P: Cognitive social learning mediators of aggression, *Child Dev* 57:700-711, 1986.

Peters, SD, Wyatt, GE, and Finkelhor, D: Prevalence. In D Finkelhor, ed: *A Sourcebook on Child Sexual Abuse*, Sage Publications, Newbury Park, CA, 1986, pp. 15-59.

Piaget, J: *The Moral Judgement of the Child*, Free Press, New York, 1965.

Radbill, SX: Children in a world of violence: A history of child abuse. In RE Helfer and RS Kempe, eds: *The Battered Child*, ed 4, University of Chicago Press, Chicago, 1987, pp. 3-22.

Reidy, TJ: The aggressive characteristics of abused and neglected children, *J Clin Psychol* 33:1140-1145, 1977.

Rieker, PP, and Carmen, E: The victim-to-patient process: the disconfirmation and transformation of abuse, *Am J Orthopsychiatry* 56:360-370, 1986.

Roscoe, B, Goodwin, MP, and Kennedy, D: Sibling violence and agonistic interactions experienced by early adolescents, *J Fam Violence* 2:121-137, 1987.

Rosenthal, PA, and Doherty, MB: Serious sibling abuse by preschool children, *J Am Acad Child Psychiatry* 23:186-190, 1984.

Rush, F: *The Best Kept Secret: Sexual Abuse of Children*, McGraw-Hill Book Co, New York, 1980.

Russell, DEH: The prevalence and incidence of intrafamilial and extrafamilial sexual abuse of female children, *Child Abuse Negl* 7:133-146, 1983.

Russell, DEH: *Sexual Exploitation*, Sage Publications, Newbury Park, CA, 1984.

Rutter, M: Normal psychosexual development, *J Child Psychol Psychiatry* 11: 259-283, 1971.

Ryan, G, Lane, S, Davis, J, and Isaac, C: Juvenile sexual offenders: Development and correction, *Child Abuse Negl* 11:385-395, 1987.

Sargent, DA: The lethal situation: Translation of the urge to kill from parent to child. In J Fawcett, ed: *Dynamics of Violence*, American Medical Association, Chicago, 1972, pp. 105-114.

Scherzer, LN, and Lala, P: Sexual offenses committed against children, *Clin Pediatr* 19:679-685, 1980.

Shengold, LL: Child abuse and deprivation: Soul murder, *J Am Psychoanal Assoc* 27:533-559, 1979.

Showers, J, and Johnson, CF: Child development, child health and child rearing knowledge among urban adolescents: Are they adequately prepared for the challenges of parenthood? *Health Educ* 16:37-41, 1985.

Silverman, FN: The roentgen manifestations of unrecognized skeletal trauma in infants, *AJR* 69:413-426, 1953.

Snow, B, and Sorenson, T: Ritualistic child abuse in a neighborhood setting, *J Interpersonal Violence* 5:474-487, 1990.

Sonsonnet-Hayden, H, Haley, G, Marraige, K, and Fine, S: Sexual abuse and psychopathology in hospitalized adolescents, *J Am Acad Child Adolescent Psychiatry* 26:753-757, 1987.

Spinetta, JJ, and Rigler, D: The child-abusing parent: A psychological review, *Psychol Bull* 77:296-304, 1972.

Sroufe, LA, and Waters, E: Attachment as an organizational construct, *Child Dev* 48:1184-1199, 1977.

Stark, R, and McEvoy, J, III: Middle class violence, *Psychol Today* 4:52-65, 1970.

Steinmetz, S: *The Cycle of Violence: Assertive, Aggressive, and Abusive Family Interaction*, Prager, New York, 1977.

Straus, MA: Ordinary violence, child abuse, and wife beating: What do they have in common? In D Finkelhor, RJ Gelles, GT Hotaling, and MA Straus: *The Dark Side of Families: Current Family Violence Research*, Sage Publications, Newbury Park, CA, 1983, pp. 213-234.

Straus, MA, Gelles, RJ, and Steinmetz, S: *Behind Closed Doors: Violence in the American Family*, Doubleday, Garden City, NY, 1980.

Straus, MA, and Gelles, RJ: Societal change and change in family violence from 1975 to 1985 as revealed by two national surveys, *J Marriage Fam* 48:465-479, 1986.

Summit, RC: The child sexual abuse accommodation syndrome, *Child Abuse Negl* 7:177-193, 1983.

Terr, L: What happens to early memories of trauma? *J Am Acad Child Adolescent Psychiatry* 1:96-104, 1988.

Tooley, KM: The small assassins: Clinical notes on a subgroup of murderous children, *J Am Acad Child Psychiatry* 14:306-318, 1975.

Tooley, KM: The young child as victim of sibling attack, *Soc Casework* 58:25-28, 1977.

van der Kolk, B, Herman, J, and Perry, J: Childhood trauma and self-destructive behavior in adulthood. Unpublished data. In B van der Kolk: Compulsion to repeat the trauma, *Psychiatr Clin North Am* 12:398-411, 1988.

Wasserman, GA, Green, A, and Allen, R: Going beyond abuse: Maladaptive patterns of interaction in abusing mother-infant pairs, *J Am Acad Child Psychiatry* 22:254, 1983.

Wheeler, JR, and Berliner, L: Treating the effects of sexual abuse on children. In GE Wyatt and GJ Powell: *Lasting Effects of Child Sexual Abuse*, Sage Publications, Newbury Park, CA, 1988, pp. 227-247.

Widom, CS: The intergenerational transmission of violence. In NA Weiner and ME Wolfgang, eds: *Pathways to Criminal Violence*, Sage Publications, Newbury Park, CA, 1988, pp. 137-201.

Widom, CS: The cycle of violence, *Science* 244:160-166, 1989a.

Widom, CS: Child abuse, neglect, and adult behavior: Research design and findings on criminality, violence, and child abuse, *Am J Orthopsychiatry* 59:355-367, 1989b.

Widom, CS: Does violence beget violence? A critical examination of the literature, *Psychol Bull* 106:3-28, 1989c.

Wolfe, DA, Jaffe, P, Wilson, SK, and Zak, L: Children of battered women: The relation of child behavior to family violence and maternal stress, *J Consult Clin Psychol* 53:657-665, 1985.

Wright, K: Sociocultural factors in child abuse. In BA Bass, GE Wyatt, and GJ Powell: *The Afro-American Family Assessment: Treatment and Research Issues*, Grune & Stratton, New York, 1982, pp. 237-261.

Wyatt, GE: The sexual abuse of Afro-American and white American women in childhood, *Child Abuse Negl* 9:507-519, 1985.

Wyatt, GE, and Powell, GJ, eds: *The Lasting Effects of Child Sexual Abuse*, Sage Publications, Newbury Park, CA, 1988.

Zuravain, SJ: Unplanned pregnancies, family planning problems and child maltreatment, *Fam Relations* 36:135-139, 1987.

REVIEW PROCESS

JAMES A. MONTELEONE, M.D.

An 18-month-old boy was admitted to the hospital from a small downstate community. The child was first seen with symptoms of abdominal discomfort, anorexia, and vomiting. A chest film revealed old, healed, fractured ribs. Liver enzymes were elevated, and CT scan of the abdomen revealed a lacerated liver. With the diagnosis of blunt trauma to the abdomen and child abuse, the case was reported to the Division of Family Services via the abuse hot line. Social Services found that the mother, a 21-year-old, was single and living with a paramour.

The Division of Family Services substantiated abuse. On recovery the child was sent home with the mother with the understanding that the paramour was no longer in the home.

Two weeks later, the Child Protection Team was called by the physician who had initially referred the child to the hospital. She had learned that, shortly after the child returned home, he was taken to a different emergency room. The mother stated she had found him motionless in his crib. He was pronounced dead at that hospital. The coroner/undertaker was out of town and the sheriff was called to see the child. He declared the cause of death crib death and the child was buried.

Despite requests by the Child Protection Team, the local physician, and medical examiner, the local authorities refused to exhume the body or to open a case.

♦THE DEATH REVIEW PROCESS

Society has a responsibility to protect those who cannot protect themselves, but it does not always do this. Research conducted by the National Committee for the Prevention of Child Abuse found that 25% to 50% of fatal child abuse victims had prior involvement with child protective services. The National Committee For the Prevention of Child Abuse (NCPCA) estimated that in 1991 1,383 children in the United States died from child abuse and neglect, or 2.15 per 100,000 children. This is almost four child fatalities per day. It has been estimated that an additional two deaths per day go undetected (Robinson & Stevens, 1992). In Missouri between 1983 and 1986, 334 children between birth and age four died as a result of injury (Ewigman & Kivlahan, 1990). Twenty percent of these children (68) died of inflicted injuries: 48% inflicted by their mothers, 24% by their fathers, and 16% by the mother's boyfriend. The perpetrator was unknown for 11 of the children. More than 30% of the children in this study died because they were exposed to hazards, 5% from neglect, and 3% from unrecognized hazards. The records were not adequate to determine the cause of death in 39% of the cases. Several explanations exist for inaccurate records: inadequate death scene investigations, failure to order autopsies, limited coordination among agencies, inconsistency in the quality of medical records, and a lack of personnel with specialized training in the area of suspicious child fatalities.

Ewigman and Kivlahan assert that fatal child abuse is a threat to the health and welfare of our children. National data show a rise in the number of reported child abuse and neglect fatalities. According to data collected by the National Center for the Prevention of Child Abuse, in 1989 child maltreatment-related fatalities increased by 5% over the number reported in 1988. Since 1985, reported child fatalities have increased by 57% nationwide. The number of overall reports of child abuse and neglect grew to almost 2.7 million in 1991, a 31% increase since 1985. This increase may represent an actual increase in the number of fatalities or a more accurate count of the problem. These figures represent the lowest estimate of the problem. A number of studies show that many child abuse and neglect fatalities are not reported.

Homicide is the leading cause of injury death for children under age 1. The National Center of Health Statistics reported that the homicide rate for children under 1 rose 55% between 1985 and 1988, climbing from 5.3 per 100,000 to 8.2 per 100,000.

In 1991 approximately 36% of the child fatality victims died from neglect and 64% due to physical abuse. The average age of the victim of fatal abuse was under 5 with 54% of them under age 1. The average age of the victim of non-fatal child abuse was seven years of age.

Victims of child abuse often fall through the cracks. Injuries are mistakenly declared accidental because they occur suddenly and are considered unpredictable and uncontrollable. But injuries do not just happen; they are caused, they are predictable, and they should be controllable.

Childhood deaths due to violence and unintentional injury occur more frequently in the United States than in any other industrialized country. Injuries due to motor vehicle accidents are the leading cause of death. Homicide is second, suicide is third, and drowning, fourth. Minorities are disproportionately affected in most categories, especially homicide.

For homicide victims, there are patterns with respect to perpetrators and methods. The usual perpetrator in the newborn period is the mother and the cause of death is frequently suffocation or drowning. For infants, a parent is usually the perpetrator and bodily force is most often the cause. For adolescents, strangers and occasional acquaintances are frequent perpetrators. Adolescents are killed by guns, knives, and cars.

Many states have adopted procedures to review child fatalities. The development of child fatality review teams is a positive step toward accurate identification and future prevention of such deaths. These teams, generally multidisciplinary and interagency, review child deaths to gain insight into the actual cause of the death and, more importantly, to suggest actions that need to be taken in the future to prevent such deaths.

In 1978 Los Angeles County formed the nation's first interagency child death review team involving criminal justice and health and human service professionals. By the end of 1992, 33 states had some form of death review team, at the state level, throughout the state in counties or cities, or only in limited local areas. The number of review teams in a state is usually determined by whether such teams are statutorily mandated. In California, there is no California statute mandating review teams— it is up to each individual county to form a team. In Georgia and Missouri, laws were passed that mandate a team in each county, in addition to a State board with oversight responsibility. Most review teams are not authorized by state statute. As of 1992 only eight states had passed statutes mandating child abuse death review teams.

Georgia provides for local child abuse review committees to evaluate medical examiners' reports regarding the death of any child and make their own investigations and reports regarding those deaths. Georgia requires a medical examiner's inquiry of all unexpected or unexplained deaths of children under 7. Georgia has also established a state-wide Fatality Review Panel to evaluate child death reports delivered by child abuse protocol committees and make its own report and recommendations. The committees, after reviewing details surrounding the fatalities, provide information and recommendations for policy changes to prevent future fatalities.

Several states have implemented or are considering new policies as a result of review committee findings and recommendations. Maine, because of the large number of children dying in neglectful families, has developed guidelines employing a broader definition of risk factors, with an emphasis on substance abuse. Connecticut, after a review committee report stressed the need for comprehensive, face-to-face investigations of all reports and a more critical evaluation of the child's extended family for placement, improved training for school, medical, and criminal justice personnel. New York responded by making efforts to better educate workers regarding substance abuse and domestic violence, among other areas, by including these topics in their child abuse training.

It is important to identify child abuse/neglect fatalities. Families in which these deaths occur often need services such as counseling and treatment, and the siblings in the home may be at risk of harm and need to be removed from the home. Also, criminal prosecution may be warranted.

The American Bar Association has stressed the need for accurate, systematic reviews of child deaths (Kaplan, 1992). *The reasons given are:*

1. We do not know the number of children who die each year and the accurate causes of their deaths.
2. We do not know the number of children who die each year from child abuse and neglect.
3. There is an underreporting of deaths from abuse and neglect in state vital records systems and there is a significant difference between the causes of death on children's death certificates and the causes of deaths indicated in police and child protective services records.
4. There are no nationwide accepted and used standards for child autopsies or death investigations.

5. In many states, child protective services have no involvement in a death suspected to result from child abuse or neglect unless there are surviving siblings. In other states, child protective services are not notified of the death even if there are surviving siblings.

6. Many states operate with a coroner system. Coroners are often elected officials who have no medical training or training in forensic pathology. Some medical examiners have no training in pathology or training in evaluating child deaths due to abuse or neglect.

◆STUDIES OF CHILDHOOD DEATHS AND CATASTROPHIC INJURIES

A number of states have conducted studies of childhood fatalities (see Bibliography at the end of the chapter). The author, because of his familiarity with the studies and procedures in his state and the availability of the results of these studies, has included some of the results of those studies. In the mid-1980s and early 1990s two studies of childhood fatalities and catastrophic injuries were conducted in Missouri. One study was done by the St. Louis Child Abuse Network and the other by Ewigman and Kivlahan.

The St. Louis Child Abuse Network study had two components. The first phase of the study reviewed the cases of 37 children who died or had catastrophic injuries believed to be due to abuse. The second phase of the study compared these children to two matched control groups—one of children with histories of mild abuse and one group with no history of abuse (Monteleone et al., 1988; Dodson et al., 1988).

The Ewigman and Kivlahan study reviewed death certificates of children who had died as the result of injury.

THE ST. LOUIS CHILD ABUSE NETWORK STUDY, PHASE ONE

In 1983 a group of child abuse professionals in St. Louis, represented by the state Division of Family Services, local juvenile court and law enforcement, and two pediatric hospitals, organized and initiated a review process to study severe child maltreatment in the area (referred to as the Board of Inquiry). The project was entitled the *St. Louis Board of Inquiry to Investigate Fatal and Catastrophic Injuries Due to Child Abuse and Neglect.* The purpose of the Board's review was to determine how to prevent severe child maltreatment. This study is particularly significant because it is one of few, if any, studies comparing abusive families with matched nonabusive families.

BACKGROUND STATISTICS

The association between child abuse and neglect and violent crime as reported in the literature was verified by the crime statistics in St. Louis in the years before the study; these trends were confirmed over time. Reports show that 3.5% of Missouri's children have been reported as abused or neglected. Fifteen percent of these abuse reports originated in the St. Louis metropolitan area. Approximately 2.5% of the state's children receive services related to abuse and neglect. Deaths caused by abuse and neglect are estimated at more than 30 per year statewide. Over a three-year period before the study, the number of deaths resulting from maltreatment known through St. Louis Children's Hospital ranged from four to 11 per year and totaled 22. Severe maltreatment with permanent intellectual handicaps occurred in at least 15 cases. The statistics concerning abused children seen at the second hospital, Cardinal Glennon Children's Hospital, were similar.

DATA SOURCE

The Board of Inquiry reviewed all available information about fatal or nearly fatal cases of child maltreatment available from Division of Family Services records and medical records, including the medical examiner's findings. They also heard testimony from case workers, hospital social service workers, and police.

CRITERIA FOR CASE REVIEW

The cases reviewed included all those in which children either died, had burns over 50% of their body surface, or had objective medical evidence of severe head injury as noted on skull X-ray or CT brain scan. In the St. Louis metropolitan area, all children with severe injuries of these types were known to personnel at the hospitals of the medical examiner's office.

APPROACH OF THE BOARD OF INQUIRY

When reviewing the cases, the Board of Inquiry asked several questions, which formed an outline of information to be collected for each case.

Specific judgments that the board tried to render included the following:

Was the case potentially preventable? If so, how?

Did the public and private agencies function as intended? If not, where did the malfunction occur?

In addition, the Board of Inquiry carefully examined family structures that contained paramours. It looked for evidence of other family violence and considered possible intervention for families that were isolated relative to community services in general and the child health delivery system specifically. The answers to all these questions were tabulated on summary forms and computerized for analysis and compilation of summary results.

The decision to include severe but nonfatal cases in the review process enhanced the project. There were no differences in demographic features between the survivors and those who died. However, by including the nonfatal cases, the Board of Inquiry was able to define the extreme morbidity in the injuries that would have been fatal except for medical intervention. This approach also provided a sample allowing statistically meaningful comparisons of severely abusive families as compared to other groups. The Board of Inquiry was able to determine the degree of handicap among the survivors. The degree of handicap information allowed one to project the long-term dollar costs for the future care of the handicapped victims. Furthermore, the participation of the hospitals allowed retrospective tabulation of the acute medical costs.

BOARD OF INQUIRY FINDINGS

Over a period of 18 months (October 1983 to May 1985), the Board of Inquiry reviewed 37 cases, the equivalent of one year's local experience. Four cases were judged not to be the result of abuse. Eleven were fatal cases and 22 nonfatal. The average age in the nonfatal cases was 10 months. The average age of the children who died was 1 year, 8 months. The major findings are summarized in **Table 17-1**.

The victims' ages, the type of abuse, and the injury are listed in **Table 17-2**. Whiplash shaking injuries were present in 8 children and were concentrated among the very young. These injuries were associated with a high incidence of permanent

Table 17-1. Board of Inquiry Summary of Findings

Summary of Case Results	
Number of cases reviewed	37
Judged nonabuse	4

Died	
	11/33
Average age	10 mos.
Recovered	1 yr, 8 mos.

Human Outcomes	
Death	11/33
Recovered	11/33
Permanent severe handicap	11/33

Children	
Incomplete immunizations	14/33
Lack of routine medical care	9/33
Prior medical problems	9/33
"Shaken infant" injury	8/33

Families	
Family violence	9/33
Substance abuse	8/33
Hostile to DFS worker	9/33
Known to DFS	16/33
Paramour	15/33

Acute Fiscal Outcomes	
Total acute costs	$550,000
Average survivor costs	$22,391

Future Costs	
Care for each impaired child	$2,000,000

Other Features	
Judged "preventable"	10/33
Perinatal risk factors	13/33

injury. The most frequent perpetrators were live-in boyfriends, who were involved in 14 cases and were perpetrators or co-perpetrators in 10 cases. These boyfriends were involved in five of the fatal cases and usually injured toddlers and older children. Although they had fathered children, none had been married. Mothers were perpetrators in four fatal cases, and biological fathers were perpetrators in two cases.

Table 17-2. Description of Abuse and Neglect Cases, Type of Maltreatment, and Injuries

Victim Age	Case Number	Type of Abuse	Type of Injury
0.12	35	N	Skull FX, Neglect, Lack of Supervision
0.15	5	A	Multiple Injuries/Strangulation
0.21	17	A	SIS
0.21	28	A	CNS/POSS SIS
0.23	26	A	CNS
0.24	6	A	SIS
0.25	37	N	CNS
0.31	9	A	WSIS & Broken Ribs
0.32	32	A	Head Injury/Skull FX
0.33	33	A	SIS, Beating/Shaking
0.35	20	A	Neglect/Hypoglycemia
0.41	2	N	Exposure/Pneumonia
0.45	6	A	SIS/Subdural
0.46	21	A	SIS/Subdurals
0.47	23	A	Head Injuries +
0.51	10	A	SIS, Shaking, Possible Strangulation
0.62	11	A	Malnutrition, Bilateral Subdural Hematomas
0.80	14	A	CNS/Multiple Injuries
1.05	29	A	CNS, New & Old Arm FX
1.25	24	A	Burns—Immersion
1.29	4	A	Spinal Cord, Multiple Bruises
1.34	15	A	Head Injury, Beating
1.41	27	A	Multiple Injuries
1.59	1	N	Drowning
1.72	19	A	Beating/Ruptured Duodenum
1.74	22	A	CNS/Liver
1.75	3	A	Skull FX, Meningitis, Multiple FX, Malnutrition
1.76	7	A	Multiple Injuries-Beating SIS-Plus
1.97	13	A	Trauma/Unilateral Skull FX
2.30	8	A	Beating/Ruptured Duodenum
2.52	25	A	CNS
4.71	30	A	CNS
5.66	12	A	Head Injury, Beating

(The four cases determined to be non-abusive are not listed)

Abbreviations: * A/N =Abuse or Neglect. In all other fields: Y = yes, N = no, X = not applicable, U = unknown, SIS = Shaken Infant Syndrome, CNS = Central nervous system injury, FX = fracture.*

In 18 cases the panel judged that the overall system had malfunctioned. Recommendations for change were made in 20 of the 33 abuse cases (**Table 17-3**).

Table 17-3. Recommendations
General
1. Education for prevention, parenting skills—coping mechanisms, discipline techniques, normal child behavior, toilet-training techniques, prevention of shaken infant syndrome, babysitter recommendations.
2. Delineate lay (non-mandated reporter) responsibility to report abuse. (3*)
Juvenile Court
1. Juvenile Courts should have participated in board of injury. (29)
2. More expeditious action by Juvenile Court in cases involving injured children. (9)
3. Change law regulating court agreements for custody. (25)
4. Juvenile Court investigation records should be available to DFS case workers responsible for family. (29)
5. Workers (DFS, MEDICAL) need clear understanding of Juvenile Court's requirements to protect children. (29)
6. Juvenile Court should be involved in cases with serious injuries, other than those cases in which the child is dead or dying. (29)
State Social Services
1. *Develop guidelines* for DFS workers to assess risk to child, other children in the household, and subsequent children when abuse has been substantiated. (29)
2. *Develop guidelines* for DFS workers dealing with families in which one of the parents is mentally ill. (29)
3. In those cases with mentally ill parent, worker should be given proper psychiatric diagnosis and evaluation of parent and his/her potential to do harm to the child. (29)
4. Cases should be kept open longer in those families known to have been severely abusive. (32)
5. DFS should perform computer check of *babysitter* in all cases in which a sitter is involved. (32)
6. When multiple workers are involved with a family, there should be *continuity of care* and a presented plan and assurance that the plan will be carried out after initial worker has changed. (33,34)
7. Adequate *respite care* should be provided. (33)
8. Workers should concentrate and emphasize parenting skills and coping mechanisms. (33,34)
9. DFS should stay involved longer after child is placed in foster care. (5)
10. Develop special foster care facilities for run-away, difficult adolescents. (37)
11. Adolescent mothers getting state funds for child support should be carefully supervised to assure that these funds are being spent as intended—for child support. (37)
Medical
1. Medical personnel should realize the necessity to report, to the hot line, fractures in infants that could not have been self-inflicted. (1)
2. Better tracking of medical neglect cases (missed appointments). (1,2)
3. Medical doctors need education to recognize abuse and willingness to report abuse. (8)
Police
1. Clarify and simplify jurisdiction problems involving police of different municipalities, cities, counties, etc. (28)
2. Better *coordination and cooperation* between police and DFS. (9)
* *The number in parentheses refers to the specific case as noted in Table 17-2.*

The high medical costs for care were also a major finding. The total acute hospital care costs were more than $550,000. The acute care costs among survivors averaged more than $22,000 each. For each child who died, approximately one child was permanently and severely disabled. In addition to the personal tragedies, these cases were also expensive. A lifetime of custodial care costs $2,000,000 per child. The ten disabled children found in this study will accrue $20,000,000 in future costs.

Eighteen of 33 cases were either judged preventable or had perinatal risk factors detectable by the High Risk Infant Follow-up Program of the St. Louis Regional Maternal and Child Health Council. In 1985 the network created a targeted prevention program, Project First Step, to link public health nurses who do high-risk newborn infant follow-up screening with social service case workers to help families deal with intense risk factors.

RISK FACTORS IDENTIFIED BY CASE STUDIES

Risk factors identified by the study included health care, housing, family structure, and family violence.

THE VICTIMS

Seven children had not received standard immunizations. Nine children had special medical problems before the injury. Among these, six had not received appropriate follow-up treatment. Eleven children had not received routine well baby care. In total, 12 children lacked either immunizations or routine well baby care. Growth was normal in 17 children, abnormal in three.

Only two of 33 victims were known to survive their injuries with no apparent physical sequelae, although the outcome was unknown in four. Twenty-one victims either died or suffered permanent severe neurological impairment, including mental retardation. Among these 21, the average age was 1.37 years, similar to the average age of the entire population, which was 1.17 years.

CRIMINALITY

In 14 of 33 families with severe abuse or neglect, at least one of the primarily involved adults had a criminal record. This is exclusive of any criminal proceedings that occurred after the severe injury.

PREVENTABILITY

The panel judged that 10 cases were preventable. Eighteen cases were either preventable or had perinatal risk factors that would have allowed early detection of risk. As already noted, recommendations were made for system change in 20 cases.

CONCLUSIONS

The conclusions drawn by the Board of Inquiry are as follows:

1. Severe child maltreatment is expensive.

2. Severe child maltreatment is concentrated among very young children.

3. A large proportion of cases have detectable risk factors and even more should be preventable.

4. Live-in boyfriends are especially dangerous to toddlers.

5. The large number of families with criminal backgrounds indicates that preventive programs should be directed at criminal populations.

6. There is approximately one permanently handicapped survivor for each child who dies. Half of the survivors are permanently disabled and lost from the ranks of productive citizenship.

7. A large proportion of cases involve perinatal risk factors that could facilitate early recognition of risk for severe maltreatment.

8. If even a small number of severe but nonfatal cases were prevented, a preventive program would be highly cost-effective.

9. *Prevention programs should be targeted toward:*
   Newborns and very young children
   Newborns with perinatal risk factors
   Infants who are not receiving medical care
   Infants who are not brought for follow-up medical treatments
   Families with live-in boyfriends
   Families with criminal records

THE ST. LOUIS CHILD ABUSE NETWORK STUDY, PHASE TWO

In addition to the first phase case review that was done by the Board of Inquiry, the second phase of the St. Louis Child Abuse Network Study was a case-control study of fatal versus mild versus nonabusive families.

APPROACH

The cases evaluated by the Board of Inquiry were subjected to further analysis. This consisted of having the investigating case worker complete a lengthy family assessment questionnaire. Because this data form was designed before the Board of Inquiry's review, the lessons learned in that review were not incorporated. It was, however, based on modifications of a comprehensive family assessment data form developed at Brandeis University and considered as a means of computerizing social service information by the Missouri Division of Family Services.

Control subjects were selected as follows. The Missouri Division of Vital Statistics provided a list of birth-date-matched and zip-code-matched children and addresses for cases substantiated as mild abuse cases plus similarly matched cases with no record of abuse. There were three groups for comparison: severe abuse, mild abuse, and no abuse.

Investigations were done by off-duty investigators. They completed the same family assessment questionnaires used for severe abuse families. The nonabuse families were requested to give informed consent. The families were approached in sequential order according to their rank on the list. The nonabuse control families were paid for their time and were highly cooperative.

The data forms were subsequently entered into a computerized database (Dbase III) and analyzed with Abstat, a commercially available statistical package, using an IBM/AT personal computer.

RESULTS

Overall, there were few differences found between the mild and severe abuse cases. However, the information regarding arrest records and the presence of paramours was incomplete. Among the severe cases, 15 of 33 families were known to contain a paramour from the Board of Inquiry's case review, whereas in the long data form, only two of 24 families had a paramour designated.

SOCIAL CLASS

Even though the controls were matched by the child's date of birth and zip code, differences in social class were apparent in the early analyses. The parents' educational levels differed significantly ($p<0.0206$). The educational levels were 11.4, 9.7, and 13.8 years for the severe, mild, and nonabuse groups, respectively. The total income of control cases was also significantly higher than among abuse cases. There were no significant differences between mild and severe abuse cases. Food stamps were received by 16 of the severe abuse families, 17 of the mild abuse families, and only one of the nonabuse families. Medicaid distribution was similar, with 52% of severe families, 76% of mild families, but only 3% (1/34) of nonabuse families receiving this entitlement (p<0.0000). This raises the question of why more of the severely abusive families did not have Medicaid. Based on average income, they all should have qualified.

PERINATAL ISSUES

The parents of the nonabuse controls were older than the abusive parents (p<0.0008). The ages of the parent groups were 24.40 years for the severe, 24.94 for the mild, and 30.18 for nonabuse groups, respectively. Even though teenage parents were rare among abusive parents, more abusive parents first became parents during their teens.

Only one mother who perpetrated severe abuse did not receive prenatal care. Although this variable did not achieve statistical significance, it should be retained for comparison with future studies. The prenatal care of nonabusive mothers typically began earlier in the pregnancy (mean = 1.9 months) than did the care of abusive mothers. The related variable length of prenatal care corroborated the findings from the month of onset of prenatal care.

THE CHILDREN

The section that provided a problem scale for children revealed few differences. Significant differences were found in only two of 42 items.

CAREGIVER PROBLEMS

Adult problems were readily detected and there were many significant differences. Items considered included childhood, isolation, anxiety, depression, somatic complaints, substance abuse, and history of arrest. Areas of job training and employment were also considered.

Childhood

A surprising number of abusive caretakers reported living away from their parents during childhood. In fact, this was one of the most strongly significant findings (p<0.0002) with 4/20 of the severe, 9/15 of the mild, and 2/30 nonabusive caregivers living away from their parents during childhood.

Isolation

Isolation of the caregiver was readily identified, but did not indicate the extent of risk. Significant differences were found for the question regarding membership in a church, social club, or similar organization. This differentiates between abusive and nonabusive families (p<0.0008), but not between mild and severe abusive situations.

The question "Have you requested help from an agency?" elicited a high frequency of *yes* responses from both severe (11/16) and mild (17/22) abusive groups versus nonabuse controls (7/30) and was highly significant (p<0.0002). Interestingly, 11 of the severe abuse group, 19 of the mild abuse group, and six of the nonabuse group answered *yes* to the question "Did you receive help from an agency?" (p<0.0001). This indicates inconsistency in the data collection, but it also raises the possibility that the severe abuse group was less successful in getting help than the mild abuse group.

Substance Abuse

Inquiry regarding drinking problems for the primary caregiver had a unique pattern. There were no differences between the severely abusive group and nonabusive controls, but the mildly abusive families reported more problems than the other two groups. Confirmation is required to ensure that this discrepancy was not a statistical (random) artifact. The differences in reported drug use among primary caregivers did not reach statistical significance, but most of the severely abusive families indicated that this was a problem. There was no difference in the drug use inquiries among the primary caregivers.

Employment

The items phrased "(Do you) have trouble getting or keeping a job?" revealed marked differences between abusive and nonabusive groups. For primary caregivers, no differences were seen between mild and severe abuse groups, but both groups reported much more difficulty than nonabusive primary caregivers. The mild abuse group reported the most trouble keeping a job, the severe abuse group was intermediate, and the nonabuse group had the least trouble.

Arrests and Convictions

Questions regarding arrests for assault showed significant differences among primary but not secondary caregivers. *This item was the single major difference between severe and mildly abusive families.* Although there were no differences on *yes/no* items to the question "Have you ever been arrested for disturbing the peace?" there were differences in the number of times that individuals had been arrested for this problem (p<0.0351) with the severely abusive group having been arrested most often. Data on arrests for drunk and disorderly conduct did not differ, nor did the data for sex offenses. Combining the arrest variables added little. The variable "any arrest" was mildly significant (p<0.0311).

Total convictions among primary caregivers did not achieve statistical significance (p<0.1249) because several of the controls had been convicted. There were no differences among the secondary caregivers. Similarly, the factor "served time" was not significant (p<0.1226). A more discriminating item might be advisable.

Family violence in the caregiver's family was highly significant, even when "don't know" responses were excluded. Family violence was found in 4/14 of the severe, 6/10 of the mild, and 7/34 of the nonabusive groups. Caregivers' mothers had criminal records in one severe case and two mild cases but in none of the controls.

The item "physical fight" was based on the question "Have you ever had a physical fight with your mate?" This also generated significant differences (p<0.0001) between abusive and nonabusive families but not between mild and severe abuse groups. A majority of both mild and severe abusive couples reported having physical fights.

Conclusions From Case Control Study

The conclusions drawn by the Board of Inquiry from the control phase were as follows:

1. Abusive families differ statistically from nonabusive families in many regards. Poverty-related, social class differences are most prevalent and obvious.

2. Severely abusive and mildly abusive families share the same demographic features and are largely indistinguishable. In fact, mildly abusive families often had more adverse scores than severely abusive families.

3. Currently, there are no criteria that allow one to differentiate degrees of risk for severe versus mild abuse. The most promising items seem to relate to caregivers' previous demonstrations of aggression and physical violence, especially arrests for assault. More items that reflect aggressive behaviors during the caregivers' childhood should amplify this set of factors.

The Ewigman and Kivlahan Study

Ewigman and Kivlahan (1990) investigated the causes of death due to injury of children ages birth through 5 years in Missouri and suggested a new way to classify child injury fatalities, and the childhood surveillance system. The study excluded occupant motor vehicle fatalities and children who were injured in other states and died in Missouri. They reviewed the records of 314 children whose deaths were attributed to injury as noted on death certificates and the deaths of 20 children who were determined to be victims of child abuse or neglect (substantiated by the

Missouri Division of Family Services), but whose deaths were determined to be of natural causes on the death certificate. The study was to determine how children in Missouri die from injuries and whether child abuse was underreported or misclassified.

The study reviewed death certificates, birth certificates, Division of Family Services records, Federal Bureau of Investigation statistics, autopsy records, medical records, and legal records, and also reviewed arrest, charge, or prosecution records.

"Accident" was listed as the manner of death on the death certificate of 222 of the 334 children in the study. Twenty cases had "natural" and 58 had "homicide" listed as the cause of death. Twenty-four cases had "undetermined" as the cause of death.

Ewigman and Kivlahan stated that death certificates do not provide the necessary information about child injuries or child abuse and cited two sample cases.

A 4-year-old boy was struck by a motor vehicle on a residential street while riding his bicycle. He had a skull fracture and severe brain injury. The death was listed as an accident on the death certificate. The codes listed on the death certificate included skull fracture and motor vehicle traffic injury. No other information was on file with Division of Family Services or the State Bureau of Investigation, and there was no legal follow-up. Further investigation revealed that the 4-year-old had been allowed to ride his bicycle in the street, unsupervised, while the caregiver was several houses away from the event, drinking alcohol. This injury was not the result of an accident. The event was predictable, caused by neglect and lack of supervision.

A 2-year-old died from severe burns sustained in a residential fire. The manner of death listed on the death certificate was accidental and the codes included house fire and burns. Further investigation revealed that the mother had left the child alone with a 6-year old sibling while she went to the store for cigarettes. The trailer was heated by leaving the lit gas oven door open. The mother was convicted of endangering the welfare of a child and was sentenced to several years' probation. This event was also predictable and caused by neglect and lack of supervision.

Ewigman and Kivlahan assigned a behavioral cause of death to all of the cases studied. The categories assigned were inflicted injuries, unmet needs, exposure to hazards, unrecognized hazards, and inadequate information. Forty percent of the cases could not be given a behavioral cause of death because they were inadequately investigated, inadequately documented, or both. The authors felt that this, alone, was an indictment of the system of investigating and classifying child fatalities.

About one-third of the cases fell under the category "exposure to hazards," which included electrocution by unsafe appliances, drownings, fire hazards, and gun hazards. Many of the children who died as a result of exposure to hazards were unsupervised or were supervised by caregivers who were influenced by mind- or mood-altering substances.

One-fifth of the deaths resulted from inflicted injuries or homicides. The injuries were inflicted by caregivers, 71% of whom were arrested. Two-thirds of those arrested were found guilty. Most were charged with murder, one with abuse of a child, and six with endangering the welfare of a child. One-third of the perpetrators were sentenced to five years or less, one-third six to 20 years, and one-third to more than 20 years.

Five percent of the deaths resulted from unmet needs, involving children left without food and protection. Three percent of the deaths resulted from unrecognizable hazards. The deaths were unpredictable and uncontrollable, even with adequate supervision.

This study demonstrated that many childhood deaths are inadequately investigated. Many children are dying from common household hazards resulting from inadequate supervision, and more are dying from child abuse and neglect.

Ewigman and Kivlahan made three recommendations as a result of their study:

1. All child fatalities must be reviewed to gain an understanding of child abuse-related deaths.

2. These reviews must arise at the state level so as to identify and correct systemic deterrents that failed to protect a child and to ensure a coordinated approach to the problem.

3. The review committee must have access to all relevant records, including social services reports, court documents, police records, autopsy records, mental health records, and hospital- or medical-related data.

RECOMMENDATIONS OF TASK FORCE ON FATAL CHILD ABUSE

Based on the Ewigman and Kivlahan study, a task force was formed to make recommendations about what can be done to decrease the death rate from homicides and injuries due to neglect of children in Missouri.

The Missouri Department of Social Services' Task Force on Fatal Child Abuse reviewed procedures followed by other states and heard testimony from numerous experts.

As a result they made the following recommendations (Steinmetz, 1990):

1. Establish child death review teams in every county of the state to determine the cause of suspicious deaths of children under 15 years of age.

2. The cases investigated by the team are referred by the coroner/medical examiner.

3. A protocol defining suspicious circumstances is established by the department of social services.

4. The county team includes the coroner/medical examiner, prosecutor, sheriff or police officer, and representatives of the Division of Family Services, the juvenile court, and the county health department. The prosecutor chairs the team.

5. Establish regional death review teams, with expertise in child death review, to aid local teams in detecting child abuse.

6. Establish a state death review team to review reports from the county teams, identify system problems, and suggest ways to prevent child abuse deaths. The state-wide team gathers data from the local and regional teams and submits an annual report to the governor.

7. Require autopsies of children in all deaths not attributed to well-documented accidents or to previously diagnosed fatal illnesses.

8. Require all health practitioners, law enforcement officials, social service personnel and any other person with responsibility for the care of children to report the death of any child under the age of 15 to the coroner/medical examiner.

9. Allow unsubstantiated reports of abuse and neglect to remain available to the Division of Family Services and to law enforcement authorities for a period of 10 years. The records would be closed to all other persons.

10. Relax confidentiality restrictions between certain parties when it is in the best interests of the child.

11. Require the department of health to develop guidelines for physicians and hospitals to identify suspicious deaths.

MISSOURI CHILD FATALITY REVIEW PROJECT

In 1991 Missouri legislators enacted House Bill #185, which created the Child Fatality Review Project. The bill mandates multidisciplinary investigations of deaths of children (**Table 17-4**). The aim of such legislation is to establish a multidisciplinary approach to investigating child fatalities. It provides for improved investigations of child deaths, which improves accuracy in reporting the cause of death, and offers advice regarding means of preventing childhood injuries and fatalities.

Table 17-4. Mandated Activities for Child Fatalities

Every county must have a multidisciplinary child fatality review panel (114 counties and City of St. Louis).

The county panel must consist of at least the following six core members: prosecuting attorney, coroner/medical examiner, law enforcement representative, Division of Family Services representative, public health representative, and juvenile officer.

All deaths age birth to 14 must be reported to the coroner/medical examiner.

Children, age one week to one year, who die in a sudden, unexplained manner must have an autopsy.

A state child fatality review panel must meet at least two times per year.

Panels must use uniform protocols and data collection forms.

Certified child-death pathologists must perform the autopsies.

PROGRAM ACCOMPLISHMENTS

The program established, under the Department of Social Services, a State Technical Assistance Team (STAT) to coordinate activities, train panel members, develop protocols, collect data, and determine the criteria for child fatality review (**Table 17-5**). STAT developed a fatality data collection system that gathers detailed information not previously available regarding childhood deaths and links data from the county panels with birth and death certificates. In addition, STAT trained a large group of professionals to use a multidisciplinary approach to investigate children's deaths and trained selected panel members in skills such as forensic interviewing and death scene investigation. STAT developed tools for panel members to use during investigations. These included a crime scene checklist to ensure that pertinent aspects of an investigation are performed consistently, and protocols to improve photography and sketches of the scene and improve interviewing victims, witnesses, and suspects.

Table 17-5. Criteria for Child Fatality Review

Possible inflicted injury.	Unexplained death or death in an undetermined manner.
Any firearm injury.	Suspected sexual assault.
Injury not witnessed by person in charge of child at time of the injury/event.	Other suspicious findings (describe).
Possible inadequate supervision.	Death due to confinement.
Sudden, unexplained death of a child under age 1.	Bathtub/bucket drowning.
Natural cause of death possibly due to malnutrition or to delay in seeking medical care.	Suffocation/strangulation.
	Any poisoning.
Open DFS protection service case on victim.	Severe unexplained injury.
Victim in DFS custody.	Prior DFS substantiation of child abuse or neglect on the victim or other children in the residence for similar circumstances.
Pedestrian driveway injury.	

They improved the appropriate use and availability of autopsies. The Missouri Medicaid program paid for autopsies on eligible children and thereby assured that a county's financial status or a victim's socioeconomic status did not affect the quality or availability of this crucial component of the death investigation. In addition, program facilitators organized a state-wide group of pathologists specially trained to ensure the appropriate performance of autopsies. They arranged annual education programs to keep members informed of policies, provide current practice updates, and offer a forum for professional interchange.

Finally, the Department of Social Services appointed an eight-member state advisory panel to review all of the data and to recommend systemic improvements. The advisory group met every six months.

CHILD FATALITY FINDINGS (JANUARY TO SEPTEMBER 1992)

The following is the first report from the Division of Family Services and the Commissioner of Health.

The Missouri Child Fatality Review Project has produced important information about the causes of childhood deaths and revealed details of child abuse deaths.

It has successfully addressed the problem of unreported childhood deaths caused by abuse or neglect. The panels reviewed 172 child deaths in the first nine months of 1992. The number of deaths of children under 14 years of age in which officials have confirmed abuse or neglect nearly doubled since enactment of the bill. Investigators confirmed 84% more child deaths from abuse and neglect in 1992 than for the same period in 1989.

During the first nine months of 1992, 765 Missouri children under the age of 15 years died. Most of the deaths (566) had nonsuspicious cause and were not referred for further review.

Seventy-nine percent of all deaths resulted from sudden infant death syndrome and other natural causes. A majority (335 infants) died in the first month of life, primarily of natural conditions such as premature birth. While approximately one-third of Missouri's children are less than 5 years old, 80% of those who died were in this age group. Among injury-related deaths for children less than 1 year of age, homicide was the leading cause of death (52%). For all children under the age of 15, motor vehicle accidents were the most common cause of injury-related deaths (39%).

Lack of supervision was a major factor leading to death in reviewed cases. For example, 41% (70) of children among reviewed cases were not supervised by adults at the time of injury leading to death.

Of the children who died, 40% were Medicaid eligible, while only 25% of all Missouri children are eligible for Medicaid.

Most of the children who died from injuries, homicide, and sudden unexplained death were living with unmarried parents, with mothers having less than a high school education, and in environments with conspicuous alcohol or drug abuse.

Homicide was the number one cause of injury deaths in children younger than 1. Homicide victims are more likely to be poor and racial minorities.

CHILD ABUSE AND NEGLECT DEATHS

The program's most striking finding was the sharp increase in the number of child abuse and neglect fatalities confirmed by the Division of Family Services. The number of substantiated fatalities rose from 25 cases in 1989 to 46 cases in 1992, an 84% increase. This increase reflects more cases being brought to official attention through the panel review process. During this period, the Division of Family Services did not change the investigative criteria for substantiation of abuse or neglect.

Of the fatal child abuse cases substantiated by the Division of Family Services, 36% of the children died of physical abuse, 53% died as a result of neglect, 9% were medically neglected, and 2% were sexually maltreated.

AUTOPSIES

The autopsy is a critical component in determining the cause of death. For example, diagnosing sudden infant death syndrome (SIDS) requires an autopsy to exclude other causes of death, such as intracranial bleeding from shaken infant syndrome. Since the law mandated that all children 1 week to 1 year of age who died in a sudden, unexplained manner have an autopsy performed, for the first time, 100% of Missouri children dying from SIDS had an autopsy. In past years, as many as 13% of the deaths attributed to SIDS (in 1987) were not autopsied.

Although the law mandated autopsies in certain cases, the overall number of autopsies for children from birth through age 14 did not change significantly from 1989 to 1992. Rather than causing more autopsies to be performed, this legislation fostered more appropriate use of this procedure. The autopsy rate for SIDS, accidents, and reviewed deaths increased, while the rate for motor vehicle accidents decreased. The majority (81%) of cases requiring panel review were autopsied, while 40% of nonreviewed cases were autopsied.

The review process and the reimbursement incentive significantly increased the number of autopsies performed on Medicaid children. While Medicaid reimbursement for autopsies ensured that eligible children who die will receive autopsies when necessary, there is a need to fund autopsies for children not covered by Medicaid. Autopsy cost is a significant burden on counties with few financial resources. The performance of autopsies should be based on the needs in each specific case, not on county or family finances.

OTHER BENEFITS OF THE PROJECT

Although the project was initiated to detect deaths due to child abuse and neglect, the program has made the state aware of, and has precipitated interest in, other major causes of childhood mortality, such as SIDS, unintentional injuries, and infant deaths due to premature births.

As a result of this review, more than 2,500 county and state workers have better knowledge and skills for reviewing cases of childhood deaths, hopefully increasing the likelihood that future children's deaths will be appropriately explained.

The number and quality of autopsies performed on children have improved through the organization of a group of specially trained pathologists.

The availablity of autopsies for low-income children has increased through Medicaid reimbursement for eligible children. This ensures that economic status is no barrier to investigations of child deaths.

The Child Fatality Review Project links many data sources into a single comprehensive system, which depicts deaths caused by child abuse or neglect better than any previous system did.

RECOMMENDATIONS

The state advisory panel reviewed all of the data accumulated by the review panels and recommended the following improvements:

1. The state should continue allotting resources to facilitate community change.

   Consideration should be given to extending the comprehensive, multidisciplinary approach used for reviewing child deaths to other social and health problems such as cases of sexual abuse.

2. Improve caregiver supervision through education and better access to child care services.

To prevent injuries and deaths due to lack of supervision, parents and caregivers need age-appropriate information on the behavior and needs of children, access to day care, and parent training.

3. Educate investigators about the importance of accurately recording the level of supervision and circumstances surrounding the death of the child.

   A significant number of children's deaths were investigated without determination of supervision status. Without this crucial knowledge, neglectful situations may be missed.

4. Monitor families at risk of a second preventable death or injury and provide them with services.

   Surviving children in the same family or household are often at risk for morbidity and mortality. Case coordinators should be trained to follow through on services recommended by county panels for high-risk families.

5. Fund autopsies for the highest risk children.

   Medicaid reimbursement for autopsies increased the utilization of this important procedure for eligible children. The state should provide additional funds to finance autopsies for children not covered by Medicaid.

6. Implement a strategy aimed at reducing injuries and preventable deaths.

   The data from this project define how and why children are dying in Missouri. The state should develop prevention strategies with the collaboration of hospitals, health departments, schools, social service agencies, and community organizations to reduce injuries and preventable deaths in children.

THE MANUAL ON THE FOLLOWING PAGES WAS PREPARED BY THE MISSOURI STATE TECHNICAL ASSISTANCE TEAM AS A GUIDE IN INVESTIGATION. THE ENCLOSED PROTOCOLS AND CHECKLISTS WERE DEVELOPED AS INVESTIGATIVE AIDS.

MISSOURI DEPARTMENT OF SOCIAL SERVICES
STATE TECHNICAL ASSISTANCE TEAM
Multi-disciplinary Trainers/Investigators of Child Abuse

BASIC INVESTIGATION PROTOCOLS

CONTENTS

Serious Crime/Event Scene Checklist

Scene Investigation Checklists

Sudden, Unexplained Deaths of Infants
Scene Investigation Checklist for Children Age 1 - 14

Joint Investigations with the Division of Family Services

Role, Responsibility and Authority of the Division of Family Services
and Understandingthe Child Abuse and Neglect "Hotline" (Central Registry Unit)
Role & Responsibilities of Law Enforcement and Coroner/Medical Examiners
Child Abuse & Neglect Legal Excerpts

Investigative Guides

Basic Interviewing Techniques

— Victim Interviewing Techniques
— Witness Interviewing Guidelines
— Interviewing Alleged Perpetrator

Basic Scene Photography
Basic Scene Sketching and Investigative Note Taking
Scene Reconstruction Using Dolls and Silhouettes

Case Summary Checklists

Victim Abuse/Neglect Interview Summary
Child Abuse/Neglect Investigation Summary

Investigative Aids and Sample Forms

Sample Forms

— Search Warrant
— Consent to Search
— Miranda Rights Waiver
— Chain-of-Custody Evidence Log
— Photo Log
— Body Diagrams

SERIOUS CRIME/EVENT SCENE CHECKLIST

■ **ASSIGNMENT OR NOTIFICATION**:

Record time of assignment and arrival at scene. Attempt to obtain all available information from reporter.

■ **UPON ARRIVAL**:

■ 1. **Preserve and Protect Life**. Determine if there are injuries or imminent dangers that require immediate attention. If there is **any** possibility of life, seek medical help immediately (obtain names of medical personnel and other responders). Normally, the injured should not be moved prior to medical assistance unless in immediate danger (fire, water, etc.). Call for other assistance, as necessary (law enforcement, coroner/medical examiner, Division of Family Services, juvenile officer, fire department, utility company, etc).

■ 2. **Determine what Crime and/or Event has occurred**. Identify victim(s) and witnesses, and make a preliminary determination of what has occurred and what actions are required.

■ 3. **If Appropriate, Identify and/or Arrest Alleged perpetrator(s)**. If an alleged perpetrator(s) is identified, but is not on the scene, obtain and broadcast a complete description:

- Name/Nickname (if available)
- Race
- Sex
- Age and Date of Birth
- Address
- Physical Description (height, weight, hair, eyes, complexion, scars, tatoos, etc.)
- Clothing Description
- Any other Identifiers
- Vehicle
- Direction of Flight
- Weapon Description (if any)

Broadcast the description and what the person is wanted for as soon as possible, and update with new information.

If the alleged perpetrator is on the scene, and is believed to be armed, or is concealed and/or barricaded, request assistance and follow your agency's policy.

If an immediate arrest is required, secure and search the alleged perpetrator as quickly as possible. For your protection, search for anything that could cause harm. While conducting this search of the alleged perpetrator, any weapons, evidence or contraband is seizable and usually admissible as evidence.

NOTE: Safety and the protection and preservation of life are paramount. Do not take unnecessary risks.

■ **4. Establish and Protect the Crime/Event Scene**. Once identified, "freeze" the scene and everything in it. With the exception of assisting the injured, the crime/event scene should remain untouched pending appropriate processing and photographing. If possible, secure and protect the perimeters with rope, tape or other markers.

Within manpower limits, identify, separate and isolate witnesses prior to interviewing.

NOTE: In the case of an obvious death (no possibility of life), do not move the body or anything surrounding it prior to the arrival of the coroner/medical examiner. Photograph the body and scene prior to other processing. While conveying a body to the morgue or other facility, take necessary measures to protect the head and extremities from accidental damage (paper bags on hands and feet, etc.).

If the victim appears near death (and it doesn't interfere with medical assistance), attempt to obtain a dying declaration of what occurred.

SPECIAL NOTE: If the event involves the fatality of a child (birth through 14 years), the coroner/medical examiner **must** be notified immediately. A multi-disciplinary investigation including law enforcement and the coroner may be required.

The **sudden, unexplained death of an infant (one week to one year)** is commonly referred to as SIDS (Sudden Infant Death Syndrome). The cause of SIDS remains unknown, but criteria for its diagnosis have been established by the National Institute of Child Health and Human Development. For the death of an infant to be diagnosed as SIDS, an **autopsy**, a **clinical history review** and a thorough **death-scene investigation** must be performed. To assist you in conducting these very sensitive and complex investigations, we have developed a separate investigative guide (enclosed). This completed checklist is invaluable to the pathologist who performs the autopsy, thus it is important to complete the investigation and checklist form as soon as possible. Obviously, all parts of the crime/event scene protocol are not appropriate to most of these cases. You may also wish to seek the assistance of the Division of Family Services or other community agencies better equipped to offer appropriate services and support to the family.

■ **5. Processing the Scene**. When in doubt, "freeze" the scene and do nothing until you are prepared to do it correctly. Do not hesitate to ask for outside advice and assistance. Develop investigative goals and objectives.

— Determine the legal basis for any search and seizure, particularly beyond the immediate crime/event scene. Considering your agency's policy and procedures, the prosecuting attorney should be consulted on specific legal questions; e.g., consent to search versus the need for a search warrant and other "search and seizure" issues (see attached samples).

— Establish a "chain-of-custody log" (who found what and where) to be maintained by a single officer. Designate that person to receive and take charge of all physical evidence at the scene.

NOTE: Prior to seizing, all evidence should be photographed and logged as found (see attached sample).

— Only designated persons should search the crime scene and handle evidence. All others, excluding emergency medical assistance, should remain outside the protected area.

— Take measurements and make sketches that will relate directly to the photographs. Indicate North in all sketches.

— Take a complete photographic set of the entire scene area including a "landmark" photo (front of house, vehicle license, etc.). Complete and use photo cards when appropriate (most close-ups; sample attached).

— Photographs and corresponding sketches should be taken from the "general" to the "specific"; e.g., an overall room shot, to the bed, to a blood stain on the pillow.

— Body pictures should be taken from at least two views and be full-length. Close-up photos of wounds and abnormalities should be visible in the full-length pictures. If the body has been moved, use "body silhouettes" to reconstruct the scene. In the case of an infant, a doll may be more appropriate.

— Prior to seizure, **if appropriate**, evidence should be examined for latent fingerprints. Weapons and non-traditional surfaces (paper, cardboard, leather, masonry, etc.) are best processed at the laboratory. Such evidence should be handled with care and is usually best transported in a paper or cardboard container.

NOTE: All recovered and seized weapons should be considered **loaded and dangerous** until examined by a qualified person familiar with firearms.

— All seized evidence should be properly marked, packaged and placed in a secure evidence locker or conveyed to the appropriate laboratory for processing. A "chain-of-custody" log should track the handling of every piece of evidence.

■ **6. The Interview/Interrogation Process**.

— If the person(s) to be interviewed is a child, consider requesting the assistance of someone experienced in "child interviewing." The Division of Family Services and the Juvenile Officer are mandated to participate in some investigations. Seek advice.

— Alleged perpetrator(s) and witnesses should be separated and interviewed individually.

— Alleged perpetrator(s) should be interrogated relative to his/her part in the crime/event. Improbabilities and inconsistencies should be noted and used to enhance the questioning process. Contradicting statements can be an important part of the case.

NOTE: Follow your agency's policy and procedures for advising alleged perpetrators of their Miranda rights and obtaining verbal and written waiver of these rights (see attached sample).

— Witnesses should be questioned regarding their first-hand knowledge of the event; e.g., what they actually saw or hard. To obtain the most detail, **ask specific questions** concerning the event and the persons involved. Always ask for and look for more detail. As an investigative tool, second-hand information can be valuable if it leads you to an unidentified witness or alleged perpetrator; by itself, the information has very limited value. Always attempt to obtain names and specific verifying facts.

— If appropriate, initiate a canvas of the entire neighborhood or area. Many people will divulge information if asked but will not voluntarily come forward as a witness.

— **Make Note of Spontaneous Statements**. From the moment you arrive on the scene, be alert to spontaneous statements made by witnesses, family and/or alleged perpetrators. These **unsolicited**, voluntary utterances usually do not require that the subject have prior warning of his/her Miranda rights. These initial statements can be a very important part of the investigation; e.g., they may contradict a later statement; implicate a person(s) in a particular action; or indicate remorse for an act later denied.

— Record all investigative results (interviewing, disposition of evidence, names of responders and what they did, etc.) in some way. Following the policy and procedures of your agency, take hand-written notes, record electronically, video tape, or use a combination of all these methods. Whatever the means, **record and document** every step of the investigation.

■ 7. **Report Preparation.** Assemble all obtained information into a logical sequence of events. Your report should accurately reflect the results of the entire investigation. All persons, observations, statements, evidence, sketches, photographs, medical and technical findings should be prepared to clearly portray all the known facts of the case. If new or additional information becomes available, a **supplemental** report should be prepared and distributed to all the participating agencies (multi-disciplinary team members, including prosecutor, etc.).

■ 8. **Resources, Support and Assistance.**

— In cases involving children, when local assistance is not available (child fatalities, serious and complex sexual abuse and the ritualistic abuse of children), you may contact the State Technical Assistance Team by calling: 314-751-5980 or 800-487-1626 (24-hour assistance). We will make every attempt to answer your questions or direct you to an available resource.

NOTE: The protocol for accessing STAT assistance is available by calling the phone numbers listed above.

SCENE INVESTIGATION CHECKLISTS

■ For Sudden, Unexplained Deaths of Infants (birth-one year).

■ Death Scene of Children (one year-14 years).

These checklists may be prepared as attachments to the investigative report. If possible, they should also **accompany the body to the Certified Child-Death Pathologist** to be used as reference during the autopsy. Information obtained concerning the history and circumstances of death will contribute to a better autopsy result.

NOTE: Any section **not completed** should be marked accordingly in the left-hand column.

■ Death-scene checklists are an evaluation/investigation aid to assist in making a more accurate determination of the cause of death. In interviewing parents, caregivers and witnesses, NEVER assume criminality.

■ BE OBJECTIVE. An empathetic non-confrontational approach is both appropriate and effective. Explain that the information is necessary to accurately determine the cause of death.

■ If a RECONSTRUCTION of the scene is appropriate, make every effort to obtain first-person information (see Use of Dolls and Silhouettes, page 366).

COMPLETED / NOT COMPLETED	**MISSOURI CHILD FATALITY REVIEW PROJECT** **615 HOWERTON COURT** **JEFFERSON CITY, MO 65109** **314-751-5980 800-487-1626** **SCENE INVESTIGATION GUIDE FOR SUDDEN, UNEXPLAINED DEATH OF INFANTS** Adapted from the St. Louis City Medical Examiner's Model
1. ❒ ❒	Name of deceased: _____Race: _____ Sex: M ❒ F ❒ Date of Birth:_____Date of Death:_____Time of Death _____ Scene Address:_____ Agency/Department:_____Investigator(s): _____ Report Number: _____Date/Time of Scene Investigation: _____
	PART I: ASSESSMENT OF INFANT AND POSITION (FOR USE WITH NARRATIVE REPORT)
2. ❒ ❒	Assess for birthmarks or injuries of any type including bruises, scrapes, cuts, burn marks, diaper rash. Include colors, shapes, sizes, locations; fully describe in narrative:
3. ❒ ❒	Hemorrhage of eyes or lips present? No ❒ Yes ❒
4. ❒ ❒	Body Temp? Time? Method? Sweaty? Atmospheric? Time?
5. ❒ ❒	Liver Mortis? (Where Observed? Fixed Time?) Consistent with position when found? No ❒ Yes ❒
6. ❒ ❒	Rigor Mortis? (Where Observed? Fixed Time?)
7. ❒ ❒	Well nourished & well cared for? (If No, explain fully in narrative) No ❒ Yes ❒
8. ❒ ❒	Body and Clothing Clean? No ❒ Yes ❒ Right Size? No ❒ Yes ❒ Dressed in?_____
9. ❒ ❒	Describe bed/crib/bassinet/couch/floor/water mattress/bean bag or other sleeping structure including all sheets, pillows, plastic covers, blankets, defects or misc. objects in bedding.
10. ❒ ❒	**A.** Body position when discovered: on stomach ❒ left side ❒ pinned vertically ❒ on back ❒ right side ❒ pinned horizontally ❒ seated upright ❒ other wedging ❒ **B.** Usual sleeping position: on stomach ❒ left side ❒ on back ❒ right side ❒ seated upright ❒

INSTRUCTIONS: Complete each numbered item by providing the appropriate response, and by marking the completed or _not_ completed box in the left-hand margin. Make every attempt to obtain as much information as possible, use additional pages as necessary for comments section. For assistance, call 1-800-487-1626.

11. ❐ ❐	Sketch position of infant and identify if in crib, bed or other (Indicate direction of child's head; circle one): N W E S
12. ❐ ❐	Photographs of infant, silhouette or doll taken by: _____Time: _____Date:_____
13. ❐ ❐	Anything covering nose or mouth? No ❐ Yes ❐ What _____
14. ❐ ❐	Position of face (nose-mouth) when discovered: Face directly Up ❐ Both Nostrils Unobstructed ❐ Object Covering Mouth ❐ Face directly Down ❐ Both Nostrils Blocked ❐ Object Covering Nose ❐ Face to Right ❐ Right Nostril Blocked ❐ Objects Near Face ❐ Face to Left ❐ Left Nostril Blocked ❐
15. ❐ ❐	Photos of Above Obtained? No ❐ Yes ❐
16. ❐ ❐	If infant found face down, was there a visible cup, pocket depression in the bedding? No ❐ Yes ❐ Depth _____ Diameter _____ No ❐ Yes ❐
17. ❐ ❐	Is there a visible crease on face, neck or head from pillows or bedding? No ❐ Yes ❐ Photograph? No ❐ Yes ❐
18. ❐ ❐	Position of Head/Neck when originally found: Head tilted to left No ❐ Yes ❐ Neck extended backwards No ❐ Yes ❐ Head tilted to right No ❐ Yes ❐ Neck flexed to chin No ❐ Yes ❐
19. ❐ ❐	Material found in nose? No ❐ Yes ❐ Unknown ❐ Mucus ❐ Vomit ❐ Bloody Froth ❐ Blood Tinged Secretion ❐ Food ❐ Saliva ❐ Dried Secretion ❐ Other ❐ Formula ❐ Froth ❐
20. ❐ ❐	Material found in mouth? No ❐ Yes ❐ Unknown ❐ Mucus ❐ Vomit ❐ Bloody Froth ❐ Blood Tinged Secretion ❐ Food ❐ Saliva ❐ Dried Secretion ❐ Other ❐ Formula ❐ Froth ❐
21. ❐ ❐	Secretions noted on following? Pillow ❐ Blanket ❐ Sheet ❐ Mattress ❐ Clothing ❐ Other ❐ Mucus ❐ Vomit ❐ Bloody Froth ❐ Blood Tinged Secretion ❐ Food ❐ Saliva ❐ Dried Secretion ❐ Other ❐ Formula ❐ Froth ❐ Urine or Stool ❐ Infant's face in contact with wet materials? No ❐ Yes ❐
22. ❐ ❐	Resuscitation attempted? No ❐ Yes ❐ Unknown ❐ By Whom _____

23. ☐☐	Name, age, marital status, employment and health status of natural parents? Mother (include maiden name):_____ Employer: _____ Father:_____ Employed: _____
24. ☐☐	What does baby live with?
25. ☐☐	If parents employed, who babysits?
26. ☐☐	Do siblings ever watch baby unattended or could they have accidentally injured child without parents' knowledge? No ☐ Yes ☐
27. ☐☐	Name, age and health status of siblings?
28. ☐☐	Any history of SIDS or other infant death involving either parent? No ☐ Yes ☐ If yes, describe details including date of death and location of occurrence.
29. ☐☐	When was the baby last seen alive; by whom?
30. ☐☐	What was the condition of the child at the time?
31. ☐☐	Was the child sleeping alone? No ☐ Yes ☐ If no, who was child sleeping with?
32. ☐☐	Was an Apnea monitor in the room? No ☐ Yes ☐ Was the child on the monitor at the time of death? No ☐ Yes ☐
33. ☐☐	Any possibility of overlying, i.e., recent alcohol consumption or drugs by person sleeping with child, too little room for too many people, etc.? No ☐ Yes ☐
34. ☐☐	Who found infant?
35. ☐☐	Medical assistance summoned? No ☐ Yes ☐ By whom?_____
36. ☐☐	Was baby moved from original position? No ☐ Yes ☐ Why?
37. ☐☐	Was death witnessed? No ☐ Yes ☐ Fully describe details in narrative section.
38. ☐☐	Conveyed to medical facility? No ☐ Yes ☐ By whom?_____ Name and address of facility _____
39. ☐☐	Who pronounced infant dead? _____
40. ☐☐	Time last fed? What was fed? Amt. in oz? Any difficulties?
41. ☐☐	Breast fed? No ☐ Yes ☐ Formula fed? No ☐ Yes ☐
42. ☐☐	Any known food intolerance? No ☐ Yes ☐ What? Poor feeder? No ☐ Yes ☐
43. ☐☐	Has baby received any of the following? Circle one. Cow's milk Goat's milk Honey Watered down formula Other_____ Unknown ☐
44. ☐☐	Has baby had an illness within the last two weeks? No ☐ Yes ☐ Since when? _____ Appetite Changes ☐ Wheezes ☐ Fussy ☐ Sniffles ☐ Cough ☐ Fever ☐ How high _____ Diarrhea ☐ Cold ☐ Irritability ☐ Other: _____ Runny Nose ☐ Vomiting ☐ Congestion ☐
45. ☐☐	Was baby taken for treatment for above symptoms? No ☐ Yes ☐ Where? _____ If yes, what diagnosis was rendered?_____
46. ☐☐	Has baby been under routine care of a pediatrician? No ☐ Yes ☐ Who? _____ Clinic Name:_____
47. ☐☐	Well Baby visits/immunizations received? No ☐ Yes ☐ If yes, physicians's name/clinic:
48. ☐☐	Any known allergies or any known reaction to baby shots? No ☐ Yes ☐ If yes, explain? _____

49. ☐ ☐	Has baby been exposed to any contagious disease recently? No ☐ Yes ☐ If yes, explain: _____ _____
50. ☐ ☐	What pets are in the house?
51. ☐ ☐	Has family traveled recently? Where?
	PRENATAL HISTORY
52. ☐ ☐	Regular prenatal visits? No ☐ Yes ☐ Number: Where:_____
53. ☐ ☐	Known complications of pregnancy? No ☐ Yes ☐ Explain:
54. ☐ ☐	Special diet during pregnancy? No ☐ Yes ☐ What? _____
55. ☐ ☐	Maternal alcohol or street drugs: No ☐ Yes ☐ Unknown ☐ Alcohol Cocaine Heroin Marijuana Other:_____
56. ☐ ☐	Maternal smoking during pregnancy? No ☐ Yes ☐ Unknown ☐ Packs per day:_____ How many other adults in household smoking _____
57. ☐ ☐	Known maternal health problems? (diabetes, hypertension, etc.) No ☐ Yes ☐ If yes, please describe: _____ _____
58. ☐ ☐	Was mother taking prescription medication for above medical condition? No ☐ Yes ☐ What? _____
	BIRTH HISTORY
59. ☐ ☐	What hospital: _____Difficulty with delivery? No ☐ Yes ☐ Type of delivery: _____
60. ☐ ☐	Birth Weight: _____ Apgar Scores at 1 and 5 minutes?_____ Gestational age or full term? _____
61. ☐ ☐	Birth defects or other abnormalities of infant at birth?
62. ☐ ☐	Number of previous pregnancies and outcome?
	PART III-ENVIRONMENTAL AND SOCIOECONOMIC CONDITIONS
63. ☐ ☐	Conditions of residence: _____ Overcrowding: No ☐ Yes ☐ Describe:
64. ☐ ☐	Quality of dwelling? Below average Average Above average Other:
65. ☐ ☐	Unusual conditions seen? No ☐ Yes ☐ If yes, explain:
66. ☐ ☐	Number of children living at this address? Number of adults living at this address:
67. ☐ ☐	Building Type: _____ Neighborhood Type:_____
68. ☐ ☐	Welfare: No ☐ Yes ☐ Monthly Amount $_____ Food Stamp Amount: $_____ WIC Program? No ☐ Yes ☐
69. ☐ ☐	Estimated family income per year? Less than $5,000 _____ $5,000 to $10,000 ——————— $10,000 to $20,000 _____ $20,000 to $25,000 _____ $25,000 to $30,000_____ $30,000 to $35,000 ——————— Over $35,000 _____
70. ☐ ☐	Reminder: Has this family been hotlined in the past for abuse or neglect? No ☐ Yes ☐ If yes, describe known details in narrative section.
71. ☐ ☐	Have appropriate medical records, including birth record, been requested? No ☐ Yes ☐

	PART IV-OPTIONAL CHECKLIST FOR DEFECTIVE CRIBS POSSIBLY RELATING TO DEATH
72. ❑ ❑	Location of crib in room? Manufacturer?
73. ❑ ❑	Examine for obvious cracks, splits, toe hold, old paint:
74. ❑ ❑	Space between mattress and sides of crib? (should be less than 1")
75. ❑ ❑	Space between rails (should be less than 2 3/8")
76. ❑ ❑	Distance between mattress position and top of rails (should be greater than 26")
77. ❑ ❑	Distance from floor to mattress?_____ Distance from top of railing to floor with railing up?_____ and down _____
78. ❑ ❑	Floor surface? What is supporting matttress?
79. ❑ ❑	Sturdiness of rails; Do they fall down when shaken or pressure is applied? No ❑ Yes ❑
80. ❑ ❑	Can rails be pulled away from side of crib: No ❑ Yes ❑ How far?
81. ❑ ❑	Does plastic mattress fit securely or is it loose?
82. ❑ ❑	Toys or objects in Crib? Describe?
83. ❑ ❑	Additional Comments (to include name and pedigrees of all persons and responders at scene):

Signature of Investigator _____   Date _____

COMPLETED / NOT COMPLETED	
	MISSOURI CHILD FATALITY REVIEW PROJECT 615 HOWERTON COURT JEFFERSON CITY, MO 65109 314-751-5980 800-487-1626 **SCENE INVESTIGATION GUIDE FOR CHILD FATALITIES OVER AGE 1**
1. ☐☐	Name of deceased: _____Race: _____ Sex: M ☐ F ☐ Date of Birth:_____Date of Death:_____Time of Death _____ Scene Address: _____ Agency/Department: _____Investigator(s): _____ Report Number: _____Date/Time of Scene Investigation: _____
	ASSESSMENT OF POSITION AND CIRCUMSTANCES
2. ☐☐	Describe in detail injuries of any type including bruises, scrapes, cuts, burn marks, swelling, etc. Include colors, shapes, sizes, locations. If a burn, describe what caused it (hot water, cigarette lighter, etc.).
3. ☐☐	If any injury, how did it occur?
4. ☐☐	Has child been injured in any way during the last month? No ☐ Yes ☐ How? _____
5. ☐☐	Hemorrhage of eyes or lips present? No ☐ Yes ☐
6. ☐☐	Body Temp? Time? Method? Sweaty? Atmospheric Temp? Time?
7. ☐☐	Livor Mortis? (Where Observed? Fixed Time?) Consistent with position when found? No ☐ Yes ☐
8. ☐☐	Rigor Mortis? (Where Observed? Fixed Time?)
9. ☐☐	Is the child well nourished and well cared for? (If No, explain fully in narrative) No ☐ Yes ☐
10. ☐☐	Body and Clothing Clean? No ☐ Yes ☐ Right Size? No ☐ Yes ☐ Dressed in?_____
11. ☐☐	**A.** Describe location where child was found (bed, floor, yard, etc.). **B.** Describe anything unusual found on or around the body.

INSTRUCTIONS: Complete each numbered item by providing the appropriate response, and by marking the completed or <u>not</u> completed box in the left-hand margin. Make every attempt to obtain as much information as possible, use additional pages as necessary for comments section. For assistance, call 1-800-487-1626.

12. ❑ ❑	**A.** Body postion when discovered: on stomach ❑ on back ❑ seated upright ❑ left side ❑ right side ❑ **B.** Sketch postion of child and identify if in bed or other identification location (Indicate direction of child's head; cirlce one): N W E S
13. ❑ ❑	Photographs of child or silhouette taken by: _____ Time: _____ Date: _____
14. ❑ ❑	Anything covering nose or mouth? No ❑ Yes ❑
15. ❑ ❑	Material found in nose? No ❑ Yes ❑ Unknown ❑ Appears to be: Mucus ❑ Vomit ❑ Bloody Froth ❑ Blood Tinged Secretion ❑ Food ❑ Saliva ❑ Dried Secretion ❑ Other _____ ❑ Formula ❑ Froth ❑
16. ❑ ❑	Material found in mouth? No ❑ Yes ❑ Unknown ❑ Appears to be: Mucus ❑ Vomit ❑ Bloody Froth ❑ Blood Tinged Secretion ❑ Food ❑ Saliva ❑ Dried Secretion ❑ Other _____ ❑ Formula ❑ Froth ❑
17. ❑ ❑	Secretions noted on following? Pillow ❑ Blanket ❑ Sheet ❑ Mattress ❑ Appears to be: Clothing ❑ Other _____ ❑ Mucus ❑ Vomit ❑ Bloody Froth ❑ Blood Tinged Secretion ❑ Food ❑ Saliva ❑ Dried Secretion ❑ Other _____ ❑ Formula ❑ Froth ❑ Urine or Stool ❑ Childs face in contact with wet materials? No ❑ Yes ❑
18. ❑ ❑	Resuscitation attempted? No ❑ Yes ❑ Unknown ❑ Who?_____
19. ❑ ❑	Name, age, marital status, employment and health status of natural parents? Mother (include maiden name): _____ Employer:_____ Father: _____ Employer:_____
20. ❑ ❑	Who does child live with if different than parent?
21. ❑ ❑	If parents employed, who babysits?
22. ❑ ❑	Do siblings ever watch child or could they have accidentally injured child without parents knowledge? No ❑ Yes ❑
23. ❑ ❑	Name, age and health status of siblings _____ _____ _____

24. ❑❑	Who are the child's regular playmates?_____
	_____
	_____
	_____
25. ❑❑	When was the child last seen alive; by whom?
26. ❑❑	What was the condition of the child at the time?
27. ❑❑	What was the child's activity at the time of death?
28. ❑❑	If sleeping, was the child sleeping alone? No ❑ Yes ❑ If no, who was child sleeping with?
29. ❑❑	Who found child?
30. ❑❑	Medical assistance summoned? No ❑ Yes ❑ By who? _____
31. ❑❑	Was baby moved from original position? No ❑ Yes ❑ Why?
32. ❑❑	Was death witnessed? No ❑ Yes ❑ Fully describe details in narrative section.
33. ❑❑	Conveyed to medical facility? No ❑ Yes ❑ By who? _____
	Name and address of facility _____
34. ❑❑	Who pronounced child dead? _____
35. ❑❑	When had child last eaten? _____What?
36. ❑❑	Any known food intolerance? No ❑ Yes ❑ What? Poor feeder? No ❑ Yes ❑
37. ❑❑	Has child had an illness within the last two weeks? No ❑ Yes ❑ Since when?
	Appetite Changes ❑ Wheezes ❑ Fussy ❑ Sniffles ❑ Cough ❑
	Fever ❑ How high? _____ Diarrhea ❑ Cold ❑
	Irritablility ❑ Runny Nose ❑ Congestion ❑ Other:_____ ❑
38. ❑❑	Was child taken for treatment for above symptoms? No ❑ Yes ❑ Where? _____
	If yes, what diagnosis was rendered?
39. ❑❑	Has child been under routine care of a pediatrician? No ❑ Yes ❑ Who? _____
40. ❑❑	Has child been on medication? No ❑ Yes ❑ What? _____
41. ❑❑	Child visits/immunizations received: No ❑ Yes ❑
	If yes, physician's name/clinic:_____
42. ❑❑	Any known allergies or any known reaction ot shots or medications? No ❑ Yes ❑
	If yes, explain: _____
43. ❑❑	Has child been exposed to any contagious disease recently? No ❑ Yes ❑
	If yes, explain: _____
44. ❑❑	What pets are in house?
45. ❑❑	Has family traveled recently? Where?
	PRENATAL HISTORY
46. ❑❑	Regular prenatal visits? No ❑ Yes ❑ Number: Where:
47. ❑❑	Known complications of pregnancy? No ❑ Yes ❑
	Explain:
48. ❑❑	Special diet during pregnancy? No ❑ Yes ❑ What?
49. ❑❑	Maternal alcohol or street drugs: No ❑ Yes ❑ Uknown ❑
	Alcohol cocaine Heroin Marijuana Other:

50. ☐☐ Maternal smoking during pregnancy?   No ☐   Yes ☐   Unknown ☐   Packs per day:_____
How many other adults in household smoking _____

51. ☐☐ Known maternal health problems? (Diabetes, hypertension, etc.)   No ☐   Yes ☐
If yes, please describe:
_____
_____

52. ☐☐ Was mother taking prescription medication for above medical condition?   No ☐   Yes ☐   What? _____

BIRTH HISTORY

53. ☐☐ What hospital: _____Difficulty with delivery?   No ☐   Yes ☐
What type of delivery: _____

54. ☐☐ Birth weight: _____   Apgar Scores at 1 and 5 minutes? _____   Gestational age or full term?_____

55. ☐☐ Birth defects or other abnormalities of child at birth?

56. ☐☐ Number of previous pregnancies and outcome?

ENVIRONMENTAL AND SOCIOECONOMIC CONDITIONS

57. ☐☐ Conditions of residence: _____   Overcrowding   No ☐   Yes ☐
Describe:

58. ☐☐ Quality of dwelling?   Below average   Average   Above average   Other:

59. ☐☐ Unusual conditions seen?   No ☐   Yes ☐   If yes, explain:

60. ☐☐ Number of children living at this address?   Number of adults living at this address:

61. ☐☐ Building Type: _____   Neighborhood Type:_____

62. ☐☐ Welfare: No ☐   Yes ☐   Monthly Amount $ _____   Food Stamp Amount: $ _____
WIC Program?   No ☐   Yes ☐

63. ☐☐ Estimated family income per year:

Less than $5,000 _____ $5,000 to $10,000 _____ $10,000 to $20,000 _____ $20,000 to $25,000_____
$25,000 to $30,000_____ $30,000 to $35,000 _____   Over $35,000 _____

64. ☐☐ **REMINDER**: Has this family been hotlined in the past for abuse or neglect?   No ☐   Yes ☐
If yes, describe known details in narrative section.

65. ☐☐ Have appropriate medical records, including birth record, been requested?   No ☐   Yes ☐

66. ☐☐ Maternal smoking during pregnancy?   No ☐   Yes ☐   Unknown ☐   Packs per day:
How many other adults in household smoking _____

67. ☐☐ Additional Comments (to include names and pedigrees of all persons and responders at scene):

_____
_____
_____
_____
_____

NOTE: Use additional pages as necessary.

Signature of Investigator _____   Date _____

ROLE, RESPONSIBILITY AND AUTHORITY OF THE
DIVISION OF FAMILY SERVICES

The Missouri Division of Family Services (DFS) has statutory responsibility and authority for accepting and investigating all reports of child abuse and neglect of children under age 18, as defined in RSMo Chapter 210.

Each report shall be immediately communicated to the local county office and shall contain information on previous reports on the alleged victim, siblings, or the alleged perpetrator, and relevant dispositional information regarding the previous reports.

Upon receipt of a report that, if true, would constitute a violation of section 568.060 (sexual abuse, serious physical abuse or child endangerment), the local DFS office shall contact the appropriate law enforcement agency. DFS will provide them with a detailed description of the report received and request their assistance in all aspects of the investigation. Within a reasonable length of time, the local DFS office shall provide information to the local prosecuting attorney regarding the agency's involvement with the law enforcement agency involved in the co-investigation.

The local DFS office shall cause a thorough investigation to be initiated immediately or no later than within 24 hours of the receipt of the report. If the report indicates that the child is in danger of serious physical harm or child's life is threatened, the investigation shall include immediate direct observation of the alleged victim. All alleged victims must be seen within 24 hours. If the only allegation is educational neglect and if there is no suspicion of any other type of abuse or neglect, the investigation must be initiated within 72 hours of the report.

When a mandated reporter makes a hotline report, the local DFS office shall contact the mandated reporter within 48 hours of the receipt of the report in order to ensure that full information has been received and to obtain any additional information or medical records that may be pertinent. The mandated reporter shall be informed of his right to obtain information on the general disposition of his report, upon his request.

If DFS determines that a report was made maliciously or for the purpose of harassment, the local office shall refer the report and any evidence of malice or harassment to the local prosecuting attorney.

At the time of the initial investigation, the DFS employee conducting the investigation shall provide the alleged perpetrator with a written description of the investigation process.

If the investigation conducted by the local office reveals that the only basis for action involves a question of an alleged violation of section 167.031 RSMo. (which deals with home schooling), the report shall be sent to the school district in which the child resides.

Protective social services shall be provided by the local office to the victim(s) and his family to prevent further abuse or neglect, to safeguard their health and welfare, and to help preserve and stabilize the family whenever possible.

Multidisciplinary services shall be utilized whenever possible in making child abuse or neglect investigations and in providing protective social services. The Division shall cooperate with the highway patrol and juvenile courts to develop training programs for Division staff, juvenile officers, and law enforcement officers to assist them in conducting investigations.

The Division shall, on a continuing basis, undertake and maintain programs to inform all mandated reporters and the general public of the nature, problem, and extent of abuse and neglect, of the services available to children and their families, and to encourage self-reporting and the voluntary acceptance of such services. Those persons in professions which are mandated to report shall be informed of their duties, options, and responsibilities in making reports.

The Division shall conduct ongoing training programs in relation to the child abuse law for agency staff. This shall include not less than 40 hours of preservice training on the identification and treatment of child abuse and neglect, and not less than 20 hours of inservice training each year on the identification of child abuse and neglect. This training shall be prepared and offered by the Division in cooperation with an institution of higher learning in the state of Missouri which offers an accredited social work program.

The Division shall also continuously publicize to mandated reporters and to the public the existence and the number of the 24 hour, toll-free telephone service (800-392-3738).

As a result of its investigation, DFS shall report a child's injuries or disabilities which resulted from abuse or neglect to the juvenile office and may make such report to the appropriate law enforcement authority. Within 30 days of the report, the local office shall finalize the report and update the central registry with the outcome of the investigation.

All identifying information shall be retained by the Division for the following time frames:

— Court adjudicated reports shall be retained indefinitely, but are only available to appropriate law enforcement agencies and child death review panels after ten years from the date of the report or from the date a court substantiated the abuse or neglect.

— Reason to suspect reports are retained for ten years.

— Unsubstantiated reports are retained for five years and are only available to appropriate law enforcement agencies and child death review panels.

The local office shall notify, in writing, the alleged perpetrator and the parents of the child named in the report, the outcome of the investigation, how long the information shall be retained, and that the alleged perpetrator has 30 days to seek reversal of the Division's determination by a court appeal.

Other statutes (RSMo 207 and RSMo 211) charge the Division with the responsibility for serving the needs of Missouri's children by providing remedial treatment services and, where needed, alternative placement outside the family home when such placement is in the best interest of protecting the child.

STATE OF MISSOURI
CHILD ABUSE AND NEGLECT HOTLINE
1-800-392-3738

The Division shall maintain a toll-free, statewide telephone number which operates at all times, and which is capable of accepting reports pursuant to Chapter 210. The Division shall maintain a central registry capable of receiving and maintaining reports in a manner that facilitates rapid access to the information. Anonymous reports may be accepted, but Division staff shall attempt to obtain the name and address of the person making the report.

The Child Abuse and Neglect Hotline is staffed by experienced and trained employees of the Division of Family Services (DFS) who receive calls of suspected child abuse or neglect.

When a person calls the Hotline, the DFS social worker:

- Interviews the reporter (caller) to determine the following:

    — Is the alleged victim under age 18 years of age?

    — Does the alleged perpetrator have care, custody or control of the child (e.g., parent, caretaker, etc.)?

    — Has the alleged victim been injured or adversely affected by action or inaction of the caretaker?

    — Names, addresses or other information which will allow DFS to identify, locate and interview the alleged victim, family and alleged perpetrator.

- If these criteria are met, the report will be accepted as a child abuse and neglect report, and the Hotline social worker will forward it to the county DFS office where the alleged incident occurred. During the interview with the reporter, the social worker taking the hotline call will ask if the child is in immediate danger.

- If these criteria are not met, an official child abuse and neglect report is not taken. However, in some cases where the child has been assaulted by a person not having care, custody or control, the information will be taken and referred to the DFS county office for discussion with law enforcement or the juvenile court.

The abuse and neglect of Missouri children is cause for concern and action. Child abuse prevention cannot be accomplished by one individual or agency. Collaboration and a community-wide coalition that includes both the public and private sectors is critical. When you suspect child abuse or neglect, it is important that you report it promptly so that, if abuse or neglect is occurring, it can be addressed before it escalates into a tragic incident.

THE ROLE AND RESPONSIBILITIES OF LAW ENFORCEMENT AND THE CORONER/MEDICAL EXAMINER

Law enforcement officers are often the first responders to events where child abuse and neglect has or may be occurring. As mandated reporters, officers should evaluate and investigate all circumstances where abuse or neglect is a possibility.

Law enforcement shall (RSMo 566, 568 & 573, et al):

- Determine if the child is in immediate danger or risk, necessitating emergency removal from the home or caregiver.

- Establish the presence of criminality.

- If child abuse or neglect is suspected, report the allegation to the DFS Central Registry (Child Abuse Hotline, 800-392-3738) or the local DFS office.

- Participate in co-investigations with DFS and multi-disciplinary teams, and:

  — when necessary, place children in protective custody;

  — investigate criminal allegations;

  — arrest perpetrators;

  — prepare appropriate reports and documents;

  — support prosecution and juvenile proceedings.

Coroner/Medical Examiners are responsible for determining the cause and manner of death of ALL persons who die due to sudden, unexplained and/or suspicious circumstances. The Child Fatality Review Project (section 210.193, et al) adds specific requirements regarding deaths of children under 15 years of age. The coroner/medical examiner shall:

- Obtain reports of ALL deaths of children birth through age 14.

- Confer with a certified child-death pathologist to determine the need for an autopsy.

  NOTE: Infants one week to one year of age that die suddenly and unexplained, must be autopsied.

- Evaluate the known circumstance of death, and if they match the established criteria, refer the case to the local child fatality review panel.

- Coordinate with law enforcement and the multi-disciplinary panel members to facilitate the death investigation.

- Prepare death certificates and other forms (including the CFRP Form 1) as required by law.

EXCERPTS FROM MISSOURI LAWS RELATING to CHILD ABUSE AND NEGLECT

CHILD ABUSE

210.110. Definitions.-As used in sections 210.110 to 210.165, unless the context clearly indicates otherwise, the following terms mean:

(1) **"Abuse"**, any physical injury, sexual abuse, or emotional abuse inflicted on a child other than by accidental means by those responsible for his care, custody, and control except that discipline including spanking, administered in a reasonable manner shall not be construed to be abuse;

(2) **"Child"**, any person, regardless of physical or mental condition, under eighteen years of age;

(3) **"Director"**, the director of the Missouri division of family services;

(4) **"Division"**, the Missouri division of family services;

(5) **"Neglect"**, failure to provide, by those responsible for the care, custody, and control of the child, the proper or necessary support, education as required by law, nutrition or medical, surgical, or any other care necessary for his well-being; and

(6) **"Those responsible for the care, custody, and control of the child"**, those included but not limited to the parents or guardian of a child, other members of the child's household, or those exercising supervision over a child for any part of a twenty-four hour day.

(L 1975 H.B. 578 § 1, A.L. 1982 H.B. 1171, 1173, 1306 & 1643, A.L. 1985 H.B. 366, et al.)

210.125. Protective custody of child, who may take, reports required-temporary protective custody defined.—1. A police officer, law enforcement official, or a physician who has reasonable cause to suspect that a child is suffering from illness or injury or is in danger of personal harm by reason of his surroundings and that a case of child abuse or neglect exists, may request that the juvenile officer take the child into protective custody under chapter 211.RSMo.

2. A police officer, law enforcement official, or a physician who has reasonable cause to believe that a child is in imminent danger of suffering serious physical harm or a threat to life as a result of abuse or neglect and such person has reasonable cause to believe the harm or threat to life may occur before a juvenile court could issue a temporary protective custody order or before a juvenile officer could take the child into protective custody, the police officer, law enforcement official or physician may take or retain temporary protective custody of the child without the consent of the child's parents, guardian or others legally responsible for his care.

3. Any person taking a child in protective custody under this section shall immediately notify the juvenile officer of the court of the county in which the child is located of his actions and notify the division and make a reasonable attempt to advise the parents, guardians or others legally responsible for the child's care. The jurisdiction of the juvenile court attaches from the time the juvenile is taken into protective custody. Such person shall file, as soon as practicable but no later than twelve hours, a written statement with the juvenile officer which sets forth the identity of the child and the facts and circumstances which gave such person reasonable cause to believe that there was imminent danger of serious physical harm or threat to the life of the child. Upon notification that a child has been taken into protective custody, the juvenile officer shall either return the child to his parents, guardian, or others responsible for his care or shall initiate child protective proceedings under chapter 211, RSMo. In no event shall an employee of the division, acting upon his own, remove a child under the provisions of this act.*

4. Temporary protective custody for purposes of section shall not exceed twenty-four hours. Temporary protective custody for a period beyond twenty-four hours may be authorized only by an order of the juvenile court.

5. For the purposes of this section, **"temporary protective custody"**, shall mean temporary placement within a hospital or medical facility or emergency foster care facility or such other suitable custody placement as the court may direct; provided, however, that an abused or neglected child may not be detained in temporary custody in a secure detention facility.

(L. 1975 H.B. 578 § 4, A.L. 1982 H.B. 1171, 1173, 1306 & 1643)
*Original rolls contain words "this act". This act, H.B. 1171, 1173, 1306 & 1643 contained numerous sections. See Disposition of Sections Table, Vol V.

210.140 Privileged communications not recognized, exception.—Any legally recognized privileged communication, except that between attorney and client, shall not apply to situations involving known or suspected child abuse or neglect and shall not constitute grounds for failure to report as required or permitted by sections 210.110 to 210.165, to cooperate with the division in any of its activities pursuant to sections 210.110 to 210.165, or to give or accept evidence in any judicial proceeding relating to child abuse or neglect.

(L. 1975 H.B. 578 § 7, A.L. 1980 S. B. 574).

210.145.

5. Upon receipt of a report pursuant to sections 210.110 to 210.165, which, if true, would constitute violation of section 568.060, RSMo, the local office shall contact the appropriate law enforcement agency and provide such agency with a detailed description of the report received. In such cases, the local division office shall request the assistance of the local law enforcement agency in all aspects of the investigation of the complaint. The local division office making such a request shall within a reasonable time report in writing the following information to the local prosecuting or circuit attorney:

9. Multidisciplinary services shall be utilized whenever possible in making the investigation and in providing protective social services, including the service of the juvenile officer, the juvenile court, and other agencies, both public and private. The division shall cooperate with the highway patrol and juvenile courts to develop training programs to increase the ability of division personnel, juvenile officers and law enforcement officers to investigate suspected cases of abuse and neglect.

568.045. Endangering the welfare of a child, in the first degree--1. A person commits the crime of endangering the welfare of a child in the first degree if he knowingly acts in a manner that creates a substantial risk to the life, body, or health of a child less than seventeen years old.

2. Endangering the welfare of a child in the first degree is a class D felony unless the offense is committed as part of a ritual or ceremony, in which case the crime is a class C felony.
(L 1990 H.B. 1370, et al.)

568.050. Endangering the welfare of a child in the second degree.--1. A person commits the crime of endangering the welfare of a child in the second degree if:
(1) He with criminal negligence acts in a manner that creates substantial risk to the life, body or health of a child less than seventeen years old; or
(2) He knowingly encourages, aids or causes a child less than seventeen years old to engage in any conduct which causes or tends to cause the child to come within the provisions of paragraph (d) of subdivision (2) of subsection 1 or subdivision (3) of subsection 1 of section 211.031, RSMo; or
(3) Being a parent, guardian or other person legally charged with the care or custody of a child less than seventeen years old, he recklessly fails or refuses to exercise reasonable diligence in the care or control of such child to prevent him from coming within the provisions of paragraph (c) of subdivision (1) of subsection 1 or paragraph (d) of subdivision (2) of subsection 1 or subdivision (3) of subsection 211.031, RSMo; or (4) He know-

ingly encourages, aids or causes a child less than seventeen years of age to enter into any room, building or other structure which is a public nuisance as defined in section 195.130 RSMo.

2. Nothing in this section shall be construed to mean the welfare of a child is endangered for the sole reason that he is being provided nonmedical remedial treatment recognized and permitted under the laws of this state.

3. Endangering the welfare of a child in the second degree is a class A misdemeanor unless the offense is committed as part of a ritual or ceremony, in which case the crime is a class D felony.
(L. 1977 S.B. 60, A.L. 1984 H.B. 1616, A.L. 1988 H.B. 1340 & 1348 A.L. 1990 H.B. 1030 and H.B. 1370, et al.)

CHILD DEATH REVIEW TEAMS

210.192. Child death review team to investigate deaths--qualifications--prosecutors and circuit attorneys to organize--report on investigations--immunity from civil liability--program for prevention. 1. the prosecuting attorney or the circuit attorney shall impanel a child death review team for the county of city not within a county in which he serves to investigate the deaths of children under the age of fifteen years of age. The team shall be formed and shall operate according to the rules, guidelines and protocols provided by the department of social services.

210.194. Teams, coroners and medical examiners--rules authorized for protocol and identifying suspicious deaths.--2. The director shall promulgate guidelines and protocols for coroners and medical examiners to use to help them to identify suspicious deaths of children under the age of fifteen years.

**CHILD SEXUAL ABUSE CASES
TRAINING--INVESTIGATION--TREATMENT**

660.520. Special team for child sexual abuse cases, assist in training, investigation, and prosecution--counties may develop team, members--division of family service duties.--1. There is hereby established in the department of social services a special team which shall: (1) Provide training, expertise and assistance to county multidisciplinary teams for the investigation and prosecution of child sexual abuse cases; (2) Assist in the investigation of child sexual abuse cases, upon the request of local law enforcement agencies, prosecutors, or division of family services staff; (3) Assist county multidisciplinary teams to develop and implement protocols for the investigation and prosecution of child sexual abuse cases.

660.523. Uniform rules for investigation of child sexual abuse cases--training provided for division of family services staff.--2. The department of social

services shall develop separate protocols for multiple-suspect and multiple-victim cases.
(L. 1190 H.B. 1370, et al. § 2)

REFER TO LATEST EDITION OF THE MISSOURI REVISED STATUTES CUMULATIVE SUPPLEMENT FOR COMPLETE STATUTE REVIEW.

VICTIM INTERVIEW TECHNIQUES

PREPARING FOR THE INTERVIEW:

If a child abuse/neglect case, contact the reporter for additional information.

Gather background information on the victim including (do not contact alleged perpetrators to gain this information):

■ Victim's age, grade level
■ Victim's level of physical, mental and emotional development
■ Ability to read, write, count and recall events
■ Any physical or behavioral problems
■ Knowledge of anatomy and sexual behavior
■ Family terminology for genital areas if sexual abuse alleged (may be obtained from family members if not suspected to be the offender)
■ Family composition and stability
■ Relationship between victim and offender (if known)
■ Length of time involved with offender (if known)
■ Past history of abuse or neglect

Gather background information on the alleged perpetrator including:

■ Arrest record
■ Criminal history
■ Other relevant information

NECESSARY ACTION:

■ Ensure the child's safety.
■ Determine if emergency medical attention is needed.
■ Arrange for medical exam when physical or sexual abuse alleged. If there is any physical evidence (clothing, etc.) don't allow the child to change or bathe until examined by physician.
■ Notify parents.

SETTING:

■ Should occur in a safe, non-threatening neutral environment, not where alleged abuse took place.

■ Should be conducted in private, with no outside distractions or interruptions.

■ Interviewing tools should be present (dolls, drawings, paper, crayons, doll house, etc.)

INTERVIEW TECHNIQUES:

■ Don't interview young children if they are hungry, sleepy or otherwise physically uncomfortable. Be aware of their eating and sleep schedules.

■ Keep questions and sentences simple.

■ Relate to the child on his/her developmental level.

■ Use words that are familiar to the child.

■ Do not assume that your meaning of a word is the same as the child's.

■ Be careful using pronouns (like he or she) and words like "there" and "that". The child may be unable to follow your meaning.

■ Be careful with touching and inappropriate posturing of your body.

■ Don't use the child's or the interviewer's body parts to evaluate the child's knowledge of anatomy.

■ Be careful of non-verbal communication (i.e., touching, facial expressions, eye contact, posture, hand gesturing, body distance).

■ Be aware of the child's non-verbal communication.

■ Avoid why questions...they imply blame.

■ Guard against using leading gestures and questions.

■ Minimize size differential between investigator and child by getting on the same physical level as the child.

■ Allow the child time to respond.

■ Allow enough time to conduct the interview.

■ Reassure the child that you believe him/her and that they are not to blame for what has happened.

■ Tell the child it's okay to answer "I don't know" or "I don't understand," rather than guess.

■ Do not make promises that you may be unable to keep.

INTERVIEW:

■ Introduce yourself to the child. Give a simple explanation of your job.

■ Take time to establish rapport with the child.

Some sample questions (general):

■ What is your name?
■ How old are you?
■ Where do you live?
■ What is your mother's name?
■ What is your father's name?
■ Who lives with you? visits you?
■ What school do you go to?
■ What grade are you in?
■ What is your favorite subject? least favorite?
■ What is your teacher's name?
■ Who was your teacher last year?
■ Have the child recall past events (other than the abuse incidents).
■ What makes you happy? sad? mad? scared?
■ What do you like best about the people you live with? least?
■ What kind of things do you like to do alone?

Some sample questions (specific):

(NOTE: It is best to ask as few direct questions as possible. When a child begins to disclose, you may prompt them with questions such as: What happened next? What else do you remember? What else do I need to know? Could you tell me what you mean by? I need to understand a little more here.)

■ Where did it happen?
■ When did it happen? Time of day? Month? Year? With a younger child you may need to link this with the clothes they were wearing, before or after a meal, TV show, the weather, etc.
■ Who was there?
■ What did he or she do?
■ Did he or she touch you? Where?
■ Did you touch him or her? What part of your body touched him or her?
■ What did he touch you with? (May be an object.)
■ Did he or she hurt you?
■ What were you wearing? What was offender wearing?
■ What happened to your clothes? Offender's clothes?
■ What did he or she say?
■ Did you say anything to him or her?
■ Did anyone take pictures?

- Where are the pictures?
- Did he or she ask you not to tell anyone? (Use of threats or bribes.)
- Did anyone see you?
- Did you tell anyone?
- Has this happened before? When? Where? (If sexual abuse alleged, look for grooming and events leading up to the act.)
- Did this happen to anybody else?
- What is his name?
- How do you know him or her?
- Was anyone else at home? Where were they?
- Was anyone else in the room when this happened?
- Has anyone else done this to you?

RISK ASSESSMENT:

Assessment of whether the child is at risk should be an ongoing process during the course of the investigation. Possible factors to consider include:

- Was the child physically abused and/or neglected?
- Does the child have a prior history of abuse?
- How severe was the abuse? How frequent? How recent?
- Was the child coerced? force or threats used?
- Does the child have a support system?
- How vulnerable is the child?
- What is the child's age? Look at mental, emotional and physical development.
- Is the child fearful or unwilling to remain in the home?
- Does the alleged perpetrator still have access to the victim?

ENDING THE INTERVIEW:

- Ask the child if he/she has any questions and answer honestly.

- Comfort the child without making unreasonable promises.

- Ask the child what he or she expects will happen and explain what will happen next.

- State whether there will be further contacts or interviews. (If additional interviews are needed, remember it is less traumatic for the child to use the same interviewer.)

- If the child has not revealed any abuse, you may wish to refer them to a qualified person for education or awareness discussions.

- If prosecution is a possibility, counseling, therapy or other abuse-related discussions could be destructive to the case. Discuss with the prosecutor.

WITNESS INTERVIEWING GUIDELINES

BASIC REQUIREMENTS OF WITNESSES:

Some of the more important factors which must be considered by the investigator conducting an interview are discussed below. However, before attempting to weigh their effect upon the witness' story, the interviewer first must determine that the witness meets the three essential requirements of a witness:

- That he/she was present during the event or a portion of it.
- That he/she was conscious (awake) of what was happening.
- That he/she was attentive to what was happening. This final element is the most difficult to establish.

All witnesses must be properly identified in the investigator's notes and reports.

- Correct spelling of witness' name.
- Telephone - both work and home.
- Home address - the apartment number, floor and location (front or rear).
- Dates of birth and social security numbers.
- Other contact person: Name, address, phone (both work and home).

Attempt to interview the witness away from other witnesses or alleged perpetrator(s).

Interviews should take place as soon as possible after the event has occurred so that witness' stories are not affected by memory loss, influenced by talking to others, etc. Immediate gathering of information enables the investigator to prepare for interrogation of alleged perpetrator(s).

WHERE TO INTERVIEW THE WITNESS:

- At a place convenient and familiar to the subject.
- In a neutral setting. (The most undesirable place for a witness interview is at the police station.)
- Any other place where privacy is assured.

METHOD OF INTERVIEWING:

- Interview should be low pressure and conducted in an informal atmosphere.
- Allow subject first to tell what happened or what they observed in a narrative style.
- Specific questions should be used to gather more detail and to jog the witness' memory.

- Ask the witness for the correct spelling of names and for the addresses and phone numbers of other persons they talked about.
- Ask if there is anything that you (the investigator) failed to ask.
- Ask if there is anything else they (the witness) want to discuss.

Never tell the witness that by talking now they will not have to appear in court.

At the end of the interview tell the witness that you do not have any more questions, but as the investigation continues, you may need to talk to them about new information or clarify what they have just told you. Encourage the witness to contact you with any additional information.

If the interview involves a child, refer to "Victim Interview Techniques" for suggested techniques and procedures.

You must remain focused on the event/injury you are investigating. Keep your questions directed toward the alleged offense. Never assume guilt or innocence. Every event should be evaluated and investigated on its own merits.

INTERVIEWING ALLEGED PERPETRATORS

FOREWORD:

Always follow your local dictates. Procedures or practices should be guided by your department's rules and regulations and applicable local, state and federal laws. A background check on those involved can be valuable.

INTERVIEW PREPARATION:

An interview is simply the process of one person obtaining information from another person by the question and answer method.

- Communicate your thoughts clearly and accurately.
- Do not display bias in your non-verbal communication.
- Be professional.
- Gather as much background information as possible prior to interviewing the alleged perpetrator:
  - Criminal history
  - Social history
  - Medical history
  - Driving record
  - Credit history
  - Family, friends, hobbies, likes, dislikes and personal history
  - Read original reports (e.g., police, etc.)
  - Check with other professionals - (e.g., social worker, etc.)

- Make sure you know the offense and what happened to the victim.
- Revisit the scene.
- Review photographs.
- All interviews **must** be conducted in a **private**, comfortable and non-threatening environment.
- You may want to use the control of cigarette smoking, restroom breaks, soda refreshments, use of telephone, etc. as a tool to enhance communication.

Remember, most of the time the person being interviewed is looking for help or a release from their guilt. They are remorseful if you can trigger the correct emotional response.

INTERVIEW

- Introduce yourself.
- State the reason for the interview.
- Be candid, honest and polite. You are setting the stage. <u>First impressions are lasting impressions. Shake the person's hand</u>.
- If two interviewers are present, one should conduct the interview. The other interviewer may take notes and show support by displaying positive gestures.
- If dealing with a person in custody, begin your interview with the Miranda Rights.
- Advise them of Miranda and obtain signed and dated waiver. Let this be guided by your policy and procedure.
- If the person starts making incriminating statements and has not been previously advised, you should advise them of their Miranda Rights and then continue on with your interview.
- Look for their verbal and non-verbal responses.
- Treat this person like a <u>human being</u>. Use empathy.
- During the interview process you are building rapport. Show understanding. Do not exhibit feelings of anger or disgust.
- Let the offender talk about themselves.
- Pay attention to their fantasies and their dreams.
- Display through your actions and words that you are interested in the offender as a person.
- Help the suspect look at the problem with a lowered level of personal threat, i.e., "I understand how these things can happen, sometimes we just lose control," etc.
- Appeal to the person's emotions. You may want to show photos of the victim. Don't allow the suspect to show disrespect for the victim.
- You may want to say things like this to an alleged perpetrator:
- How did it feel when_____?
- How do you feel when _____?
- Do you like _____?
- When dealing with the subject, don't ask the direct question, "Did you do it?"
- Keep in mind you must obtain: Who, What, When, Where, Why, and How if possible.
- Provide a face-saving situation for alleged perpetrator, if applicable.
- Distinguish between denials and objections. Guilty people often object; innocent people use denial or profess guilt.
- Don't take objections personally.
- Recognize the importance of attending to verbal and non-verbal cues.
- If you are going for criminal prosecution, you need to look beyond probable cause to reasonable doubt.
- Encourage openness by sharing <u>non-critical</u> information about the suspect or case.
- Be attentive at all times. (Really listen. Maintain eye contact.)
- Be patient; make sure you have scheduled sufficient time for the interview.
- To lower the threat, emphasize positive characteristics to bolster his/her ego. Be open minded and empathize with the weaknesses and defects of the suspect.
- Always ask if they photographed, video-taped, etc., if applicable.
- Always ask if drugs or alcohol were used.

■ Consult with your prosecuting attorney during the investigative process.

■ Talk on the same communication level as the person you are interviewing. Don't use big words or difficult words to impress or embarrass the other person.

■ Don't be judgmental.

■ Use reflective listening - mirror back to the person what they said.

■ Don't let your personal feelings or emotions control your action or reactions to the investigation.

■ Close the interview on a cooperative note. Remember you are the <u>professional</u>.

Special Note:

The use of videotape and tape recording has been purposely omitted. You may want to use these as monitoring devices. Follow your local dictates and check with the prosecutor.

BASIC SCENE PHOTOGRAPHY

The purpose of crime/incident scene photography is to provide a photograph to record the facts and offer viewers a better understanding of the scene. Photographs should show how the crime was committed, the manner in which particular evidence is related to the incident or crime and the setting in which the crime/incident occurred.

NOTE: Whenever possible, evidence should be photographed <u>before</u> seizing.

IDENTIFYING THE PHOTOGRAPH:

Use plain sheet of paper or Photo ID Card that includes:

- Case #
- Victim
- Location
- Date and time
- Name of person taking the picture
- Remarks

NOTE: This Photo ID should be the first picture taken on each role of film. This identifies the role of film to this particular case. Each time you change location use a new Photo ID Card to show the new location, i.e., front living room, left rear bedroom, etc. It is desirable to take pictures with and without Photo ID cards.

GENERAL VIEW:

- Front of building (showing house numbers) or other location.
- Landmark, i.e., street signs, etc.
- Terrain adjoining scene.
- Overall view of each room, show all sides.
- Environmental photo showing current living conditions.

MEDIUM VIEW:

- These pictures show specific objects with relationship to the rest of the room.
- A measuring device to show relative size is also suggested.

CLOSE-UPS:

- Close-ups are photographs of individual items or small sections of a larger surface; i.e., weapon, bullet holes, blood, etc.
- Measuring device used on each photo
- Different angles
  <u>Always have a medical person or family member remove the clothing of children or other victims if photographs are to be taken of private body parts. Witnesses should always be present. Use extreme discretion before taking evidence photographs of the genitalia.</u>

NOTE: DFS has specific policy concerning photographing private body parts.

FIELD USE SUMMARY:

- Photo slate or ID.
- General view of location exterior.
- Point of entry - a medium view shows actual point of entry.
- General view of the interior (all rooms).
- Overall view of the scene and adjacent area.
- Medium and close-up photographs of the victim taken from various angles, including overhead shots.
- Close-up photographs of all wounds with instrument of death visible (if known) while the body is in its original position.
- If body has been removed, use cutouts or other marker to show body location.
- Medium range and close-ups of blood stains, fire marking, broken furniture, bullet holes and other evidence.
- The object pictured must be material or relevant to the point in issue.
- The photograph must be free from distortion and not misrepresent the scene or the object it purports to reproduce.

The investigating person has the responsibility to direct the photographer at the scene. The pictures should set the scene, provide information concerning the manner in which the incident occurred and may show whether the incident was connected to another crime or was a deliberate act.

NOTE: YOU HAVE ONLY ONE CHANCE TO GET AN INITIAL SCENE COMPLETELY PHOTOGRAPHED. BE SURE TO TAKE PLENTY OF PHOTOGRAPHS.

Photo ID Cards also provide space on the back for drawing a rough scene sketch. Sketches provide a record of each item photographed in relation to its location from known points, and makes the report more complete. Photo ID Cards should be kept with the photo negatives as part of the case evidence.

HANDLING EXPOSED AND DEVELOPED FILM:

- Indicate on Photo Log where and when film was developed and printed.

- Developed prints should be dated, appropriately marked (to correspond with the photo log) and signed by the photographer.

FIGURE 1.
Coordinate method of a rough sketch using a base line

FIGURE 2.
Coordinate method of a rough sketch using fixed points

FIGURE 3.
Rough sketch

FIGURE 4.
Finished projection sketch

ALWAYS INDICATE THE DIRECTION OF NORTH

BASIC SCENE SKETCHING AND INVESTIGATIVE NOTE TAKING

SKETCHES:

■ Sketches and properly prepared notes may be useful to the investigator as a reference in questioning witnesses, suspects and victim(s); in preparing the investigation reports; and for refreshing memory when presenting information in court. They are also very useful when used in combination with scene photographs.

■ A Sketch is used to portray graphically the scene of an incident or crime and items within the scene that are of interest to the investigation. Several methods may be used to establish the location of evidence and other important items on a sketch.

COORDINATE METHOD:

■ In one form of the coordinate method, a base line is drawn between two known fixed points on the sketch (fig. 1). A measurement is then made from left to right along the base line to a point from which a vertical line at right angles to the base line may be projected to the object that is to be plotted. The distance on the base line is indicated in the legend in parentheses following the name of the object. The distance from the point on the base line to the object is measured and recorded next to the dotted line that is inserted from the base line to the object.

■ In another more accurate form of the coordinate method, measurements of the distances of an object from two (2) known fixed points are made (fig. 2).

■ Each sketch should incorporate the following elements:

  • Reasonably accurate measurements.
  • Relative locations of objects of interest.
  • Measurement verified by an assistant before its insertion.
  • A conventional system of consistent measurement (English or metric system). Paces or steps to do not represent accurate measurements and should be avoided.
  • The compass direction of North.
  • A legend that explains all symbols or letters used to identify objects on the sketch.
  • The scale, if drawn to scale.
  • A title block that includes the following:
    – Report or incident number
    – Name of victim(s) or the scene portrayed
    – Location of the scene
    – Date and hour sketch started and completed
    – Name of the person(s) who made the sketch

The Photo ID Card has space on the back for drawing a rough scene sketch. Sketches provide a record of each item photographed in relation to its location from known points, and makes the report more complete.

A new ID Photo Card should be used each time you change location.

EXAMPLE: You move from the front living room to the left rear bedroom. A new Photo ID Card should be completed showing current room location. The photographer should take a photograph of the ID card first, capturing on film an indicator of the next set of photographs to follow.

By using this method, you will have a complete scene record which can easily be reconstructed later.

If circumstances do not allow for a detailed sketch, prepare a rough sketch without measurements, based on contents and/or other fixed objects (fig. 4).

SCENE RECONSTRUCTION USING DOLLS AND SILHOUETTES

When appropriate, the death scene of an infant or child can be recreated to document specific facts relevant to the investigation (e.g., body positioning, location of body relative to other objects; location of injuries or other marks on the body).

INFANT DOLLS - When appropriate, infant death scenes can be recreated using a life-like toy doll with moveable arms, legs and head. Based on the parents/caregivers recollection of how the infant was found, the doll can be used to accurately reconstruct the scene at the time of death. Photographs can permanently record the recreated scene.

NOTE: The doll should be introduced to the parent/caregiver as a "toy," and every effort should be made to not personalize the object, or infer that it represents a "baby."

PAPER SILHOUETTES - Water resistant paper silhouettes come in various sizes to represent different age groups (infant, child and adult). While they are single dimensional, silhouettes can be used to recreate death or other event scenes when it is important to record body position and other factors relevant to the scene investigation.

To indicate injuries, marks or other information, use a wide-line marking pen. As silhouettes are disposable, they may be used at trauma scenes if the victim has been removed prior to scene processing.

LAW ENFORCEMENT
CHILD ABUSE/NEGLECT INTERVIEW SUMMARY

Location:_____Date:_____Time:_____

_____D.O.B._____
Last Name   First   Middle

Physical Appearance: _____

_____

Eating Schedule:_____Nap time:_____

Persons Present: _____

_____

DFS Present: Yes_____No _____   Notified: Yes____No____

Interviewer(s): _____

Allegations:_____

_____

Victim's name for body parts (if sexual abuse):

Penis_____Vagina_____Anus/Rectum_____

Child's name for abuse: _____

Interview tools used:

Anatomical Dolls_____Drawings _____Other_____

Date and Time of Last Incident: _____

Incident Address: _____

Frequency: _____

Other Reports: _____

Who did child reveal this to? _____

Any evidence identified by victim?   Yes____No____

Explain: _____

Location of Evidence: _____

Photos or videos taken during abuse?   Yes_____No_____

When were the photos or evidence last seen and location? _____

Witness to the abuse:_____

Any other children involved? _____

Was protective custody taken? _____

Were audio/video recordings made? _____

LAW ENFORCEMENT
CHILD ABUSE/NEGLECT INVESTIGATION SUMMARY

Case Number _____Date/Time_____

Was this a DFS Referral from Local Office/Hotline?   Yes ____No ____

Hotline Investigator/Local Worker _____

If this is a caretaker abuse case, was DFS hotline made?   Yes _____No _____

Was the juvenile officer notified?   Yes _____No _____

CA/N check on Victim _____

CA/N check on Alleged Perpetrator _____

CA/N on other Family Members_____

If multi-victim and/or multi-perpetrator, was the State Technical Assistant Team contacted?
Yes _____ No _____

Was the county prosecutor notified? Yes _____No _____

Victim Identification:

Last Name	First Name	Middle Name

Address   Phone Number

D.O.B.   School Attended   Grade

Protective Custody: Yes ____No_____Date _____Time _____

Physical appearance _____

Victim Photographed: Yes ____No_____

Mother:

Last Name	First Name	Middle Name	Maiden

Address   Telephone #

Employer   Telephone #

D.O.B._____Social Security #_____ At Home: Yes____No____

Father:

Last Name   First Name   Middle Name

Address   Telephone #

Employer   Telephone #

D.O.B._____Social Security #_____ At Home: Yes____No____

Guardian/Caretaker:

Last Name   First Name   Middle Name

Address   Telephone #

Employer   Telephone #

          At Home: Yes _____No _____

Siblings in Home:

Yes _____ No _____ Number_____

Were the siblings abused? Yes _____No _____

Protective Custody: Yes _____No Date/Time_____

OTHER HOUSEHOLD MEMBERS:

NAME	RELATIONSHIP	D.O.B.
1.		
2.		
3.		
4.		

Suspect:

Last Name   First Name   Middle Name

Address   Telephone #

Employer   Telephone #

D.O.B.   Social Security Number   Relationship with Victim

Height   Weight   Eyes   Hair   Build

Physical Appearance: _____

_____

Arrested: Yes_____   No _____   Miranda Warning? Yes _____   No _____

Criminal History:

MULES _____   NCIC _____

SID _____   FBI _____

Statement: _____

Complaintant/Reporter:

Last Name   First Name   Middle Name   Maiden

Address   Telephone #

Employer   Telephone #

D.O.B.   Relationship to Victim

Date/Time Reported: _____

Statement: _____

Witness:

Last Name   First Name   Middle Name   Maiden

Address   Telephone #

Employer   Telephone #

D.O.B   Relationship to Victim

Evidence:

Photographs taken: Yes _____ No _____   Color _____ B&W _____

Audio/Video recordings made: Yes _____ No _____

_____ Victim _____ Scene _____ Perpetrator _____ Evidence _____ Other

Evidence recovered:

Inventory Number: _____Destination: P.D._____ Lab_____

Consent to Search Signed and Executed: Yes_____ No_____

Search Warrant Signed and Executed: Yes_____ No_____

SAFE or Other Physical Examination:

Has the victim had a medical or SAFE exam? Yes_____ No_____

Doctor_____SAFE Doctor? Yes_____ No_____

NOTE: Complete a DSS and CA/N check on all parties involved.

THE FINAL REPORT

Prepare a **narrative summary** of the investigative results. If it is a multi-disciplinary investigation, **coordinate** the information and evidence obtained by the various participating agencies and departments. All summaries, individual and multi-disciplinary, should be assembled into a single, sectioned and indexed document (e.g., all official reports from each agency; interview statements; checklists and forms; evidence lists; photographs and other exhibits, etc.).

Summaries should be complete, concise and accurate.

NOTE:

Before use, sample forms should be

reviewed by your agency and

local prosecutor.

Missouri Department of Social Services
State Technical Assistance Team
Multi-disciplinary Trainers/Investigators of Child Abuse
(314) 751-5980
800-487-1626

Search Warrant

THE STATE OF MISSOURI TO ANY PEACE OFFICER IN THE STATE OF MISSOURI:

Whereas, a complaint in writing, duly verified by oath, has been filed with the undersigned Judge of this court, stating upon information and belief, and personal belief, that the following (contraband), (property) to-wit:

_____
_____
_____
_____
_____
_____
_____

believed to have been used as means for committing the felony of:

_____
_____
_____

and/or

_____

(believed to be stolen) is being kept or held in (town/city/county),

_____

address/location _____

_____

building/vehicle/other_____

Whereas, the Judge of this Court from the sworn allegations of said complaint and from the supporting written affidavits filed therewith has found that there is probable cause to believe that allegations of the complaint to be true and probable cause for the issuance of a search warrant therein;

Now, therefore, these are to command you to search the said premises described above within 10 days after the issuance of this warrant by day or night and take with you, if need be, the power of your jurisdiction and if said property described above or any part thereof be found on said premises by you, that you seize the same and take same into your possession, making a complete and accurate inventory of the property so taken by you in the presence of the person from whose possession the same is taken, if that be possible, and giving to such person, a receipt for such property, together with a copy of this warrant, or, if no person be found in possession of said property, leaving said receipt and said copy upon the premises searched, and that you thereafter return the property so taken and seized by you, together with a duly verified copy of the inventory thereof and return this warrant to this Court to be herein dealt with in accordance with law.

Witnessed my hand and seal of this Court on this _____ day of_____,
19_____.

_____
Judge

Missouri Department of Social Services
State Technical Assistance Team
Multi-disciplinary Trainers/Investigators of Child Abuse
(314) 751-5980
800-487-1626

RETURN AND INVENTORY

I,_____, being a peace officer within and for the aforesaid county, to-wit: _____, do hereby make return to the above and within warrant as follows: that on the _____day of _____, 19_____, and within ten days after issuance of said warrant, I went to the location and premises described therein, and that upon said premises I discovered the following property, which I then and there took into my possession:

that I made this inventory in the presence of the person from whose possession I took said property (that there was no person present from whose possession said property was taken); that I delivered to such person a receipt for the property taken, together with a copy of this warrant, (that there were no persons in possession of said property present on said premises, I left a copy of this warrant with a receipt for the property taken, in a conspicuous place on said premises); that I have now placed said property so taken in the possession of this court.

(Officer)_____

Time:_____A.M./P.M.

Subscribed and sworn to me before this _____day of _____, 19_____

_____
Judge

AFFIDAVIT ATTACHMENT

Affidavits in support of search warrants should be as complete and detailed as possible. Any information that will authenticate the contents of your request should be included. You should also make every attempt to establish the credibility of your informant/witness by detailing your personal knowledge of the subject and the circumstances that would make it likely that this person has credible information.

AFFIDAVIT IN SUPPORT OF A SEARCH WARRANT

I, S_____, am a member of the St. Louis Metropolitan Police Department. I have been a police officer for twenty-five years and have been assigned to the Homicide Division for sixteen and a half years.

In January of 1983, I conducted an investigation into the fatal shooting of _____ which occurred on January 28, 1983 at _____. During the course of this investigation, I interviewed _____ on several occasions. On December 6, 1983, _____ made a taped statement concerning his knowledge of the death of _____. In May of 1984, _____ directed Homicide detectives to the _____ in _____, Missouri, where the barrel of the murder weapon had supposedly been thrown in the lake.

On August 23, 1984, _____ escaped from Custody and has been At-Large since that time. On September 2, 1984, an unidentified white male was found in the Shelby National Forest in Memphis, Tennessee. The victim had been shot and stabbed and had been partially eaten by animals.

On October 22, 1985, _____ obtained hospital x-rays and mailed them to the Shelby County Sheriff's Office in Memphis, Tennessee. On October 25, 1985, the unidentified body was identified as _____.

An investigation revealed that at the time of the escape _____ was seen entering an automobile occupied by a white male and a white female. These persons were later identified as _____, the wife of _____, and _____ who is the boyfriend of _____. _____formerly resided in Memphis, Tennessee.

_____stated that about 3:30 p.m., on August 28, 1984, he was at the resident of _____ at _____.

_____stated that _____ and _____ became involved in an argument in the hallway on the first floor.

_____ stated that he heard someone screaming in pain

Missouri Department of Social Services
State Technical Assistance Team
Multi-disciplinary Trainers/Investigators of Child Abuse
(314) 751-5980
800-487-1626

377

and he observed _____ laying on the floor holding his back. _____ was standing over _____ and was holding a knife and said he was going to kill him (_____). _____stated that he turned around to leave and went back in the hallway and saw _____ dragging _____ down the hallway and into his room. _____stated that _____ then ordered him into the bedroom and fired a shot into the wall just north of the door. _____ stated that he was forced to wrap the body up and was also forced to draw directions on a Rand-McNally Road Atlas from St. Louis to Memphis, Tennessee which was left in the house. _____ also stated that he helped _____ place the body of _____ into the trunk of a Lincoln Continental which is owned by _____, the father of _____. _____ also stated that there was blood on the floor of the bedroom and he also saw blood on the hands of _____.

It is respectfully requested that a search warrant be issued for the residence of ____ at _____ to search for the Rand-McNally Road Atlas, the bullet in the wall and blood on the floor. The residence consists of a living room, a kitchen, a hallway and a bedroom which is located on the east wall of the building. It is also respectfully requested that a search warrant be issued to search the trunk of a 1973 Lincoln Continental for blood, fibers, and hair. The automobile bearing VIN _____ and Missouri License for _____. The auto is issued to _____ at _____, St. Louis, Missouri.

_____
Signature

_____
Signature

Subscribed and sworn to before me this _____ day of _____ 19____ at _____a.m./p.m.

_____
JUDGE

PERMISSION TO SEARCH AND SEIZE

I,_____, have been informed by

_____ and _____

who made proper identification as (an) authorized law enforcement officer(s) of the

_____

of my CONSTITUTIONAL RIGHT not to have a search made of the premises and property owned by me and/or

under my care, custody and control, without a search warrant.

Knowing of my lawful rights to refuse to consent to such a search, I willingly give my permission to the above-

named officer(s) to conduct a complete search of the premises and property, including all buildings and vehicles,

both inside and outside of the property located at_____'

_____.

The above-named officer(s) further have my permission to take from my premises and property, any letters,

papers, materials or any other property or things which they desire as evidence for criminal prosecution in the

case or cases under investigation.

This written permission to search without a search warrant is given by me to the above-named officer(s) vol-

untarily and without any threats or promises of any kind, at _____ ___.m. on this _____ day of

_____, 19_____, at _____.

Signed:_____

Witness:_____Witness:_____

Address:_____Address:_____

Phone (H)_____(B)_____Phone (H)_____(B)_____

Missouri Department of Social Services
State Technical Assistance Team
Multi-disciplinary Trainers/Investigators of Child Abuse
(314) 751-5980
800-487-1626

STATEMENT OF RIGHTS

Before we ask you any questions, it is my duty to advise you of your constitutional rights.

■ You have the right to remain silent.

■ Anything you say can and will be used against you in a court of law.

■ You have the right to talk to a lawyer and have him present with you while you are being questioned.

■ If you cannot afford to hire a lawyer, one will be appointed to represent you before any questioning, if you wish.

■ You can decide at any time to exercise these rights and not answer any question or make any statements.

I have read (or have been read) the above statement of my rights and I understand each of those rights.

Date _____

Time _____

Place _____

_____
Signature

_____
Address

_____
Social Security Number

_____
Advising Officer

_____
Witness

_____
Witness

Missouri Department of Social Services
State Technical Assistance Team
Multi-disciplinary Trainers/Investigators of Child Abuse
(314) 751-5980
800-487-1626

Property/Evidence Log

Owner _____   Address _____

Town/City _____   Phone _____

Victim _____   Address _____

Town/City _____   Phone _____

Type of Case_____   Date Occurred _____

Property Status: Evidence ❑   Recovered ❑   Safekeeping ❑   Date Received_____

Location seized or recovered _____

Property Description (include model, serial number or other descriptors)

Seized and packaged by: Name:_____
Agency: _____   Date:_____

Post-Event Chain of Custody		
From:	To:	Date:
From:	To:	Date:
From:	To:	Date:
From:	To:	Date:
From:	To:	Date:
From:	To:	Date:

Released/Returned to Name: _____

　　　　　Signed: _____   Date:_____

Released/Returned to Name: _____

　　　　　Signed: _____   Date:_____

NOTE: If evidence must be mailed to a laboratory for processing, send by registered mail, and keep the mail receipt as part of the chain-of-evidence.

Missouri Department of Social Services
State Technical Assistance Team
Multi-disciplinary Trainers/Investigators of Child Abuse
(314) 751-5980
800-487-1626

PHOTO LOG

Agency_____

Investigator/Photographer _____

Case #_____Type Case _____

Victim_____

Address/Location_____

Date_____Time _____

Camera_____Lens Type_____Film_____ASA Rating _____Light Source_____

Where film developed & printed:_____Date _____

Photo Frame Number	Distance from Camera to Subject Ground	Direction Camera Pointed	Shutter Speed	Lens Opening	Subject

Missouri Department of Social Services
State Technical Assistance Team
Multi-disciplinary Trainers/Investigators of Child Abuse
(314) 751-5980
800-487-1626

INFANT DIAGRAM

INCIDENT NO: _____

CHILD: _____ BIRTHDATE: _____ INVESTIGATOR: _____

DATE VIEWED: _____ WITNESS: _____

DESCRIPTION OF INJURIES: _____

CHILD DIAGRAM

INCIDENT NO:_____

CHILD:_____ BIRTHDATE:_____

INVESTIGATOR:_____

DATE VIEWED:_____

WITNESS: _____

DESCRIPTION OF INJURIES:_ _____

_____

_____

_____

_____

Indicate location of described injuries.

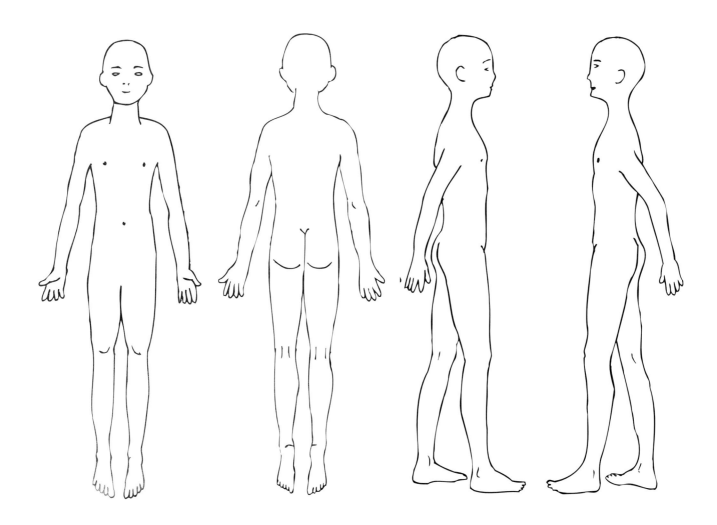

♦ BIBLIOGRAPHY

Block, S, and Tilton, D: ICAN multi-agency child death review team, Report for 1992, ICAN, 1992.

Children's Services, State of Oregon: A report of Oregon child fatalities due to abuse and neglect, 1985-1989.

Colorado Department of Health, Colorado Department of Social Services, March 1993.

Dodson, WE, Monteleone, JA and Edwards, D: The St. Louis Case Control Study of Severe Child Abuse, VII International Congress on Child Abuse and Neglect, Sept. 25-28, 1988, Rio de Janeiro, Brazil.

Durfee, M: Fatal child abuse: Intervention and prevention, *Protecting Child* Spring:9-12, 1989.

Durfee, MJ, Gellert, GA, and Tilton-Durfee, D: Origins and clinical relevance of child death review teams, *JAMA* 267:3172-3175.

Ewigman, B, and Kivlahan, C: Final Recommendations of the Department of Social Services Task Force on Fatal Child Abuse, 1990.

Kaplan, SR: Child fatalities and child fatality review teams, unpublished document, ABA Center on Children and the Law.

Monteleone JA, Edwards, D, and Dodson, WE: The St. Louis Board of Inquiry Into Severe Child Abuse, VII International Congress on Child Abuse and Neglect, Sept. 25-28, 1988, Rio de Janeiro, Brazil.

Robinson, DH, and Stevens, GM: Child abuse and neglect fatalities: Federal and state issues and responses, CRS Report for Congress, Congressional Research Service, The Library of Congress, April 16, 1992.

Smith, P, and Durfee, MJ: Child death review: A review of unpublished reports by states, stabstract/NEWSTAT 1/10/92.

Stangler, G, and Kivlahan, C: Missouri Child Fatality Review Project, interim progress report, Missouri Departments of Social Services and Health, April 1993.

Witherspoon, D: Organizing a multi-agency child death review team (draft).

LEGAL ISSUES

JESSE A. GOLDNER, M.A., J.D.
CASSANDRA K. DOLGIN, B.A., J.D.
SANDRA H. MANSKE, R.N., M.A., J.D.

The identification and investigation of alleged child abuse and neglect for purposes of medical treatment, social service intervention, or criminal prosecution are likely to involve some aspect of the legal system. First, various state statutory provisions provide definitions of "child abuse" and "child neglect," although they may differ both from state to state and within a given state, depending on the objective in making the identification: for reporting to child protection agencies, for establishing a standard for juvenile court intervention, and for denominating behavior deemed unlawful and meriting punishment through the criminal justice system.

Second, state laws and regulations, as well as other legal rules, prescribe the manner in which child abuse and neglect cases are handled. They address both the method of reporting the incident to the appropriate state agency and how that agency is to respond to the report. Third, the legal system not only controls what may transpire in a juvenile, criminal, or divorce court setting, but also dictates some of what should occur in the physician's office or hospital.

♦ AN HISTORICAL PERSPECTIVE

The United States initially adopted the legal view that children were a form of property of their parents from English common law (Horowitz & Davidson, 1984). Although the law did recognize the parental obligation to maintain, educate, and protect one's own child, the widely accepted maxims, "a man's home is his castle" and "spare the rod and spoil the child," reflected the reality that parental duties were relatively free from legal restrictions. Consequently, only cases of severe child abuse, involving cruel and merciless punishment or permanent physical injury, resulted in intervention and criminal prosecution (*State v. Jones*, 1886).

During the Industrial Revolution there was a greater willingness to recognize the need for child protection. This was manifested by legislation that limited child labor and provided for other forms of child protection. The early 19th century witnessed the limited adoption of state statutes authorizing the removal of children from neglectful environments. It was not until 1874, however, with the founding of the Society for the Prevention of Cruelty to Children, an outgrowth of the Society for the Prevention of Cruelty to Animals, that a significant push for legislative reform in the area of child maltreatment came into its own (Radbill, 1987).

State juvenile court systems, modeled after the Illinois Juvenile Court Act of 1899, emerged in the early 1900s. The development of these courts represented a direct exercise of the state's *parens patriae* authority, which justifies state intervention over parental objection in order to protect children (Bross, 1988). The exercise of such state power over a child is generally controlled by three principles:

> *First, the power is based, primarily, on the presumption that children lack the mental competence and maturity possessed by adults. Second, before intervening the state must show that the child's parents or guardians are unfit, unable, or*

unwilling to care for the child. Finally, the state should exercise the parens patriae power solely to further the best interests of the child (Rosenberg & Hunt, 1984).

The development of juvenile courts corresponded with the movement towards professionalism in social work and increased social services directed at child protection. Today, the juvenile court exercises jurisdiction over minors brought within the system due to alleged abuse, neglect and abandonment, as well as incorrigibility and delinquency.

These courts, as opposed to those that are part of the criminal justice system, afford the judge broad discretion in addressing the problems encountered by invoking state coercion to effectuate the social welfare system's goal of rehabilitation and treatment of abusive parents and other caretakers. The court's determination that a child is in need of supervision or assistance may result in court-ordered family services, placement of the child in foster care or a state youth facility, or, in extraordinary circumstances, termination of parental rights.

Differentiating between physical abuse and symptoms or injuries resulting from disease processes or accidents often proved to be a difficult task. The work of two physicians provided guidance. Radiologist Dr. John Caffey, in the early and mid-20 century, related previously unexplained X-ray findings to trauma which may have resulted from parental action. In the 1950s and early 1960s, Dr. C. Henry Kempe and his colleagues at the University of Colorado Medical School defined the "battered child syndrome" as an observable clinical condition capable of medical diagnosis. Together, these discoveries had legal as well as medical significance (Kempe et al., 1962; Radbill, 1987).

Medical identification of certain nonaccidental physical injuries contributed not only to increased criminal prosecutions but also to legislative efforts to require reporting of suspected cases of child abuse. In 1963, the U.S. Department of Health, Education, and Welfare's (now Health and Human Services) Children's Bureau developed a model child abuse reporting statute. By 1967, each state had enacted such a law. These first reporting statutes were narrow in purpose and scope. Their aim was simply to identify suspected child abuse, and only physicians were designated as mandatory reporters. As knowledge regarding child abuse increased, however, states refined these laws, expanding their purpose beyond mere identification to investigation and intervention, and broadening the group of mandated reporters (Fraser, 1978).

Recently, the rehabilitative approach to dealing with child abuse and neglect cases, which has been favored in the treatment of physical and sexual abuse, has been subject to extensive attack. Some critics have cited frustrations with the courts' ability to effectively intervene in many cases where such intervention seems necessary. Other critics point to the inability of professionals working in the area of mental health and child protection to change deviant behavior, particularly in a cost-effective way.

Consequently, at least to some extent, attention is shifting in two other directions. On the one hand, over the last decade, in an effort to increase the success of reliance on the judicial system to aid in the handling of these cases, many jurisdictions have passed statutes or issued judicial rulings that are designed to make testimony by a child easier and less traumatic in some or all of the different types of proceedings involving child abuse. These generally involve efforts to minimize the need for the child to be in the presence of the alleged abuser, while at the same time protecting the rights of defendants and others involved in these cases. These include, for example, the possible use of closed circuit cameras, videotaped testimony and courtroom screens, and the increased admissibility of hearsay evidence (Myers, 1986). Some limitations on the use of such techniques are reviewed later in this chapter. At the same time, increased efforts are being made to focus on prevention as perhaps the most cost-effective way of dealing with child abuse and neglect in the long run (Daro, 1988).

Generally, it is the state that responds to child maltreatment, but during the past quarter century federal legislation has greatly influenced the states' legal response to child maltreatment. Beginning in 1974, the National Center on Child Abuse and Neglect was established by congressional mandate (Child Abuse Prevention and Treatment Act, 1974). The law imposed various requirements on the states as a condition for receiving federal funds for "developing, strengthening, and carrying out child abuse and neglect prevention and treatment programs." Presently, eligibility for funding under the legislation requires the establishment of state reporting laws, statutory immunity provisions for those who report suspected cases of abuse and neglect under state law, a state agency responsible for carrying out investigatory and treatment procedures, a state-wide central child abuse registry, provisions for confidentiality of registry records, and the appointment of a *guardian ad litem* for the child in cases involving judicial proceedings (Child Abuse Prevention and Treatment Act, 1974; Rosenberg & Hunt, 1984).

In 1980, the passage of additional federal legislation (Adoption Assistance and Child Welfare Act, 1980) required states to make reasonable efforts to avoid removing maltreated children from parental custody and mandated court or administrative review of state-supervised foster care placement at least every six months. This review determines the continuing necessity for and appropriateness of the placement, the compliance with an established case plan, and the extent of progress made towards alleviating or mitigating the cause of the placement. The review must also include a projected date for the child's return home, or, when return to the biological parent's home is unlikely, recommend placement for adoption or legal guardianship (Cunningham & Horowitz, 1989). The enactment of federal statutes concerning Native Americans (Indian Child Welfare Act, 1978) requires state agencies to make "active efforts" to provide services "designed to prevent the breakup of the Indian family."

Finally, federal legislation has enhanced intervention in child sexual abuse cases. Recent statutory measures impose criminal sanctions upon any person who uses, or assists another in using, a minor to engage in sexually explicit behavior for the purpose of producing physical depictions of this behavior with the intent to distribute the material in interstate commerce (Federal Protection of Children Against Sexual Exploitation Act, 1986).

♦ REPORTING STATUTES AND CHILD PROTECTIVE SERVICES

The identification of abuse and neglect, the assessment of family social service needs, and the implementation of treatment programs and other intervention strategies for abused children and their families are carried out predominantly by state and county child protective service (CPS) agencies. Authorization for such action typically is found in state laws that establish and provide funding for these agencies and define the criteria for, and mode of, intervention. The primary purposes of CPS agencies are "(1) to protect and insure the safety of children who have been or are at risk of maltreatment, and (2) to provide services to alter the conditions which create risk of maltreatment in the future" (Cunningham & Horowitz, 1989).

A report to the state's child abuse and neglect hotline, made either by a professional involved with the child or by a neighbor or other nonmandated reporter, generally results in a referral to a CPS agency. Often, such a referral results from a report to the local police. Occasionally, the report is initiated by one parent with respect to the other in the context of a child custody dispute.

Child abuse and neglect reporting laws dictate the manner in which referrals are made to the CPS agency and also how the agency is to respond. Additionally, the statutes mandate other duties and rights of health care personnel and other reporters. These laws govern the central registries that maintain information regarding cases which have previously been investigated by the CPS agency. Finally, the laws often define the relationship between the CPS agency, the juvenile court, and various law enforcement agencies.

REPORTING STATUTES

Each state, as well as the District of Columbia, Puerto Rico, and the Virgin Islands, has enacted its own child abuse and neglect reporting legislation. As a result, there is a lack of uniformity in statutory language and in the effect of the various laws. In particular, the statutes vary as to the precise definition of child abuse and the standards and procedures used for reporting suspected cases (Fraser, 1978). All of the statutes, however, share a common purpose and tend to follow a similar format based on the federally mandated requirements (Meriwether, 1986).

The purpose of every child abuse and neglect reporting statute is to protect the child from additional injury. Accordingly, statutes are written to encourage and facilitate reporting of suspected abuse or neglect. They are designed to promote early identification of the child in peril so that adequate investigation and treatment of the child, as well as of the family, when appropriate, can begin.

Every state reporting statute contains essentially the same elements, including: (1) what must be reported (reportable conditions/definition of child abuse); (2) who must or may report; (3) when a report must be made (including the degree of certainty a reporter must have); (4) reporting procedures; (5) the existence and operation of a central registry; (6) rules regarding protective custody; (7) immunity for good faith reporters; (8) the abrogation of certain privileged communication rights that might otherwise apply; and (9) sanctions for failure to report. In addition, many child abuse reporting statutes provide for the taking of photographs or X-rays of the child when physical abuse is suspected, even in the absence of parental consent *(see Tables 18-1 to 18-4)*.

WHAT MUST BE REPORTED

Every state reporting statute requires that mandated reporters report suspected child abuse and neglect (**Table 18-1**). Each state, however, defines child abuse and neglect differently; therefore, reportable conditions vary among the states (Table 18-1). In general, reportable conditions include nonaccidental physical injury, neglect, sexual abuse, and emotional abuse.

WHO MUST REPORT

Each state reporting statute designates who is required to report suspected child abuse and neglect (**Table 18-2**). Typically, these individuals include physicians, health care professionals, educators, and law enforcement personnel. Many states, however, have an even broader base of mandated reporters, including such professionals as coroners, dentists, probation officers, social workers, or other persons responsible for the care of children. Over twenty states require "any person" to report (Blue, 1988). In addition, the majority of state reporting statutes also provide for permissive reporting by nonmandated reporters.

STATE	Mandatory Reporting Required	Permissive Reporting Allowed	Immunities	Civil Penalty	Criminal Penalty	Definition of Neglect	Definition of Emotional Injury	Definition of Medical Neglect	Definition of Physical Abuse	Definition of Sexual Abuse	Temporary Protective Custody	X-Ray/Photo	Emergency Treatment	Interagency Reporting
Alabama	X	X	X		X	X	X	X	X	X			X	X
Alaska	X	X	X		X	X	X	X	X	X	X	X		X
Arizona	X		X		X				X		X	X	X	X
Arkansas	X	X	X	X	X	X	X	X	X	X	X	X	X	X
California	X	X	X		X	X	X	X	X	X		X		X
Colorado	X	X	X	X	X	X			X		X	X	X	X
Connecticut	X		X		X	X	X	X	X	X	X		X	X
Delaware	X		X		X	X	X	X	X	X	X			X
District of Columbia	X		X		X	X	X	X	X	X	X	X		X
Florida	X		X		X	X	X	X	X	X	X	X	X	X
Georgia	X	X	X		X	X						X		X
Hawaii	X	X	X		X	X			X	X				X
Idaho	X		X		X	X	X	X	X	X	X			X
Illinois	X	X	X			X	X	X	X	X	X	X	X	X
Indiana	X	X	X			X	X	X	X	X	X	X		X
Iowa	X	X	X	X	X	X			X	X	X	X		X
Kansas	X	X	X		X	X	X	X	X	X	X	X	X	X
Kentucky	X	X	X			X	X	X	X	X	X	X	X	X
Louisiana	X	X	X		X	X	X	X	X	X	X		X	X
Maine	X	X	X			X	X	X	X	X	X	X	X	
Maryland	X		X						X	X	X		X	X
Massachusetts	X	X	X	X	X						X	X	X	
Michigan	X	X	X	X	X	X		X	X	X	X	X	X	X
Minnesota	X	X	X	X	X	X	X	X	X	X	X	X		X
Mississippi	X		X	X		X	X	X	X	X	X		X	X
Missouri	X	X	X		X	X	X	X	X	X	X	X	X	X
Montana	X	X	X	X	X	X	X	X	X	X	X	X	X	X
Nebraska	X		X		X	X	X	X	X	X	X	X	X	X
Nevada	X	X	X		X	X	X	X	X	X	X	X	X	X
New Hampshire	X		X		X	X	X	X	X	X	X	X	X	X
New Jersey	X		X		X	X	X	X	X	X	X		X	X
New Mexico	X		X		X	X	X	X	X	X	X		X	X
New York	X	X	X	X	X	X		X	X	X	X	X		
North Carolina	X		X			X	X	X	X	X	X	X	X	X
North Dakota	X	X	X		X	X	X	X	X	X	X	X	X	X
Ohio	X	X	X		X	X	X	X	X	X	X	X	X	X
Oklahoma	X		X		X	X	X	X	X	X	X	X	X	X
Oregon	X		X		X	X	X	X	X	X	X	X	X	X
Pennsylvania	X	X	X		X	X	X	X	X	X	X	X	X	X
Rhode Island	X		X	X	X	X	X	X	X	X	X	X	X	X
South Carolina	X	X	X		X	X	X	X	X	X	X	X	X	X
South Dakota	X	X	X		X	X	X	X	X	X	X	X	X	X
Tennessee	X		X		X			X			X	X	X	X
Texas	X		X		X			X	X	X	X	X	X	X
Utah	X		X		X	X		X	X	X	X	X	X	X
Vermont	X	X	X		X	X	X	X	X	X	X	X	X	
Virginia	X	X	X		X	X	X	X	X	X	X	X	X	X
Washington	X	X	X		X	X			X	X	X	X	X	X
West Virginia	X	X	X		X	X	X		X	X	X	X	X	X
Wisconsin	X	X	X		X	X	X	X	X	X	X	X	X	X
Wyoming	X		X			X	X	X	X	X	X	X	X	

Table 18-1 General Provisions of Reporting Statutes. *Derived from tables in Myers JEB and Peters WD: Child Abuse Reporting Legislation in the 1980's, Denver, Colorado: American Humane Association, 1987. Used with permission.*

STATE	Alcohol/Drug Abuse Counselor	Neighbor, Relative, Friend	Firefighter/Inspector	Physician/Surgeon	Osteopath	Dentist	Resident/Intern	Commercial Film & Photo Processor	Hospital/Institution Personnel	Health Practitioner or Professional	Chiropractor	Pharmacist	Nurses	Teachers/School Counselors	Other School Personnel/Administrator	Social Worker or Social Wk. Technician	Law Enforcement/Judge	Coroner/Medical Examiner	Psychologist/Mental Health Profes.	Optometrists	Podiatrist	Christian Science Pract. Religious Healers	Lic. Day Care Providers/Workers	Clergymen	Attorneys	Any Person Lic. to Practice Healing Arts	Emergency Medical Technician	Parole/Probation Officer	Foster Care/Child-Care Personnel	Homemaker	Any Public or Private Official	Any other person/Any Person
Alabama				X	X	X			X		X	X	X	X	X	X	X	X	X	X	X		X				X					
Alaska				X	X	X							X	X	X	X	X		X	X		X	X			X	X	X	X			
Arizona				X	X	X	X	X			X		X	X	X	X	X	X	X		X		X	X					X			
Arkansas				X	X	X		X			X		X	X	X	X	X	X	X				X						X			
California				X		X	X	X			X	X	X	X	X			X			X		X	X			X		X			
Colorado				X	X	X		X			X		X	X	X	X		X	X	X	X		X						X			
Connecticut				X	X	X					X		X	X	X	X	X	X	X	X	X		X	X					X			X
Delaware				X	X	X					X		X	X	X	X	X	X	X				X			X			X			X
District of Columbia				X							X		X	X	X	X	X	X	X				X									
Florida				X	X				X	X	X		X	X	X	X	X	X	X		X		X						X			X
Georgia				X	X	X	X		X				X	X	X	X		X	X		X		X						X			
Hawaii				X		X			X	X	X	X	X	X		X	X	X	X				X			X		X	X			
Idaho				X			X						X	X		X		X					X									X
Illinois				X	X	X		X		X		X			X	X	X	X	X		X	X	X						X	X		
Indiana				X	X	X		X		X		X			X	X	X		X		X		X						X			X
Iowa				X	X	X		X	X	X		X	X	X	X	X	X		X				X									
Kansas			X		X	X		X			X	X	X	X	X	X		X	X		X	X			X	X			X			X
Kentucky			X	X	X	X			X	X		X	X	X	X	X	X	X	X										X			X
Louisiana				X			X		X			X	X		X	X		X											X			
Maine			X	X	X	X	X		X	X		X	X	X	X	X	X		X	X		X	X				X		X	X		
Maryland									X				X		X	X	X															X
Massachusetts		X	X	X	X	X		X			X		X	X	X	X	X	X	X		X		X				X	X	X			
Michigan				X		X					X		X	X	X	X	X		X				X						X			
Minnesota									X				X	X	X	X		X							X				X			
Mississippi				X		X	X					X	X	X	X		X		X					X	X				X			X
Missouri				X		X	X	X	X	X	X	X	X	X	X	X	X	X	X	X	X	X							X	X		
Montana				X	X	X	X		X	X	X		X	X	X	X	X	X		X	X	X	X						X			
Nebraska				X					X				X	X	X	X																X
Nevada	X			X		X	X		X		X		X	X	X	X	X	X	X	X	X	X	X	X	X		X	X	X			
New Hampshire				X	X	X	X		X		X		X	X	X	X	X	X	X		X		X	X	X				X			X
New Jersey																																X
New Mexico				X			X						X	X		X	X															X
New York				X	X	X	X		X		X		X		X	X	X	X	X	X	X	X	X						X			
North Carolina																																X
North Dakota				X		X				X			X	X	X	X	X	X	X	X			X	X								
Ohio				X		X	X			X			X	X	X		X		X	X		X	X	X		X			X			
Oklahoma				X	X	X	X				X		X	X																		X
Oregon																																X
Pennsylvania				X	X	X	X		X		X		X	X	X	X	X	X	X	X	X	X	X						X			X
Rhode Island																																X
South Carolina				X		X			X				X	X		X	X	X	X		X		X	X					X			
South Dakota				X	X	X	X			X			X	X	X	X	X	X	X	X	X	X	X						X			
Tennessee		X		X	X				X		X		X	X	X	X	X	X	X				X	X					X			X
Texas																																X
Utah																																X
Vermont				X	X	X	X		X		X		X	X	X	X	X	X	X				X					X				
Virginia					X		X				X		X	X	X		X		X				X	X			X		X	X		
Washington									X	X		X	X	X	X	X		X														
West Virginia											X		X	X	X	X	X		X				X	X		X	X	X	X			
Wisconsin	X			X	X	X			X	X		X	X	X	X	X	X	X	X	X				X					X	X		
Wyoming																																X

Table 18-2 Who Must Report Child Abuse and Neglect. Derived from tables in Myers JEB and Peters WD: *Child Abuse Reporting legislation in the 1980's, Denver, Colorado: American Humane Association, 1987. Used with permission.*

WHEN MUST A REPORT BE MADE

Child abuse reporting statutes dictate when a report must be made. Most statutes require reporters to make an immediate oral report by telephone, followed shortly thereafter by a written report to the appropriate state agency. This procedure facilitates an immediate investigatory response by the CPS agency, ensuring that the child is protected. It also establishes a permanent record of the alleged incident.

The degree of suspicion a reporter must reach before making a report is set out in the reporting statute and likewise varies from state to state. The original child abuse reporting statutes provided for a report to be made when there was "reason to believe" that a child had been abused (Fraser, 1978). Many states have expanded the requirement and now use language such as "cause to believe" or "reasonable cause to suspect" that a "child has been or may be subjected to abuse or neglect or observes a child being subjected to conditions or circumstances which would reasonably result in abuse or neglect." Practically, "cause to believe" and "reasonable cause to suspect" mean essentially the same thing for reporting purposes. As noted below, however, there may be a distinction in cases where civil liability for failure to report is at issue.

REPORTING PROCEDURES

Each state statute specifies at least one agency to receive reports of suspected child abuse and neglect (**Table 18-3**). Traditionally, four different agencies have served as potential recipients for child abuse reports: social service agencies, police departments, health departments, and juvenile courts.

Most states have designated the department of social services, or a division within that department, as the appropriate agency to ultimately receive these reports. Some states designate only the department of social services, while other states designate two or more agencies such as the police and the department of social services to receive reports. These states generally require that all reports ultimately flow into the department of social services. A few states, however, permit the reporting to two or more agencies without requiring the coordination of information by any agency.

In many states the reporting statute specifies what information is to be included in the report. In other states the receiving agency determines, on a case-by-case basis, what information is required. Required information typically includes name, age, address, present location of the child, type and extent of the injuries, name and address of the parent(s) and/or caretaker(s) if known, and any other information that the reporter believes might be relevant. Most states require a mandated reporter to divulge his or her name and position, but permit a permissive reporter to remain anonymous.

Reporting statutes generally prescribe the time within which the CPS agency must initiate its investigation. In most instances this is within 24 hours of the receipt of a report.

CENTRAL REGISTRIES

Reports received by a state's child abuse hotline are recorded in a central registry. Central registry records usually contain additional case information such as prior reports of child abuse and neglect and CPS case outcomes, treatment plans, and final dispositions at the CPS level. Nearly every state has established a central registry of child protection cases. Current exceptions include Minnesota, New Mexico, and Utah.

State law generally deems central registry records confidential and regulates their disclosure because they contain highly private data about individuals and families. Three general statutory approaches govern record accessibility: (1) Only individuals

STATE	Department of Social Services	Law Enforcement	Central Register
Alabama	X	X	
Alaska	X	X	
Arizona	X	X	
Arkansas	X		
California	X		
Colorado	X	X	
Connecticut	X	X	
Delaware	X		
District of Columbia	X	X	
Florida	X		
Georgia	X		
Hawaii	X	X	
Idaho	X	X	
Illinois	X		
Indiana	X	X	
Iowa	X	X	
Kansas	X	X	
Kentucky	X		
Louisiana	X	X	
Maine	X		
Maryland	X	X	
Massachusetts	X		
Michigan	X	X	
Minnesota	X	X	
Mississippi	X		
Missouri	X		
Montana	X	X	
Nebraska	X		
Nevada	X		
New Hampshire	X		
New Jersey	X		
New Mexico	X		
New York			X
North Carolina	X		
North Dakota	X		
Ohio	X	X	
Oklahoma	X	X	
Oregon	X	X	
Pennsylvania	X		
Rhode Island	X	X	
South Carolina	X	X	
South Dakota	X	X	
Tennessee	X	X	
Texas	X		
Utah	X	X	
Vermont	X		
Virginia	X		
Washington	X	X	
West Virginia	X		
Wisconsin	X	X	
Wyoming	X	X	

Table 18-3 Mandated Recipients of Child Abuse and Neglect Reports. *Derived from tables in Myers JEB and Peters WD: Child Abuse Reporting Legislation in the 1980's, Denver, Colorado: American Humane Association, 1987. Used with permission.*

within a CPS agency may have access; (2) the CPS agency may issue regulations authorizing access by certain persons outside of the agency; or (3) state law may enumerate precisely which persons may have access. This third approach is most prevalent today. Those typically having access are law enforcement personnel investigating a report of child maltreatment, the treating physician, the CPS agency, the court, and persons conducting bona fide research (Besharov, 1978). In addition, the child's attorney or guardian ad litem generally is permitted to review registry records in instances when the CPS agency or law enforcement personnel refers the case to juvenile court and court involvement ensues. Registry information often is available for purposes of screening applicants for licenses to establish child care facilities, agencies/services/applicants for employment or volunteer work with such operations or with schools. Almost all states provide that prohibited disclosure is punishable as a misdemeanor (Horowitz & Davidson, 1984).

PROTECTIVE CUSTODY

Nearly every state authorizes certain categories of individuals to take a child into protective custody if the individual concludes that the child would be seriously endangered if he or she remained with or was released to the parent or other caretaker. The child abuse reporting statutes designate who may take the child into custody, when, and under what circumstances. Depending on the particular statute, such individuals may include one or more of the following: police officers, physicians, juvenile or probation officers, and CPS professionals.

Some states require a court order, at least over the telephone if not in writing, before taking the child into custody against the parent's wishes. Other states directly authorize protective custody, provided that written notice or another document is filed with the juvenile court within 24 to 48 hours after the action is taken. In either case, a custody hearing will typically be held at the juvenile court within a short period of time thereafter to review the initial decision to hold the child. Some states provide for protective custody when an authorized individual deems that there "is an imminent danger to the child's life or health." Other states allow protective custody when returning the child to his parent "would endanger his health or welfare" (Meriwether, 1986).

IMMUNITY FOR GOOD FAITH REPORTERS

Individuals may be reluctant to report suspected child abuse. Potential reporters may fear that the suspected perpetrator will bring a lawsuit against them if the abuse is unconfirmed. To encourage reporting and alleviate this fear, every state's reporting statute extends some type of immunity from civil and criminal liability to persons making reports. Although such immunity provisions may not completely insulate the reporter from a lawsuit (that is, they cannot prevent the filing of an action against a reporter), they can make the successful litigation of such suits nearly impossible.

Some jurisdictions grant absolute immunity to mandated reporters (*Storch v. Silverman*, 1986). This means that the mandated reporter is protected even if the report was false and the reporter knew it to be false. Most jurisdictions, however, provide immunity only to an individual making a good faith report. In these states, a reporter is liable only when the plaintiff can prove that the reporter made a false report and that the reporter knew that the report was false, or otherwise acted in bad faith or with a malicious purpose (*Gross v. Myers*, 1987).

ABROGATION OF PRIVILEGED COMMUNICATIONS

Certain professionals owe their patients or clients a duty of confidentiality. This duty is incurred by virtue of the ethical obligations which the individual undertakes on becoming a professional and adopting the standards of that profession (Stromberg, 1988). Any breach of this obligation would ordinarily lead to a malpractice suit against the professional in which money might be awarded to the patient or client as compensation for damages sustained as a result of the breach of confidentiality. If the disclosure is mandated by a state statute, as in the instance of child abuse, however, no liability will result. Moreover, as discussed below, in such instances, the failure to make the disclosure, even in the face of an otherwise existing obligation of confidentiality, may, in fact, result in liability.

In addition to this obligation of confidentiality, certain professional communications are protected by a judicially or legislatively created testimonial privilege. Generally, a privilege operates to exclude information obtained in the course of a particular relationship from being presented as evidence at judicial proceedings.

The most common types of privileged communications are those between doctor-patient, husband-wife, attorney-client, social worker-client, and priest-penitent. States differ, however, as to which communications are protected by testimonial privilege. Most states abrogate all types of privileged communications in a child abuse case, except attorney-client (**Table 18-4**). Many states also refuse to intrude on the priest-penitent relationship.

Mandatory reporters must report suspected abuse or neglect, regardless of whether the abuse or neglect became apparent as a result of a confidential communication with the patient or client. Also, the professional must testify in juvenile court child protection cases when subpoenaed. In many jurisdictions, this requirement to testify may also exist in criminal cases and in child custody cases in which allegations of child abuse are involved. Failure to testify when a judge orders that the testimony be given is likely to result in holding the witness in contempt and jailing the witness. In some states, however, if a claim of privilege is appropriately made, the testimony may be limited to information required to be reported under the reporting statute rather than to more extensive information about which the witness may have become aware (Stromberg, 1988).

CRIMINAL SANCTIONS FOR FAILURE TO REPORT

Most states have provisions in their reporting statutes that make it a crime for a mandated reporter to knowingly fail to report suspected child abuse. Almost all of these statutes classify the offense as a misdemeanor and specify a maximum fine and or jail sentence. Although criminal prosecutions for failure to report are rare, courts have ruled that physicians, including psychiatrists, may be subject to criminal penalty under the child abuse statute for failure to report suspected child abuse (*Groff v. State,* 1980; *Capaldi v. State,* 1988). The inclusion of a penalty provision serves a useful function for some reluctant professionals. They may find it more palatable to report suspected child abuse if they can explain to the child's family or caretaker that it is a crime for them not to make the report.

SOCIAL SERVICE AND LAW ENFORCEMENT RESPONSE

A report of suspected child abuse or neglect to a state maintained telephone "hotline" or to a local office in accordance with the state's child abuse reporting statute usually initiates the CPS process. At this early stage of the process, child abuse and neglect are often broadly defined. Individual local CPS offices and workers exercise wide discretion in how the agency will respond to individual reports of child maltreatment.

VALIDATION OF REPORTS

As noted in the preceding discussion of reporting procedures, each state has enacted legislation prescribing criteria for case follow-up, which generally requires an investigation within a limited period of time. The primary aim of the investigation is to determine the validity of the report. If the case is "substantiated," "founded," or "indicated," a decision must be made regarding how to proceed.

STATE	Physician/Patient	Professional/Patient	Elem./Second School Counselor/Student	Dentist/Patient	Husband-Wife Interspousal	Chiropractor/Patient	All Privileges except Atty/Client	Registered Nurse	Optometrist/Patient	Similar Privileges	Anyone Required to Report	Clergy/Penitent	Psychologist/Psychiatrist/Client	Social Worker/Client	Psychotherapist/Patient	Health Practitioner	Surgeon	Staff Members of Schools	Family Violence & Sexual Assault Advocate/Client
Alabama							X												
Alaska	X				X														
Arizona							X												
Arkansas							X												
California	X														X				
Colorado	X	X			X														
Connecticut					X														
Delaware							X												
District of Columbia	X				X														
Florida							X												
Georgia																			
Hawaii	X				X														
Idaho							X												
Illinois											X								
Indiana	X				X														
Iowa					X												X		
Kansas	X												X	X					
Kentucky	X	X																	
Louisiana	X	X			X							X							
Maine	X				X										X				
Maryland																			
Massachusetts														X	X				
Michigan							X												
Minnesota	X		X		X	X		X						X				X	
Mississippi	X																		
Missouri							X												
Montana	X									X									
Nebraska	X				X														
Nevada											X								
New Hampshire							X												
New Jersey																			
New Mexico	X									X									
New York																			
North Carolina	X				X														
North Dakota							X												
Ohio	X																		
Oklahoma	X									X									
Oregon	X				X			X						X	X			X	
Pennsylvania											X								
Rhode Island							X												
South Carolina		X			X														
South Dakota	X		X		X														
Tennessee		X			X									X					
Texas							X												
Utah	X																		
Vermont																			
Virginia	X				X														
Washington	X								X				X	X					
West Virginia							X												
Wisconsin	X				X														
Wyoming	X				X									X					

Table 18-4 Evidentiary Testimonial Abrogation of Privileges in Child Abuse Cases. *Derived from tables in Myers JEB and Peters WD: Child Abuse Reporting Legislation in the 1980's, Denver, Colorado: American Humane Association, 1987. Used with permission.*

If the child is not in the protective custody of a physician, the police, or the juvenile court at the time of the investigation, the CPS investigator must determine if there is imminent risk of harm to the child that would warrant the child's immediate removal from the home. If such action is needed, the police or the juvenile court may be contacted to facilitate this removal.

If the available evidence is insufficient to merit a finding of abuse or neglect, or if the investigation could not be completed, the case may be deemed "unsubstantiated" or "unfounded." The case may then be closed and all references to the report and case deleted from the central registry within a designated period of time, if no additional reports are made (Iverson & Segal, 1990). Central registries involve state collection of potentially inflammatory personal information. This gives rise to constitutional concerns regarding the rights to privacy and due process. Accordingly, many states have enacted procedures, by statute or state regulation, for the expungement of registry records. Expungement of records is based either on the child's attainment of a certain age, passage of a designated period of time since services were terminated, or a finding by the CPS agency that the report was unsubstantiated. In some states individuals may formally challenge information contained in the registry through administrative or court procedures for the expungement or modification of records (*Roth v. Reagen*, 1988).

INVESTIGATIVE PURPOSES AND PROCEDURES

Reporting statutes often detail the purpose of the investigation. Generally the goal is to evaluate the nature, extent, and cause of the abuse or neglect, and to identify the person responsible. Efforts are also made to ascertain the names and conditions of other children in the home, the nature of the home environment, and the relationship of the child to the parents or other caretakers.

The investigative caseworker typically begins the process by contacting the individual who made the hotline report to confirm the information originally provided and to obtain additional information. The investigation consists of a series of interviews. Often the child is the next person interviewed. Preferably, this takes place in a neutral setting. The parents are also interviewed, often during a home visit. Thereafter, other persons named in the report who may have relevant information are questioned. These persons typically include teachers, physicians, neighbors, and other relatives (Hechler, 1988; Levine, 1973).

The CPS purpose when responding to a report of child maltreatment is distinct from the objectives of the criminal justice system. Yet, as noted, law enforcement personnel may be contacted by the CPS worker during the investigatory stage or they may already be otherwise involved. This is true in cases involving serious abuse, where there is a reason to believe that the parents are or may likely be resistant to CPS intervention, or if the CPS caseworker is concerned for his or her own safety.

State law provides the authority for CPS home visits, either expressly or through implication, but if individuals refuse to cooperate, a warrant or court order may be needed to gain access to a home. In addition, many state statutes, regulations, or case laws authorize CPS or law enforcement investigators to conduct examinations of the child or to refer the child for evaluation by medical personnel.

CONSTITUTIONAL CONCERNS

Constitutional considerations are raised in the CPS investigative stage, because the constitution protects individuals against state action. CPS caseworkers act under "color of state law" (i.e., they carry out their investigative tasks pursuant to legislative authority). Protection under both federal and state constitutions may be implicated in such areas as home visits, child and parent interviews, and examinations of the child.

Search warrants are generally not required to conduct such visits or examinations. The burden of obtaining a warrant would seriously impair, if not frustrate, the state's effort to protect the child, particularly in emergency situations. There may, however, be constitutional limits on the nature and circumstances under which investigatory visits take place (*Daryl H. v. Coler*, 1986; Hardin, 1988). Usually the parent or guardian consents to the caseworker's or police officer's entry into the residence. Absent consent, or if the search exceeds the scope of the consent, any evidence found may be deemed inadmissible in any subsequent criminal proceeding. Similarly, statements made to investigators by a parent or other perpetrator may be inadmissible if a court finds that at the time of the questioning the individual was in custody or otherwise deprived of his freedom in some significant way (*People v. Hagar*, 1987; Hardin, 1988).

TREATMENT AND REFERRAL OPTIONS

Following a determination of the validity of the allegation of abuse or neglect, a report is made to the agency's central registry. If the hotline referral is substantiated, a CPS caseworker, who may or may not have been involved in the initial investigation of the report, is usually assigned to the case. The caseworker develops a treatment plan and presents it to the family. CPS agencies offer various mental health and social services and seek voluntary acceptance of these recommended services. If the parent or guardian does not cooperate with the CPS agency, or if such voluntary treatment will not adequately protect the child, the investigative or treatment caseworker will request that a juvenile or probation officer file an abuse or neglect petition with the juvenile or family court or file such an action himself. Such an action will seek court intervention with the child and his or her family. Intervention may include temporary removal of the child from the home, court-ordered treatment, or, in some circumstances, termination of parental rights.

When the police have not been involved in the investigation, referral to a local law enforcement agency upon completion of the CPS investigation may be mandated under state law, when the abuse is "substantiated" or meets the statutory requirements for criminal child or sexual abuse. In the absence of legislative direction, CPS regulations may require referral to prosecuting authorities or the police.

CIVIL LIABILITY AND CHILD MALTREATMENT

Health care professionals and others engaged in protective services may be exposed to civil liability during the identification and investigation of alleged child abuse (Sprague & Horowitz, 1991).

FAILURE TO REPORT BY MANDATORY REPORTER

Violation of a statutory duty, such as the duty imposed on a mandated reporter to report suspected child abuse or neglect, is negligence *per se* (negligence in itself). Under this theory, an injured child and his or her family could successfully sue a doctor or another mandated reporter for willingly or negligently failing to detect and report known or suspected child abuse. The suit could result in a judgment awarding monetary damages to compensate the patient for all injuries that occurred as a result of abuse or neglect after the time when a report should have been made. In the leading case on this issue, the California Supreme Court held that a physician and his hospital employer may be liable for medical malpractice for failure to properly diagnose and treat the battered child syndrome when subsequent injuries occur (*Landeros v. Flood*, 1976).

In another case, which eventually settled out of court for $600,000, the child's mother and her boyfriend brought the child to the hospital with severe injuries twice within a 12-hour period. The hospital did not make a report of suspected child abuse at either time. The next day the mother and her boyfriend took the child to another hospital. The child was diagnosed with permanent brain damage.

The child's father sued the first hospital and others for negligence based on the first hospital's failure to report suspected child abuse (*Robinson v. Wical*, 1970).

It is in situations such as these that the precise language of the reporting statute may be of great legal significance. Seemingly minor differences in statutory language could have major implications for the outcome of a case. If the reporting statute's language mandates reporting when there is "cause to believe" that abuse has taken place, the statute is adopting a subjective standard. Under this standard, proof that the health care professional actually believed that abuse or neglect had occurred would be necessary. If "cause to suspect" was the applicable language, the standard would still be subjective, but a lesser degree of certainty would be required. Under either of these subjective standards, the plaintiff must establish that the reporter actually held the belief or suspicion and failed to report for liability to result.

Some jurisdictions require "reasonable cause to believe" or "reasonable cause to suspect." Here, the jurisdiction is adopting an objective standard. Under the objective standard, the test is what a reasonable person in the same situation as the professional would believe or suspect, regardless of the actual mindset of the professional (Fraser, 1978). Generally, the subjective standard is a more difficult one to meet.

OTHER BASES OF LIABILITY OF REPORTERS AND POTENTIAL DEFENSES

In rare instances, civil actions may also be brought against health care professionals or others based on their conduct in connection with a child abuse or neglect case. Typically these lawsuits allege that the physician, social worker, or police officer, and their respective agencies negligently acted under the reporting statute, thereby causing harm to the parent or the child. A parent or child may bring an action seeking monetary damages for a wrongful report of child abuse, defamation and slander, negligent diagnosis or treatment, breach of confidentiality, over-intrusive investigation, wrongful removal of a child from his or her home, wrongful institution or prosecution of an alleged offender, and wrongful examination of the child for signs of abuse (Sprague, 1991; Besharov, 1984). Willful conduct may also be alleged, including battery, false imprisonment, and/or malicious prosecution.

These claims are usually based on state tort (private or civil wrong or injury) law which, through statute or common law (judicial precedent), recognizes that individuals in certain situations owe duties to one another. Violation of these duties can form the basis of an action for monetary damages. Similarly, an alleged violation of constitutional rights, either federal or state, may form the basis of a claim for damages (Sprague & Horowitz, 1991).

As previously noted, all jurisdictions provide absolute or limited immunity for the reporting of suspected child abuse. The same immunity provisions typically apply to other authorized actions taken by any individual in connection with the making of the report. Such actions include, for example, the taking of photographs and X-rays, the removal or retaining of the child, the disclosure of otherwise confidential or privileged information to CPS investigators, and the participation in any judicial proceedings that result from the reporting. Immunity provisions may preclude liability, but they cannot prevent the initiation of a civil action.

Initially, the court assumes that the plaintiff's allegations in the petition or complaint regarding the defendant's actions are true, without hearing any testimony. The court then determines if the immunity granted by the child abuse reporting statute was applicable. In jurisdictions that have adopted a rule of "absolute" immunity for statutorily prescribed activities of the defendants, the judge will dismiss the proceeding.

If, however, the jurisdiction has adopted a rule of "qualified" immunity (i.e., immunity only for actions undertaken in "good faith"), the court will allow the case to go to trial. The jury, or the judge acting as the finder of fact, will then hear testimony on behalf of each party from various witnesses regarding the allegations of the petition. If the alleged actions are proved to be true, but the trier of fact concludes that they were taken in good faith, the proceeding will be dismissed. Liability attaches only if the facts adduced at the trial prove both that the defendants engaged in the alleged behavior and that the defendants did not act in good faith.

ADDITIONAL CAUSES OF ACTION BASED ON FAILURES TO PROTECT THE CHILD AND RELATED DEFENSES

In situations involving state-employed child protection workers that resulted in the death or additional serious injury to the child, the child and an innocent parent or guardian may bring an action alleging that the public employees should have taken various steps to protect the child. The lawsuits may allege a failure to accept reports for investigation, a failure to adequately investigate reports, a failure to remove the child from the home, a failure to protect the child following return to the home or to foster care or a child care facility, or a failure to provide services leading to the return of the child (Sprague, 1991). These actions are also typically brought under state tort law.

Similar suits for damages have been brought charging violations of the federal constitution. The typical allegation is that the officials' failure to act deprived them of their liberty in violation of the Due Process Clause of the Fourteenth Amendment to the United States Constitution. Specifically, the plaintiffs assert that substantive due process requires state agents to protect children referred as abused to child protection agencies. Nevertheless, in 1989, the United States Supreme Court limited the type of suit that could be brought in some of these cases (*DeShaney v. Winnebago County Dept. of Social Servs.*, 1989). The Court concluded that a state's failure to protect a child, not in the actual custody of the state, against violence generally will not constitute a violation of the Due Process Clause, because the Clause imposes no duty on the states to provide members of the general public with adequate protective services. While the Clause forbids the state from depriving individuals of life, liberty, and property without due process of law, it only limits the state's power to act and does not impose an affirmative obligation to insure any minimal level of safety and security. Thus, the constitutional issue is not whether the CPS agency, or another public actor, was aware of the danger to the child, but rather whether it limited or prevented the child from acting on his or her own behalf. Liability still could be found, however, under state rather than federal law, based on negligent conduct, or in instances where a child is within the custody of a state agency.

In addition to any immunity provided under the reporting statute, civil liability may also be precluded by the "public duty" doctrine or rule (Prosser & Keeton, 1984). This rule generally applies only to health care professionals or other child care workers who are state employees. The rule provides that a public official is generally not liable to individuals for his or her negligence in discharging public duties. The rationale behind the rule is that the duty is owed to the public at large, rather than to any one individual.

Liability will attach, however, where the duty is specifically owed an individual under state tort law. A special relationship between an individual and a public official or agency may be sufficient to give rise to liability for negligence in carrying out that duty (Prosser & Keeton, 1984). State reporting laws may be viewed as creating such a duty. Consequently, the public duty doctrine generally will not protect a physician or other health care professional employed by a public agency who undertakes to treat a child, but then fails to report child abuse or otherwise fails to comply with the specific requirements of the reporting statute.

Finally, in addition to legislating a statutory immunity for actions taken by reporters under the child abuse reporting laws, a number of states have enacted general immunity statutes that protect public employees from liability for injuries caused while acting within the scope of their employment (Prosser & Keeton, 1984). The underlying rationale is that the fear of being sued will infringe on the individual's discharge of his or her duty. In addition, even in the absence of a statutory provision, as a matter of common law, immunity may be affirmatively pled and judicially invoked by public employees.

As with the immunity provisions under the reporting statutes, "absolute immunity" applies to "public officials whose special functions or constitutional status requires complete protection from suit" (*Harlow v. Fitzgerald*, 1982), and extends to judges, legislators, and prosecutors, acting within their official capacity. Only "qualified" or "good faith immunity," on the other hand, is available to officials performing discretionary functions. But even such limited immunity may be sufficient to terminate a lawsuit based on insubstantial claims involving bare allegations of malice by government employees (*Harlow v. Fitzgerald*, 1982).

◆ THE LITIGATION OF CHILD ABUSE AND NEGLECT CASES

Court involvement in child abuse or neglect cases may occur in the form of a civil proceeding under specific child abuse or neglect statutes in a juvenile or family court; or in a criminal proceeding for homicide, assault or battery, or criminal child abuse or neglect. The issue may also be litigated in a child custody case related to a dissolution of marriage proceeding. A recent study examined more than 800 substantiated cases of intrafamilial child abuse and neglect reported in three counties across the country in the mid 1980's. Statistical analyses indicated that juvenile court proceedings were brought in just 21% of the cases and criminal prosecutions in only 4%, although treatment plans developed in some 75% of the cases and out-of-home placement occurred in 50% of the sample. Thus, it is apparent that criminal prosecutions of the perpetrator remain relatively infrequent (Tjaden & Thoennes, 1992). Usually, the state's goal of protecting the child in peril is met in a civil proceeding that takes place in a juvenile court or a family court.

This section reviews how child abuse cases generally proceed in juvenile, criminal, and divorce courts. It concludes with a discussion of the evidentiary rules that may arise in any trial dealing with child abuse.

THE ROLE OF THE JUVENILE COURT AND ITS PROCEDURES

The role of the juvenile court or family court in child abuse cases is to (1) protect the child from further injury; (2) provide a fair and impartial hearing on the allegations in the petition; (3) consider recommendations of the child protection agency and other social service agencies; (4) implement a treatment plan for the child and/or the parent(s) when appropriate; and (5) protect the constitutional rights of both the child and the parents. The function of the court is not to punish but rather to work closely with the social service agencies to effect a treatment plan designed to protect the child. Generally, the court attempts to improve the family situation so that the family is preserved (Fox, 1984; Johnson, 1975; Hertz et al., 1991), unless the child has suffered serious harm and would continue to be endangered if allowed to remain within that family.

Statutory provisions give these courts their specific powers. Typically, juvenile courts are authorized to adjudicate proceedings involving claims of abuse and neglect, dependency, and delinquency, as well as requests for the termination of parental rights (Johnson, 1975; Fox, 1984). There has been a long-standing debate, however, on whether the focus of juvenile court jurisdictional statutes, from a policy perspective, should be directed to intervention where there has been a showing of potentially harmful behavior of the parents or caretaker (Besharov, 1988) or only where there is a showing of harmful effects of such behavior on the child (Wald, 1975).

Some states have structured their juvenile justice system around family courts. Family courts generally have a broader jurisdiction than juvenile courts. This includes divorce and child custody, intrafamily assaults, and juvenile traffic offenses. Juvenile courts and family courts are courts of limited jurisdiction, and thus are involved only in those types of cases which the state's statutes specifically authorize the court to hear. Moreover, these courts can issue orders only as specifically authorized by statute (Fox, 1984). Separate sets of state and local court rules may also govern the conduct of juvenile and family court procedures.

Child abuse and neglect proceedings usually involve bifurcated hearings. In order for the court to take any action with respect to the child, it first must determine that the child has, in fact, been abused or neglected and thus qualifies to be a "ward" of the court or "dependent" on the court for care and protection. This is often referred to as the "adjudicatory" stage or phase of the proceeding. If the court concludes that abuse or neglect has taken place, the child is considered to be under the "jurisdiction" of the juvenile court and the second phase or dispositional hearing is held. The dispositional hearing is designed to determine the appropriate intervention and to initiate a treatment plan.

The court may then order one or more of a variety of dispositions for the child. Additionally, the court may order dispositions for one or both of the parents. Generally, if the parent fails to comply with the juvenile court's order, the court cannot punish the parent by fines or imprisonment, but is restricted to conditioning the child's return to the home on the parent's obeying the court's order (Hertz et al., 1991). In very limited instances, in which the remedy of changing custody is not available or appropriate, the court may be authorized to hold the parent in contempt and jail the parent until the parent complies with the court's order.

Juvenile court proceedings generally are confidential and closed to the public and the press. In most instances, only those individuals directly involved are allowed access.

PARTICIPANTS IN THE JUVENILE COURT PROCESS

Participants in a juvenile court child abuse proceeding may include the judge, the petitioner, the child, the parent or parents, an attorney for the petitioner, an attorney for the parent, a *guardian ad litem*, and sometimes an attorney for the child (Fox, 1984; Johnson, 1975).

Judge

Child abuse cases in juvenile court are heard by a judge assigned to the juvenile court on a permanent or a rotating basis or by an attorney who is appointed to hear cases in juvenile court. These attorneys are called commissioners, masters, or referees.

The judge's initial responsibility in juvenile court child abuse cases is to protect the child's well-being, and in seeking to attain that goal, to see to it that proper procedures are observed. In addition, the judge is the trier of fact. Generally, there are no juries. The judge rules on the admissibility of evidence and then decides, based on the evidence admitted, whether the child should be adjudicated and placed under the jurisdiction of the juvenile court. In the dispositional hearing, the judge reviews the various recommendations and determines the appropriate disposition for the child.

Petitioner

State statutes often restrict who may bring actions in juvenile court. Generally, a suit may be filed by probation officers, juvenile officers, officials of the state or local social service agency, or local county or prosecuting attorneys. In some states "any interested person" can initiate a proceeding. The decision to initiate juvenile court proceedings is based on a variety of factors, including: (1) the nature of injury involved; (2) the attitude of the family toward voluntary cooperation with social service agencies; and (3) prior history of abuse or neglect within the family.

Child

The child is the subject of the juvenile court proceeding. The case is often named or "styled" "In the Interest of John Doe, a Child." The child may be called as a witness at the hearing by any of the parties and may be subject to cross-examination by other parties.

Parents

Each parent of the child is entitled to notice of the hearing and in most jurisdictions is considered a party in the case. The parent, too, can be called as a witness and would then be subject to cross-examination. A parent can claim his or her constitutional right under the Fifth Amendment to refuse to respond to any question that might tend to be incriminating. Such a right may be limited if the state grants immunity to the parent whereby testimony given by the parent cannot then be used against him or her. In addition, the U.S. Supreme Court has held that, even without such a grant of immunity a parent can be required to produce a child, in his or her custody, for a court hearing, at least in those instances where a parent has custody of a child pursuant to a court order resulting from child protection proceedings. Such action can be mandated even though it might tend to incriminate the parent and aid the state in criminally prosecuting the parent (*Baltimore City Dep't of Social Serv. v. Bouknight*, 1990).

Attorney for the Petitioner

In most juvenile courts, there will be a county, city, or corporation attorney who is employed full-time to represent the party instituting the court action. In some jurisdictions, CPS agencies have their own attorneys whose functions include bringing such juvenile court actions. In some localities the government contracts with private attorneys for representation. The petitioner's attorney drafts and files the petition and other necessary pleadings or motions. At the adjudicatory hearing the attorney for the petitioner attempts to establish, through the presentation of evidence, that the allegations in the petition are true. Then, at the dispositional hearing, the attorney attempts to convince the court to follow the recommendations of the petitioner regarding the child's future.

Attorney for the Parent(s)

Because it is often the parent who is suspected of inflicting the harm or neglecting the child, the parent will typically want to be represented by an attorney in the juvenile court proceeding. In every state the parent has a right to be represented. In most jurisdictions the state will appoint an attorney if the parent is indigent, although this is not required by the U.S. Constitution. The right of a parent to appointed counsel may be granted by state statute. The U.S. Supreme Court has held that the Constitution does not require the appointment of counsel for parents in every parental termination proceeding (*Lassiter v. Department of Social Services*, 1981). The Court ruled that in the absence of an applicable state statute or rule regarding the appointment of an attorney for indigent parents, the decision to do so must be made by the trial judge on a case-by-case basis.

The attorney for the parent, of course, is required to protect the interests of the parent. In the adjudicatory hearing, the parent's attorney usually tries to persuade the court that no abuse or neglect occurred, that any injury sustained was accidental, or alternatively that the perpetrator was someone other than the parent and the parent cannot be faulted for the perpetrator's conduct.

If the child is adjudicated to be within the jurisdiction of the juvenile court, the parent's attorney in a dispositional hearing will typically seek to have the child remain in the custody of his or her client or otherwise minimize the extent of official intervention in the family. The attorney must also protect the other interests of his client. The attorney must caution the client not to make statements that could be used against the parent in a later criminal prosecution. If there is a conflict of interest between the parents, it may be necessary for each parent to have his or her own attorney.

Representation for the Child

Many states have enacted statutes that provide representation for the child in child protection proceedings. State laws vary, however, as to whether the child is to be represented by a *guardian ad litem* (guardian for this particular law suit), an attorney, or both. Frequently, one individual is appointed to both positions although the responsibilities of the two differ.

Both the *guardian ad litem* and the attorney may present evidence and question witnesses at the adjudicatory hearing and both may offer recommendations regarding the child's placement and treatment at the dispositional hearing.

The *guardian ad litem* represents the child's best interest in the child abuse or neglect proceeding. He or she must use independent judgment to determine the best interest of the child. The *guardian ad litem* is not the child's legal guardian and has no duties after the proceeding. An attorney must be an advocate for his client, in this case the child, and when the child is mature enough to express an opinion, counsel must generally advocate what the child determines to be in his or her own best interest.

JUVENILE COURT PROCEDURES

Petition

A juvenile court case involving abuse or neglect usually begins with the filing of a petition or complaint that alleges one or more specific instances of child abuse, neglect, or dependency. The petitioner is usually a juvenile probation officer or a representative of the state's department of social services charged with the investigation of allegations brought to the court by social service personnel, police, or other individuals. With the assistance of the attorney, the petitioner decides whether or not to file the action.

Custody Hearing

The juvenile court will typically conduct a custody or detention hearing within a short time after a petition is filed. This allows the judge to review the initial decision to hold the child and to authorize continued placement outside the home. The hearing occurs only if the child has not been returned to his or her home pending further proceedings but rather remains in a hospital, other temporary shelter, or with relatives without the parents' consent. The temporary placement may have been authorized or arranged by the juvenile court, a probation officer, or a CPS worker. Before ordering the continuation of the protective custody, the judge generally must ascertain, pending a full hearing, that there is a substantial risk of immediate harm to the child and that there is no viable alternative for reducing that risk.

Adjudicatory Hearing

In an adjudicatory hearing the state presents the evidence of abuse or neglect to the court. The only issue to be resolved is whether the child has been abused, neglected, abandoned, or otherwise comes within the jurisdiction of the court. In many instances the parent will admit the allegations or at least a sufficient part of them for the court to conclude that it is authorized to "take jurisdiction" or to "adjudicate" the child to be a ward of the court. In other situations, however, it is necessary for the attorney representing the petitioner to call witnesses to substantiate the facts alleged in the petition. Typical witnesses are doctors, police, teachers, child protection workers, relatives, parents, or other individuals who possess relevant information. Often, a subpoena is issued to compel the witnesses' attendance at the proceedings.

The burden of proving child abuse or neglect in a juvenile court is on the party asserting the abuse or neglect, typically the state. The petitioner does not have to prove that a specific individual committed a certain abusive act, but only that the child's environment is injurious to his or her welfare or that those legally responsible for the child's care did not carry out their legal responsibility.

The standard of proof refers to the level of certainty by which the trier of fact must be convinced that the allegations in the petition are true. In a juvenile court child abuse case the standard is not that of "beyond a reasonable doubt," as in a criminal matter. State laws differ, however, as to whether the petitioner must prove child abuse or neglect by the standard of a "preponderance of the evidence" or by "clear and convincing evidence." Clear and convincing is higher than preponderance but lower than beyond a reasonable doubt. Proof by a "preponderance of the evidence" means that the petitioner must convince the judge that it is more likely than not that certain facts are true, by a 51% degree of certainty. A "clear and convincing evidence" standard requires proving that it is highly probable that the existence of those facts is true. The U.S. Supreme Court has concluded, however, that a burden of proof of at least "clear and convincing evidence" is constitutionally necessary when the petitioner seeks to terminate parental rights. Some states, however, do require the higher standard of proof of "beyond a reasonable doubt" for termination of parental rights (*Santosky v. Kramer*, 1982).

In most jurisdictions the judge has the authority to exclude individuals from the courtroom upon a finding that this is in the best interests of the child to do so. A judge may, for example, exclude a parent when the child is testifying to acts of abuse or neglect. Similarly, the judge may exclude a child, who might otherwise be entitled to be present, during medical or other testimony.

Rules of evidence do apply in juvenile court proceedings, but their application may be less strict and court procedures less formal than in criminal cases. Direct evidence (i.e. evidence by an eyewitness to the incident) is not necessary to prove child abuse or neglect. Rather, abuse or neglect can be proven by circumstantial evidence. The inference of abuse or neglect can be drawn from a combination of evidence, such as the nature and extent of the injuries, the lack of explanation for the injuries consistent with medical knowledge, the age of the child, and the fact that the parent was the custodian of the child at the time of the alleged abuse.

If the state fails to establish child abuse or neglect by the requisite standard of proof, the case is dismissed and no further action is taken. If, however, the child is adjudicated and the court takes jurisdiction over the child, the case proceeds to disposition.

Dispositional Hearing

The appropriate placement for the child and the appropriate treatment, if any, for the child and the parent are determined at the dispositional hearing. The hearing may take place immediately after the adjudication or may be scheduled for a later date, pending the collection of additional information that might aid the judge in deciding the terms for the court order. Evidence submitted at the hearing usually focuses on the recommendations made to the judge by a court social worker, and in some situations by the *guardian ad litem*, regarding placement and treatment. Generally, state statutes give juvenile courts the authority to order a broad range of dispositions, but the specific powers granted to the court differ from state to state. Additionally, some states add a phrase such as "and such other orders as the court deems necessary." Common dispositional powers include: (1) returning the child to the home with or without supervision; (2) giving physical custody to a relative; (3) placing the child in foster care; or (4), in severe cases, terminating the rights of the parent to the child.

Once a child has been adjudicated a ward of the juvenile court, the court retains "jurisdiction" or control over the child until the child either reaches the age of majority (as defined by state law, usually 18) or until the jurisdictional status is otherwise terminated by the court. Most juvenile courts hold periodic reviews to measure the progress of the case and to determine the need to modify previous orders. Review hearings are usually scheduled every six months to a year.

The most drastic measure a state may take to protect an abused or neglected child is the termination of parental rights. In essence the court orders that the parent(s) no longer have any rights or duties with respect to the child (Wadlington et al., 1983). Termination of parental rights may be either voluntary or involuntary. State statutes specify the grounds and the specific circumstances under which parental rights may be terminated. Usually involuntary termination is a disposition of last resort.

The most common grounds for termination of parental rights are abandonment, child abuse, or neglect. Statutes specify what conditions constitute abandonment for termination purposes. In some states termination of parental rights is not an authorized disposition in the initial child abuse or neglect proceeding. Rather, it can only be ordered in situations where there is chronic failure to support the child or a consistent pattern of specific unacceptable parental behavior with respect to the child. Ordinarily, the parent must be given sufficient time and opportunity to become a more adequate parent before termination. In some states a parent's severe chronic mental illness rendering him or her unable to adequately care for the child may also be grounds for termination of parental rights.

CHILD ABUSE AND NEGLECT IN CRIMINAL COURT

The prosecution of individuals accused of crimes perpetrated against children, while not necessarily commonplace, has increased in recent decades, particularly in the area of child sexual abuse (Smith & Goretsky, 1992). This increase is due, in part, to advances made in identifying battered and sexually abused children and to the relaxation of evidentiary rules relating to victim competency, in-court testimony, and certain out-of-court statements (Bulkley, 1985; MacMurray, 1989; Attorney General, 1984; Kempe et al., 1962).

Although the juvenile court's involvement in these cases is based on the state's role as *parens patriae*, the criminal justice system's (CJS) involvement is exercised under the state's police power, which authorizes official action to prevent identified harms to society. The use of this power serves to dissuade private retribution on the part of victims by placing responsibility for prosecuting alleged violations of the criminal law solely within the government's ambit. CJS activities include law enforcement investigations, criminal prosecutions, and sentencing proceedings. The substantive criminal law defines what conduct is criminal and provides the punishment to be imposed upon an adjudication or finding of guilt.

SUBSTANTIVE CRIMINAL LAW

State legislatures are responsible for declaring what conduct within their own jurisdictions is deemed criminal and subject to punishment. Similarly, the U.S. Congress provides for the punishment of activity determined to be harmful to society that occurs within certain territories under federal supervision.

In most jurisdictions, "child abuse" or "child neglect" is viewed as violating the prohibition of one or more of the following statutory crimes: murder, homicide, manslaughter, felonious restraint, false imprisonment, assault, battery, rape, statutory rape, deviant sexual assault, sexual assault, indecent exposure, child endangerment, reckless endangerment, and corruption of minors. A majority of jurisdictions do, however, have specific crimes of child abuse and child neglect. Depending on the alleged conduct and resulting harm to the victim, a criminal prosecution may be sought for one or more of these offenses. Conviction of more than one substantive crime arising from the same series of actions may be authorized, if the proof of each particular crime differs or overlaps (LaFave & Scott, 1986; Perkins & Boyce, 1982).

Crimes are further differentiated as felonies and misdemeanors. The boundary between which offenses constitute felonies and misdemeanors varies from state to state. In some jurisdictions, the distinction between the two is based on whether ordered incarceration will take place in a local jail or in a state penitentiary, but more frequently the difference in the prescribed minimum penalty in the event of a conviction. In general, a felony offense typically is punishable by one year or more of imprisonment. Sanctions imposed for a misdemeanor conviction usually involve incarceration for less than a year and/or a fine of $500 or less (LaFave & Scott, 1986). The distinction between misdemeanors and felonies is not only relevant to the potential punishment, but also to the resulting procedural consequences. Greater constitutional protection is offered to defendants in felony prosecutions, such as the right to a trial by jury (Perkins & Boyce, 1982). Defendants are entitled to appointed counsel for all felonies and in misdemeanors where the convicted defendant's punishment involves confinement (Whitebread & Slobogin, 1986).

PROCEDURE IN CRIMINAL CASES

The precise procedure in criminal cases varies somewhat from state to state, but the sequence is basically the same (**Figure 18-1**) (Kamisar et al., 1986; Whitebread & Slobogin, 1986). Most frequently, the initial stage in the CJS process is the police investigation. In cases of alleged child abuse, police involvement may (1) precede reporting to the CPS agency; (2) coincide with or accompany the CPS investigation; or (3) follow the CPS agency's substantiation of a reported allegation of maltreatment and referral to juvenile court and/or the law enforcement agency. Regardless of the time and manner in which law enforcement officers are notified of a suspected case, the police investigation is directed at goals separate from those of child protection investigations. The law enforcement agency's primary function is to determine whether a crime has occurred, and if so, whether there is sufficient evidence indicating the guilt of a particular person to justify arresting and charging the individual. CPS agencies are concerned with the identification of abuse for prevention and intervention purposes in furtherance of child protection.

Investigation

Police officers use a variety of investigative techniques, including: pre-arrest questioning of possible suspects, interviewing witnesses or others with pertinent information, and collecting physical evidence. Care must be taken, however, to insure that a health care professional does not breach the obligation of confidentiality in an effort to cooperate with law enforcement personnel. Access to an individual's medical records or information should not be given to law enforcement personnel without a valid release of information, specific statutory authority, or a court order (Stromberg, 1988).

Medical Records and Information

Health care professionals may wish to obtain a release of information authorizing the disclosure of information to police and prosecutors. Only half of the state statutes explicitly authorize and require the reporting of child abuse cases to the police. Such statutes may permit disclosure to certain law enforcement agencies or personnel of either specific facts or general medical or other reliable information known to health care personnel. In the absence of such specific authority, on occasion, police sometimes attempt to gain access to this information by threatening the health care professional with criminal charges based on other statutes. Such threats ought to be resisted.

Police Prosecution Courts Corrections

Figure18-1 A General View of the Criminal Justice System. This chart seeks to present a simple yet comprehensive view of the movement of cases through the criminal justice system. Procedures in individual jurisdictions may vary from the pattern shown here. The differing weights of line indicate the relative volumes of cases disposed of at various points in the system, but this is only suggestive since no nationwide data of this sort exist.

Reprinted from: The Challenge of Crime in a Free Society, The President's Commission on Law Enforcement and the Administration of Justice, Washington, D.C., 1967.

1. May continue until trial.

2. Administrative record of arrest. First step at which temporary release on bail may be available.

3. Before magistrate, commissioner, or justice of peace. Formal notice of charge, advice of rights. Bail set. Summary trials for petty offenses usually conducted here without further processing.

4. Preliminary testing of evidence against defendant. Charge may be reduced. No separate preliminary hearing for misdemeanors in some systems.

5. Charge filed by prosecutor on basis of information submitted by police or citizens. Alternative to grand jury indictment; often used in felonies, almost always in misdemeanors.

6. Reviews whether Government evidence sufficient to justify trial. Some States have no grand jury system; others seldom use it.

7. Appearance for plea; defendant elects trial by judge or jury (if available); counsel for indigent usually appointed here in felonies. Often not at all in other cases.

8. Charge may be reduced at any time prior to trial in return for plea of guilty or for other reasons.

9. Challenge on constitutional grounds to legality of detention. May be sought at any point in process.

10. Police often hold informal hearings, dismiss or adjust many cases without further processing.

11. Probation officer decides desirability of further court action.

12. Welfare agency, social services, counseling, medical care, etc. for cases where adjudicatory handling not needed.

409

A few states still have misprision of felony statutes, which create an affirmative obligation to report a felony on the part of anyone with knowledge of its occurrence. Although some jurisdictions have statutes prohibiting the obstruction of justice or the hindering of prosecution, these, as well as misprision of felony laws, generally require an affirmative interference with an officer's lawful discharge of duties in order for the statute to apply (Perkins & Boyce, 1982; LaFave & Scott, 1986). Thus, it would be permissible for the health care professional to refuse to disclose to the police otherwise confidential or privileged information.

On occasion health care personnel may be presented with a *subpoena duces tecum* commanding the production of medical records (Stromberg, 1988). Subpoenas are generally issued in the name of a court clerk at the request of an attorney, but at this stage there has been no judicial determination that the record should, in fact, be disclosed without consent. In the absence of a release of information from an authorized individual such as a parent, a judge should be asked to rule on the question of whether the medical record should be released to avoid the possibility of liability for breach of confidentiality.

Questioning of Suspects

As the police proceed with their investigation, possible suspects may be questioned. If an individual has been taken into custody or otherwise deprived of his freedom of action in any significant way, prior to questioning by law enforcement officials, the suspect must be given his "Miranda warnings" (*Miranda v. Arizona*, 1966; Whitebread & Slobogin, 1986). These warnings contain specific cautionary language informing the individual that he has a right to remain silent, that anything he says may be used against him in a court of law, that he has a right to an attorney, and that if he can't afford an attorney one will be appointed for him. If the warnings are not given, or if any statement or confession made was not voluntary, then the information may be excluded from evidence in any subsequent related criminal trial.

Arrest and Booking

Prior to making an arrest (i.e., formally taking an individual into custody), law enforcement officers must have probable cause to believe that the arrestee is committing or has committed a felony, or that the arrestee committed a misdemeanor in the officer's presence (Whitebread & Slobogin, 1986). If, however, the crime is a misdemeanor not committed in the officer's presence, the policeman will have to obtain an arrest warrant from a magistrate or other judicial officer.

Once the police have probable cause to justify an arrest, they usually take the suspect into custody and process or "book" him or her. Fingerprints are made and "mug shots" or booking photos are taken. How long the suspect can be held without judicial review is determined by state law. If an arrest warrant is not issued by a court before the termination of the prescribed time period, the police must release the suspect. In many jurisdictions, an individual arrested has the right to have a bond commissioner or judge decide if he or she is to be released on personal recognizance or if a bail amount is to be set, pending prosecutorial review of the case and the possible issuance of formal charges.

Prosecutorial Discretion

The investigating police officer presents the case to the prosecutor's office. The prosecutor possesses broad discretion regarding whether or not to file formal charges. This latitude finds support historically in American law. A number of factors generally influence the decision to file charges, including the strength of the available evidence, the harm caused by the offense, the victim's attitude toward pressing the case, the arrestee's prior criminal record, and the adequacy of alternative remedies apart from prosecution (LaFave & Israel, 1985).

Prosecutors sometimes are particularly reluctant to prosecute child abuse cases. Sometimes there is the belief that a criminal prosecution of a parent may impede treatment and reunification of the family. More importantly, quite frequently a young child is the victim or otherwise is the primary or sole witness and concerns arise regarding both the child's credibility and the absence of other admissible evidence. Extensive cross-examination of a child witness may lead to confusion. Fears also exist that the child may be highly suggestible to influence by the perpetrator or other family members, causing an alteration of the content of the child's testimony at trial from the description of events provided earlier to the police and prosecutors. Sex abuse cases generate concerns that the jury will view the child as being prone to fantasy or being curious about sexuality and therefore apt to be confused. The extent to which these notions are valid is debatable. Many prosecutors, however, believe that the jury's possible concerns make it difficult to establish the elements of a criminal offense to the satisfaction of a jury "beyond a reasonable doubt" (Lloyd, 1981; Melton, 1981). Those relatively few cases in which prosecutions are brought generally involve sexual abuse, severe maltreatment, a nonparent perpetrator, an ethnic minority perpetrator, a female victim, or a victim who is 7 to12 years of age (Tjaden & Thoennes, 1992).

Over the past decade, many prosecution offices have organized special units or assigned a limited number of prosecutors to pursue these cases. In such instances expertise with these cases is developed and successful prosecutions may be more likely to occur.

If the prosecutor elects to bring criminal charges, a complaint is filed and if an arrest warrant has not previously been obtained, the court generally will issue one upon the filing of the complaint. Further screening out of cases may occur as a result of a preliminary hearing of grand jury action, as described below.

Initial Appearance

The arrestee, now referred to as the defendant, is presented before the court and advised of the formal charges contained within the complaint. This proceeding must occur within a specified period of time after arrest, as prescribed by law. At this hearing bail and other possible conditions of release will be set or reviewed if initial determinations on these issues were made earlier. In felony cases a date will be set for a preliminary hearing on the charges, as described later, unless such a hearing is waived by the defendant or a grand jury issues an indictment in the interim. Defendants charged with misdemeanors are generally not entitled to preliminary hearings or grand jury indictments and the case will be brought based solely on the prosecutor's charge (LaFave & Israel, 1985).

Right to Counsel

At the initial appearance, the court will generally inquire whether the defendant has retained counsel or wishes to do so. If the defendant is indigent, the court will appoint an attorney to represent the defendant. The attorney will either be a public defender or an attorney in private practice who has agreed to represent indigents. In either instance, the attorney will be paid by the state (LaFave & Israel, 1985).

Bail

Bail is usually viewed as a means of securing the defendant's presence at subsequent proceedings, and it also has come to be viewed as a way of helping to ensure the safety of the community. State and federal statutes may specify factors for the court to consider in determining whether bail should be set and in what amount. Typically, these factors include the seriousness of the offense, the strength of the case, the defendant's prior criminal record, and the defendant's background. The court may impose additional conditions of release. Appropriate conditions in child abuse cases may include a prohibition on contact with the victim, other members of the victim's family, or other witnesses.

Sometimes, particularly in homicide cases, the court will refuse to set bail or other conditions of release and instead will order that the defendant be held in jail pending the trial. Such preventive detention may be warranted upon a finding of future dangerousness or when there is a serious likelihood that the defendant will flee or otherwise attempt to obstruct justice (Whitebread & Slobogin, 1986). This measure may be appropriate in child abuse cases when there are concerns that the perpetrator will return to the child's home and either engage in further abuse or attempt to influence the child to recant accusatory statements.

Preliminary Hearing

The preliminary hearing or grand jury is the next stage in the process. In many jurisdictions, individuals accused of crimes have a right to an adversarial preliminary hearing before a magistrate or judge. There based on the evidence presented the court determines whether probable cause exists to believe that a crime was committed and that the defendant was the perpetrator. Both the prosecution and the defense have the right to present evidence by subpoenaing witnesses and questioning them, as well as by the submission of documentary evidence such as medical and other reports.

The government carries the burden of proof. The defendant rarely presents affirmative evidence on his own behalf at this stage, although prosecution witnesses may be rigorously cross-examined. Probable cause will be found in practically all cases because the magistrate or judge generally does not have to weigh the credibility of the various witnesses unless the testimony is implausible or incredible. The only question is whether or not a jury, if it believed even some of the evidence presented, could find that a crime was committed and the defendant did it. If the judge concludes that a jury could so find, then the case is "bound over" for trial. The prosecutor will then issue a charge, usually called an information, based on what took place at the preliminary hearing. If no probable cause is found, the case must be dismissed and the defendant released (LaFave & Israel, 1985; Whitebread & Slobogin, 1986).

The preliminary hearing gives the defendant an opportunity to review the likely testimony to be presented against him. This may play a significant role in inducing him to enter a guilty plea. The defendant, of course, is entitled to attend the proceedings, although as described below, in some cases involving child abuse, limits may be placed on this right.

Grand Jury

In federal felony prosecutions, the Fifth Amendment to the U.S. Constitution requires that the case proceed only upon issuance of a grand jury indictment. A number of state constitutions contain comparable provisions. In some of those jurisdictions the preliminary hearing may be bypassed by the presentation of the case to a grand jury.

Grand jury review, whether or not subsequent to a preliminary hearing, also serves to provide a means of determining whether there is probable cause to proceed with prosecution against the defendant. But, unlike a preliminary hearing held before a judicial officer, the grand jury consists of a selected group of private citizens who review cases over a legislatively-determined period of time.

The grand jury screening process differs fundamentally from the preliminary hearing in the manner in which it is conducted. The grand jury meets in closed session and only hears testimony from witnesses whom it or the prosecutor subpoenas. Members of the grand jury and the prosecutor may question the witnesses, but the defendant and his counsel are not permitted to attend the proceeding (LaFave & Israel, 1985; Whitebread & Slobogin, 1986). The grand jury mechanism may be preferable in cases involving child maltreatment, because if the child is to be a witness, the grand jury procedure protects the child victim from the trauma of an additional confrontation with a perpetrator and an additional cross-examination by defense counsel. In some jurisdictions it may not even be necessary for the child victim to appear before the grand jury because a parent or law enforcement officer may be permitted to testify to what the child has stated or a videotape of the child's statement may be used in lieu of live testimony.

Upon a majority of the grand jurors finding sufficient evidence to justify prosecution, an indictment is signed by the members of the grand jury and designated a "true bill." The indictment, which sets forth a description of the offense, is then filed with the trial court. Return of a "no true bill" requires dismissal of the charges against the defendant.

Arraignment

After the filing of either the prosecutor's information or the grand jury indictment with the court, the defendant is formally arraigned. The defendant appears before the court and is informed of the charges now pending against him or her. The defendant then enters a plea of not guilty or guilty. The question of the propriety of bail and other release procedures may again be explored.

Pretrial Motions

Between entering a plea and the commencement of trial, the criminal defendant will typically make one or more pretrial motions, challenging such technical matters as the institution of the prosecution; the sufficiency of the indictment; the admissibility of expected physical evidence, statements, or confessions; the court's jurisdiction; and the physical location of the trial. In addition, the defendant will seek to "discover" certain materials from the prosecution and otherwise obtain information from witnesses who may testify against him. The extent to which this occurs is dependant on applicable law.

Plea Bargaining, Guilty Pleas, and Dismissals

Before arraignment, plea bargaining between the prosecutor and defendant frequently occurs. Agreements derived from plea negotiations may take various forms. Such agreements can involve a plea of guilty to a less serious offense, a plea of guilty to the charged offense with a promise by the prosecutor to recommend a reduced sentence, or a plea of guilty to one or more charges in exchange for dismissal of other charges or a promise not to file additional charges. Justification for plea bargaining is found in the notion that it provides a quick disposition of cases necessitated by a system of justice that is already heavily overburdened. Plea bargaining is an important tool for the prosecutor when the child witness is reluctant to testify or the physical evidence of the crime is less than compelling.

The vast majority of criminal cases are disposed of by a guilty plea or by the dismissal of charges. In one study that examined a set of criminal filings in three counties across the country during the mid 1980s, 68% of the defendants entered guilty pleas to some or all of the charges and another 20% were dismissed prior to trial (Tjaden & Thoennes, 1992). These figures are consistent with national trends for all felony cases where only 10% to 15% of the cases that reach the trial court actually go to trial (LaFave & Israel, 1985).

Diversion

Diversion programs have emerged as a possible alternative to adjudication within the CJS. Diversion involves halting or suspending formal criminal proceedings against a defendant without a formal conviction and requiring his or her participation in a therapeutic program. Diversion programs are a response to the difficulties in successfully prosecuting child maltreatment cases, particularly those involving sexual abuse.

Diversion generally is used only for misdemeanors or less serious or first felony complaints, and typically when the victim and the accused are family members. It may begin before the arrest or at any other stage before to the commencement of the trial. Individuals selected for diversion are generally viewed as likely to participate in treatment and likely to benefit from it. Typically they are offered counseling directed at the abusive behavior, as well as career development, education, and supportive treatment services. If the participant responds favorably for a specified period of time, the court or the prosecutor or both will dismiss the case. If the defendant fails to meet the program's obligations, prosecution is resumed on the original criminal charge.

Jurisdictions vary in their use, if any, of diversion programs. Some states, by statute, specifically authorize diversion for particular crimes if certain criteria are met, while other jurisdictions provide for some degree of prosecutorial discretion or specific court involvement (Kamisar et al., 1986; LaFave & Israel, 1985). Similar schemes may be used as part of a condition of probation after a guilty plea or conviction at trial (Giarretto, 1976).

Constitutional and Related Issues at Trial

The trial of any criminal case raises a broad array of constitutional and related issues, practically all of which are designed to protect the defendant and ensure a fair and impartial trial.

Presumption of Innocence and Burden of Proof

The defendant is entitled to a presumption of innocence. This means that the prosecution has the burden of producing evidence of guilt and must persuade the trier of fact (the jury or the judge alone in a "bench trial") of the truth of each of the elements or legally significant facts of the offense with which the defendant is charged. Moreover, each of the elements must be proven by a high degree of evidence "beyond a reasonable doubt." Although it is difficult to define this standard, it is usually said that there must be "an abiding conviction, to a moral certainty, of the truth of the charge" (*Commonwealth v. Webster*, 1850).

Privileges

The Fifth Amendment to the U.S. Constitution protects the defendant against compelled self-incrimination. This protection includes the right of the defendant not to take the witness stand and be forced to testify against himself.

In addition, statements admitting responsibility for abuse which are made to spouses, physicians, and other health care professionals may be excluded as a result of a claim of privilege (McCormick, 1984). The privilege may apply in criminal cases with respect to at least some of the information provided to health care professionals, even in the face of an abrogation of the privilege for civil child protection proceedings under a state's reporting statute (Stromberg, 1988).

Searches, Seizures, and Confessions

As briefly noted in the discussion of social service and police response to reports of child abuse and neglect, an investigation of alleged child maltreatment may implicate a variety of constitutional issues which affect the admissibility of evidence at trial. These concerns are commonly based on activities such as the examination of the child, a search of a perpetrator's home, and statements obtained from the child's parent(s), guardian(s), or other possible perpetrators. The constitutional issues come into play not only in the context of potential civil liability of health care and child protection professionals, but also in criminal cases involving charges brought against perpetrators of child abuse and neglect.

Generally, constitutional provisions protect against intrusions by state authorities. Such authorities may include the police, child care workers, and even medical personnel employed by or acting on the direction of law enforcement or other state agencies. If such constitutional violations do occur, evidence that is obtained as a result of the violation may not be admitted in criminal prosecutions. Thus, physical evidence that implicates a defendant may be excluded if it was seized in violation of the defendant's rights to be free from unreasonable searches and seizures under the Fourth Amendment to the U.S. Constitution. Similarly, confessions made in the absence of required Miranda warnings or as a result of police coercion may not be admissible at a criminal trial.

Confrontation Clause

The Confrontation Clause of the Sixth Amendment to the U.S. Constitution is an area of constitutional law that has recently attracted attention from the U.S. Supreme Court. The Clause often impacts upon the trial of criminal cases involving allegations of child abuse. The Clause provides, in part, that "[i]n all criminal prosecutions, the accused shall enjoy the right ... to be confronted with the witnesses against him." The Clause confers on a criminal defendant a right to confront witnesses at trial, both face-to-face and through cross-examination, and is designed to increase the defendant's ability to challenge the charges against him and to ensure an adversarial proceeding at trial (Whitebread & Slobogin, 1986). Confrontation Clause rights are also buttressed by rights under the Fourteenth Amendment's Due Process Clause, which prohibits a state from depriving an individual of liberty without due process of law.

The tension between the right to confrontation and attempts both by legislatures and individual judges to protect child victims from the potential trauma of confronting the abuser at trial or in pre-trial proceedings is evident. Unlike the situation that may occur in both juvenile court and divorce-related hearings, where the court may be authorized in some circumstances to allow a child to testify "in camera" or in chambers and outside the presence of the alleged perpetrator, such testimony in a criminal case may violate the defendant's right to a public trial under the Sixth Amendment to the Constitution. It may also violate his or her right to confront witnesses and be present at trial under the Confrontation Clause. Finally, the First Amendment rights of the press and related rights of public access to trials may likewise be implicated (Whitebread & Slobogin, 1986).

A number of states have passed legislation providing for closed circuit and videotaped testimony in an effort to balance the competing interests of the child victims and the rights of criminal defendants. In addition, as discussed in the evidentiary section below, the Confrontation Clause may play a role in connection with the creation of various exceptions to the hearsay rule.

A violation of the Confrontation Clause may occur when the defendant is denied face-to-face confrontation with the witness. Although the defendant's right to be present extends to every stage of the trial, some exceptions do exist. The Supreme Court failed to find a violation of the Confrontation Clause when the defendant (but not his lawyer) was denied access to a pretrial hearing to determine the competency of two children who were victims of an alleged sex offense (*Kentucky v. Stincer*, 1985). The Court noted, however, that the questions asked did not relate to the crime itself and therefore the lack of the defendant's participation did not bear a substantial relationship to the defendant's opportunity to defend himself at trial. Moreover, the same questions were asked at trial where the defendant was present and there was full and complete cross-examination (LaFave & Israel, 1985).

The problem surrounding face-to-face confrontation is more likely when a child victim gives live testimony at trial, out of the presence of a defendant. In another case, the U.S. Supreme Court reversed the conviction, when a state law permitted a trial judge to order the placement of a large screen between the defendant and two

13-year-old girls who testified that he had sexually assaulted them. The Court noted that the screen improperly prevented the witnesses from seeing the defendant and only allowed him to dimly perceive them. Justice O'Connor, who agreed with the reversal but filed a separate opinion, pointed out that the statute presumed that trauma would occur any time a young victim testified. She suggested that had there been an individualized finding by the trial judge that the child witnesses needed special protection, a different result might have ensued (*Coy v. Iowa*, 1988; Whitebread & Slobogin, 1986).

Soon thereafter, the Supreme Court upheld a conviction under somewhat similar circumstances. In a 1990 case, a state statute provided for a one-way television procedure if the trial judge decided that face-to-face testimony "will result in the child suffering serious emotional distress such that the child cannot reasonably communicate" (*Maryland v. Craig*, 1990). The statute provided that once this finding was made, the witness, prosecutor, and defense counsel would withdraw to a separate room, while the judge, jury, and the defendant remained in the courtroom. The defendant could watch direct and cross-examination of the child over a video hookup and remain in electronic communication with his counsel.

The Court concluded that the central concerns regarding the Confrontation Clause were addressed under such a procedure. The Court acknowledged the "growing body of academic literature documenting the psychological trauma suffered by child abuse victims who must testify in court." It concluded that as long as the trial judge decided, on a case-by-case basis, that such trauma would result if the child was faced with the defendant, and procedures such as those provided were followed to ensure the defendant's rights were respected, there was no constitutional violation (Whitebread & Slobogin, 1986).

Trials

Defendants charged with felonies or misdemeanors punishable by more than six months in jail are entitled to jury trials. Juries generally comprise 12 persons, but in some jurisdictions, in certain cases, a jury of six is permissible. A defendant can waive his right to a jury trial and be tried by a judge alone. A jury verdict either of guilt or acquittal, at least in felony trials, must be unanimous. If the jury cannot come to a unanimous agreement, a mistrial results and the prosecution is terminated without a decision on the merits of the case. The state may not retry the defendant after an acquittal, but a subsequent prosecution may follow a mistrial.

Sentencing

Following a guilty verdict, a sentencing hearing is scheduled. Before the hearing, a pre-sentence report is completed, usually by the state's probation and parole department, to guide the judge in the sentencing decision. The report includes information about the defendant based on interviews with a variety of individuals who have had contact with the defendant. The report may include the results of psychological testing or interviewing.

Both state and federal law define the range of permissible sanctions that may be imposed for the offense committed, including whether probation is available. In some jurisdictions, in some circumstances, the jury will recommend a punishment, which the judge can follow or choose to ignore in favor of a less severe penalty (Campbell, 1978).

In some situations, the defendant may receive a prison sentence, but the sentence may be suspended with the defendant being placed on probation (with or without some limited period of incarceration) under the supervision of the probation department. A typical condition of probation in child abuse cases is a requirement of treatment of the defendant. The defendant's failure to attend or to participate in the treatment program can be viewed as a violation of probation and the court might then reinstate the prison term originally decreed. Other conditions of probation may include an order to stay away from the victim and required payment to the victim of his or her treatment costs.

Appeals and Post-conviction Actions

Following a criminal conviction, direct appellate review is limited to a statutorily defined period of time and allows challenges to any alleged errors committed by the judge that occurred at trial. These include the judge's rulings on various motions that the defendant's attorney made before or at trial, on objections which were made to the admissibility of evidence, and on instructions which the judge gave to the jury regarding the applicable law in the case. If the defendant's appeal is unsuccessful, he may make a "collateral attack" on the conviction. A collateral attack is usually based on constitutional challenges, such as a claim of ineffective assistance of counsel at trial or on appeal. The state, however, may not appeal from an acquittal.

CHILD CUSTODY DISPUTES AND ALLEGATIONS OF ABUSE

ARENAS OF LITIGATION

Sometimes allegations of child abuse arise in child custody disputes. Often they include claims of sexual abuse (Nicholson, 1988; Fahn, 1991). The parents may have been residing together as a family unit at the time, or the alleged behavior may have occurred subsequent to the break-up but pending judicial resolution of custody and visitation rights. Alternatively, the alleged incident might have taken place after a temporary or final custody decree, while the child was in the custody of a custodial parent, or during the course of visitation by the child with the noncustodial parent.

If no dissolution of marriage action has been filed, but there is a dispute concerning child custody, its resolution is likely to take place in the context of a juvenile court child protection proceeding as described above. In addition, most states have enacted legislation that provides for "civil orders of protection" for victims of domestic violence. Many of these statutes provide for judicial determination of custody rights with respect to the children of the parties involved in the context of such litigation (Finn, 1989).

Finally, the issue of child abuse may appear in any one of a number of stages of a court action related to the dissolution of a marriage of the child's parents. For example, together with or shortly after the filing of a petition for divorce, a motion may be filed requesting the court to issue an order providing for temporary custody and visitation pending the final hearing on the petition for a decree of divorce. At the final hearing, in which the court must determine provisions for joint or sole custody and visitation rights, the issue of child abuse may also be contested. Subsequent to the court issuing a final custody order, one or both of the parents may file motions to modify that order, alleging a change in the circumstances of the child or custodial parent. There, too, the question of child abuse may be litigated. State law or state or local court rules will determine whether it will be a juvenile or family court or a court of general civil jurisdiction which will rule on the custody issue in each of these contexts (Edwards, 1987).

Litigation of child custody disputes in each of these situations differs from that in the juvenile court/child protection context or the criminal context. The court here is engaging in a private dispute settlement function where it must choose between two or more individuals, each of whom claims an associational interest with the child. In the other situations described previously, the court is enforcing standards of behavior believed necessary to protect the child or the greater society at large and, perhaps, to punish a wrongdoer (Mnookin, 1975).

PROCEDURAL AND EVIDENTIARY RULES

The state's power to adjudicate private custody disputes, like its power in child protection cases, derives from the common law concept of the state as *parens patriae* (Cunningham & Horowitz, 1989). Each state, through legislation and judicial precedent, has prescribed both procedural and evidentiary rules which regulate how the issue is to be litigated as well as substantive rules that guide the court in determining what its orders regarding custody should be (Clark, 1988; Goldner, 1987).

Depending upon the particular state, rules exist that permit or require the appointment of a guardian ad litem in child custody disputes. Similarly, under more or less restrictive circumstances, the trial judge may order that an investigation and report regarding custodial arrangements for the child be made by employees of public or private social service agencies or by other competent individuals. The child may be referred to professionals for diagnosis by the court or by the individual conducting the custody investigation. The investigator may consult with and obtain information from medical, psychiatric, or other experts who have previously dealt with the child. The judge may conduct in-chambers interviews with the child to ascertain custodial preferences or seek the advice of professional personnel in an effort to elicit such information most effectively. Some jurisdictions require the consent of all parties, in some circumstances, for the application of one or more of these unique procedural devices in a given child custody case. The manner in which a given state approaches these issues affects the court's ability to ascertain whether or not abuse or neglect has taken place. This, in turn, will control the extent to which the abuse or neglect then plays a role in the court's ultimate determination of contested custody questions.

Evidentiary rules control the extent to which professional privileges such as that between physician and patient, psychologist and client, and husband and wife, limit the amount of information available to a court in making a child custody determination. Although most state reporting statutes seem to abrogate these privileges in child custody situations involving known or suspected child abuse or neglect (Stromberg, 1988), the precise language of the statutory provision that abrogates the privilege in a given state and possible judicial interpretations of that language could still affect whether or not related evidence is deemed admissible.

SUBSTANTIVE STANDARDS

A majority of states currently provide that custody decisions turn upon "the best interests of the child" or comparable language, as the substantive standard for making custody determinations (Clark, 1988). Likewise, visitation rights may be subject to a similar analysis. "The best interests of the child," however, can be an ambiguous standard. This standard essentially requires that a prediction be made in relation to the child's needs and each parent's ability to meet them.

The analysis of the phrase, when specified by the legislature, may provide guidelines that take into account a lengthy list of factors. These include matters such as (1) the wishes of the child's parents as to custody; (2) the wishes of the child; (3) the interaction and interrelationship of the child with his parents, siblings, and any other person who may significantly affect the child's best interest; (4) the child's adjustment to his home, school, and community; (5) the mental and physical health of all individuals involved, including any history of abuse of any individuals involved; (6) the needs of the child for a continuing relationship with both parents and the ability and willingness of parents to actively perform their functions as mother and father for the needs of the child; (7) the intention of either parent to relocate his residence outside the state; (8) which parent is more likely to allow the child frequent and meaningful contact with the other parent; and (9) other considerations of environment, physical and emotional needs, intellectual stimulation, financial resources, moral development, and family makeup (Clark, 1988; Goldner, 1987).

When custody is contested, the judge must choose among various alternative arrangements, allocating between the two parents the rights and obligations relating to the child that were formerly shared by them. Although most jurisdictions now authorize awards of "joint custody" under which the parents continue to share rights and responsibilities with respect to the child after divorce, such an award is not required (Clark, 1988). In cases where child maltreatment is alleged, the court necessarily seeks to determine the truth of the accusations. When the allegations are substantiated, the judge should, of course, choose a custody arrangement that will maximize the child's safety.

REVIEW AND MODIFICATION

Custody decisions are generally viewed as matters best left to the sound discretion of the trial court because of the fact-sensitive nature of the determinations, combined with the general lack of firm guidelines controlling "the best interests of the child" analysis (Pace, 1973; Oster, 1965). The wide latitude traditionally afforded to a trial court allows for a necessarily individualized case-by-case decision (Pearson & Ring, 1982). It does, however, limit the scope of review of an appellate court to that of reversal only for an "abuse of discretion." Thus, on appeal, a higher court generally will not re-evaluate the facts to determine whether, in its own view, a finding of child abuse perpetrated by the accused should have been made.

Legislation providing for modification of a child custody or visitation order commonly requires a showing of a "substantial or material change of circumstances" and that a modification will be in "the best interests of the child" (Atkinson, 1986). Allegations of abuse, formerly raised when custody was initially decided, will generally not constitute a change of circumstances without new evidence of abuse.

EVIDENTIARY ISSUES

The law of evidence is the system of rules and standards which regulates the admission of proof at the trial of any lawsuit (McCormick, 1984). In response to efforts to introduce various types of evidence, in the nature of both testimony and physical exhibits (sometimes called "real" evidence), objections may be made by opposing counsel. The trial judge must then rule on these objections and determine what actual evidence the finder of fact (which may be the jury, as in criminal cases, or the judge in juvenile court child protection cases or divorce cases) will be allowed to consider. The judge will rely on established rules that are part of the law of evidence in making these determinations.

General rules of evidence may affect virtually any question that is asked of a witness during the trial. Particularly unique and difficult evidentiary issues do arise, however, in cases involving child abuse and neglect, and these warrant specific attention here. These issues include the possible use of circumstantial evidence, the competency of child witnesses, the use of hearsay testimony, limits regarding the scope of admissible expert testimony, and the use of various types of demonstrative evidence such as photographs and anatomically correct dolls.

Generally, the applicable rules of evidence in criminal child abuse prosecutions, civil juvenile court child protection proceedings, and child custody cases are the same. The rules may be somewhat "relaxed" in noncriminal proceedings in juvenile court or in divorce cases, because a judge rather than a jury is the fact finder and, at least theoretically, has been trained to ignore inadmissible evidence in making his or her determination.

DIRECT AND CIRCUMSTANTIAL EVIDENCE

Child abuse often does not yield a great deal of evidence that, under American rules of evidence, would be admissible in any of the trials or hearings related to child abuse. Most cases of child abuse occur in the child's home and often the only people present are the child and the perpetrator. Even when others are present at the time of the incident, in many instances it is a member of the immediate family, such as a spouse who may be unwilling to testify or to testify truthfully, or a young child who is too immature to take the witness stand. Frequently the victim is too young or too immature to testify. Even if the child is mature enough to testify, he or she may be reluctant to do so or will change or recant his or her story. The alleged adult perpetrator typically contends that the child's injuries were accidental. Therefore direct evidence is usually sparse or nonexistent. Direct evidence is evidence which, if believed, resolves the matter in issue (McCormick, 1984).

Most of the available evidence in child abuse cases is circumstantial. Circumstantial evidence is evidence that is not based on actual personal knowledge or observation of facts or events in controversy. Rather, it is based on facts from which deductions may be drawn, showing indirectly that certain events did take place or that certain other facts sought to be proved are true. Circumstantial evidence, even if believed, does not resolve the matter at issue. Additional reasoning must be applied to reach the proposition to which it is directed (McCormick, 1984).

For example, a witness' testimony that he saw X beat a child with a belt is direct evidence of whether X did, indeed, beat the child. Testimony that the child had belt marks on his back and legs, that the child was in X's custody, and that no one else had access to the child during the time when the marks were acquired, would be strong circumstantial evidence that X beat the child. A case of child abuse may be proven entirely by circumstantial evidence, but there still must be sufficient evidence to convince the trier of fact.

In juvenile court proceedings some courts have applied the doctrine of *res ipsa loquitur* to support an inference of child abuse. *Res ipsa loquitur* means "the thing speaks for itself." For example, child abuse may be inferred from the mere fact that the child sustained a particular injury, given the character of the injury and the surrounding circumstances (*S., In re*, 1965).

COMPETENCY

An individual must be competent to testify as a witness at any trial or hearing (Melton et al., 1981). Competence to testify involves four factors: (1) a present understanding of the difference between truth and falsity and an appreciation of the obligation to speak the truth; (2) the mental capacity, at the time of the occurrence in question, to observe or receive accurate impressions of the event; (3) memory sufficient to retain an independent recollection of the observations; and (4) the capacity to communicate into words that memory and to understand questions about the event (Melton, 1981).

Historically, courts and legislatures created presumptions, depending upon age, regarding the competency of children to testify. More recently, however, the trend has been to presume that all witnesses are competent to testify and to resolve doubts as to the credibility of the witness in favor of allowing the testimony and having the trier of fact decide what weight to give that testimony. A party can still challenge a witness, however, and the trial judge may prohibit the testimony if the judge finds that the witness did not meet one of the criteria listed above. Because judges would otherwise have the discretion to exclude testimony on the basis of competence, a number of jurisdictions have recently passed legislation which makes admissible *all* testimony by a child regarding evidence of child sexual abuse (Morey, 1985).

HEARSAY

In general, a witness can only testify to those facts about which he or she has personal knowledge. The witness may not testify to what others have said in an out-of-court or extra-judicial statement to prove the truth of the matter stated. Such secondhand information is called hearsay (McCormick, 1984). Hearsay evidence is usually inadmissible in a judicial proceeding. Hearsay is excluded to prevent the introduction of statements made by out-of-court declarants whose statements were not made under oath and whose credibility cannot be evaluated by the jury.

There are, however, certain recognized exceptions to the hearsay rule (McCormick, 1984). Each of these exceptions has been recognized in some or all jurisdictions. The exceptions typically have been created when the situation and the circumstances surrounding the declarant's statement increase the reliability of the out-of-court statement and thereby make the statement more trustworthy. For such statements to be admissible, however, they must meet the jurisdiction's requirements for that particular hearsay exception and, in criminal cases, not violate the Confrontation Clause of the U.S. Constitution. A number of the recognized exceptions to the hearsay rule are important in child abuse and neglect cases (Graham, 1988; Myers, 1987).

Excited Utterances and Statements of Physical and Mental Conditions

One recognized hearsay exception is that for excited utterances. This exception allows for the admission of nonreflective statements regarding a startling event made while the declarant is still in a state of excitement. For example, a statement made by a child to a neighbor or the police that her mother beat her with a belt may be admissible, if the court finds that the statement was made while the child was still excited and that the statement was impulsive and spontaneous rather than a product of reflective thought.

A related exception, recognized in most jurisdictions, is that for statements made to anyone regarding then existing physical conditions, including pain or other physical sensations. These are admissible to prove the truth of the statement. That is, they are admissible to prove that the physical condition or pain existed at the time the statement was made. Thus, a statement made by a child to its mother, while pointing to a genital area, that "it hurts," could be admissible under this exception.

Similarly, most jurisdictions admit statements of the declarant's then existing state of mind or emotion. Thus, for example, in child custody litigation incident to a divorce, a child's statement to another individual regarding affection for or dislike of a parent will be admissible. Similarly, statements indicating fear of an abusive parent may also be admitted.

Statements for Medical Diagnosis

In most jurisdictions there is a separate recognized exception authorizing the admission of statements made for purposes of medical diagnosis and treatment. Statements admissible under this exception may pertain to present or past conditions, if they are made to a physician or the physician's agent, such as a nurse, technician, or receptionist. Such statements are admissible on the assumption that one generally does not fabricate statements to health care providers because the success of the patient's treatment depends on the accuracy of the information provided. Thus, an affirmative response by a child to a question asked by a physician of whether anyone "touched you there" would be admissible as evidence to prove that the molestation had taken place.

Some courts also will admit statements that refer to the cause of the condition for which the declarant is seeking treatment, if the statements are reasonably pertinent to the diagnosis and are made in connection with the treatment. In the child abuse situation, a number of courts have reasoned that because the treatment of child abuse includes removing the child from the abusive setting, the doctor should attempt to ascertain the identity of the abuser. Therefore, a child's statement to a physician to the effect that "Daddy hurt me" would be admitted.

Present Sense Impressions

A few jurisdictions recognize an exception for "present sense impressions." These are statements describing or explaining an event or condition that are made while the declarant was perceiving the event or condition or immediately thereafter. For example, if a child was rescued while the abuse was taking place, and immediately began to describe to the rescuer what had occurred, his or her statement may be admitted.

Admissions by Parties

Another recognized exception to the hearsay rule is when the out-of-court statement is that of a party to the litigation and is relevant to the party's defense. For example, a parent-perpetrator may tell a neighbor, "I beat my child because he wet his pants." In a criminal case against the parent, the neighbor could testify to this statement. Its admission in a juvenile court proceeding may depend on whether the parent is considered a party under the state's juvenile court rules.

Business and Medical Records

Finally, an additional exception to the hearsay rule allows the introduction of business records. This generally includes medical records. When business records are used to prove the truth of their contents, this constitutes hearsay. Such records, however, often will be admitted under a recognized exception to the hearsay rule for records that are kept by a business, in the regular course of its operation. The theory being that, if the "business" itself will rely on the accuracy of such records in carrying out its operations, a court should do likewise. For the record to be admitted, there must be "foundational testimony" to the effect that the entry to the records was made accurately and promptly, in the course of usual business activity, and the person recording the information had firsthand knowledge of the matter.

In most instances, medical records may be admissible as substantive evidence of the child's diagnosis, condition, medical history, and laboratory and X-ray findings, under the business records exception to the hearsay rule. Medical records may also be used to refresh the physician's memory regarding the specific case when the physician is testifying at trial or when giving evidence in a deposition. This use is appropriate whether or not the record is otherwise admissible as a business record.

Many courts are reluctant, however, to admit prognostic statements or statements concerning the cause of a condition, which are contained in the medical record, unless the doctor who wrote the statement is available for cross-examination or the statement was based on objective data rather than on data requiring speculation. For example, it would probably not be necessary to have a radiologist testify in court that the child has a spiral fracture of the femur. In this situation the record would be admissible to show that the child had the spiral fracture. Conversely, a doctor's statement that the spiral fracture of the femur was caused by child abuse, rather than by an accidental fall, would probably not be admitted into evidence unless the doctor was available for cross-examination.

Some jurisdictions have recognized a so-called "residual" exception to the hearsay rule. This permits the receipt of "reliable" hearsay evidence, which does not fit into an established exception, under limited situations, as long as the statement has "equivalent circumstantial guarantees of trustworthiness" to the recognized exceptions. Courts have sometimes relied on this exception in litigation involving children.

Sexual Abuse Hearsay Exception

A number of jurisdictions, legislatively or by judicial decision, have created a new hearsay exception that authorizes admission of out-of-court statements by children about sexual abuse (McCormick, 1984; Note, 1985; Myers, 1987). Often the sexual abuse hearsay exception's applicability is limited to criminal or juvenile court proceedings or both. This exception is similar to the residual exception, but only applies to children's statements about sexual abuse. The time, content, and circumstances of the statement must provide sufficient guarantees of trustworthiness. In addition, the child must either testify at the hearing or must be unavailable. When unavailable, there must be additional corroborative evidence of the act which is the subject of the child's statement. These statutes allow a parent, doctor, or other individual to whom a child has made a statement regarding sexual abuse to testify to the child's description of what occurred, irrespective of whether or not the statement otherwise meets the requirements of another hearsay exception.

Videotaping Statutes

Some state legislatures have passed statutes permitting a child's testimony to be preserved on videotape for presentation to a jury, thus enabling the child to avoid repeated appearances in court (McCormick, 1984; MacFarlane, 1985; Note, 1985). The statutes exempt from the ban on hearsay an audiovisually recorded statement of a child victim or witness that describes an act of sexual abuse or physical violence if certain requirements are met. The court must find that: (1) the minor will suffer emotional or psychological stress if required to testify in open court; (2) the time, content, and circumstances of the statement provide sufficient guarantees of trustworthiness; and (3) certain other procedural requirements were met. Generally, the presence of the judge, the accused, or counsel is not required at the taping, and any person can conduct the interview. Before the statement is admitted, however, on the defendant's request, the court must provide for further questioning of the minor. The admission of the statement, however, does not preclude the court from allowing a party to call the minor as a witness, if justice requires.

In addition, these statutes authorize presenting the evidence of the statement of the child as the equivalent of testimony in the case, either by audiovisually recorded deposition or by closed circuit television. Such statutes specify who is to be present at the recording and authorize the exclusion of a party on a finding that his presence may cause severe emotional or psychological distress to the child. The use of such a recording is permitted provided the defendant can observe and hear the testimony and can consult with his lawyer.

Confrontation Clause Issues

Although the rules regarding hearsay and its exceptions are generally applicable in juvenile, criminal, and divorce cases, particular note should be made of the interplay between these hearsay rules and a criminal defendant's rights under the Confrontation Clause of the Sixth Amendment to the U.S. Constitution. As noted in the discussion of criminal trials as well as in the discussion of hearsay, state legislatures and trial courts have endeavored to reduce the trauma a child might sustain from testifying in a criminal trial. Such protective measures may, however, violate the Confrontation Clause.

The Confrontation Clause and the hearsay rules are not one and the same. Nevertheless, they advance a number of similar values. As a matter of constitutional law, the right to confrontation (1) ensures that the witness will give his statements under oath, thus impressing him with the seriousness of the matter and guarding against a lie by the possibility of a penalty for perjury; (2) forces the witness to submit to cross-examination, which aids in the discovery of truth; and (3) permits the jury to observe the demeanor of the witness in making his statement, allowing it to assess his credibility (*California v. Green*, 1970).

When the state seeks to admit hearsay evidence in a criminal case, the proper inquiry under the Confrontation Clause is said to be two-fold. First, where the declarant was available as a witness at trial, it must be asked whether the defendant was permitted an adequate opportunity for cross-examination. Second, and more important for present purposes, if the declarant was not present as a witness at trial, it must be asked whether the absence of the witness was necessary and whether there was sufficient "indicia of reliability" surrounding the out-of-court statement (Whitebread & Slobogin, 1986; McCormick, 1984). When the declarant is a child victim, the prosecutor must produce evidence of a good faith effort to obtain the presence of the witness, or establish that the witness is "not capable of testifying" as defined by state law. This may involve a showing that the witness is incompetent, or that the child should be excused from testifying because the experience will cause additional trauma.

In a 1990 U.S. Supreme Court decision, a female defendant and her companion were convicted of lewd conduct against the companion's 2 1/2-year-old daughter (*Idaho v. Wright*, 1990). The conviction was successfully challenged by the female defendant on the ground that the trial court should not have admitted the pediatrician's testimony that the victim suggested to him her father had abused her. The critical statements were made in response to the doctor asking whether her daddy touched her with his "pee-pee." The girl responded that "daddy does this with me. . ." The trial judge determined that the daughter was incompetent to testify and refused to allow her testimony, but he concluded that her statements to the pediatrician were reliable and admitted them under the state's "residual exception" to the hearsay rule.

On appeal, the Supreme Court held that incriminating statements such as these, although otherwise admissible under an exception to the hearsay rule, may be prohibited under the Confrontation Clause. To be admitted, the prosecution must produce the declarant for cross-examination or establish the declarant's unavailability, as well as demonstrate that the statement bears adequate indicia of reliability.

The Court assumed that given the incompetency finding, the child had in fact been "unavailable" for testimony. The question then became one of the reliability or trustworthiness of the statements. The Court refused to adopt any hard and fast rules for professional interviews, such as a requirement that the statements be videotaped or that leading questions could not be used. It ruled that in determining reliability, factors relating to whether the child was likely to be telling the truth when the statements were made were to be considered and that these included the declarant's mental state, spontaneity, and consistent repetition; motive or lack of motive to make up a story; and the use of terminology unexpected of a child of that age.

In this particular case, the Court pointed out that the doctor had conducted the interview in a suggestive manner. Given the presumptive unreliability of the statements, the Court concluded that there was no special reason for supposing that the statements were particularly trustworthy.

EXPERT TESTIMONY

Generally, a witness is only permitted to testify to factual matters and may not offer an opinion or conclusion regarding the meaning of those facts. An expert witness, however, is allowed to give opinions in areas related to his or her expertise when the judge determines that such testimony is beyond the common knowledge of the trier of fact and will aid the trier of fact in deciding the issues in the case (McCormick, 1984). An expert witness is someone with specialized knowledge obtained through training and/or experience. In order to qualify as an expert, the witness will be required to state facts about his or her education and experience.

The opposing attorney or the judge may ask additional questions regarding the witness' expertise. The trial judge is given great discretion in deciding whether the witness qualifies as an expert on the particular matter in issue.

Generally, physicians and perhaps other licensed or certified health care professionals have sufficient training and experience to express a medical opinion in order to help the judge or jury understand the medical aspects of the case. Therefore, in most situations, an individual with a medical degree will qualify as an expert witness. There is no requirement for subspecialization. The weight the fact finder, be it a judge or a jury, gives the physician's testimony may, however, be affected by such factors as board certification in the particular area involved, experience, publications, and the clarity of the witness' presentation on the pertinent condition.

Battered Child and Failure-to-Thrive Syndromes

When physical abuse is alleged, expert medical testimony is often essential to establish that the injury was not accidental. In child abuse cases, a physician usually qualifies as an expert who can give his opinion as to the nature of the child's injuries. Medical testimony that the child's injuries are consistent with the "battered child syndrome" is often allowed on the ground that it is an accepted medical diagnosis (*Estelle v. McGuire*, 1991; Boresi, 1989; *State v. Best*, 1975). For example, patterned abrasions (belt, cord, stick) and certain fractures in young children (posterior rib fractures in different stages of healing) are powerful evidence of nonaccidental injury and child abuse.

"Failure-to-thrive" syndrome is another diagnosis generally recognized by the medical community and the courts. The syndrome describes a condition in which a very young child's height and weight consistently fall below the third percentile on the standard growth chart (Cunningham & Horowitz, 1989). Although similar growth patterns may be indicative of certain organic disease processes, it may be due to parental neglect or deprivation, such as inadequate feeding and poor nutrition. Courts generally have accepted an expert's conclusion that the problem is due to neglect, when, subsequent to the child's hospitalization and receipt of proper nutrition, the child has gained substantial weight in a relatively short period of time (Goldner, 1979).

Other Abuse-related Syndromes

Psychologists, social workers, and other mental health professionals may be called as expert witnesses in child abuse cases to testify to matters within their competence. Such areas include testimony regarding the emotional status of the child, conditions of the child's home, and parenting techniques. "Child abuse family profile," "child sexual abuse accommodation syndrome," and the "battering parent syndrome" are terms used to denote specific behavior patterns and characteristics common to children and families where child abuse has occurred. In a very few jurisdictions, testimony regarding the presence of these characteristics and syndromes common in abused children or in families in which abuse occurs may be offered into evidence by an expert to indicate the probability that the child has been abused. Courts in many jurisdictions are reluctant, however, to admit expert testimony regarding these syndromes because such syndromes are based on psychological factors that are speculative as compared to physical factors that are either concrete or qualitative (Boresi, 1989; Cunningham & Horowitz, 1989).

DEMONSTRATIVE EVIDENCE

Demonstrative evidence consists of things rather than assertions of witnesses about things. Demonstrative evidence, such as photographs, medical illustrations or diagrams of the child's injuries, and X-rays, is frequently helpful in assisting the trier of fact in child abuse cases to understand a particular issue.

Photographs, Drawings, and X-rays

Generally, demonstrative evidence will be admitted if a proper foundation is laid. That is, it must be shown that the demonstrative object is a fair and accurate representation of the thing it purports to represent or illustrate. For example, if a physician testifies about a child's bruises and cuts observed in the hospital and then is shown a picture of the child taken at approximately the same time the doctor examined the child, the doctor will be allowed to testify that the photo is a "true and accurate representation" of what he or she saw. Consequently, the photograph can then be admitted into evidence and shown to the trier of fact. Similarly, drawings that indicate the location of injuries may be admitted when the proper foundation is laid.

In a criminal prosecution for child abuse, admission of photographs of the child's injuries is left to the discretion of the judge because such photographs may inflame and prejudice a jury. The judge must balance the probative value of the pictures against their prejudicial effect in ruling on admissibility.

Generally, the child's X-rays will be admitted into evidence if accompanied by testimony explaining their relevance. X-rays may reveal certain types of fractures that, when found in a young child, are indicative of child abuse rather than accidental injury. For example, posterior rib fractures in different stages of healing in a young child are highly suggestive of physical abuse. Conversely, an X-ray may indicate an accident rather than child abuse. A fractured clavicle accompanied by bruises on the arms is indicative of an accidental fall.

Anatomically Correct Dolls

The use of anatomically correct dolls is designed to reduce the trauma to child witnesses in sexual abuse cases. The dolls may ease the child experience of testifying and assist the child who has difficulty relating events using appropriate sexual or physiological terms to the trier of fact (Cunningham & Horowitz, 1989). Some states have enacted legislation expressly permitting the use of such dolls during children's testimony. In addition, expert witnesses are sometimes permitted to describe or comment on a child victim's interactions with the dolls. Because the use of such dolls has sometimes been viewed as controversial, some jurisdictions bar their use in the courtroom (*Amber, In re*, 1987; Ringland, 1986; Dulka, 1988).

◆ BIBLIOGRAPHY

Adoption Assistance and Child Welfare Act, 1980. 42 U.S.C. *§* 670, et seq. (Supp. 1990).

Amber, In re, 191 Cal.App.3d 682 (1987).

Atkinson, J: *Modern Child Custody Practice*, Kluwer Law Book Publishers, New York, 1986.

Attorney General's Task Force on Family Violence, Final Report, Sept 1984.

Baltimore City Dep't of Social Serv. v. Bouknight, 493 U.S. 549 (1990).

Besharov, D: The legal aspects of reporting known and suspected child abuse and neglect, *Villanova L Rev* 23:458, 1978.

Besharov, D: Child welfare malpractice, *Trial* 20:56, March 1984.

Besharov, D: The need to narrow the grounds for state intervention. In D Besharov, ed : *Protecting Children from Abuse and Neglect : Policy and Practice*, Charles C Thomas, Publisher, Springfield, IL, 1988.

Blue, W: *State v. Williquette:* Protecting children from abuse through the imposition of a legal duty, *Am J Trial Ad* 12:171, 1988.

Boresi, K: Syndrome testimony in child abuse prosecutions: The wave of the future? *St Louis U Pub L Rev* 8:207, 1989.

Bross, D: Medical diagnosis as a gateway to the child welfare system: a legal review for physicians, lawyers and social workers, *Den U L Rev* 65:213, 1988.

Bulkley, J: Introduction: Background and review of child sexual abuse: Law reforms in the mid-1980's, U *Miami L Rev* 40:5, 1985.

California v. Green, 399 U.S. 149 (1970).

Campbell, AW: *The Law of Sentencing*, Lawyers Cooperative Publishing Co, Rochester, NY, 1978.

Capaldi v. State, 763 P.2d 117 (Okl. Cr. 1988).

Child Abuse Prevention and Treatment Act, 1974. 42 U.S.C. $\mathcal{S}$ 5101 et seq. (Supp. 1990).

Clark, H: *Hornbook on the Law of Domestic Relations in the United States*, ed 2, West Publishing Co, St. Paul, MN, 1988.

Commonwealth v. Webster, 5 Cush. 295 (Mass. 1850).

Coy v. Iowa, 487 U.S. 1012 (1988).

Cunningham, C, and Horowitz, R: *Child Abuse and Neglect: Cases, Text and Problems*, American Bar Association, National Legal Resource Center for Child Advocacy and Protection, Washington, DC, 1989.

Daro, D: *Confronting Child Abuse: Research for Effective Program Design*, Free Press, New York, 1988.

Daryl H. v. Coler 801 F.2d 893 (7th Cir. 1986).

DeShaney v. Winnebago County Dept. of Social Servs., 489 U.S. 189 (1989).

Dulka, M: Raising the standard for expert testimony: An unwanted obstacle in proving claims of child sexual abuse in dependency hearings, *Golden Gate L Rev* 18:443, 1988.

Edwards, L: The relationship of family and juvenile courts in child abuse cases, *Santa Clara L Rev* 27:201, 1987.

Estelle v. McGuire, 510 U.S., 112 S.Ct. 475 (1991).

Fahn, M: Allegations of child sexual abuse in custody disputes: getting to the truth of the matter, *Fam L Q* 25:193, 1991.

Federal Protection of Children Against Sexual Exploitation Act, 1986. 18 U.S.C. 2251, et seq. (Supp 1991).

Finn, P: Statutory authority in the use and enforcement of civil protection orders against domestic violence, *Fam L Q* 23:43, 1989.

Fox, SJ: *The Law of Juvenile Courts in a Nutshell*, ed 2, West Publishing Co, St. Paul, MN, 1984.

Fraser, B: A glance at the past, a gaze at the present, a glimpse at the future: A critical analysis of the development of child abuse reporting statutes, *Chi Kent L Rev* 54:641, 1978.

Giarretto, H: Humanistic treatment of father-daughter incest. In R Helfer and G Kempe, eds: *Child Abuse and Neglect: The Family and the Community*, Ballinger Publishing Co, Cambridge, MA, 1976.

Goldner, J: *Child Abuse and Neglect and the Law: Cases and Materials for Attorneys and Law Students*, Region VII Child Abuse and Neglect Resource Center, Institute of Child Behavior and Development, University of Iowa, Iowa City, 1979.

Goldner, J: *Missouri Dissolution of Marriage, Support and Child Custody*, Harrison Co, Norcross, GA, 1987.

Graham, M: The confrontation clause, the hearsay rule, and child sexual abuse prosecutions: The state of the relationship, *Minn L Rev* 72:523, 1988.

Groff v. State, 390 So.2d 361 (Fla. App. 1980).

Gross v. Myers, 748 P.2d 459 (Mont. 1987).

Hardin, M: Legal barriers in child abuse investigations: State powers and individual rights, *Wash L Rev* 63:493, 1988.

Harlow v. Fitzgerald, 457 U.S. 800 (1982).

Hechler, D: *The Battle and the Backlash: The Child Sexual Abuse War*, Lexington Books, Lexington, MA, 1988.

Hertz, R, Guggenheim, M, and Amsterdam, A: *Trial Manual for Defense Attorneys in Juvenile Court*, American Law Institute-American Bar Association, Philadelphia, PA, 1991.

Horowitz, R, and Davidson, H: Protecting children from family maltreatment. In R Horowitz and H Davidson, eds: *Legal Rights of Children*, Shepard's/McGraw-Hill, Colorado Springs, CO, 1984.

Idaho v. Wright, U.S., 110 S.Ct. 3139 (1990).

Indian Child Welfare Act, 1978. 25 U.S.C. 1901, et seq. (Supp. 1990).

Iverson, T, and Segal, M: *Child Abuse and Neglect: An Information and Reference Guide*, Garland Publishing, Inc, New York, 1990.

Johnson, TA: *Introduction to the Juvenile Justice System*, West Publishing Co, St Paul, MN, 1975.

Kamisar, Y, Lafave, N, and Israel, J: *Modern Criminal Procedure*, ed 6, West Publishing Co, St Paul, MN, 1986.

Kempe, C, et al: The battered-child syndrome, *JAMA* 181:17, 1962.

Kentucky v. Stincer, 474 U.S. 15 (1985).

LaFave, W, and Israel, J: *Hornbook on Criminal Procedure* (with 1989 Supp), West Publishing Co, St Paul, MN, 1985.

LaFave, W, and Scott, A: *Hornbook on Criminal Law*, ed 2, West Publishing Co, St Paul, MN, 1986.

Landeros v. Flood, 551 P.2d 389 (Cal. banc 1976).

Lassiter v. Department of Social Servs., 452 U.S. 18 (1981).

Levine, R: Caveat parens: A demystification of the child protection system, *U Pitt L Rev* 35:1, 1973.

Lloyd, D: The corroboration of sexual victimization of children. In J Bulkley, ed: *Child Sexual Abuse and the Law*, American Bar Association, National Legal Resource Center for Child Advocacy and Protection, Washington, DC, 1981.

MacFarlane, K: Diagnostic evaluations and the uses of videotapes in child sexual abuse cases. In *Papers From a National Policy Conference on Legal Reforms in Child Sexual Abuse Cases*, American Bar Association, National Legal Resource Center for Child Advocacy and Protection, Washington, DC, 1985.

MacMurray, B: Criminal determination for child sexual abuse prosecutor case-screening judgments, *J Interpersonal Violence* 4:233, 1989.

Maryland v. Craig, U.S., 110 S.Ct. 3157 (1990).

McCormick, C: *Hornbook on the Law of Evidence*, ed 3 (with 1987 Supp), West Publishing Co, St. Paul, MN, 1984.

Melton, G: Procedural reforms to protect child victim/witnesses in sex offense proceedings. In J Bulkley, ed: *Child Sexual Abuse and the Law*, American Bar Association, National Legal Resource Center for Child Advocacy and Protection, Washington, DC, 1981.

Melton, G, Bulkley, J, and Wulkan, D: Competency of children as witnesses. In J Bulkley, ed: *Child Sexual Abuse and the Law*, American Bar Association, National Legal Resource Center for Child Advocacy and Protection, Washington, DC, 1981.

Meriwether, M: Child abuse reporting laws: Time for a change, *Fam L Q* 20:141, 1986.

Miranda v. Arizona, 384 U.S. 436 (1966).

Mnookin, R: Child custody adjudication: Judicial functions in the face of indeterminacy, *Law Contemp Prob* 39:226, 1975.

Morey, R: The competency requirement for the child victim of sexual abuse: Must we abandon it? *U Miami L Rev* 40:245, 1985.

Myers, J: Hearsay statements by the child abuse victim, *Baylor L Rev* 38:775, 1986.

Myers, J: *Child Witness Law and Practice*, Wiley Law Publications, New York, 1987.

Nicholson, E, ed: *Sexual Abuse Allegations in Custody and Visitation Cases*, American Bar Association, National Legal Resource Center for Child Advocacy and Protection, Washington, DC, 1988.

Note: The testimony of child victims in sex abuse prosecutions: Two legislative innovations, *Harv L Rev* 98:806, 1985.

Oster: Custody proceeding: A study of vague and indefinite standards, *J Fam L* 5:21, 1965.

Pace, P: Custody and appellate courts, *Fam L* 3:27, 1973.

Pearson, J, and Ring, M: Judicial decision-making in contested custody cases, *J Fam L* 21:703, 1982.

People v. Hagar, 513 N.E.2d 628 (Ill. App. 1987).

Perkins, R, and Boyce, R: *Criminal Law*, ed 3, Foundation Press, New York, 1982.

Prosser, W, and Keeton, WP: *Hornbook on the Law of Torts*, ed 5 (with 1988 Supp), West Publishing Co, St Paul, MN, 1984.

Radbill, S: Children in a world of violence: A history of child abuse. In R Helfer and R Kempe, eds: *The Battered Child*, The University of Chicago Press, Chicago, 1987.

Ringland, R: Child abuse evidence problems, *U Dayton L Rev* 12:27, 1986.

Robinson v. Wical, Civil No. 37607, Super. Ct. of Cal., San Luis Obispo, filed Sept 4, 1970.

Rosenberg, M, and Hunt, R: Child maltreatment. In N Reppucci et al, eds: *Children, Mental Health, and the Law*, Sage Publications, Beverly Hills, CA, 1984.

Roth v. Reagen, 422 N.W.2d 464 (Iowa 1988).

S., In re, 259 N.Y.S.2d 164 (Fam. Ct. 1965).

Santosky v. Kramer, 454 U.S. 745 (1982).

Smith, B, and Goretsky, S: The prosecution of child sexual abuse cases, *ABA Juv & Child Welf L Rptr* 11:78, 1992.

Sprague, M: Defining the risks after DeShaney. In M Sprague and R Horowitz, eds: *Liability in Child Welfare and Protection Work: Risk Management Strategies*, American Bar Association Center on Children and the Law, Washington, DC, 1991.

Sprague, M, and Horowitz, R, eds: *Liability in Child Welfare and Protection Work: Risk Management Strategies*, American Bar Association Center on Children and the Law, Washington, DC, 1991.

State v. Best, 232 N.W.2d 447 (S.D. 1975).

State v. Jones, 95 N.C. 588 (1886).

Storch v. Silverman, 231 Cal. Rptr. 27 (Cal. App. 1986).

Stromberg, C: *The Psychologist's Legal Handbook*, The Council for the National Register of Health Service Providers in Psychology, 1988.

Tjaden, P, and Thoennes, N: Legal intervention in child maltreatment cases, *Child Abuse & Negl* 16:807, 1992.

Wadlington, W, Whitebread, C, and Davis, S: *Cases and Materials on Children in the Legal System*, Foundation Press, Mineola, NY, 1983.

Wald, M: State intervention on behalf of "neglected" children: A search for realistic standards, *Stan L Rev* 27:985, 1975.

Whitebread, L, and Slobogin, C: *Criminal Procedure*, ed 2 (with 1991 Supp), Foundation Press, New York, 1986.

THE ROLE OF THE MEDICAL EXAMINER IN FATAL CHILD ABUSE

MICHAEL GRAHAM, M.D.

The medical examiner's role in deaths in which abuse or neglect may have played a part consists of (1) determining the cause and manner of death to a reasonable degree of certainty; (2) providing expert evaluation of the presence, absence, nature, and significance of injuries and disease; (3) collecting and preserving evidence; (4) correlating clinical and pathologic findings; and (5) presenting expert opinions in the proper forums. Modifications introduced by a changing society and by progressive medical technology, as in the area of transplantation, constantly redefine the extent and specifics of the medical examiner's role.

One area of expansion of the medical examiner's role involves evaluating the deaths of nonneonate, preteenage children who die because of nonaccidental injuries or neglect inflicted or permitted by their caretakers.

It is convenient and practical to divide these deaths into two subgroups, recognizing that nonidentified episodes of previous injury result in some misclassification:

1. Children who fall under the traditional definition of repeated episodes of abuse, exhibiting the results of these multiple episodes of intentionally inflicted harm. Approximately 20% of child abuse deaths fall into this category.

2. Currently a more common form of fatal abuse, children who die from injuries received during a single assaultive episode (Adelson, 1991).

Neonatal deaths (including infanticide) and deaths involving "adult" injuries, such as firearms and stabbings, are described by Adelson (1974) and DiMaio & DiMaio (1989).

The involvement of the medical examiner in child abuse and neglect traditionally begins at the time of death as specified by statute and modified by local custom. The particular statute or regulation governing each jurisdiction varies. In general, any sudden and unexpected death or one wherein an injury or "nonnatural" condition is suspected to have caused or contributed to the death must be reported to the medicolegal authority in whose jurisdiction it falls. By their very nature all deaths suspected to involve abuse or neglect must be brought to the attention of the applicable medicolegal authority.

◆ MORTALITY ATTRIBUTED TO PHYSICAL ABUSE

The incidence of deaths resulting from physical abuse is second only to the incidence of sudden infant death syndrome (SIDS) deaths in children under 1 year of age and is second only to accidents in children older than 1 year of age. An estimated 1,950 to 2,000 children ages birth to 17 years in the United States die each year as a direct result of physical abuse and neglect (McClain et al., 1993). Ninety percent of deaths occur among children less than 5 years old with 41% of these deaths occurring during infancy (McClain et al., 1993). Although these children constitute only a small subgroup of abused children, it is this group that is traditionally most extensively evaluated by medical examiners in a formal medicolegal death investigation system.

In reporting the incidence of fatal abuse or neglect, the features and investigative problems depend somewhat on the age of the population and the definition of the term "child abuse or neglect." Any death that results from intentionally inflicted injuries can be categorized as abusive, but such broad usage of the term leads to confusion and blurring of the components traditionally referred to as "child abuse." This confusion makes it more difficult to study common features and establish diagnostic criteria than when a narrower definition is used. The modalities of injury and death involved in feticide and neonaticide (first 30 days of life) differ substantially from those of other children. They often involve issues (such as identification, viability, and live birth) not usually arising in deaths beyond this stage of life. Similarly, the deaths of teenagers differ significantly from those of pre-teen children. Findings in the teenage group approach those found in adults with regard to modalities and motives. Rarely does a child over the age of 10 years die of starvation or dehydration due to neglect or die of chronic battering, since children in this age group are generally able to avoid these lethal situations (Adelson, 1991).

◆ FACTORS IMPACTING INVESTIGATION

The extent and quality of the investigation into a particular death are influenced substantially by factors such as circumstances peculiar to the death, local custom, available expertise, and resources. Unfortunately, in many jurisdictions, the offices charged with investigating these deaths operate under critical limitations of resources, both personnel and financial, and are being further strained by shrinking budgets and soaring costs. Resource considerations are increasingly significant in determining if the state-of-the-art evaluations that these types of deaths merit can, in fact, be carried out.

◆ DETERMINING CAUSE OF DEATH

Although the medical examiner's role is commonly perceived as being limited to determining the cause and manner of death, today his or her involvement is vastly more extensive and encompasses issues such as those listed in **Table 19-1**. Recent trends in child abuse investigation have also led the medical examiner into such areas as membership on multidisciplinary death review committees and evaluating cases involving nonlethally injured children when abuse is suspected. In this setting the medical examiner, usually a forensic pathologist, contributes expertise to aid clinicians and law enforcement authorities in evaluating the presence, nature, and mechanism of injuries sustained by these children.

The medical examiner must determine the cause of death as specifically as is reasonably possible. The cause of death can be defined as the disease or injury, or combination of the two, that initiates the continuous series of events, however brief or prolonged, which culminates in death (Adelson, 1974). It is important not only to recognize the immediate cause of death (what killed the child now) but also to delineate any remote or underlying cause of death (the initiator of the series of events culminating in the immediate cause of death). For example, in a child dying of pneumonia as a result of a past head injury, the immediate cause of death is pneumonia and the underlying cause of death is the head injury. Establishing the causal connection between these two entities and properly recognizing the underlying cause of death have apparent and serious far-reaching implications, especially in the courtroom. There may also be coexistent conditions, those that may not be directly related to the "cause of death" but may contribute to death by enhancing or, occasionally, diminishing the lethality of another condition. They may affect the resistance or susceptibility of an individual to a particular process, such as the interaction between dehydration and sickle cell anemia to produce a fatal sickling crisis. Some deaths result from physiologic perturbations such as cardiac concussion (commotio cordis) from a blow to the chest and demonstrate no identifiable anatomic alterations, yet are still traumatic in nature. In some cases

Table 19-1. Medical Examiner's Role

Establishing time of injury or injuries and death

Identifying the presence and nature of injuries

Evaluating modifying or contributing factors (injuries and diseases)

Documentation of pertinent findings (positive and negative)

Proper collection and preservation of evidence

Correlating findings with postinjury behavior

Presenting these issues in appropriate legal forums

a specific cause of death cannot be ascertained but other possible causes can be excluded; together with a consideration of the circumstances, the possibilities can be reduced to a single cause or category. An example of this is mechanical asphyxia. Successful resolution, including criminal prosecution, of these cases is possible even though no specific cause of death is identified if other causes have been excluded.

◆ DETERMINING MECHANISM OF DEATH

The cause of death should not be confused with the mechanism of death, which is the lethal physiologic derangement through which the cause of death acts (Adelson, 1974). Examples of mechanisms of death include hemorrhage, renal failure, anoxia, dehydration, and dysrhythmia. Multiple mechanisms can be operative in any particular case, especially in children who survive the initial injury only to die of multisystem failure after extensive therapeutic intervention. Recognition of the mechanism(s) of death is useful in establishing causal relationships and evaluating the clinical course of a process but should not be substituted for determination of the cause of death. For example, the recognition that disorders such as rhabdomyolysis (disintegration or dissolution of muscle associated with excretion of myoglobin in the urine), hyperkalemia (abnormally high potassium content of the blood), and soft tissue hemorrhage (mechanism) have led to death in the absence of visceral organ injury allows the death to be properly ascribed to soft tissue blunt trauma (cause of death) sustained in a beating.

◆ DETERMINING MANNER OF DEATH

The other major death certification issue facing the medical examiner is the manner of death, or the fashion in which the cause of death arises (Adelson, 1974). Deaths are traditionally classified as natural, homicide, accident, or suicide. If an opinion cannot be reached, the death is classified as undetermined. In some jurisdictions deaths such as drug abuse or therapeutic misadventure are placed in a special "unclassified" category. The manner of death is an opinion separate from the cause of death.

All child abuse deaths are by their nature homicidal, the killing of one person by another. A ruling of homicide does not reflect the level or even the presence of criminal culpability—"homicide" does not equal "murder." Criminality is properly determined by the criminal justice system. "Natural" causes of death can occur homicidally (Davis, 1978). For example, sickle cell crisis can be precipitated by dehydration resulting from punitive withholding of water. Certain cases of neglect also fit into this category. It must also be recognized that a manner of death can be identified even in the absence of a known cause of death if the circumstances surrounding the death so warrant. The most common example of this is attributing death to the sudden infant death syndrome (SIDS). Although a thorough investigation and postmortem examination fail to establish a specific entity responsible for death in a child in a characteristic age group, the death is considered natural and its similarity to other unexpected, unexplained deaths in similar children allows it to be categorized in a well-defined specific category (SIDS) of unexplained natural deaths. Similarly, a witnessed death clearly arising from a cardiac rhythm disturbance of unknown cause (after thorough examination) may be certified as natural notwithstanding the lack of a demonstrable underlying precipitating disorder. Nonnatural manners of death can also be reasonably ascertained in some cases where the cause of death is not demonstrable. For example, the uninjured skeleton of an abducted 2-year-old child is recovered a year later in a shallow grave. The cause of death is not apparent but the circumstances reasonably indicate the death is homicidal. The "cause of death" in such a case can be certified in a number of ways reflecting local custom including "unable to be definitively established" or "homicidal violence of undefined nature." The manner of death is homicide.

In addition to the issues of cause and manner of death, questions arise about the nature, extent, and effects of injuries sustained by these children: How did the injuries occur, when did they occur, and what effect did they have on the child? A comprehensive death investigation allows these issues to be evaluated and answered appropriately.

♦ MEDICOLEGAL EVALUATION OF DEATH

A common misconception is that the investigation of a death necessitates the performance of and is restricted to the findings obtained from an autopsy. The investigation of death has many components, of which autopsy is only one and not always a necessary one.

INVESTIGATION PROCESS

The modern medicolegal evaluation of a death suspected to involve child abuse does not differ fundamentally from the evaluation of any other death, and indeed differs little from the approach to medical evaluation of any living patient. A history is obtained, the patient is examined, ancillary tests are performed, diagnoses are rendered, and a course of action is pursued. Medicolegal opinions, like working medical diagnoses, are based on interpretation of all available information at a given point in time and are subject to reevaluation and amendment as additional information surfaces.

INVESTIGATION COMPONENTS

The components of a death investigation can be divided into examination of the history of pertinent past and present circumstances, physical evaluation of the scene and the body, and use of indicated ancillary studies such as radiography, toxicology, and other laboratory tests. Each component must be considered in the investigation, although some components can be more crucial than others.

HISTORY

Knowledge of the circumstances prior to, during, and following the death is critical to interpreting findings derived from physical observations. The medical examiner must rely on others to provide this information when evaluating the death of a child. Informants include the parents and/or other caretakers, siblings, acquaintances, neighbors, witnesses, and medical and law enforcement personnel; added information can be gathered from prior health records. Because of potential criminal and civil liability associated with child abuse, a description of the events leading up to death and reference to past events is often intentionally vague, incomplete, or fallacious. Frequently these events involved only the perpetrator and the victim. The perpetrator commonly provides a "history" that exonerates him or her from any responsibility for the death. Other witnesses or knowledgeable persons are usually family members or family acquaintances. Some could have participated in the abusive act (Adelson, 1991), and others fear retribution or view the loss of the perpetrator as detrimental to their future well-being. Often the "history" provided is based on the actual events but altered to alleviate or shift responsibility from the perpetrator. Also, characteristically, the history will be inconsistent with the observed injuries and will change, sometimes radically, as the investigation proceeds. Explanations to account for the injuries often follow the general themes of the injuries being accidental, self-inflicted, or of unknown origin (Schmitt, 1984).

The history also allows documentation of prior injuries and diseases, gives an assessment of the child's health and development, and contains information about pre-existing conditions that can influence later events. A detailed, accurate history is crucial when evaluating deaths possibly related to nutritional neglect.

PHYSICAL EXAMINATION

The second major component of the death investigation is examining, evaluating, and obtaining physical evidence. This is accomplished by assessing the alleged scene of injury and/or death and interpreting findings obtained from an autopsy.

Child abuse typically occurs in the privacy of the home. The nature of the act is reflected in the paucity of signs of environmental disturbance that accompany it. However, examination of the scene where the injuries were sustained can be rewarding in that the information derived can corroborate or refute the accuracy of the history presented to explain the child's condition. Instruments used to inflict injuries are usually typical household articles such as rods, belts, or brushes. Examination of the scene can verify the presence of instruments that could have inflicted specific injuries and may lead to the recovery of other evidence.

POSTMORTEM EXAMINATION

The postmortem examination of a child suspected to be abused includes a complete autopsy by a skilled pathologist with expertise in this area. A thorough gross examination coupled with microscopic evaluation as appropriate helps to determine and document the presence and absence of diseases or injuries as well as medical intervention. Appropriate photographic documentation is obtained for future review of the case as well as for use in legal proceedings.

A complete forensic postmortem examination should be performed when any child suffers a sudden and unexpected death or when the circumstances do not reasonably exclude an element indicative of abuse. A complete autopsy should be performed on the body of any child whose death could be attributed to abuse or neglect, either directly or indirectly. Although a detailed description of the postmortem examination of a potentially abused child is beyond the scope of this chapter, a brief overview of the procedure with particular reference to "special" techniques is presented.

GROSS EXTERNAL OBSERVATION

The first part of the examination includes documenting the general features and overall condition of the body. This includes describing the clothing as well as identifying and sealing evidentiary material. Detailed identification and documentation are performed of any external signs of injury, disease, or therapeutic intervention. In addition to a verbal description and photographic record of injuries, a diagrammatic record of injuries is often useful in identifying injury patterns, as often found in burns and scalds, where the distribution pattern is critical to the evaluation of how the injury was sustained.

EXAMINATION OF SOFT TISSUES AND VISCERAL ORGANS

Most lethally abused children have external signs of injury, although a few children have only scant externally apparent injuries but extensive underlying damage. In up to 10% of all cases of fatal child abuse due to blunt trauma no marks are visible anywhere on the external body surface (DiMaio & DiMaio, 1989). To detect and evaluate injuries in fatally abused children requires a thorough examination of the soft tissues and visceral organs for indications of hemorrhage. In the soft tissues, the presence, amount, and depth of hemorrhage are noted.

Soft tissue hemorrhage is most accurately assessed by exposing the deep soft tissues via long incisions down the back and lower extremities. These incisions are needed because significant soft tissue hemorrhage can be externally inconspicuous or inapparent, especially in dark-skinned individuals, and only revealed by direct inspection of the tissues (**Figure 19-1a,b**). Hemorrhage in the deep soft tissues indicates the application of significant force. Care must be taken not to misinterpret areas of hyperpigmentation, such as Mongolian spots, as a sign of injury (**Figure 19-2**). If in doubt, an incision into such a mark will show no hemorrhage.

Figure 19-1a,b. Soft tissue hemorrhage. The hemorrhage was not obvious before dissection.

Figure 19-2. Mongolian spot.

The visceral organs are accessed using standard bitemporal and thoracoabdominal incisions. When indicated, notably in infant deaths, the eyes are removed and examined for retinal hemorrhage and separation. The cervical spine, soft tissues, and spinal cord can be examined via a vertical posterior neck incision. The gross examination is supplemented by microscopic evaluation of appropriate tissues. An extensive postmortem examination can be performed and the body subsequently shown at the funeral home with no apparent autopsy marks visible since the face is rarely altered during the autopsy.

ANCILLARY STUDIES

The final data-yielding component of the death investigation process is the performance of appropriate ancillary studies, which can provide the key that unlocks the solution to a particular death. Routine ancillary studies in suspected child abuse deaths include radiography and toxicology. In some cases postmortem microbiologic, chemical, and other laboratory determinations are required.

RADIOGRAPHIC INPUT

The postmortem examination of the potentially abused or neglected child includes radiographic evaluation of the skeletal system using well-coned-down views of the head, trunk, spine, and extremities (Kleinman et al., 1989). The radiographic findings are useful in detecting, documenting, and detailing the presence or absence of injuries and disease, as well as determining when the injuries occurred and if the injuries reflect a series of episodes or a single incident. The radiographic studies also direct the removal and sampling of injured or diseased sites for histopathologic examination.

LABORATORY INPUT

Samples of blood, urine, vitreous fluid, and other appropriate tissues are saved for indicated toxicologic, chemical, and microbiologic analysis. Trace evidence such as hairs, fibers, and particulate material is identified and collected. Smears and swabs for sexual assault evaluation are collected. Hair and blood samples to be used for future comparison studies are obtained when indicated. Transfer of blood, hair, and other body substances can occur between victim and assailant. The identification of the source of the substance can exclude some individuals as to its origination and, using DNA techniques, can often essentially identify the contributor. Samples of blood, hair, and other tissues serve as comparison standards for questioned samples. These samples can also be used to resolve parentage issues.

◆DATA INTERPRETATION

Following the collection of all pertinent information the data are correlated and interpreted by trained individuals. Credibility is essential to ensure that the expressed opinions are reasonable, are scientifically supportable, and can be offered with a reasonable degree of medical certainty as testimony. This process is dynamic and opinions change as more data are accumulated, previously acquired data are refined, and all information is assessed according to current knowledge and experience.

The opinions formulated fall into two general categories: opinions related to what happened to the child and opinions related to what did not happen. In many cases a combination of these categories is used. It may not be possible to identify exactly how a child sustained a particular injury but it is possible to conclude whether the child sustained the injury in the context of a particular scenario of events. For example, it is possible to refute a story of a fall from an 18-inch high coffee table to a carpeted floor offered as the explanation for a massive head injury, although it may not be possible to determine exactly how the injury was sustained.

INTERPRETATION OF INJURIES

Injury interpretation begins with identifying and categorizing each injury (e.g., abrasion, contusion, laceration, cut, stab). Each one is then thoroughly examined and documented, whether major or trivial. Medically trivial injuries, such as a small scrape, can be more forensically informative than injuries of more serious physiologic consequence. For example, the physiologically inconsequential shoe print abrasion on the skin overlying the lacerated liver reveals the identity of the striking object and the point of impact. Similarly, a mark associated with the fatal blow may be nondescript whereas the instrument may leave a distinctive mark in another area. This type of information not only helps determine the nature of physiologically important injuries but can shed much light on other issues such as the nature of the instrument(s), the potential number of instruments, the site(s) of impact, and the minimum number of impacts.

The body of an allegedly abused child may be reexamined 24 hours after the original autopsy to allow further delineation of the external injuries and to allow for the appearance of other injuries which were not previously discernible. The phenomenon of "clearing" noninjured areas is due to the autopsy-enhanced passive drainage of blood from the vasculature. Since extravascular blood in areas of injury does not drain, whereas blood in blood vessels does, the injured areas become more clearly delineated.

AGING OF INJURIES

The characteristics of healing injuries aid in the assessment of how long before death they occurred. Since injury healing is progressive and predictable, the gross and microscopic appearance of the injury reflects its age. For example, contusions begin as clearly delineated red-blue marks, progress over days to become less defined yellow-green areas, and finally fade to indistinct brown marks approximately within a week to a month (Wilson, 1977). The chronology of the microscopic features of wound resolution has also been described (Raekallio, 1980). However, caution must be exercised when interpreting these timing features because a variety of factors can influence the appearance (and time course) of any particular injury (Wilson, 1977), including the victim's age and state of health; the injury site, depth, and size; the specific tissue injured; individual variations; the effects of therapy; and the development of complications such as infection. The chronology of fracture resolution has also been described (Zumwalt & Fanizza-Orphanus, 1990). The features of healing in visceral organ tissues are less well characterized than skin and bone but within limits can be utilized.

The interpretation of aging in an injury can provide absolute identification of when an injury occurred as specifically as a range of hours, days, or longer and the length of survival after the trauma was inflicted. The narrowness of the range is inversely proportional to the length of survival. This information is useful in determining who did and who did not have access to the child at the time the injury occurred, as well as evaluating the antemortem behavior of the child, for

437

Figure 19-3. *Patterned injury. Rose of punctate abrasions caused by a hair brush.*

example, the onset of irritability, loss of appetite, or change in behavior. Injury aging can aid in determining when complications may have occurred after the initial injury, such as delayed rupture of the bowel following an initial non-transmural bowel wall laceration. Injury aging can also be used in a "relative" fashion to determine whether certain injuries occurred before or after others and if the injuries indicate one or more traumatic episodes occurred. The crucial information to make these determinations can be contained in a previously surgical specimen that was removed before the death occurred, for example, a bowel resection, followed by prolonged postsurgical survival. In these cases the medical examiner makes every effort to locate and examine the pertinent tissues.

PATTERNED INJURIES AND INJURY PATTERNS

The interpretation of injuries involves the evaluation of each injury alone as well as in conjunction with coexistent wounds. This requires the recognition of patterned injuries and injury patterns. These factors must be considered in the light of historical data, findings at the scene of the injury, and the physical capabilities of the child.

PATTERNED INJURIES

Although most injuries are relatively nonspecific, some contusions and abrasions have a configuration that reveals details about the instrument used to inflict the injury (**Figure 19-3a,b,c**). Patterned injuries suggest and can be matched to a particular type of instrument or occasionally linked to a specific instrument (**Figures 19-4 to 19-7**). Parallel linear marks separated by a pale zone suggest a linear object such as a stick, rod, or belt *(see Figure 19-4a,b)*. Curved marks are often caused by loops of cord (rope or electrical wire), clothes hangers, or other curved instruments (**Figure 19-5a,b**). Some instruments create a multiplicity of patterns, reflecting variations in the striking surface(s) of the instrument. In these cases each pattern further defines the particular object (**Figure 19-6a,b,c**). Sometimes the appearance of the injuries indicates the use of multiple instruments to inflict the injuries (**Figure 19-7**).

Figure 19-4a,b. *Patterned injuries. Note linear marks (arrows) separated by a pale zone.*

Figure 19-5a,b. Patterned injuries.

Figure 19-6a,b,c. Patterned injury and object used. Forehead marks by the straw, orbital injuries by metal banding.

Figure 19-7a,b,c,d,e. *Injuries inflicted by multiple instruments.*

A particularly important patterned injury to recognize is the bite mark, which usually has little physiologic significance but has tremendous forensic significance. Thorough examination and precise documentation of bite marks offer significant evidence. Swabbing of the bite can reveal serologic characteristics of the biter. Detailed analysis of the bite by an experienced forensic odontologist can indicate if the origin of the bite is human or animal, child or adult, self-inflicted or not; the injury can also be specifically matched to the bite of a particular individual. Comparison techniques may also eliminate a particular individual as having inflicted the bite.

The presence and characteristics of some injuries may not be readily apparent under sunlight or usual indoor lighting. Further delineation of some of these injuries may be accomplished by using alternative light source photography such as ultraviolet (West et al., 1992a, 1992b). Computer enhancement of photographs may also help discern previously unseen characteristics of injuries.

BLUNT INJURY PATTERNS

Although most blunt injuries are nonspecific when considered in isolation, the overall number, location(s), and age(s) often form patterns that reveal their true nature. The sheer number of injuries can indicate abuse in the absence of a responsible contributory natural disease or other satisfactory explanation such as a motor vehicle crash.

The appearance of the wounds helps differentiate a single episode of injury from the classic pattern of repeated child battering. Injuries sustained in a single episode of violence will be at similar stages of healing, whereas those sustained during chronic battering are clearly of different ages. As mentioned previously, caution must be exercised when assessing the relative age of an injury to allow for the normal variation in healing that occurs in an individual. Influencing variations were listed previously.

The distribution of the injuries is also useful in distinguishing accidental versus intentional injuries. Unintentional injuries are sparse, tend to be superficial, and are often located on the forehead, zygoma, hands, shins, and knees—well-recognized points of impact (Norman et al., 1984). Intentional injuries tend to be multiple, often of various ages, bilateral (Laing, 1977), more extensive, of diverse types (O'Doherty, 1982), and in other locations (Pascoe et al., 1979; Hull, 1974) (**Figure 19-8a,b,c**). Specific patterns indicating the mechanics of injury production can also emerge, such as blunt head injury associated with "grip" bruises on the extremities and chest or the patterns of scalding by immersion.

Figure 19-8a,b,c. *Locations of intentional injuries.*

♦LETHAL INJURIES

HEAD INJURIES

The understanding of lethal head injuries in infants and children requires consideration of various differences between adults and children. The immature head is characterized by a flexible skull, patent sutures, incomplete myelinization, increased vasoreactivity, higher metabolic rates, larger cerebrospinal fluid space, and delicate blood vessels (Merten & Osborne, 1983). The type of head injuries resulting from accidental mechanisms in children through 24 months of age and those injuries resulting from nonaccidental infliction have been described and a differentiating algorithm devised for injury categorization (Duhaime et al., 1992).

BLUNT HEAD TRAUMA

In addition to patterns of how injuries are sustained, certain lethal patterns are also evident among abused children. In 70% to 80% of fatal child abuse, death results from or involves blunt head injury (DiMaio & DiMaio, 1989). Children less than 2 years of age are at greatest risk to sustain this type of injury (Merten & Osborne, 1983). In fatally head-injured abused children under 2 years of age the median age is 8.7 months (Duhaime et al., 1992). In these children, the external examination of the head usually reveals the presence of blunt injuries to the face, scalp, lips, buccal mucosa, or frenulum. Facial injuries, excluding superficial bruising over a zygoma or on the forehead or a superficial split lip in a mobile child, suggest abuse (Norman et al., 1984). Tears of the labial frenulum are common in children learning to walk but suggest abuse in children under the age of 6 months who are not ambulatory (Kenney, 1991). Cutaneous bruising in fatal head injuries is characteristically disproportionately less than the hemorrhage seen on the undersurface of the scalp or than the degree of craniocerebral injury. The nature of the scalp and the circumstances of the injury contribute to this phenomenon. The undersurface of the scalp must be examined to identify and localize any impact site(s) and not mistakenly exclude the presence of these injuries on the basis of the lack of visible or palpable areas on the external surface (**Figure 19-9a,b**). Subgaleal hemorrhage can also be related to hair pulling (Kempe, 1975).

Figure 19-9a,b. *Blunt head trauma. The extent of the injury was not realized until the undersurface of the scalp was examined.*

SKULL FRACTURE

A skull fracture in a fatally injured child is a very strong indicator of abuse unless the circumstances of the injury would be expected to generate a considerable amount of force, for example, a motor vehicle crash or a fall from a great height. Eighty percent of skull fractures related to abuse are found in children under the age of 1 year; these injuries are uncommon in children older than 2 years (Merten & Osborne, 1983). Although thin linear calvarial fractures, usually parietal in location, and ping-pong fractures can occasionally result from low-level falls (3 feet), such fractures are not associated with serious neurologic dysfunction except in the presence of a compression epidural hematoma (Helfer et al., 1977; Duhaime et al, 1992). More extensive and complex fractures reflecting greater translational force can be seen with falls from heights greater than 4 feet. Unless translational force is extreme, these fractures are associated with predominately focal damage and recovery of global neurologic function is usually rapid (Duhaime et al., 1992). The mildest recognizable consequence of angular deceleration to the brain, concussion, can be seen in low level falls (Duhaime et al., 1992). Concussion, skull fracture, and subdural hematoma have been described in falls from bunk beds (Selbst et al., 1990).

INTRACRANIAL HEMORRHAGE

Various intracranial injuries are found in fatally abused children. Epidural, subdural, and subarachnoid hemorrhage can be present alone or in concert. Intracranial, extraparenchymal hemorrhage can act as a space-occupying lesion; however, it is not unusual for it to be clinically insignificant but forensically important as a marker indicating that significant force has been transmitted to the intracranial contents. Epidural and localized subarachnoid hemorrhages represent impact injuries. In contrast, diffuse subarachnoid hemorrhage and subdural hematomas are features of angular deceleration and are infrequent in non–motor vehicle accidents but are common in inflicted injury (Duhaime et al., 1992).

Brain findings depend on the mechanism of injury, the length of survival, and the age of the child, reflecting the state of the brain's myelination. Before the age of 5 months, blunt force injury to the brain results in shearing separation along the junction of the gray and white matter. These slit-like tears are characteristically found in the parasagittal frontal lobes and in the temporal lobes. They are usually associated with minimal hemorrhage (Lindenberg & Freytag, 1969). Old hemorrhage is differentiated from fresh hemorrhage by the presence of hemosiderin and/or gliosis. As myelination proceeds, the brain exhibits more typical adult contusions. However, the extent and magnitude of visible contusion rarely approach what is seen in adults. Localized cortical contusions can be seen in falls greater than 4 feet. Prominent cerebral edema is common (Zimmerman et al., 1978). Microscopic examination of infant brains sustaining lethal injuries often discloses the presence of axonal varicosities reflecting diffuse axonal injury. Diffuse axonal injury, a lesion commonly leading to death, reflects the application of severe angular deceleration to the brain, resulting in global cerebral dysfunction.

SHAKING

The shaken infant syndrome typically involves children under the age of 15 months, with the median age being 3 months. In its pure form the fatal shaken infant syndrome is characterized by retinal hemorrhage, subdural/subarachnoid hemorrhage, and lethal damage to the central nervous system in conjunction with a lack of direct impact involving the head (**Figure 19-14**).

Since its characterization by Caffey (1972), the existence of this entity has been controversial. The controversy centers on whether shaking alone is sufficient to cause serious injury or death or if an impact involving the head must accompany the shaking. Using an experimental model, Duhaime and associates maintain that sufficient acceleration-deceleration forces cannot be attained via shaking alone to cause axonal tearing but require the addition of impact to account for the head injuries associated with the shaken infant syndrome (Duhaime et al., 1987). Others maintain that pure shaking can result in serious injury and death (Hadley et al., 1989; Alexander et al., 1990).

The separation of pure shaking from shaking with impact can be exceedingly difficult on clinical grounds. Significant impacts to the head, especially those involving broad and soft surfaces, may be associated with minimal or no external signs of injury. At autopsy, the majority of cases involving impact will reveal hemorrhage in the undersurface of the scalp. This hemorrhage is often much more extensive than the external surface of the scalp would suggest *(see Figure 19-9a,b)*. Some individuals note the presence of impact injuries to the head in clinically diagnosed cases of shaken infant syndrome and report never seeing a case without such an impact site identifiable at autopsy (DiMaio & DiMaio, 1989). However, I and others (Alexander et al., 1990) have seen cases where no impact site was identifiable during the autopsy. The lack of an impact site injury does not preclude an impact since striking a broad soft surface may not create an identifiable injury at

Figure 19-10. *Rib fractures.*

the point of contact. I am aware of a shaking death committed by a paramour and reportedly witnessed by two teenage siblings of the deceased. The siblings described violent to-and-fro shaking with loss of consciousness by the deceased and specifically relate the lack of any impact to or by the head. I believe that a significant impact site in the scalp or the presence of a skull fracture precludes a definitive diagnosis of a pure shaken infant syndrome. These cases may best be referred to as the "shaken impact syndrome" (Bruce & Zimmerman, 1989). The incidence of impact trauma in cases clinically diagnosed as the shaken infant syndrome suggests that at least half of deaths involving shaking are associated with impact (Alexander et al., 1990). (For a more in-depth discussion of the mechanisms of shaken infant syndrome, *see Chapter 1.*)

Although no single feature allows a definitive diagnosis of fatal shaking (with or without impact), it is convenient to reduce the syndrome to its component parts for the purposes of discussion.

The lethal component of this syndrome is injury to the brain and/or cervical spinal cord. Brain injury characteristically takes the form of brain swelling and diffuse axonal injury, which is manifest by the presence of axonal bulbs and varicosities *(see Figure 19-14a)*. The development of the morphologically recognizable markers of axonal injury is time dependent and their presence and appearance reflect the post-injury survival interval (Vowles, 1987). The lethal injury can also be a contusion of the cervicomedullary or proximal cervical spinal cord as described by Hadley et al. (1989).

The second component of this syndrome is the presence of subdural and/or subarachnoid hemorrhage. The subdural hemorrhage is characteristically located over the cerebral convexities and is generally of small volume *(see Figure 19-14c)*. Similarly, subarachnoid hemorrhage tends to be mild and patchy. The hemorrhages characteristically do not act as clinically significant space-occupying lesions but primarily serve as markers of intracranial angular energy transmission or movement.

Retinal hemorrhage, sometimes accompanied by detachment, is also characteristic of the shaken infant syndrome *(see Figure 19-14b)*. Retinal hemorrhages reportedly occur in 66% to 100% of clinically diagnosed shaken infants (Ludwig, 1984; Hadley et al., 1989). This injury is not specific for shaking and can also occur with impact injuries, birth (approximately 10% to 40% of vaginally delivered babies—Sezen, 1970; Egge et al., 1980, 1981), sudden thoracic compression during cardiopulmonary resuscitation (rare), sudden elevation of head and/or neck intravascular pressure, and other causes of increased intracranial pressure (Tomaski & Rosman, 1975; Bacon et al., 1978). Retinal hemorrhages have also been related to endocarditis and hemorrhagic diatheses (McLellan et al., 1986). Old retinal hemorrhage is marked by the presence of hemosiderin deposition. In addition to retinal hemorrhage, retinal detachment and optic nerve sheath hemorrhage can also be seen.

In some cases of shaking, sentinel injuries may be present. These include contusions on the chest and/or arms created while gripping and shaking the child. Hemorrhage in the soft tissue of the upper neck as well as long bone metaphyseal fractures can also be associated with this entity (Caffey, 1946).

INTRATHORACIC INJURIES

Injuries to the trunk account for 10% to 25% of abuse deaths; the relative incidence of death increases with the age of the child (DiMaio & DiMaio, 1989). Blunt force injuries to the surface of the trunk are seldom unintentional if multiple and nontrivial.

Significant intrathoracic injuries reflect the application of severe force. Lethal intrathoracic injuries may include internal or external cardiac rupture, pneumothorax, and, rarely, flail chest. Hydrostatic right atrial tears can be caused by thoracic impacts or by compressive abdominal forces (Cumberland et al., 1991). Rib fractures due to abuse are common and when present are nearly always (90%) found in children under the age of 2 years (Leonidas, 1983) (**Figures 19-10 and 19-11**). Posterior rib fractures have been considered characteristic of abuse. Rib fractures rarely, if ever, occur in children as a result of cardiopulmonary resuscitation (Feldman & Brewer, 1984).

Figure 19-11. Rib fractures (healing) (arrows).

Figure 19-12a,b. Liver laceration. c. Mild contusion (arrow) of external abdominal wall accompanying massive liver injury.

Figure 19-13. Mesentery contusion.

Figure 19-15. Marks on neck in strangulation.

INTRA-ABDOMINAL INJURIES

The most common lethal intra-abdominal injury is a ruptured liver (**Figure 19-12**). Half of the children with this injury display no externally visible injury to the abdominal wall (DiMaio & DiMaio, 1989). Common accompanying lesions include bowel serosal contusions, contusions and lacerations of the root of the small bowel mesentery (**Figure 19-13**), and perirenal soft tissue hemorrhage. Duodenal hematomas and lacerations occasionally occur and may not become apparent for an extended time after the injury. Death, often due to peritonitis, sepsis, or some other complication, may not occur for days or weeks.

In intra-abdominal injury cases with prolonged survival, the medical examiner must evaluate previously resected tissue to determine the age of the initial injury. Gastric laceration is rare but can occur as a result of abdominal blows, especially if the stomach is distended at the time of impact (Case & Nanduri, 1983). Pancreatic injuries and secondary pancreatitis occasionally occur as a result of blows to the abdomen or back. Splenic and renal parenchymal injuries are uncommon in child abuse. Renal injuries are more likely to result from posterior or flank blows. As noted earlier, right atrial endocardial tears can result from abdominal compressive forces.

MECHANICAL ASPHYXIA

Mechanical asphyxiation deaths of children can be particularly vexing because there can be minimal or no demonstrable injuries either externally or internally. The absence or paucity of findings is related to the size/strength disparity between assailant and victim and to the victim's inability to mount significant resistance or defense against the assault and to the ease with which mechanical asphyxia can be accomplished in this age group.

STRANGULATION

Marks on the skin or in the soft tissues of the neck are usually present in strangulation, but can be absent (**Figure 19-15**). In contrast to adults, conjunctival and orbital petechiae are rarely seen in infants and are uncommon in children. The pliable cartilaginous nature of the larynx and hyoid bone in infants and children makes fractures of these structures unusual.

SMOTHERING

Smothering is the most commonly employed method of mechanical asphyxiation used to kill infants and children. Findings, when present, can be restricted to mild facial bruising or abrasion or subtle intraoral injuries. Examination of the oral cavity,

Figure 19-14a. Diffuse axonal injury.
b. Retinal hemorrhage. c. Bilateral subdural hematomas.

including the inner aspects of the lips, gums, buccal mucosa, and tongue, is critical when evaluating this type of death. In some cases, no injuries are present, and the autopsy findings are indistinguishable from those of children dying of SIDS. In these cases the cause of death determination relies heavily on other aspects of the medicolegal investigation. Rarely, evidence such as respiratory epithelium has been recovered from the suffocating agent, such as a pillow (Luke, 1969). A few smothering incidents occurring in hospitals have been videotaped. Using smothering, it takes 70 to 90 seconds to induce a flat EEG and apnea. Unconsciousness follows a period of violent movement (DiMaio & DiMaio, 1989; Rosen et al., 1983; Southall et al., 1987).

OVERLYING

Covert mechanical asphyxia can also take the form of overlying, in which the adult's body supposedly covers the child's body. Often the adult is obese and/or under the influence of alcohol or other intoxicants. Death results from chest compression with or without associated suffocation. Fatal overlying can be associated with a lack of identifiable external or internal injuries.

CHOKING

Choking results from mechanical obstruction of the internal airway. The site of obstruction can be at the opening to the larynx or more distally in the airway. The obstruction can be caused by impacted material, tissue swelling (inflammatory or neoplastic), or both. In the case of impacted material the diagnosis rests on physically demonstrating the obstruction or documenting it by history in those cases where the material was expelled or removed during therapeutic activity.

Death due to choking is usually accidental and is rarely homicidal. Homicide cases are often related to disciplinary activities. Force feeding can result in choking from a bolus of food in a manner similar to what has been termed a "cafe coronary." In other cases, the aspiration of black pepper, usually administered as a punitive measure, has resulted in death (Adelson, 1964; Cohle et al., 1988) **(Figure 19-16a,b)**. Pepper in the airway clogs the breathing tube with its bulk and irritates the tissues chemically.

Figure 19-16a,b. *Death due to aspiration of black pepper.*

OTHER MECHANISMS

Other modes of death associated with few, if any, physical findings include drowning (Nixon & Pearn, 1977; Pearn & Nixon, 1977; Griest & Zumwalt, 1989), electrocution, hypothermia (Zumwalt & Hirsch, 1980), hyperthermia (Zumwalt & Hirsch, 1980), and poisoning.

POISONING

Another form of childhood homicide often characterized by few anatomic findings is the intentional introduction of toxic substances. This can take several forms; in classical poisoning, typical poisons are used (e.g., arsenic, fluoride, ethylene glycol); pharmaceuticals prescribed to family members or acquaintances may be administered; over-the-counter preparations, such as acetylsalicylic acid, may be given; or illicit substances such as cocaine or heroin (Shnaps et al., 1981; Rogers et al., 1976) may be provided to the child. Complete toxicologic screening coupled with specific indicated assays and a high index of suspicion are necessary to identify these agents (Case et al., 1983; Dine & McGroven, 1982; Rogers et al., 1976).

Death also can result from the administration of "nontoxic" substances in a toxic manner. Any substance can have deleterious effects if given in sufficient quantity or by an inappropriate route. For example, the administration of an excessive amount of table salt will induce hypernatremia (sodium excess with its attendant chemical imbalances), and the administration of excess water causes hyponatremia (a lack of sufficient sodium). Appropriate postmortem chemical studies of blood, vitreous fluid, and urine are necessary to evaluate these deaths. Since the substance is not always meaningfully measurable, its presence is only indicated by the physiologic aberration

447

it induces. Excess administration of potassium is virtually undetectable at the time of autopsy since a rapid rise in potassium occurs as a natural consequence of death. For further specific information about poisoning *refer to Chapter 12, Poisoning.*

◆ INJURIES TO THE EXTREMITIES AND GENITALIA

Blunt force injuries to the extremities and genitalia are rarely lethal but are commonly found in fatally abused children. Nonlethal cutaneous injuries can serve as a marker for the mechanism of the lethal injury. For example, bruises on the extremities can be "grip" or "handle" markers. Injuries to the bones of the extremities are common, and their nature may be diagnostic of abuse. The recognition of nonlethal injuries can lead to the correct interpretation of how the lethal injury was sustained. Genital or rectal injuries can indicate sexual abuse or represent injuries inflicted as a disciplinary measure, perhaps related to toilet training.

◆ BURNS

Intentionally inflicted burns account for 10% to 25% of pediatric burns and have a disproportionate mortality, 30%, when compared to accidental burns, 2%. The mean age of the abused child sustaining a burn is 1 1/2 to 2 years, with the range being 1 month to 10 years (Purdue et al., 1988). A number of criteria have been proposed to help differentiate accidental burns from nonaccidental burns. These include evidence (physical or historical) of previous or concurrent injuries, the number of injuries, evidence of delay in seeking care, historical-physical-developmental discrepancies, pattern of burns, and location of burns (Stone et al., 1970). Intentionally inflicted burns occasionally are immediately lethal, but more commonly the child comes to medical attention and survives for a period of time before dying of complications such as sepsis or pneumonia. In these cases it is important to causally relate the death to the initial insult. In one third of cases of deliberately inflicted burns of obvious medical significance the caretaker seeks medical care only after an inordinate delay (Purdue et al., 1988), stating that "I didn't realize the burn was serious" or "We thought it would get better by itself." Some contact burns can be patterned, such as those caused by heating elements, or are of characteristic appearance, such as a burn from a cigarette. This pattern usually identifies the causative source of heat.

SCALDING

Most burns in children are scalds, which account for 50% to 80% of burns up to the age of 4 or 5 years (Thomas et al., 1984; Klasen, 1979). Similarly, scalding is the most frequent form of burn abuse (Watkins et al., 1985; Hight et al., 1979). Scalding can occur at any age but typically occurs in the birth to 2-year age group (Rossignol et al., 1990). The age and motor abilities of the child must be considered when evaluating the nature of the injuries. For example, a 2 1/2- to 3-year-old unattended child could pull a pan of hot water off the stove or get into a tub of hot water but should be able to attempt to extricate himself from the water. A 6-month-old infant would not normally be expected to accomplish these tasks.

Burns due to hot water immersion have a characteristic distribution that differentiates accidental scalds from intentional scalds. Body diagrams are useful in injury pattern interpretation. The differentiation of accidental (faucet burns, dousing from an overturned pan) from intentional (immersion) scalds requires knowledge of the distribution and depth of the burn, the temperature and nature of the scalding liquid, the duration of contact, the age of the child, the abilities of the child, the normal reaction to the alleged method of scalding, and the physical environment (floor, tub, etc.). Immersion burns tend to be of uniform depth with well-defined margins, whereas splash burns tend to be less well-defined, show a "run-down" pattern, and exhibit variable intensity. The distribution of immersion burns reflects the position the child assumed on being placed in the hot liquid. Protected areas are spared.

The temperature of the liquid and the length of immersion are critical in the production of scalding burns. Full-thickness scald burns of adult skin will occur in 1 to 3 seconds in 150°F water, 7 seconds if the water temperature is 140°F, 30 seconds at 130°F, and 2 minutes at 125°F (Moritz & Henriques, 1947). A child's skin is more sensitive than an adult's, and these times should be shorter in children. The average home water heater often delivers water hotter than 130°F. As part of the medicolegal death investigation or the police investigation, measurement of the water temperature from the tap and after the water sits in a receptacle for a specified period of time can help in verifying or refuting the alleged scalding mechanism, such as "The child was in the tub for less than 5 seconds before I pulled him out."

Intentional chemical burns and microwave injuries do occur but are uncommon. In the latter, tissue damage is proportional to tissue water content (Alexander et al., 1987).

◆ NEGLECT

Our society requires that caretakers provide the necessities of life, including food, hydration, clothing, shelter, and medical care. Intentional failure to fulfill these responsibilities constitutes neglect. Neglect can be either active or passive. Active neglect entails the deliberate withholding of life's necessities from the child. In passive neglect the child's welfare is overlooked because the caretaker's focus is elsewhere, such as may occur in prolonged bingeing or with psychotic episodes.

Lethal neglect is usually due to malnutrition and dehydration (**Figure 19-17**), often accompanying a superimposed terminal process such as bronchopneumonia. Fatally starved children are typically less than 1 year old (Adelson, 1974). In these cases the nutritional history is out of line with the physical findings. "He hasn't been eating very well for the past 3 or 4 days" is offered as an explanation for marasmus, which is progressive, long-term wasting and emaciation.

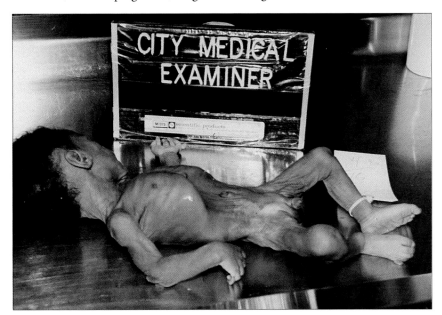

Figure 19-17. Lethal neglect due to malnutrition and dehydration.

449

PHYSICAL FINDINGS

The deceased child's weight and height must be compared to birth sizes and plotted on standard growth curves. It is also useful to compare the postmortem size with any previous growth information about the child. The presence of some chronic disease or condition that could cause or contribute to the malnourishment or dehydration must be excluded (Adelson, 1974).

Other physical findings can suggest neglect. Digestive tract contents tend to be sparse, and any fecal material present tends to be dry. Dehydration is indicated by sunken orbits, skin tenting (delayed surface restoration when skin is stretched or elevated and released), "sticky" serosal surfaces, and electrolyte abnormalities in the vitreous (Coe, 1993). Thymic involution is common. Macrovesicular steatosis may reflect protein deficiency. The overall appearance of the child will point to chronic lack of care. Poor skin condition and chronic diaper rash from soiling are common.

The neglected child's environment generally reflects poor hygienic habits, marginal food supply, and substandard care of other children in the home. Prior health care is often lacking or delinquent.

Failure to provide safe environmental conditions for the child can result in death due to extreme increases or decreases in body heat (hyperthermia or hypothermia) (Zumwalt & Hirsch, 1980; Zumwalt et al., 1976). Special care must be taken in evaluating the circumstances of these cases. Death can be due to various manifestations of these conditions, such as myoglobinuria or pancreatitis. Perimortem failure of the body's thermoregulatory system and postmortem temperature alterations must not be confused with any antemortem temperature abnormalities.

ALTERNATIVE CARE

Individuals have the right, in most cases, to refuse medical care or turn to nontraditional therapies. However, it is equally true that caretakers have a duty to provide adequate medical care to their charges. Death resulting from the intentional withholding of necessary care can be a form of neglect by omission.

A very controversial area involves the right of the parents to deny care on the basis of legitimate as opposed to convenient religious beliefs proscribing such activities or mandating nontraditional therapy such as prayer alone. This approach does not imply that the parents of these children do not care for or love their children. However, the freedom to practice their beliefs must be tempered with society's mandates regarding the welfare of their children and recognition of the consequences of spurning society's requirements.

When alternative care is involved in the death of a child, the medical examiner must obtain data to identify the cause of death, contributory conditions, and the presence and extent of any specific disease process. The nature and extent of the underlying disease process must be determined in evaluating whether the child could have been helped by current therapeutic regimens. Careful determination of the extent of the disease process can also allow an evaluation of caretaker explanations such as, "I didn't think the child was that sick."

For further information refer to Chapter 14, Neglect and Abandonment.

◆ MUNCHAUSEN SYNDROME BY PROXY

A rare variant of chronic abuse is the Munchausen Syndrome by Proxy (Meadow, 1977). In this syndrome the child is brought to medical attention with an intentionally induced "disease" accompanied by a fictitious history. The caretaker most often responsible for inducing the illness is the mother, although other caretakers, including health care personnel, are occasionally responsible. Most instances of this syndrome are nonlethal, but some children do die. In a series of 19 cases Meadow recorded 10% mortality (Meadow, 1982). Serious illness and death associated with this syndrome have been reportedly due to hypoglycemia caused by the surreptitious injection of insulin, apnea due to the administration of succinylcholine, and smothering. It is important to recognize that the assault on the child can continue during and after hospitalization.

For further information refer to Chapter 13, Munchausen Syndrome by Proxy.

♦ SEXUAL ABUSE

The forensic postmortem examination of a child includes the evaluation for possible sexual abuse. Genital and anal injuries, the presence of sexually transmitted diseases, or circumstantial evidence pointing to possible sexual abuse should prompt a full sexual abuse evaluation. The lack of genital injuries does not exclude sexual abuse. A postmortem distended anus in the absence of other injuries must be interpreted with extreme caution as it could reflect only postmortem laxity.

For further information refer to Chapters 7 and 8.

♦ CONDITIONS THAT ARE NOT ABUSE

As evidenced by the preceding discussion, fatal child abuse can take on a stunning array of appearances. However, it must be remembered that not all injuries are abusive in nature. An abused child can die of an unrelated accident or a natural condition. Various natural diseases and therapeutic measures can simulate to some degree the appearance of physical abuse and neglect. Trivial, innocently acquired scrapes and bruises must be recognized for what they are. Birth injuries need to be correctly identified.

SUDDEN INFANT DEATH SYNDROME (SIDS)

SIDS is still generally recognized as the most common cause of death among children younger than 1 year of age. It is the "sudden death of an infant under 1 year of age which remains unexplained after the performance of a complete postmortem investigation including autopsy, examination of the death scene, and a review of the case history" (Willenger, 1989). The major abuse/neglect category that is likely to be confused with SIDS is mechanical asphyxia, notably suffocation. A thorough death investigation usually allows this distinction to be made. However, in some instances, to properly ascribe death to one or the other of these conditions is impossible. Deaths in which reasonable suspicion exists that the death is not innocuous should not be certified as SIDS but should be classified as undetermined (cause and manner of death).

MONGOLIAN SPOT

Areas of hyperpigmentation such as the Mongolian spot should not be confused with injuries (Smialek, 1980) *(see Figure 19-2)*. The lack of hemorrhage in the skin and soft tissues of the Mongolian spot differentiates this lesion from an antemortem injury.

METABOLIC AND OTHER DISORDERS

Various conditions exist that may predispose a child to skeletal, cutaneous, visceral, or soft tissue damage or can manifest themselves as "pseudoinjuries," which must be differentiated from actual physical assaults. These conditions include osteogenesis imperfecti, some neoplasms, Caffey disease, congenital syphilis, kinky hair syndrome, coagulopathies, metabolic disorders, and some connective tissue diseases (Kaplan, 1986; Kirschner & Stein, 1985). Inborn errors of metabolism and poisoning share a variety of features which can make differentiation difficult (Shoemaker et al., 1992; Woolf et al., 1992).

INJURIES RELATED TO THERAPEUTIC INTERVENTION

A potential source of difficulty in evaluating the death of a child is the presence of injuries related to or allegedly explained by therapeutic or resuscitative intervention. Several types of contusions and ecchymoses can result from therapeutic endeavors (**Figure 19-18a,b**). Coagulation defects can intensify these lesions. Careful examination of areas of hemorrhage can reveal the true nature of the lesion, for example, needle or lancet punctures. The location of some contusions is also characteristic; examples include presternal contusion acquired during CPR, anterior arm and axillary fold hemorrhage caused by level of consciousness testing, and punctures on the soles of the feet related to neurologic evaluation. However, CPR–related facial bruises are distinctly uncommon (DiMaio & DiMaio, 1989).

Figure 19-18a,b. Contusions of the neck sustained during CPR.

Figure 19-19. Catheterization injury.

IATROGENIC INJURIES

In some cases, intentionally inflicted injuries will be alleged as iatrogenic. Most notable in this group are rib fractures. In contrast to adults, rib fractures caused by CPR are very rare in children without a predisposing bone disease (Feldman & Brewer, 1984). Visceral injuries such as hepatic laceration can occur during resuscitation (Thaler & Krause, 1962; Moe, 1967). Retinal hemorrhage has also been reported to occur as a result of CPR but is rare in this setting (Carter, 1983; Weedn et al., 1990; Kanter, 1986). Injuries associated with medical intervention should be noted in the clinical record and, if they are unusual, communicated to the medical examiner (**Figure 19-19**).

FOLK MEDICINE

Not only must the effects of traditional medical care be considered in evaluating an apparently injured child but injuries related to nontraditional or "home" remedies must also be recognized. Such nontraditional practices include the application of hot coins to the skin (*Cao Gio*), dermal abrasion, cupping, plumbism, moxibustion, and *Caida de Mollera* (Golden & Duster, 1977; Lock, 1978; Feldman, 1984; Kempe, 1982; Asnes & Wisotsky, 1981; Guarnaschelli et al., 1972) *(see also Chapter 1, Identifying, Interpreting, and Reporting Injuries).*

POSTMORTEM CHANGES

In addition to antemortem and perimortem artifacts, various postmortem alterations of the body can be confused with injuries that occurred before death. Included in this group are the irregular mottling of livor mortis, which can be confused with bruising, and postmortem insect bites (**Figure 19-20**) or other animal activity, which can be confused with abrasions. Careful examination of these "injuries" usually readily allows their separation from actual antemortem injuries.

Figure 19-20. *Postmortem changes. Insect bites.*

♦ORGAN AND TISSUE TRANSPLANTATION ISSUES

An expanding role for the medical examiner in deaths related to abuse is in the area of postmortem retrieval of tissue and organs for transplantation. The current major limiting factor in many types of transplant surgery is the insufficient supply of suitable donor organs and tissues. Deaths coming under the jurisdiction of the medical examiner constitute a major potential source of such material. Within this large pool of potential donors is the numerically small population of lethally abused children. These children constitute an important group since suitable pediatric organ and tissue donors are few. Legitimate concerns about the effects on pending legal proceedings frequently deter obtaining organs and tissues from allegedly abused children, curtailing access to this portion of the donor pool. To successfully fulfill society's need for these organs and tissues while at the same time meeting the requirements for potential legal actions necessitates close cooperation between all involved parties—medical, medicolegal, and legal personnel, as well as the family.

In general, no procedure can be carried out on the body of an individual whose death falls under medicolegal jurisdiction without the permission of the medical examiner. Unless otherwise specified by local statute or regulation, permission for organ and tissue retrieval must be obtained from the next of kin or legal guardian. The medical examiner cannot authorize donor harvesting, but such retrieval cannot proceed without his or her consent. The ability and willingness of the medical examiner to allow organ or tissue retrieval depends on applicable statutes and regulations, local custom, available resources, the particular organs and tissue requested, and the details of the particular death. As a general rule, the organ or tissue retrieval cannot interfere with the fulfillment of the medical examiner's statutory and professional responsibilities. However, cooperative planning among all concerned groups can lead to maximum organ and tissue utilization *and* maintain proper medicolegal evaluation of the death (National Association of Medical Examiners, 1991).

Several modifications to the usual medicolegal processing of the death can be used to facilitate satisfactory organ or tissue retrieval. Since the details of a particular death strongly influence which, if any, organs or tissues will be available for retrieval, it is advantageous when death appears likely or inevitable for the attending physician to report the impending death to the medical examiner. Such reporting facilitates harvesting of tissues and minimizes restrictions on organ and tissue retrieval. This also allows the medical examiner enough time to collect the necessary investigational information from other agencies. The intent is to allow the medical examiner to make an informed evaluation about which organs/tissues can be potentially retrieved and what further studies may be needed prior to any retrieval procedure. Following this, the family can be approached for their permission to retrieve the organs or tissues already pre-authorized by the medical examiner. In our experience this system works effectively and efficiently, and restriction of organ/tissue retrieval is minimized. Other procedures that can be indicated include examination before retrieval and photography of the victim at the hospital, preretrieval radiographic studies for medicolegal purposes, sample collection for toxicologic and other studies, medical examiner attendance at the retrieval procedure, intraoperative photographic and detailed descriptive documentation of organs or tissues before their removal, and indicated intraoperative biopsies. If the medical examiner does not attend the retrieval procedure and the operating surgeon detects an occult injury, the procedure should be halted pending further consultation with the medical examiner.

◆ BIBLIOGRAPHY

Adelson, L: Homicide by pepper, *J Forensic Sci* 9:391, 1964.

Adelson, L: *The Pathology of Homicide*, Charles C Thomas, Publisher, Springfield, IL, 1974.

Adelson, L: Pedicide revisited, *Am J Forensic Med Pathol* 12(1):16-26, 1991.

Alexander, R, et al: Incidence of impact trauma with cranial injuries ascribed to shaking, *Am J Dis Child* 144:724-726, 1990.

Alexander, RC, Surrell, JA, and Lohle, SP: Microwave oven burns to children: An unusual manifestation of child abuse, *Pediatrics* 79:255, 1987.

Asnes, RS, and Wisotsky, DT: Cupping lesions simulating child abuse, *J Pediatr* 99:267, 1981.

Bacon, CJ, Sayer, GC, and Howe, JW: Extensive retinal hemorrhage in infancy: An innocent cause, *Br Med J* 1:281, 1978.

Bite mark analysis. In D Averill, ed: *Manual of Forensic Odontology*, American Society of Forensic Odontology, 1991.

Brown, RH: The battered child syndrome, *J Forensic Sci* 21:65, 1976.

Bruce, D, and Zimmerman, R: Shaken impact syndrome, *Pediatr Ann* 18:482-494, 1989.

Caffey, J: Multiple fractures of long bones of children suffering from subdural hematoma, *Am J Radiol* 56:163-173, 1946.

Caffey, J: On the theory and practice of shaking infants: Its potential residual effects of permanent brain damage and mental retardation, *Am J Dis Child* 124:161-169, 1972.

Carter, JE: Whiplash shaking syndrome: Retinal hemorrhage and computerized axial tomography of the brain, *Child Abuse Negl* 7:279, 1983.

Case, M, and Nanduri, R: Laceration of the stomach by blunt trauma in a child: A case of child abuse, *J Forensic Sci* 28:496-501, 1983.

Case, MES, Short, CD, and Poklis, A: Intoxication by aspirin and alcohol in a child, *Am J Forensic Med Pathol* 4(2):149, 1983.

Coe, JI: Postmortem chemistry update, *Am J Forensic Med Pathol* 14:91-117, 1993.

Cohle, SD, Trestrail, JD, Graham, MA, et al: Fatal pepper aspiration, *Am J Dis Child* 142(6):633-636, 1988.

Cumberland, G, Riddick, L, and McConnell, C: Intimal tears of the right atrium of the heart due to blunt force injuries to the abdomen, *Am J Forensic Med Pathol* 12(2):102-104, 1991.

Davis, JH: Can sudden death be murder, *J Forensic Sci* 23:384, 1978.

DiMaio, DJ, and DiMaio, VJM: *Forensic Pathology*, Elsevier, NY, 1989.

Dine, MS, and McGroven, ME: Intentional poisoning of children: An overlooked category of child abuse: Report of 7 cases and review of literature, *Pediatrics* 70:32, 1982.

Duhaime, AC, Gennarelli, TA, Thibault, CE, Bruce, DA, Margulies, SS, and Wiser, R: The shaken baby syndrome: A clinical, pathological, and biomechanical study, *J Neurosurg* 66:409-415, 1987.

Duhaime, AC, et al: Head injury in very young children: Mechanisms, injury types, and ophthalmologic findings in 100 hospitalized patients younger than 2 years of age, *Pediatrics* 90:179-185, 1992.

Egge, K, Lyng, G, and Maltau, MJ: Retinal hemorrhages in the newborn, *Acta Ophthalmol* 58:231-236, 1980.

Egge, K, Lyng, G, and Maltau, MJ: Effect of instrumental delivery on the frequency and severity of retinal hemorrhages in the newborn, *Acta Obstet Gynecol Scand* 60:153-155, 1981.

Feldman, K: Pseudoabusive burns in Asian refugees, *Am J Dis Child* 138:768-769, 1984.

Feldman, KW, and Brewer, DK: Child abuse, cardiopulmonary resuscitation and rib fractures, *Pediatrics* 73:339-342, 1984.

Golden, S, and Duster, M: Hazards of misdiagnosis due to Vietnamese folk medicine, *Clin Pediatr* 10:949-950, 1977.

Griest, K, and Zumwalt, R: Child abuse by drowning, *Pediatrics* 83:41-46, 1989.

Guarnaschelli, J, Lee, J, and Pitts, FW: "Fallen fontanelle" (Caida de Mollera): A variant of the battered child, *JAMA* 222:1545, 1972.

Hadley, M, et al: The infant whiplash-shaken injury syndrome: A clinical and pathological study, *Neurosurgery* 24:536-540, 1989.

Helfer, RE, Slovis, TL, and Black, M: Injuries resulting when small children fall out of bed, *Pediatrics* 60:533-535, 1977.

Hight, D, Bakalar, N, and Hoyd, J: Inflicted burns in children, *JAMA* 242:517-520, 1979.

Hull, D: Medical diagnosis in the maltreated child. In J Carter, ed, Priory Press Ltd, London, 1974, Chapter 6.

Kanter, R: Retinal hemorrhage after cardiopulmonary resuscitation or child abuse, *J Pediatr* 108:430-432, 1986.

Kaplan, JM: Pseudoabuse: The misdiagnosis of child abuse, *J Forensic Sci* 31(4):1420-1428, 1986.

Kempe, CH: Uncommon manifestations of the battered child syndrome, *Am J Dis Child* 129(11):1265, 1975.

Kempe, CH: Cross cultural perspectives in child abuse, *Pediatrics* 69:497-498, 1982.

Kenney, J: Child abuse and neglect. In D Averill, ed: *Manual of Forensic Odontology*, American Society of Forensic Odontology, 1991.

Kirschner, R, and Stein, RJ: Mistaken diagnosis of child abuse: A form of medical abuse? *Am J Dis Child* 139:873, 1985.

Kleinman, PK, et al: Radiologic contributions to the investigation and prosecution of cases of fatal infant abuse, *New Engl J Med* 320:507-511, 1989.

Laing, SA: Bilateral injuries in childhood: An alerting sign, *Br Med J* 2:1355, 1977.

Leonidas, JC: Skeletal trauma in the child abuse syndrome, *Pediatr Ann* 12(12):875-881, 1983.

Lindenberg, R, and Freytag, E: Morphology of brain lesions from blunt trauma in early infancy, *Arch Pathol* 87:298, 1969.

Lock, M: Sears of experience: The art of moxibustion in Japanese medicine and society, *Cult Med Psychiatry* 2:151-175, 1978.

Ludwig, S: Shaken baby syndrome: A review of 20 cases, *Ann Emerg Med* 13:104-107, 1984.

Luke, JL: Recovery of intact respiratory epithelium from a cloth pillowcase four days following its utilization as a smothering instrument, *J Forensic Sci* 14(3):398-401, 1969.

McClain, P, et al: Estimates of fatal child abuse and neglect, United States, 1979 through 1988, *Pediatrics* 91:338-343, 1993.

McLellan, NJ, Prasad, R, and Punt, J: Spontaneous subhyaloid and retinal hemorrhages in an infant, *Arch Dis Child* 61:1130-1132, 1986.

Meadow, R: Munchausen Syndrome by Proxy: The hinterland of child abuse, *Lancet* 2:343, 1977.

Meadow, R: Munchausen Syndrome by Proxy, *Arch Dis Child* 57:92, 1982.

Merten, DF, and Osborne, DRS: Craniocerebral trauma in the child abuse syndrome, *Pediatr Ann* 12:12, 1983.

Moe, N: Complications following resuscitation, *Acta Med Scand* 182:773, 1967.

Moritz, AR, and Henriques, FC: Studies of thermal injury. II: The relative importance of time and surface temperature in the causation of cutaneous burns, *Am J Pathol* 23:695, 1947.

National Association of Medical Examiners: *Policy and Guidelines on Human Organ and Tissue Procurement*, The Association, St. Louis, 1991.

Nixon, J, and Pearn, J: Non-accidental immersion in bathwater: Another aspect of child abuse, *Br Med J* 1:271-272, 1977.

Norman, MG, Smialek, JE, Newman, DE, and Horembala, EJ: Postmortem examination on the abuse child: Pathological, radiographic and legal aspects, *Perspect Pediatr Pathol* 8:313, 1984.

O'Doherty, N: *The Battered Child: Recognition in Primary Care,* Bailliere Tindall, London, 1982.

Pascoe, JM, Hildebrandt, HM, Terrier, A, et al: Patterns of skin injury in non-accidental and accidental injury, *Pediatrics* 64:245, 1979.

Pearn, J, and Nixon, J: Attempted drowning as a form of non-accidental injury, *Aust Paediatr J* 13:110, 1977.

Purdue, GF, Hunt, JL, and Prescott, PR: Child abuse by burning: An index of suspicion, *J Trauma* 28(2):221-224, 1988.

Raekallio, J: Histological estimation of the age of injuries. In J Perper and C Wecht, eds: *Microscopic Diagnosis in Forensic Pathology,* Charles C Thomas, Publisher, Springfield, IL, 1980.

Retinal hemorrhages in newborn infants, *Br J Ophthalmol* 55:248-253, 1970.

Rogers, D, Tripp, J, et al: Non-accidental poisoning: An extended syndrome of child abuse, *Br Med J* 1:793, 1976.

Rosen, CL, Frost, JD, et al: Two siblings with recurrent cardiorespiratory arrest: Munchausen Syndrome by Proxy or child abuse? *Pediatrics* 71:715, 1983.

Rossignol, AM, Locke, JA, and Burke, JF: Paediatric burn injuries in New England, *Burns* 16:41-48, 1990.

Schmitt, BD: Child abuse and neglect: Types, epidemiology and characteristics. In RG Sanger and DC Bross, eds: *Clinical Management of Child Abuse and Neglect: A Guide,* 1984.

Selbst, M, et al: Bunk bed injuries, *Am J Dis Child* 144:721-723, 1990.

Sezen, F: Retinal hemorrhages in newborn infants, *Br J Ophthalmol* 55:248-253, 1970.

Shnaps, Y, Frand, M, Rotem, Y, and Tirosh, M: The chemically abused child, *Pediatrics* 68:119, 1981.

Shoemaker, J, Lynch, R, Hoffmann, J, and Sly, W: Misidentification of propionic acidi as ethylene glycol in a patient with methylmalonic acidemia, *J Pediatr* 120:417-421, 1992.

Smialek, J: Signatures of mongolian spots, *J Pediatr* 97:504, 1980.

Southall, DP, et al: Apneic episodes induced by smothering: Two cases identified by covert video surveillance, *Br Med J* 294:1637-1641, 1987.

Stone, N, Rinaldo, L, Humphrey, C, et al: Child abuse by burning, *Surg Clin North Am* 50:1419-1424, 1970.

Thaler, MM, and Krause, VW: Serious trauma in children after external cardiac massage, *N Engl J Med* 267:500, 1962.

Tomaski, LG, and Rosman, P: Purtscher retinopathy in the battered child syndrome, *Am J Dis Child* 1229:1335, 1975.

Vowles, G, et al: Diffuse axonal injury in early infancy, *J Clin Pathol* 40:185-189, 1987.

Watkins, A, Gagan, R, and Cupoli, JM: Child abuse by burning, *J Fla Med Assoc* 72:497-502, 1985.

Weedn, V, Mansour, A, and Nichols, M: Retinal hemorrhage in an infant after cardiopulmonary resuscitation, *Am J Forensic Med Pathol* 11(1):79-82, 1990.

West, M, et al: The detection and documentation of trace wound patterns by use of an alternative light source, *J Forensic Sci* 37:1480-1488, 1992a.

West, M, et al: Ultraviolet radiation and its role in wound pattern documentation, *J Forensic Sci* 37:1466-1479, 1992b.

Willenger, M: SIDS: A challenge, *J Natl Inst Health Res* 1:73, 1989.

Wilson, EF: Estimation of the age of cutaneous contusions in child abuse, *Pediatrics* 60:750, 1977.

Woolf, A, Wynshaw-Boris, A, Rinaldo, P, and Levy, H: Intentional infantile ethylene glycol poisoning presenting as an inherited metabolic disorder, *J Pediatr* 120:421-424, 1992.

Zimmerman, RA, Bilaniuk, LT, Bruce, D, et al: Computed tomography of pediatric head trauma: Acute general cerebral swelling, *Radiology* 126:403-408, 1978.

Zumwalt, RE, and Fanizza-Orphanus, AM: Dating of healing rib fractures in fatal child abuse, *Adv Pathol* 3:193-205, 1990.

Zumwalt, RE, and Hirsch, CS: Subtle fatal child abuse, *Hum Pathol* 11:167, 1980.

Zumwalt, RE, Petty, CS, and Holman, W: Temperatures in closed automobiles in hot weather, *Forensic Sci Gaz* 7:7, 1976.

TESTIFYING

JAMES A. MONTELEONE, M.D.

Appearing in court to offer expert testimony is part of the process of working in child protection. The experience can be both unpleasant and confusing unless the physician is prepared for the environment of the courtroom and has researched his or her role in the situation. This chapter offers an overview of the legal environment, specific information concerning how to prepare for a courtroom experience, and the major elements of offering testimony.

◆ THE LEGAL ENVIRONMENT

Those working in medicine are accustomed to a team approach to achieve the well-being of the patient. The legal system presents an adversarial situation, where each lawyer attempts to prove the merits of his or her case and discredit the opposite view. The judge is most concerned with procedure and with ensuring that the case will be upheld under the scrutiny of courts of appeal. Finally, if there is a jury, it is largely peopled by individuals who are unschooled in technical medical matters and must see the case through the interpretative efforts of the witnesses and lawyers. It is into this arena that the physician is thrust and justice is sought.

Most child protection cases are heard in juvenile court. There is no jury, and decisions are made by the judge. Judges serving in these areas are generally sensitive to children's issues and base their decisions on achieving the best possible result for the child, yet protecting the rights of family and parents. However, it should be remembered that the trial consists of two sides presenting admissible evidence and that the better prepared, better qualified, most articulate lawyer frequently wins, whether justice is served or not.

The physician's role in this environment is quite different from the medical role normally assumed. Clinical judgments are questioned and dissected, frequently by nonphysicians, and time is just another tool, so delays and protracted proceedings are common, unlike the quick decisions needed in medicine. These aspects can make giving testimony a painful experience, although the vast majority of court appearances, even outside the juvenile court, are straightforward and professional.

It should be noted that only rarely is justice speedy. Delays and rescheduling of trial dates are normal and it is advisable to be flexible in availability. Physicians are advised to work out an arrangement with the lawyer for whom they are testifying so that they can be on call and available and not sit and wait for hours to testify. If a long trip is required to appear in court, the physician should be certain that he or she is needed before undertaking the journey.

♦ Preparation for Court Appearance

Because lawyers are motivated to do the best for their clients and obtain a favorable result, the physician will be required to adhere to their instructions regarding appearance, demeanor, and delivery of information. This section will review these areas and offer guidance based on the typical courtroom experience.

Appearance

Because the physician is being called as an expert witness, it is best to appear professional and conservative. A coat and tie or conservative suit is preferred.

Demeanor

The physician must keep his or her tone, attitude, and reactions consistent throughout testimony, whether direct questioning or cross-examination. It is best to be controlled, polite, slow to anger, humble, serious, and patient. A poor impression is left by those who are defensive, overbearing, tentative, smug, clever, amusing, or entertaining.

Delivery of Information

As in all public appearances, the physician must speak slowly and clearly, not mumbling words or sounding tentative. Credentials should be stated to establish the physician's qualifications as an expert witness. All questions should be answered honestly; if the physician does not know the answer, he or she should so state. Reluctance to answer any question may cast doubt on the physician's testimony in the minds of the judge and/or jury.

Witnesses tend to be at ease during direct questioning and then become tense on cross-examination. This change is manifest by shifts in posture and alterations in voice quality. The voice should be kept at an even tempo, and emphasis should be used in moderation to avoid giving the impression of being uncertain or anxious. Sitting quietly and in a relaxed manner is advised. This does not imply that the witness will not be nervous, but that the nervousness should be accepted and not allowed to hinder testimony.

Answers should be objective and impartial, avoiding a judgmental tone. The court will make judgments based on the testimony and presentation of material; however, if the physician feels strongly about a point, he or she should express this opinion. The role of the expert witness is to teach, and this attitude should be maintained during all questioning.

It is important to make eye contact with both the questioner and the judge or jury. The physician is there to provide information to them and should speak directly in doing this. During cross-examination, the lawyer may position himself or herself in such a way that eye contact with the jury is difficult. The physician may need to turn from the questioner to face the jury and reestablish eye contact.

The physician must listen carefully to the questions and be certain that all is understood before attempting to answer. Questions directed from the attorney for whose case the physician is testifying should be answered immediately; a delay in answering those from the opposing lawyer gives the attorney an opportunity to object if necessary. In all but one case, objections are to questions, not answers, and a witness should not be afraid of objections raised during questioning. The one exception is the objection that the witness's answer is unresponsive to the question, wherein the physician may be directed to respond more appropriately.

The terms used in testimony should be understandable to everyone present. Using highly technical or obscure terms to impress the judge or jury is inappropriate. If a technical term must be used, it should be explained without talking down to the audience, which could imply that they are unable to comprehend what is being said.

As stated earlier, the physician must not hesitate to state that he or she does not know the answer if that is the case. As an expert witness, the doctor must not go beyond the area of expertise; he or she may decline to answer or, if the physician feels able to present a reasonable answer, offer a qualified response, such as "My feeling on this is . . . . , but you should check with an expert in that field to be certain." If the physician is uncomfortable with answering any question, he or she should insist on the point of being not qualified to respond.

If a question is unclear or not understood, it is acceptable to ask that it be repeated. If the questioner points out something that should have been done and was not, it is best to admit that it was not done and avoid becoming defensive or apologize. Anger at being advised on a medical practice or procedure by someone outside of the medical field is unwise.

If the physician disagrees with authorities in the field, honestly stating this position is appropriate. However, he or she must be prepared to defend this position.

As a rule, only the information being asked for should be given; additional information should not be volunteered. Long, involved answers should be avoided, including narratives unless they are specifically required. The court and the lawyer will direct the physician when these detailed narratives are appropriate.

When the testimony is completed, the physician should wait to be excused by the court and should leave the courtroom unless requested to stay. No emotion, either positive or negative, should be shown. In addition, both before and after testimony, the physician should conduct himself or herself with circumspection because jurors, other witnesses, or investigators may be present and observing these actions.

♦ ELEMENTS OF GIVING TESTIMONY

It is essential that the physician read the case history and other materials carefully and thoroughly before the court appearance. Some lawyers expect that an expert witness will have total recall and be familiar with all elements of a case without looking at the record. Asking to see the chart during testimony to refresh memories and be certain of the facts in the case is acceptable and will enhance the chances for accurate presentation. However, the judge can forbid the witness to review the chart in court and the physician must be prepared to deal with this contingency.

The physician should review testimony with the lawyer for whom he or she is testifying before the actual court appearance. This is an opportunity to plan which questions will be asked by both sides and the physician can inquire as to why certain questions will be asked and why some will not be asked. In addition, the physician can suggest additional questions to strengthen the lawyer's case. However, in any case, the answers must be truly the physician's and not the lawyer's.

Whether or not this meeting took place can be the subject of questions by the cross-examiner. Frequently the witness is asked if he or she met with the lawyer before giving testimony, if the testimony was rehearsed, and if the answers were dictated by the lawyer. The most appropriate answer is, "Yes, we met. He [she] told me the questions that may be asked and instructed that I answer them honestly and in my own words."

The physician should review textbooks and key references to prepare to give testimony. More obscure references are generally not required; if asked to discuss an unfamiliar reference, it is appropriate to ask to see the reference being cited. It may be necessary to read the article while on the stand. The most critical points to be noted are the publication date and journal source. The material may be outdated, from a nonrefereed journal, or taken out of context and therefore not applicable. In choosing key references, the physician should be sure to choose those which are current and cite textbooks that are commonly accepted as reflecting contemporary practice.

If a deposition was taken previously, it should be reviewed in preparation for giving testimony. This will avoid the embarrassment of contradicting previous testimony without being able to offer a valid explanation of the difference. If views on a subject have changed over time, it is best to state this fact directly and not wait to have it presented in a negative light. A careful attorney will review all cases in which the physician may have testified and point out areas of seeming contradiction. The physician must be prepared to justify or clarify what has been stated previously.

In general an attorney does not ask questions to which he or she does not know the answer; the process is meant to bring information to light for the benefit of the jury or judge. Therefore it is best to avoid embellishing accomplishments or enhancing what appears in a deposition.

PLOYS USED IN QUESTIONING AND HOW TO RESPOND

When a lawyer tries to put the witness at ease and induce a smile or laugh, the physician must be aware that smiling or laughing too long may give the impression that the situation is being taken too lightly. Maintaining a professional attitude is generally the best choice for a court appearance.

If the lawyer uses the title "Mr." rather than "Dr.," the physician should ignore the mistake. It may be a purposeful attempt to precipitate a negative reaction from the witness. Any mispronunciation of a technical term should also be ignored unless the witness is specifically asked to provide an accurate rendering. Correcting the lawyer may give the impression that the physician is pompous. If a correct pronunciation is given and the lawyer continues to mispronounce the term, this again should be overlooked rather than allowed to color the testimony. As stated previously, the physician should avoid technical terms if a more recognized and understood word is appropriate.

Conversations outside the courtroom should not involve the testimony being given. It is inappropriate to offer information beyond that given on the stand in any other situation.

Lawyers may try to rephrase testimony being given by the doctor, to enhance its presentation to the jury and/or judge. The physician must listen carefully to the edited version and make certain that it is an accurate rephrasing. Another ploy is to apply the answer to a different question. The physician must again evaluate each answer and make sure that it is what he or she really means.

In discussing a case involving multiple victims, the physician should be careful to focus on one victim at a time. If the lawyer switches back and forth from victim to victim, confusion may result in everyone's mind. If this ploy is attempted, it is best to ask to begin again and talk about each victim separately.

The lawyer may also ask several simple questions requiring a "yes" response and then insert one requiring a "no" response, hoping to catch the witness off-guard. This is called a "shotgun" approach. Each question should be listened to attentively and answered individually.

An example of this technique is as follows:

While testifying in a child pornography case in which the expert testified to the ages of children in videos, these questions were asked:

Question: Doctor, I am sure you have seen pictures of better quality than were present in that video. Is that correct?

Answer: Yes.

Question: Do different races and ethnic groups vary in the onset of puberty?

Answer: Yes.

Question: Are there differences between the sexes?

Answer: Yes.

Question: Is it true that pubertal changes will show as early as 8 years of age?

Answer: Yes.

Question: And as late as 16 years?

Answer: Yes.

Question: Even as late as 18 years?

Answer: Yes, but that is out of the range of normal.

Question: But, possible?

Answer: Yes.

Question: It's possible that the children in the video could be 18 years old?

Answer: No. Though the videos were not of the best quality, there were a number of times where I could easily ascertain the development and age of the children. I feel confident the children were prepubertal and about 9 to 12 years of age.

Another multiple question ploy to beware of is the two-in-one question in which the response to the first part of the question differs from that to the second part. The witness tends to answer the second part of the question and leave the impression that it is appropriate for the entire question.

This is an example:

Question: Doctor, can gonorrhea be transmitted from objects, such as toilet seats and towels—you are aware of research which demonstrated that potential?

Answer: There are two parts to your question. Let me answer the second part first. Yes, there have been controlled studies in which a specimen carrying gonorrhea was placed on objects such as toilet seats and researchers were able to successfully transfer the organism to an agar plate over a number of hours. However, answering the first part of that question, no one has ever been able to demonstrate that gonorrhea is spread to humans in that manner. The literature clearly states that gonorrhea is sexually transmitted.

Regarding questions about references, if the physician is asked if he or she considers a particular reference or journal to be authoritative, or is asked to supply references considered authoritative, a correct response would be, "No reference is absolutely authoritative. No single source is the final word. Although previous reports play a role in making decisions, other important factors also play a part." If the physician declares that a particular reference is authoritative, he or she may be asked to agree with everything in that reference and even expected to justify all actions against that standard.

The questioner may try to imply or state that the physician's opinion is based on speculation or guesswork. The physician should not agree. Particular words to be wary of are *conjecture, supposition, theory,* and *assumption.* A recommended response is "No, my opinion is based on reasonable medical certainty."

The questioner may also try to minimize the findings being presented.

For example, after testifying in a sexual abuse case and describing anal findings, the following cross-examination of one physician took place:

Question: In your testimony you stated that you found a 2 to 3 millimeter tear of the anus. Is that correct?

Answer: Yes.

Question: How big is a millimeter?

Answer: One-tenth of a centimeter.

Question: And how big is a centimeter? Give it in terms we can relate to.

Answer: A centimeter is not quite a half an inch. The width of my little fingernail is 1 centimeter. (He held up his little finger to demonstrate.)

Question: Then we're talking about one-tenth of that, is that correct?

Answer: Yes.

Question: Here is a pen, Doctor. Would you show the jury on that piece of paper at the easel what 2 to 3 millimeters would be?

Answer: (The witness went to the board and drew two lines.) The space between those lines would be about 2 to 3 centimeters. The dimensions are relative . . .

Question: Never mind, Doctor, just answer the questions asked. The area you are speaking about is not much wider than the tip of the pen. I have had chapped lips with breaks larger than that.

At this point, the opposing attorney should have picked up on the witness' attempt to expand on the answer and, during reexamination, asked questions whose answers would put the injury in perspective.

In sexual abuse cases, the legal proceedings frequently concentrate on physical findings. Yet the most important component in determining whether a child has been sexually abused is a credible disclosure. The physical findings should be put into perspective with statements during testimony such as, "The most important component in determining whether a child has been sexually abused is the disclosure. It must be remembered that the majority of children who have been sexually abused show no physical findings and many have no behavioral indicators. The physical findings and behavioral indicators can only support what the child says. If there are no witnesses, only two persons know what took place—the perpetrator and the victim. It comes down to whether or not you believe the child."

The opposing lawyer may try to set up a hypothetical situation and attempt to persuade the witness that it represents the case at hand when it, in fact, does not. The witness must be wary of questions starting with "What if . . ." and trying to make the witness believe that the lawyer knows something about the case that the witness does not. It is acceptable to ask if this is a hypothetical situation and answer within that context. The following is an exchange involving a hypothetical situation that was postulated during a case involving sexual abuse.

The alleged perpetrator was the baby sitter, and the individual who had interviewed the child was cross-examined as follows:

Question: You stated that after you interviewed the child you felt that the child gave a credible statement and that, based on what the child said, you believed that she had been sexually abused by her baby sitter. Is that correct?

Answer: Yes.

Question: What if I told you that the father and mother were in the process of a divorce? That the police had been called to the home by neighbors because of loud arguments between the mother and father. Would that change your conclusion?

Answer: I wasn't aware of that information. Is that true?

Question: Just answer the question. Would that change your conclusion?

Answer: No such information was in the chart when I interviewed her.

Question: Would that change your conclusion?

Answer: No. I still believe that the child was credible.

Although the witness stood by her original conclusion, that the child was credible, her reaction to the "what if" question left a different message.

The situation would have been better handled, even if the hypothetical were true, by answering the question as follows:

> "A divorce and custody situation could influence a child's disclosure. I was not aware of any such situation in this case, but had there been, I still feel the child gave a credible disclosure. I base that on the characteristics of a credible disclosure, which I discussed earlier."

Many questions cannot be properly answered with a *yes* or *no*, yet lawyers and the judge may demand they be answered that simply. A possible response might be the following:

> "I cannot answer that question with a yes or no. All things are not black and white; there are grays. May I expand on that answer?"

If the witness is not allowed to expand on the answer given, the lawyer for whom he or she is testifying should return to the question during redirect questioning and expose the entire answer.

In rebutting an answer from another expert, it is best to respond professionally and without rancor. An appropriate response might be, "Doctor _____ has a fine reputation. We do not agree on all issues."

Finally, the physician is trained to evaluate a patient and assess the merits of differential diagnoses as well as the primary diagnosis. In the witness chair the presentation of a differential diagnosis can imply doubt. If the physician is sure of the diagnosis offered and feels that there are no appropriate differential diagnoses, this should be stated clearly and defended upon cross-examination.

QUESTIONS DESIGNED TO PUT THE WITNESS ON THE DEFENSIVE

Although there are difficult questions, as outlined above, not every question is a maneuver to entrap the witness. If the physician approaches testifying by regarding each question as a potential trap, the jury and judge may derive the impression that the witness is guarded and tentative, which can be detrimental to the case for which he is testifying.

There are sensitive issues that the physician may be called upon to discuss in testimony. Among them are the awarding of a fee for participation in the case, the charge of child advocacy, and the demand for documentation. These will be addressed with specific guidelines on how to handle them.

FEE

The physician should not be embarrassed to admit when he or she is being paid for the time spent on the case. If the physician is asked if he or she is being paid to **testify** and how much, a proper response would be, "I am being paid **for the time I spend** on the case. Testifying is just one part of that time." In regard to the amount, giving the hourly fee that has been set is appropriate. Asking for compensation for the time spent on a case is perfectly acceptable.

CHILD ADVOCACY

The physician, pediatrician, or family practitioner most often appears to protect the child, the victim in a case. Therefore, usually the legal testimony offered will be to help the prosecution. However, the guiding principle should be to facilitate justice; this can be accomplished on the defendant's side in the case of misdiagnoses or conditions mistaken for abuse, as noted throughout this text. There should be no restriction as to working for the prosecution or defendant put on the work of testifying and offering expert review.

DOCUMENTATION

In caring for any patient it is necessary to make the effort to document what has been done, clearly, in the patient's chart. While following a standard protocol is helpful, it is no guarantee that everything was accomplished in order or that all the elements of the protocol applied in the case under review. In testimony, if the physician states that he or she followed the standard protocol, the opposing attorney may attempt to present the physician as sloppy or careless by pointing out areas where there are deviations from that protocol. Another tactic is to give the jury or judge the impression that if something was not documented, it was not done. The jury, as less knowledgeable individuals, may not understand explanations offered by the physician and derive an unfavorable impression from this line of questioning. The lawyer may even attempt to portray an obscure incident or finding as a grave oversight, when the physician sees it as trivial and seemingly unworthy of mention.

It is important to remember to answer all questions calmly and with control. It is possible to explain that in standard procedure in medicine you document the positive and significant negative findings, but not necessarily the unimportant negative findings. If something is not documented, this does not necessarily mean that it was not done. An important observation to make to the jury is that if all thoughts, events, and negative findings were documented, the chart would be cumbersome and charting would require more time than would have been spent on caring for the patient.

◆ BIBLIOGRAPHY

Danner, D: Do's and don'ts for experts. In NT Shayne, Chairman: *Medical Evidence*, Practising Law Institute, 1980, pp. 347-351.

Horsley, JE, and Carlova, J: *Testifying in Court*, Medical Economics Books, Oradell, NJ, 1988.

Prevention of Child Abuse

Peggy S. Pearl, Ed.D.

Child abuse prevention depends on neither a program nor a system of services, but must be founded on a society valuing its children. Within such a context the society will be willing to fund preventive services, programs, and policies rather than merely "attempting" to solve the crises caused by the lack of interest in children's welfare. **Table 21-1** lists some of the indicators that are apparent when a nation makes its children a high priority.

Table 21-1. Indicators of a Nation with Children as a High Priority

Outraged citizens are motivated to action when they hear that children are being maltreated.

Adequate and affordable housing is available for all families.

Recreation and esteem-building activities are available to all children and families.

Mental health, medical, and dental care are accessible to all families.

Social service delivery systems are accessed by families in need of assistance before maltreatment occurs rather than systems that treat after abuse occurs or punish for maltreating.

Universal instruction in the care and guidance of children is found in the curriculum of all public and private schools (kindergarten to grade 12 as well as adult continuing education).

Instruction in interpersonal communications, nonviolent conflict resolution, and resource management is provided for all students (kindergarten to grade 12 as well as adult continuing education).

Job training and education programs provide all workers with access to jobs as an avenue out of poverty.

Workplace policies support families (i.e., parental leave; job sharing; flextime; employee assistance programs; dependent care assistance programs; mental health, medical, and dental insurance; career ladders; and employee wellness programs).

Nonviolent societal role models are highly visible.

All parents have access to self-help and support groups.

Adequate funding exists for research to build the database regarding environments that facilitate optimal development of individuals throughout the life span.

Legal systems, both criminal and civil, are properly funded, staffed, and trained to promptly and fairly resolve maltreatment cases.

Culturally and ethnically sensitive home-based parent education programs are available to all new parents.

Adequate salaries are provided for professionals who work in all child-related professions to attract and retain the best and the brightest in jobs caring for the nation's priority—children and their families.

♦ PROGRAMS INVOLVING GOVERNMENT, THE JUDICIAL SYSTEM, AND THE PRIVATE SECTOR

The prevention of child abuse involves providing all parents with the necessary resources for successful parenting. The basic national commitment to children and the prevention of their maltreatment begins when the nation's leaders take the initiative to support families. However, society cannot assume that child abuse prevention is a function of government alone (U. S. Advisory, 1990; Daro, 1988b). The leaders must represent both the public and the private sectors (Recommendations, 1991; Kempe & Kempe, 1978; U. S. Advisory, 1990). The private sector must support families through interventions and programs offered in the workplace as well as encourage and fund community-wide efforts on behalf of children. Workplace policies supportive of families include job sharing, flextime, mental health, medical, and dental insurance, parental leave, employee assistance programs, and dependent care assistance programs (Cohn, 1987). Recognizing the correlation between unemployment and child abuse and neglect, job training and full employment are important segments of a societal commitment to children (Daro, 1988b).

Comprehensive child abuse prevention includes action taken within the judicial system. The legal system—criminal, civil, and juvenile courts—must support laws and procedures both to ensure the protection of children and to support families. Judicial procedures should be sensitive to the needs of children and families. Additionally, there must be adequate numbers of well-trained judges, lawyers, and court support staff, as well as manageable caseloads, to address the complex and demanding nature of child abuse and neglect litigation. The legal system must be sensitive to the needs of abuse victims to prevent additional maltreatment of these vulnerable individuals within the system as well as to protect children from continuing in abusive, dysfunctional families (Recommendations, 1991; U. S. Advisory, 1990). To continually monitor the effectiveness of the legal and protective service systems, each community should have an active citizen advocacy group (Donnelly, 1991; Recommendations, 1991; Martin, 1976). This group continually works to ensure that the policies of the private and public sectors offer the most appropriate support for families and children.

♦ PROGRAMS AND SERVICES NEEDED BY FAMILIES

To prevent child maltreatment, it is necessary that a wide range of training, services, resources, and policies be available to parents. These preventive strategies are commonly classified as *primary, secondary,* or *tertiary:*

Primary prevention: provides training, resources, and policies to all parents to enhance their parenting and keep abuse from occurring. Examples include health care, adequate child care, supportive workplace policies, and life skills training for children.

Secondary prevention: provides training, resources, and policies to targeted high-risk populations to enhance their parenting skills, including training and services to victims to keep abuse from occurring in the next generation. Secondary prevention includes self-help groups for parents who consider themselves at risk for maltreating their children, home visitor programs for new parents, and parent education programs for adolescent parents.

Tertiary prevention: provides training, resources, and policies to enhance parenting to keep abuse from recurring once it has been identified. Among the programs included are respite day care for parents, treatment for abused and neglected children, crisis intervention services, counseling, and stress management training.

Within our society basic prevention programs should be available to all parents before any maltreatment begins (Martin, 1976). All parents require access to parenting information, especially when they have their first children. Perinatal coaching, home visitor, and parent aide programs have proven effective for parents with young children. Additionally, all parents must have access to health care both for themselves and for their children. All schoolchildren require life skills education, and all parents need stress management training and access to positive support services to help them cope with the stress of parenting. In our highly mobile society, many families lack the positive support of family and friends and, consequently, this support must be supplied by other sources, for example, the church, social organizations, or mental health agencies (U. S. Advisory, 1990; Taylor & Beauchamp, 1988; Olds & Henderson, 1989). Accessible and affordable child care must be available to all working parents, but especially to single parents and the "working poor" (Daro, 1988b). Additionally, all programs must be respectful of cultural issues in order to be effective.

In both private and public schools, children need instruction regarding positive ways to interact with others as much as they need instruction in math, English, and science. Life skills education should be integrated into the curriculum beginning with kindergarten and continuing into adult education. Life skills education includes nonviolent conflict resolution, stress management skills, resource management, effective decision making, and effective interpersonal communication, as well as information regarding child development and guidance (Donnelly, 1991; Kempe & Kempe, 1978; Daro, 1988a; Martin, 1976). Additionally, the basics of substance abuse prevention education currently advocated must be a component of education for parenting or life skills.

Every community must make the accessibility of parent education classes part of a comprehensive adult education program. Topics suggested for these parent education classes include principles of child development, positive child guidance, and basics in child care, such as child nutrition and safety. One vital area that should be addressed with parents of children at any age is techniques to improve the parent-child interaction. Learning to play with and enjoy their children enhances both this interaction and the parents' pleasure in their parental role (Daro, 1988b).

Corporal punishment can easily become abuse when administered by parents who are angry and under stress. Therefore, instruction in the positive methods of child guidance is required. Additionally, parents need to know constructive methods of coping with stress. Self-help groups such as Parents Anonymous (PA) give parents alternatives to abusing their children, emotionally or physically, and provide positive support networks when stress occurs. PA uses the Alcoholics Anonymous (AA) model of self-help, which has proven successful. Both primary and tertiary support groups should be developed to prevent and combat abuse.

To enhance parenting skills and competence as well as prevent child abuse, new parents benefit from various instruction and support services. The specific content and structure of these programs will vary, as well as the sponsoring agency or institution; however, *the goals of programs for new parents should include:*

1. Increasing the parent's knowledge of child development and the demands involved in parenting

2. Enhancing the parent's skill in coping with the stresses of infant and child care

3. Enhancing parent-child bonding, emotional ties, and communication skills

4. Increasing the parent's skill in coping with the stress of caring for children with special needs

5. Increasing the parent's knowledge about home and child management

6. Reducing the burden of child care

7. Increasing access to social and health services for all family members (Daro, 1988b)

Parent education offered as tertiary prevention for various types of maltreatment differs in informational need from primary or secondary programs and responds to separate service delivery systems. Group parent education that emphasizes impulse control and alternative methods of discipline is particularly successful with physically abusive parents, whereas one-on-one, home-based services founded on individual counseling and problem solving techniques are more effective with neglectful parents. Neglectful parents need instruction in practical child care tasks, for example, diapering and feeding an infant or distracting and communicating with a 2-year-old. Programs successful in preventing emotional abuse include group-based services that define nonphysical methods of discipline; emphasize the need for consistency in determining and implementing rules; and offer parents ways of demonstrating affection toward their children (Daro, 1988a; Golub et al., 1987).

♦ROLE OF THE MEDIA

The media must play a key role in the prevention of child abuse. As a major force in shaping public opinion, the media can offer responsible programming and reporting to de-emphasize the current societal acceptance of violence. Additionally, through judicial programming, the media can reverse the current trend toward a desensitization of individuals to the horrors of violence. As the acceptance and glamorization of violence are removed, a new message can be sent, that violence in all forms is inappropriate. The media can depict nonviolent methods of conflict resolution. The media has been involved in and should continue to play a role in educating the public as to the magnitude of the consequences of violence in the lives of families and possible alternatives. The media may also advocate policies beneficial to children and families. One important step involves portraying parenting as the important and valued job in our society it is and thereby increasing parental esteem and helping prevent child abuse.

♦PROGRAMS TO PREVENT NEGLECT AND SEXUAL ABUSE

Although different in form, child maltreatment practices share common causes and therefore the societal approaches to prevention impact most types of maltreatment. However, specific mention should be made about prevention programs for neglect and sexual abuse, since the causes of these types of maltreatment differ slightly from those of physical and emotional abuse.

PREVENTION OF NEGLECT

To prevent child neglect, parents require the basic resources to provide proper care for their children. At some income levels parents cannot provide the necessary food, shelter, clothing, or mental health, medical, and dental care for their children (Recommendations, 1991; Helfer, 1987; U. S. Advisory, 1990). At this poverty level of existence, parents are also experiencing stress and are usually without adequate support systems. Currently in our society many individuals are employed full time at jobs that do not pay enough to provide the basic needs for the family. Many more parents lack the job skills necessary for entry-level jobs; even if they had these skills, many entry-level jobs fail to provide medical and dental insurance. At the same time, national and state governments provide fewer mental health, medical, and dental services for citizens. The consequences of these two trends is that growing numbers of children are without adequate health care services (Daro, 1988b).

When society makes adequate child care a national priority, it ensures, through various public and private sector means, that all parents have access to the basic resources to care for their families. To care for our nation's children, all parents must have access to decent and affordable housing; adequate mental health, medical, and dental care; nutritious food; and developmentally appropriate child care services (Recommendations, 1991; U. S. Advisory, 1990; Daro, 1988b; Olds & Henderson, 1989; Fink & McCloskey, 1990). The cycle of poverty that results in the disintegration of families and an atmosphere of chronic violence must be interrupted with culturally sensitive programs that work, addressing housing, jobs, substance abuse treatment, family support, and so on (Donnelly, 1991).

To prevent neglect, parents must also function at optimal levels so they can focus on their children's needs. Many parents are impaired in their ability to parent because of substance abuse or psychopathologic disorders. To prevent child maltreatment these adults must have access to substance abuse prevention and treatment programs and mental health services. These services must be available to all parents either free, at fees based on ability to pay, along sliding scales, or under provisions of employee insurance or employee assistance programs (U. S. Advisory, 1990; Daro, 1988b).

PREVENTION OF SEXUAL ABUSE

In the last decade many programs to prevent sexual abuse were developed and widely implemented. Generally these sexual abuse prevention programs teach children how to protect themselves from abuse. Researchers and clinicians caution that the major responsibility for prevention of sexual abuse cannot be placed on the victims or potential victims because they are children. Sexual abuse prevention programs must focus on the perpetrator (Swift, 1979). The National Committee for the Prevention of Child Abuse developed a comprehensive strategy for preventing adults from becoming child sexual abusers.

This prevention strategy includes the following:

1. Education for adolescents and young children that provides all adolescents with quality sex education, including healthy sexuality, during the preteen and teenage years to enhance their knowledge of what is normal and abnormal.

2. Training for professionals and volunteers who work with children that teaches these individuals how to identify and help children who are being abused, how to teach children to protect themselves from abuse, and how to detect those who may be potential molesters.

3. Education for parents that provides all new parents with quality education and support to enhance early attachment and bonding when their first babies are born. This should include information about appropriate and inappropriate touch and what to do about it. Parents need to know how to detect and handle in their own children symptoms that may indicate sexual abuse has occurred.

4. Institutional changes that ensure that all child-serving institutions and programs (e.g., schools, boys clubs, Girl Scouts, day care, etc.) train children in self-awareness and self-protection. Guidelines and regulations must be in place to screen, train, and monitor all volunteers and staff.

5. Media messages that create an environment in which the prevention programs and concepts just outlined will be effective by communicating two messages.
    First, for adolescents and adults, messages that say:
    Child sexual abuse is a crime.
    Help is available.
    Abuse is a chronic problem unless you get help.
    Children get hurt when you sexually abuse them.
    Children cannot consent to this kind of behavior.
    Second, messages to children, including:
    It's okay to say no.
    It's not your fault.
    Reach out for help if this begins to happen to you.
    Help is available for you (Cohn, 1986).

The comprehensive child sexual abuse prevention strategy just outlined, like all prevention programs, strengthens individuals and families by enhancing parenting skills.

♦ SUMMARY

All parents should have available to them the resources, education, and services needed to parent effectively. A comprehensive multidisciplinary approach to prevention is needed. No specific program or plan is most effective with all parents. A mix of family support programs is needed in both the private and public sectors to enhance parenting. Once abuse has occurred, various resources, educational programs, and services are needed to prevent additional abuse. Each family needs an individualized approach, with some requiring intense and ongoing services to prevent maltreatment (Daro & Gelles, 1992). Research has shown specific gains in the following areas after parental participation in secondary and tertiary prevention programs: improved mother-infant bonding and maternal capacity to respond to the child's emotional needs; demonstrated ability to care for the child's physical and developmental needs; fewer subsequent pregnancies; more consistent use of health care services and job training opportunities; and decreased reliance on welfare use, higher school completion rates, and higher employment rates (Donnelly, 1991; Daro, 1988b).

Prevention requires society's commitment to the welfare of children. This commitment must be backed by both the public and the private sectors and must extend beyond mere rhetoric to include allocating resources as well as changing existing policies that do not conform to this commitment. Society must recognize the importance of parenting and then commit resources to assist parents in performing this challenging and rewarding job.

♦ BIBLIOGRAPHY

Cohn, AH: Preventing adults from becoming sexual molesters, *Child Abuse Negl* 10(4):559-562, 1986.

Cohn, AH: Our national priorities for prevention. In RE Helfer and RS Kempe, eds: *The Battered Child*, University of Chicago Press, Chicago, 1987.

Conte, JR, Rosen, CR, and Saperstein, L: An analysis of programs to prevent the sexual victimization of children (paper presented at the Fifth International Congress on Child Abuse and Neglect), Montreal, 1984.

Daro, D: *Confronting Child Abuse: Research for Effective Program Design*, Free Press, New York, 1988a.

Daro, D: Intervening with new parents: An effective way to prevent child abuse (working paper 839), National Committee for the Prevention of Child Abuse, Chicago, 1988b.

Daro, D: Child sexual abuse prevention: Separating fact from fiction, *Child Abuse Negl* 15(1/2):1-4, 1991.

Daro, D, and Gelles, RJ: Public attitudes and behaviors with respect to child abuse prevention, *J Interpersonal Violence* 7(4):517-531, 1992.

Donnelly, AC: What we have learned about prevention: What we should do about it, *Child Abuse Negl* 15(1)99-106, 1991.

Fink, A, and McCloskey, L: Moving child abuse and neglect prevention programs forward: Improving program evaluation, *Child Abuse Negl* 14(2):187-206, 1990.

Golub, JS, Espinosa, M, Damon, L, and Card, J: A videotape parent education program for abusive parents, *Child Abuse Negl* 11(1):255-265, 1987.

Helfer, RE: The developmental basis of child abuse and neglect: An epidemiological approach. In RE Helfer and RS Kempe, eds: *The Battered Child*, University of Chicago Press, Chicago, 1987.

Kempe, CH, and Kempe, RS: *Child Abuse*, Harvard Press, Cambridge, MA, 1978.

Martin, HP: Suming up and moving on. In HP Martin, ed: *The Abused Child: A Multidisciplinary Approach to Developmental Issues and Treatment*, Ballinger Publishing Co, Cambridge, MA, 1976.

Olds, DL, and Henderson, CR, Jr: The prevention of maltreatment. In D Cicchetti and V Carlson, eds: *Child Maltreatment: Theory and Research on the Causes and Consequences of Child Abuse and Neglect*, Cambridge University Press, Cambridge, England, 1989.

Recommendations for the 21st century, *Child Abuse Negl* 15(1):39-50, 1991.

Swift, C: The prevention of sexual abuse: Focus on the perpetrator, *J Clin Child Psychol* 133-136, 1979.

Taylor, DK, and Beauchamp, C: Hospital-based primary prevention strategy in child abuse: A multi-level needs assessment, *Child Abuse Negl* 12(3):343-354, 1988.

Trundell, B, and Whatley, MH: School sexual abuse prevention: Unintended consequences and dilemmas, *Child Abuse Negl* 12(1):103-113, 1988.

US Advisory Board on Child Abuse and Neglect: *Child Abuse and Neglect: Critical First Steps in Response to a National Emergency*, Health and Human Services, Washington, DC, 1990.

INDEX

A

AA; *see* Alcoholics Anonymous

Abandonment, 246-248
 emotional, 246, 247-248
 fatal or near-fatal, 246
 neglect and, 241-258
 with physical needs provided by others, 247
 termination of parental rights and, 407

Abandonment infanticide, 246

Abdomen, dynamics of blunt trauma to, 60, 61

Abdominal injuries, radiology of, 44-50

Abnormal responses, emotional abuse and, 274

Abrasions, 78
 injuries caused by fall including, 8

Absolute immunity, reporting statutes and, 400-401, 402

Abstat, St. Louis Child Abuse Network Study and, 317

Abuse
 allegations of, child custody disputes and, 417-419
 breeds abuse, 290
 child; *see* Child abuse
 children as abusers and; *see* Child(ren) as abusers
 conditions that are not, medical examiner and, 3-4, 50-52, 451-452
 of discretion, child custody disputes and, 419
 elder, 286
 emotional; *see* Emotional abuse
 factors in altering cycle of, children as abusers and, 297-298
 fetal; *see* Fetal abuse
 physical; *see* Physical abuse
 repeated episodes of, 440-441
  medical examiner and, 431
 ritualistic; *see* Ritualistic abuse
 sexual; *see* Sexual abuse
 single episode of, 440-441
  medical examiner and, 431
 spouse, 16, 286
 substance; *see* Substance abuse
 traumatizing, children as abusers and, 294-295

Abused-to-abuser cycle, children as abusers and, 297

Abusers, children as; *see* Child(ren) as abusers

Abusive acts, sexual abuse and, 114

Abusive burn; *see* Burns, abusive

Acceleration-deceleration phenomena, shaken infant syndrome and, 12, 83-86, 313-314

Access to children by pedophile, 120

Accident
 as cause of death, Ewigman and Kivlahan study and, 320
 classification of death as, 433
 head injuries and, 81

Accident Facts, 90

Accidental burn, 94

Accidental drowning, differentiating nonaccidental drowning from, 15

Accidental injuries
 versus inflicted injuries, 4-5, 50-52, 451-452
 involving frontal plane, 4

Accidental scalds, 448

Acetylsalicylic acid, poisoning from, 447

Acid phosphatase, 149

Acquired immunodeficiency syndrome (AIDS), 205, 214

Active inducer, Munchausen Syndrome by Proxy and, 235

Active neglect, 449

Acyclovir in treatment of sexually transmitted diseases, 207, 211

Addict, doctor, Munchausen Syndrome by Proxy and, 235-236

Adhesions, labial, physical examination in sexual abuse and, 145

Adjudicatory hearing in juvenile court, 405-406

Adjudicatory stage of proceeding, juvenile courts and, 403

Admissions by parties, evidentiary issues and, 422

Adolescents
 behavioral indicators of sexual abuse in, 166, 167
 causes of death of, 310-311

Adoption Assistance and Child Welfare Act of 1980, 389

Adult criminality, neglect and, 252

Affect, negative, emotional abuse and, 273

Affidavit attachment, search warrant and, 376, 377-378

Age of majority, 407

Age specificity of pedophile, 119

Aggression
 children as abusers and, 288-290, 291, 292, 297
 emotional abuse and, 274
 sibling, 287

Aging of injuries, medical examiner and, 437-438

AIDS; *see* Acquired immunodeficiency syndrome

Alanine amino transferase (ALT), liver injury and, 63

Alcohol
 and drugs, neglect and, 251
 poisoning from, 217, 219, 220, 224

Alcoholics Anonymous (AA) model of self-help, 469

Alexithymia, emotional abuse and, 276

Alleged perpetrators, interviewing, 357-359

Alopecia, 7-8

Alopecia areata, 8

ALT; *see* Alanine amino transferase

Amber, In re, 426

American Academy

    of Child and Adolescent Psychiatry, 170

    of Pediatrics, 170

American Bar Association, death review process and, 311-312

American Humane Association, 115

American Medical Association, guidelines of, to assist physicians in evaluating and reporting child abuse and neglect, 254

American Professional Society on the Abuse of Children, 170

Ammonia burns, diaper rash and, 18

Amnesia, dissociation and, 196

Amoxicillin in treatment of sexually transmitted diseases, 207, 209

Amphetamines, effect of, on fetus, 250-251

Anal asymmetry when dilated, physical examination in sexual abuse and, 156

Anal canal, 136

    anal sexual abuse and, 152

    shortening or eversion of, physical examination in sexual abuse and, 153

Anal dilatation, physical examination in sexual abuse and, 153

Anal pruritus, anorectal gonorrhea and, 206

Anal sexual abuse, physical findings associated with, physical examination in sexual abuse and, 152-157

Anal sphincter

    anal sexual abuse and, 152

    laxity and reduced tone of, physical examination in sexual abuse and, 153

Anal verge, 136

Anal verge skin, changes in, anal sexual abuse and, 155

Anal warts, physical examination in sexual abuse and, 155-156

Analytic orientation, emotional abuse and, 272

Anatomically detailed dolls

    evidentiary issues and, 426

    use of, in interview with victim of sexual abuse, 180-181

Ancillary studies, medical examiner and, 436

Anemia, iron deficiency, 63

Angulation of hymenal edge, physical examination in sexual abuse and, 144

Animal bites, 19

Anion gap metabolic acidosis, elevated, drugs associated with, 222

Aniridia, 70

Anogenital warts, physical examination in sexual abuse and, 155-156

Anorectal gonorrhea, 206

Anterior chamber injury, traumatic, 70-71

Anterior column of rugae, 136

Anterior disk herniation, 37

Anterior hymenal cleft, 139

Antifreeze, poisoning from, 224

Antihistamines, poisoning from, 218

Apnea

    Munchausen Syndrome by Proxy and, 232

    poisoning and, 221

    sudden infant death syndrome and, 18

Appeals in criminal court, 417

Appearance, testifying and, 460

Appointed counsel, criminal court and, 408

Arraignment in criminal court, 413

Arrest and booking in criminal court, 410

Arrest warrant, criminal court and, 410

Arrestee, criminal court and, 411-412

Arrests, St. Louis Child Abuse Network Study, Phase Two, and, 319

Arrow-shaped configuration of burns, 94, 101-102

Arsenic, poisoning from, 447

ART; *see* Automated reagin test

Arthritis, 206, 208

Asher, R., 230

Aspartate amino transferase (AST), liver injury and, 63

Asphyxia, mechanical

    medical examiner and, 446

    sudden infant death syndrome and, 451

Assault, sexual abuse and, 114

Assaultive acts, sexual abuse and, 114

AST; *see* Aspartate amino transferase

Atlas of Roentgenographic Measurement, 37

Atresia, biliary, 52

Atrial tears, right, 444-445, 446

Attachment, children as abusers and, 288

Attachment disorders

    emotional abuse and, 278-279

    neglect and, 246-248

Attack as defense of pedophile, sexual abuse and, 120

Attorney

    juvenile court and, 405

    for parent(s) in juvenile court, 404-405

    for petitioner in juvenile court, 404

Audiotaping, use of, in interview with victim of sexual abuse, 183

Auditory hallucinations, dissociation and, 197

Automated reagin test (ART), 210

Automobile restraint systems, infant, burns and, 98

Autopsy

    indirect ophthalmoscopy and, 71

    medicolegal evaluation of death and, 434-436

    Missouri Child Fatality Review Project and, 322

    postmortem examination and, 435

Avium-intracellularae, 213

Avulsion of tooth, 11

Axonal injury, diffuse, shaking injuries and, 84

Azidothymidine (AZT) in treatment of HIV infection, 213

Azithromycin in treatment of sexually transmitted diseases, 209

AZT; *see* Azidothymidine

B

Babygram, 28

Bacteremia, 208

Bacterial vaginosis, 209

Bail in criminal court, 411-412

Baltimore City Dep't. of Social Serv. v. Bouknight, 404

Barbiturates, poisoning from, 218

Bargaining, plea, in criminal court, 413

Baron von Munchausen's Narrative of His Marvelous Travels and Campaigns in Russia, 230

Bartholinitis, 206

Basic investigation protocols, 326-384

Battered child, 2

    evidentiary issues and, 425

Cardiac rupture, internal or external, 444-445
Cardinal Glennon Children's Hospital, St. Louis Child Abuse
    Network Study and, 312
Cardiopulmonary assessment in thoracoabdominal injuries, 62
Cardiopulmonary resuscitation (CPR)
    contusions acquired during, 452
    ocular injuries as result of, 68
    rib fractures and, 38, 445
Care standards, inadequate, neglect and, 245
Caretaker
    indicators of abuse by, 22
    interview of, sexual abuse and, 170-174
    problems of, St. Louis Child Abuse Network Study, Phase Two,
      and, 318
Carnitine deficiency, sudden infant death syndrome and, 18
Caruncle, urethral, mistaken for sexual abuse, 159
Case history, testifying and, 461
Catastrophic injuries, studies of, review process and, 312-317
Cauliflower ear, 11
Cause
    to believe
      reasonable, reporting statutes and, 400
      reporting statutes and, 393
    of death
      determining, medical examiner and, 432-433
      undetermined, sudden infant death syndrome and, 451
    probable, criminal court and, 412
    reasonable, to suspect, reporting statutes and, 393, 400
    to suspect, reporting statutes and, 400
CBC; *see* Complete blood count
CDC; *see* Centers for Disease Control
Cefixime in treatment of sexually transmitted diseases, 207
Cefotaxime in treatment of sexually transmitted diseases, 207
Ceftizoxime in treatment of sexually transmitted diseases, 207
Ceftriaxone in treatment of sexually transmitted diseases, 207, 208
Cefuroxime axetil with probenecid in treatment of sexually
    transmitted diseases, 207
Centers for Disease Control (CDC), 204, 218
Central nervous system hemorrhages mistaken for abuse, 3
Central registries, reporting statutes and, 393-395
Centrality of violence, children as abusers and, 292
Cephalhematoma, 44
Cerebral edema
    radiology and, 42
    strangulation and, 40
Cervicitis, 206, 207, 208, 209, 211, 212
Chain of custody, toxicology screening and, 223
Chancroid, 213
Character disorder parent, emotional abuse and, 262
Charcot's hystero-epilepsy, multiple personality disorder and, 193
Chemical burns, 90, 449
Chest
    flail, 444-445
    radiology of, 37-39
Cheyne-Stokes breathing, 14
Child(ren)
    under 12 years of age, sexual abuse and, 184
    abused; *see* Child abuse
    as abusers, 285-307
      abuse and, 293
      abused-to-abuser cycle and, 297

Child(ren)—cont'd
    as abusers—cont'd
      aggression and, 290, 291, 292, 297
      attachment and, 288
      centrality of violence and, 292
      child maltreatment and aggression and, 288-290
      definition of, 287
      effects of physical abuse and, 290-292
      effects of sexual abuse and, 295-297
      experimentation and, 293
      factors in altering cycle of, 297-298
      family violence and, 285-286
      impact of sexual abuse and, 294-297
      physically abusive children and, 286-287
      prevalence of, 287-288, 293-294
      self-destructiveness and, 291-292
      sexual behavior problems and, 295-296
      sexually abusive children and, 292-293, 296-297
      sexually reactive children and, 296
      social learning and, 289-290
      traumatizing abuse and, 294-295
      traumatizing family precursors and, 294
      traumatizing family responses and, 295
      treatment perspectives and, 298-299
    access to, by pedophile, 120
    assessment of, emotional abuse and, 274-275
    battered; *see* Battered child
    behavioral indicators of sexual abuse in, 166-169
    best interests of, child custody disputes and, 418, 419
    causes of death of, 310-311
    credibility of, factors that enhance, sexual abuse and, 184
    endangered, neglect and, 243
    fantasies focusing on, of pedophile, 119, 120
    indicators of nation placing high priority on, 467
    interview of, in sexual abuse, 163-190
    in juvenile court, 404
    normal development and behavior of, 2-3
    parents maltreated as, emotional abuse and, 275
    physically abusive, children as abusers and, 286-287
    representation for, in juvenile court, 405
    at risk, failure to thrive and, 250
    sexually abusive, children as abusers and, 292-293, 296-297
    sexually reactive, children as abusers and, 296
    showing sexually explicit material to, by pedophile, 120
    significant others' view of, emotional abuse and, 277
    St. Louis Child Abuse Network Study and, 312-325
    starvation of, 449
    surveillance of, Munchausen Syndrome by Proxy and, 237
    vulnerabilities of, sexual abuse and, 116
Child abuse
    accidental versus inflicted injuries and, 4-5
    bruises and; *see* Bruises
    closed head injury and, 12-14
    conditions that may be confused with, 3-4, 50-52, 451-452
    cutaneous injuries and, 5-8
    definition of, 2
    differential considerations in, radiology and, 50-52
    drowning and; *see* Drowning
    external head injuries and, 9-12
    facial injuries and; *see* Facial injuries

Coagulopathies, 451
Cocaine
crack, 219, 220
effect of, on fetus, 250-251
freebase, 220
poisoning from, 220-221, 224, 447
Cognitive development, Piaget's stages of, emotional abuse and, 271
Cognitive functioning, delayed, emotional abuse and, 278
Cognitive indicators of emotional abuse, 273
Cognitive interview, 177
Coining, 99
Coitus, ectopic, 157
Collateral attack, criminal court and, 417
Colon, radiology of, 49-50
Colonic hematoma, 50
Color of state law, child protection services caseworkers and, 398
Colposcopy, physical examination in sexual abuse and, 144
Coma, poisoning and, 220, 221
Commissioners, juvenile court and, 403
Commotio cordia, 432
Communications, privileged, abrogation of, reporting statutes and, 395-396, 397
Companions, imaginary, dissociation and, 197
Competence to testify, evidentiary issues and, 420
Complete blood count (CBC), thoracoabdominal injuries and, 63
Compression epidural hematoma, 442
Computed tomography (CT), 29, 30
abdominal trauma and, 50
central nervous system injury and, 14
hepatic injury and, 45
intracranial injuries and, 44
pancreatic injury and, 46
skull fractures and, 43
Computer enhancement of photographs, examination of injuries and, 440
Computer programs tabulating number of visits to emergency rooms, 61-62
Condyloma, 149
Condyloma acuminatum, 211, 212
Confessions in criminal court, 414-415
Confidentiality, abrogation of privileged communications and, 395-396
Confrontation, Munchausen Syndrome by Proxy and, 237
Confrontation clause
in criminal court, 415-416, 421, 423
evidentiary issues and, 423-424
Congenital glaucoma, 70
Congenital hemangiomas mistaken for sexual abuse, 159
Congenital HIV infection, 149
Congenital insensitivity to pain, 51
Congenital syphilis, 51, 451
Congestion, venous, physical examination in sexual abuse and, 155
Conjunctivitis, 206
gonococcal, 71, 206
Connective tissue diseases, 451
Consanguinity, 113
Consciousness, level of, head injury and, 86
Constipation mistaken for sexual abuse, 152, 159
Constitutional concerns, reporting statutes and, 398-399
Constitutional issues at trial in criminal court, 414-416
Contact burns, 90, 103-106

Contusion(s), 78, 81-83
aging of, 437
hepatic, 45
pulmonary, 38
Contusion tears, 82, 83
Conventional orientation, emotional abuse and, 271-272
Convictions, St. Louis Child Abuse Network Study, Phase Two, and, 319
Copper absorption, Menkes' kinky hair disease and, 52
Corner fracture, 32, 51
Coronary, cafe, 447
Coroner
death review process and, 312
role and responsibilities of, 347
Corporal punishment, 286, 469
Corrupting, emotional abuse and, 260, 267-268
Cortical pathways injury, shaken baby syndrome and, 71
Cosmetic practices, hair loss and, 7-8
Counsel
appointed, criminal court and, 408
right to, in criminal court, 411
Countertransference, child abuse and neglect and, 254
Court
criminal; *see* Criminal court
juvenile; *see* Juvenile court
Court appearance, preparation for, testifying and, 460-461
Court order, protective custody and, 395
Cousin incest, 165, 294
Cousin sexual abuse, 294
Coy v. Iowa, 416
CPK isoenzymes; *see* Creatinine phosphokinase isoenzymes
CPR; *see* Cardiopulmonary resuscitation
CPS; *see* Child Protective Services
Crack cocaine, 219, 220
effect of, on fetus, 251
Craniofacial injuries, radiology of, 39-44
Creatinine phosphokinase (CPK) isoenzymes with MB bands, cardiac injury and, 64
Credentials of physician, in testifying, 460
Credibility of child, factors that enhance, sexual abuse and, 184
Cribriform hymen, 138
Criminal behavior, mental illness and, emotional abuse and, 275
Criminal court
appeals and post-conviction actions in, 417
arraignment in, 413
arrest and booking in, 410
bail in, 411-412
child abuse and neglect in, 407-417
confrontation clause in, 415-416
constitutional and related issues at trial in, 414-416
dismissals in, 413
diversion in, 413-414
grand jury in, 412-413
guilty pleas in, 413
initial appearance in, 411-412
investigation in, 408
medical records and information in, 408-410
plea bargaining in, 413
preliminary hearing in, 412

Neglect—cont'd
drugs and alcohol and, 251
education and, 245
effects and outcomes of, 251-253
emotional growth and, 245
environmental hazards and, 244-245
excessive hot water temperature and, 244-245
failure to thrive and, 248-250
fetal, 250-251
fire hazards and, 244
future neglecting parent and, 252
health care and, 245
housekeeping problems and, 244
inadequate care standards and, 245
inadequate shelter and, 244
inadequate sleeping arrangements and, 244
incidence and definitions of, 242-243
lack of supervision and, 247
lethal, 449
long-term effects of, 252-253
malnutrition and, 245, 252
medical, 19
medical examiner and, 449-450
nutrition and, 245
ocular manifestations of, 71
parent education classes and, 470
parental custody refusal and, 247
passive, 449
personal hygiene and, 245
physical environment and, 244
physician roles in prevention of, 254
poisoning and, 219
prevention of, 253-254, 470-471
psychopathology and, 252
regional centers and, 254
structural hazards and, 244
substance accessibility and use and, 244
substantive criminal law and, 407-408
supervision and, 245
termination of parental rights and, 407
throwaways and, 246
types of, 243-245
unsanitary conditions and, 244
Neglecting parent, future, neglect and, 252
Negligence per se, reporting statutes and, 399
Neisseria gonorrhoeae, 147, 148, 203, 205, 207, 208
Neonaticide, fetal abuse and, 17
Neurogenic patulous anus mistaken for sexual abuse, 159
Neuroimaging, 44
New parent programs in prevention of child abuse, 468-470
NIS-1; *see* National Study of the Incidence and Severity of Child Abuse and Neglect
No true bill, criminal court and, 413
Nolo contender plea, sexual abuse and, 121
Nonabused girls, findings in, physical examination in sexual abuse and, 137-142
Nongonococcal urethritis, 208
Nonorganic failure to thrive, 248-250
emotional abuse and, 261
Nonspecific vaginitis, 209

Nonsuppurative regional lymphadenopathy, 210
Normal child development and behavior, 2-3
Norms orientation, emotional abuse and, 271-272
Nuclear medicine, 28-29
Nutrition, neglect and, 245

O

"O" sign, anal sexual abuse and, 153
Observation, physical examination in sexual abuse and, 135
O'Connor, S.D., 416
Ocular injuries
abusive, 68-71
nonabusive, 68
Offenders, regressed, sexual abuse and, 118
Operation, mock, ritualistic abuse and, 266
Ophthalmic manifestations of child abuse, 67-73
abusive ocular injuries and, 68-71
anterior chamber injury and, 70-71
cortical pathways injury and, 71
lens dislocation and, 70
lens subluxation and, 70
neglect and, 71
nonabusive ocular injuries and, 68
ocular injuries as a result of birth process and, 68
ocular injuries as a result of CPR, 68
ocular manifestations in sexual abuse and, 71
periorbital edema and, 68
presenting signs of, 67
retinal hemorrhage and, 68, 69
shaken baby syndrome and, 69
subconjunctival hemorrhage and, 68
team approach to, 71
vitreous hemorrhage and, 70
Ophthalmologist, ophthalmic manifestations of child abuse and, 67-73
Ophthalmoscopy, indirect, autopsy and, 71
Opiates, poisoning from, 219
Optic atrophy, 71
Optic nerve sheath hemorrhages, 71
Oral injuries, 9-12
Organ transplantation issues, medical examiner and, 453-454
Osteogenesis imperfecti, 50-51, 451
Osteomyelitis, 51
Osteopenia, rickets and, 51-52
Osteopetrosis, 52
Overlying, medical examiner and, 447
Overpressuring, emotional abuse and, 260, 269
Overreporting, neglect and, 243

P

PA; *see* Parents Anonymous
Pain, congenital insensitivity to, 51
Palmar hand injuries, 4
Pancreas, radiology of, 46-47
Pancreatic injuries, 446
Pancreatic pseudocyst, 46
Pancreatitis, 46, 47, 450
pleural effusions and, 38
secondary, 446
traumatic, 63

Physical examination—cont'd
 in sexual abuse—cont'd
  genital examination in, 135-137
  gymnastics and, 160
  healed lacerations in, 148
  hematoma in, 155
  horseback riding and, 160
  hymen and, 159
  hymenal tears in, 146
  increased friability in, 144
  increased vascularity in, 144
  inflammation in, 144
  labial adhesions in, 145
  laxity and reduced tone of anal canal in, 153
  masturbation and, 159, 160
  new lacerations in, 148
  normal examinations in sexually abused children in, 156-157
  normal female anatomy in, 135-137
  observation in, 135
  perianal erythema in, 153
  physical findings associated with anal sexual abuse in, 152-157
  physical findings in rape victims in, 157
  pigmentation in, 156
  presence of sperm in, 133, 149-150
  providing reassurance in, 134
  questions often asked about, 159-160
  reviewing previous records in, 134
  sexually transmitted diseases in, 149, 160
  shortening of anal canal in, 153
  skin changes in, 155
  swelling of perianal tissues in, 153
  tears in anal canal in, 154
  urethral dilation in, 145-146
  urinary tract infections and, 159
  use of tampons and, 159
  vaginal findings in sexually abused girls, 144-151
  vaginal tears in, 146
  venous congestion in, 138, 155
Physical fight, St. Louis Child Abuse Network Study and, 319
Physical findings associated with anal sexual abuse, physical examination in sexual abuse and, 152-157
Physical indicators of emotional abuse, 273
Physical needs provided by others, abandonment with, 247
Physically abusive children, children as abusers and, 286-287
Physician
 protective custody and, 395
 role of
  in prevention of neglect, 254
  in testifying, 459
  Piaget's stages of cognitive development, emotional abuse and, 271
Pigmentation, physical examination in sexual abuse and, 156
Pine oil intoxication, 224
Ping-pong fracture, 442
Pinworms, fissures and, 154
Planchette, multiple personality disorder and, 192-193
Play, sex
 sexual abuse and, 115
 sexually abusive children and, 293, 296

Plea, guilty, in criminal court, 413
Plea bargaining in criminal court, 413
Pleural effusions, pancreatitis and, 38
Pneumatosis intestinalis, 49
Pneumocystis carinii, 213
Pneumoperitoneum, 47
Pneumothoraces, rib trauma and, 38
Pneumothorax, 444-445
Podophyllin in treatment of sexually transmitted diseases, 207, 212
Poisoning, 217-228, 451
 alcohols and, 217, 219, 220, 224
 characteristics of perpetrator and, 218-219
 cocaine intoxication and, 220-221, 224
 electrolytes in, 222
 examples of agents used in, 223-224
 glycols and, 224
 history in management of, 221
 hydrocarbons and, 224
 illicit drug use and, 220-221
 intentional, 218-228
 laboratory data in, 222
 management of, 221-223
 medical examiner and, 447-448
 Munchausen Syndrome by Proxy and, 219
 neglect and, 219
 pepper aspiration, 224
 physical examination in, 222
 radiologic studies in, 223
 salt, 218, 223-224
 serum osmolality in, 222
 signs and symptoms of, 221
 toxicology screening in, 223
Police
 protective custody and, 395
 recommendations for, St. Louis Child Abuse Network Study and, 315
 reporting statutes and, 393
Pornography, child, collection of, by pedophile, 120
Positive methods of child guidance, instruction in, in prevention of child abuse, 469
Post-conviction actions in criminal court, 417
Posterior column of rugae, 136
Posterior fourchette, 135
Posterior rib fractures, 38, 425, 426, 445
Posterior rim hymen, 138
Posterior vestibule, 136
Post-hypnotic suggestion, multiple personality disorder and, 192
Postimmersion syndrome, 15
Postmortem anal dilation mistaken for sexual abuse, 159
Postmortem changes, medical examiner and, 452, 453
Postmortem examination, medical examiner and, 435-436
Postmortem insect bites, 452
Postpartum depression and grief, emotional abuse and, 270
Post-traumatic stress disorder (PTSD)
 multiple personality disorder and, 193, 195
 sexual abuse and, 138
Potassium, poisoning from, 448
Potassium perchlorate administration, nuclear medicine and, 28
Potty training, age-inappropriate, emotional abuse and, 100, 105, 106, 269-270

Scalds, 89, 90, 91, 94, 100-101, 448-449

Scapular injuries, 39

Scars, 78

    anal sexual abuse and, 155

Scene investigation checklists, basic investigation protocols and, 333

Scene photography, basic, 360-362

Scene reconstruction using dolls and silhouettes, 366

Scene sketching, basic, and investigative note taking, 363-365

Schizophrenia, multiple personality disorder and, 193

Schizophrenic parent, emotional abuse and, 262

School-aged children, behavioral indicators of sexual abuse in, 167

Screening and referral process, sexual abuse and, 168-170

Screening patients for regional centers for abuse management, sexual
        abuse and, 129-130

Scurvy, 52

Search and seize, permission to, sample form for, 379

Search warrant

    affidavit in support of, sample form for, 377-378

    child protection services caseworkers and, 399

    sample form for, 374-375

Searches in criminal court, 414-415

Secondary prevention of child abuse, 468-470

Sedation

    magnetic resonance imaging and, 30

    nuclear medicine and, 28

    ultrasound and, 30

Seduction, sexual abuse and, 118

Seize, search and, permission to, sample form for, 379

Seizures

    in criminal court, 414-415

    multiple personality disorder and, 195

    Munchausen Syndrome by Proxy and, 232

    poisoning and, 220, 221

    shaking injuries and, 86

Self-destructiveness, children as abusers and, 291-292

Self-image, negative, emotional abuse and, 274

Self-inflicted injuries mistaken for abuse, 3

Self-orientation, emotional abuse and, 271

Sentencing in criminal court, 416-417

Sentinel injuries, shaken infant syndrome and, 444

Separation, sexual abuse and, 115

Septate hymen, 138

Serious crime/event scene checklist, basic investigation protocols
        and, 328-332

Serum osmolality, poisoning and, 222

Sex play

    sexual abuse and, 115

    sexually abusive children and, 293, 296

Sex ring, sexual abuse and, 115

Sexual abuse, 21, 22, 113-131

    abusive acts and, 114

    allegations of, in divorce and child custody disputes, 183-184

    anal, physical findings associated with, physical examination in
        sexual abuse and, 152-157

    anatomically detailed dolls in interview in, 180-181

    appropriate concern for, 185

    assault and, 114

    assaultive acts and, 114

    attack as pedophile's defense and, 120

Sexual abuse—cont'd

    audiotaping in interview in, 183

    in background of pedophile, 119

    behavioral indicators in, 126, 166-168

    caregiver interview in, 170-174

    child interview guidelines in, 174-182

    child interview outline in, 178-180

    child vulnerabilities and, 116

    classification of, 114-115

    colon involvement in, 49

    crisis centers for, 128-130

    definition of, 114-115

    denial as pedophile's defense and, 120

    developmentally appropriate interview in, 175-176

    differentiating normal from abnormal sexual behavior in, 168

    documentation of, 182-183

    drawings in interview in, 181-182, 185-187

    effects of, children as abusers and, 295-297

    emergency room responsibilities and, 126-127

    emotional abuse and, 266-267

    evaluation of information obtained in interviews in,
        170, 171, 184-185

    evaluation of victims of, guidelines for, 204-205

    exploitation and, 115

    fabrication as pedophile's defense and, 120

    fear in victimization process and, 165

    guilty plea and, 121

    history of, 123-126, 163

    identifying pedophiles and, 119-120

    inadequate individuals and, 118

    incest and, 114-115

    initial interview with child in, 176-177

    insufficient information to document, 185

    interview of victim of; *see* Interview of victim of sexual abuse

    introversion and, 118

    justification as pedophile's defense and, 120

    lies by children about, 125-126

    male victims of, 116

    medical evaluation and, 123-126

    medical examiner and, 451

    mental illness as pedophile's defense and, 120

    minimization as pedophile's defense and, 120

    morally indiscriminate individuals and, 118

    no evidence of, 185

    nolo contender plea and, 121

    ocular manifestations of, 67, 71

    parent/caregiver interview outline in, 170-174

    patterns of, 121-123

    pedophile's defenses and, 120

    perpetrator of, 116-121

    philosphy of care for children who are victims of, 127-128

    physical examination in; *see* Physical examination in sexual abuse

    preferential child molesters and, 118

    prevalence of, 163-164

    programs to prevent, in prevention of child abuse, 470-471

    protocol for victims of, in crisis centers, 129

    regional centers for management of, 128-129

    regressed offenders and, 118

    reliable history of, 185